ECHOCARDIOGRAPHY REVIEW GUIDE

Companion to *Textbook of Clinical Echocardiography*

FOURTH EDITION

ECHOCARDIOGRAPHY REVIEW GUIDE

Companion to *Textbook of Clinical Echocardiography*

Catherine M. Otto, MD
J. Ward Kennedy-Hamilton Endowed Chair
   in Cardiology
Professor of Medicine
University of Washington School of Medicine
Director, Heart Valve Disease Clinic
Associate Director, Echocardiography Laboratory
University of Washington Medical Center
Seattle, Washington

Rosario V. Freeman, MD, MS
Professor of Medicine
Director, Training Programs in Cardiovascular
   Disease
University of Washington School of Medicine
University of Washington Medical Center
Seattle, Washington

Rebecca Gibbons Schwaegler, BS, RDCS
Adjunct Professor
Diagnostic Ultrasound Department
College of Nursing
Seattle University
Cardiac Sonographer
University of Washington Medical Center
Seattle, Washington

Jason P. Linefsky, MD, MS
Associate Professor of Medicine
Emory University
Assistant Section Chief, Cardiology
Atlanta VA Healthcare System
Decatur, Georgia

ELSEVIER

Previous editions copyrighted 2016, 2011, 2008 by Saunders, an imprint of Elsevier Inc.

Executive Content Strategist: Robin Carter
Senior Content Development Specialist: Jennifer Ehlers
Publishing Services Manager: Catherine Albright Jackson
Senior Project Manager: Doug Turner
Designer: Maggie Reid

Printed in India

Last digit is the print number: 9 8 7 6 5 4

ELSEVIER

1600 John F. Kennedy Blvd.
Ste 1600
Philadelphia, PA 19103-2899

  Working together
to grow libraries in
developing countries

www.elsevier.com • www.bookaid.org

Preface

Echocardiography Review Guide, Fourth Edition: Companion to Textbook of Clinical Echocardiography, Sixth Edition

The fourth edition of *Echocardiography Review Guide* complements the sixth edition of *Textbook of Clinical Echocardiography*, providing a review of basic principles, additional details of data acquisition and interpretation, and a step-by-step approach to patient examination for each diagnosis. In addition, self-assessment questions, with detailed explanations of the correct answers, allow the reader to be actively involved in the learning process.

This book will be of interest to practicing cardiologists and sonographers as a quick update on echocardiography and will be of value for cardiology fellows and cardiac sonographer students who are mastering the material for the first time. Cardiac anesthesiologists will find helpful information about details of the examination and a chapter dedicated to intraoperative transesophageal echocardiography. In addition, primary care, emergency department, and intensive care physicians using point-of-care ultrasound can refer to this book to get started and to improve their echocardiography skills. Multiple-choice questions provide a review and self-assessment for anyone preparing for an echocardiography examination and can be used in echocardiography laboratories for continuous quality improvement.

The chapters are arranged in the same order as those in the *Textbook of Clinical Echocardiography*, and we recommend that these two books be used in parallel. As in the textbook, there are introductory chapters on basic principles of image acquisition, transthoracic and transesophageal echocardiography, other echocardiographic modalities, and clinical indications. Each of the subsequent chapters focus on a specific clinical diagnosis, including ventricular systolic and diastolic function, ischemic cardiac disease, cardiomyopathies, valve stenosis and regurgitation, prosthetic valves, endocarditis, cardiac masses, aortic disease, adult congenital heart disease, and procedural transesophageal echocardiography.

Every chapter includes the Echo Exam review guide from the *Textbook of Clinical Echocardiography* for quick reference. In addition, there is a detailed step-by-step approach to the echocardiographic examination for each diagnosis. Information is conveyed in bulleted points, with a short list of important basic principles followed by a list of key points. Potential pitfalls are identified and approaches to avoiding errors are provided.

Data measurements and calculations are explained with specific examples. Numerous illustrations with detailed figure legends demonstrate each major idea and guide the reader through the teaching points.

Along with a review of basic principles, step-by-step approaches, and clinical examples, carefully structured multiple-choice questions allow the reader to consolidate the information and identify areas where further study is needed. In addition to providing the correct answer for each question, a discussion is provided to explain how the answer was determined and why the other potential answers are not correct. The questions are based on information presented in both the textbook and in the review guide; in effect, this review guide is the "workbook" that accompanies the textbook.

Any book on echocardiography is only a supplement to formal training; no book can replace hands-on training or practical experience. We fully endorse the current requirement for education and training of physicians in clinical cardiac ultrasound as provided by the Accreditation Council for Graduate Medical Education (ACGME), including training programs in Cardiovascular Disease, Critical Care Medicine, Emergency Medicine, Cardiovascular Anesthesiology, and other specialties. We also support the additional recommendations for training, depending on physician specialty and scope of practice, as proposed by the American College of Cardiology, Society for Cardiovascular Anesthesiology, American Society of Echocardiography, and other organizations. In addition, we support sonographer training in accredited programs with formal certification, evaluation of competency, and ongoing continuing education as established by the American Registry of Diagnostic Medical Sonography, Cardiovascular Credentialing International, and other similar organizations.

The material in this book reflects the clinical practice of echocardiography at one point in time. Cardiac imaging is a rapidly changing field, and we encourage our readers to stay up to date by reading journals and other online sources and by attending national meetings and continuing medical education courses.

Catherine M. Otto, MD
Rosario V. Freeman, MD, MS
Rebecca Gibbons Schwaegler, BS, RDCS
Jason P. Linefsky, MD, MS

Acknowledgments

It is never possible to fully acknowledge all those who help make a book possible; however, we would like to thank some of those who helped us along the way. First, the cardiac sonographers at the University of Washington and Atlanta VA Medical Center deserve our special appreciation for the excellence of their imaging skills and the time they dedicated to acquiring additional images for us and discussing the finer points of data acquisition. These sonographers include Debra Anderson; Pamela Clark, RDCS; Maurizio Corona, RDCS; Sarah Curtis, RDCS; Caryn D'Jang, RDCS; Margaret Falkenreck, RDCS; Alicia Feracho; Michelle Fujioka, RDCS; Carolyn Gardner, RDCS; Deanna Hanson, RDCS; Yasmin Hickman, RCS; Dylan Johnson, RDCS; Yelena Kovalenko, RDCS; Carol Kraft, RDCS; Carin Lodell, RDCS; Chris McKenzie, RDCS; Irina Nesterova, RDCS; Hoang Nguyen, RDCS; Amy Owens, RDCS; Brian Pearson, RDCS; Joannalyn Shephard, RDCS; Karl Skinner, RDCS; Yu Wang, RDCS; and Todd Zwink, RDCS. Special thanks are due the many readers who provided comments and input on the text and questions. Our appreciation extends to Dolores Meloni, Robin Carter, Jennifer Ehlers, and Doug Turner at Elsevier and to the editorial and production teams who supported this project and helped us make it a reality.

Finally, we all sincerely thank our spouses—Steve, Jack, Brooke, and Robert—for their unwavering and continual encouragement, as well as the younger members of our families—Vea, Remy, Brendan, Sarah, Claire, Jack, Anna, Fiona, Micah, and Eric—for their support of and patience with the book-writing process. This book would not have been possible without their helping us find the time to bring this project to fruition.

Catherine M. Otto, MD
Rosario V. Freeman, MD, MS
Rebecca Gibbons Schwaegler, BS, RDCS
Jason P. Linefsky, MD, MS

Contents

Glossary

Abbreviations Used in Figures, Tables, and Equations

2D = two-dimensional
3D = three-dimensional

A = late diastolic ventricular filling velocity with atrial contraction
A' = diastolic tissue Doppler velocity with atrial contraction
A2C = apical 2-chamber
A4C = apical 4-chamber
AcT = acceleration time
A_{dur} = transmitral A-velocity duration
a_{dur} = pulmonary vein a-velocity duration
AF = atrial fibrillation
A-long = apical long-axis
A-mode = amplitude mode (amplitude versus depth)
AMVL = anterior mitral valve leaflet
ant = anterior
Ao = aortic or aorta
AR = aortic regurgitation
AS = aortic stenosis
ASD = atrial septal defect
ATVL = anterior tricuspid valve leaflet
AV = atrioventricular
AVA = aortic valve area
AVR = aortic valve replacement

BAV = bicuspid aortic valve
BP = blood pressure
BSA = body surface area

c = propagation velocity of sound in tissue
CAD = coronary artery disease
cath = cardiac catheterization
CI = cardiac index
C_m = specific heat of tissue
cm/s = centimeters per second
CMR = cardiac magnetic resonance (imaging)
CO = cardiac output
cos = cosine
CS = coronary sinus
CSA = cross-sectional area
CT = computed tomography
CW = continuous-wave (Doppler)
Cx = circumflex coronary artery

D = diameter
DA = descending aorta
dB = decibel
dP/dt = rate of change in pressure over time
DSE = dobutamine stress echocardiography
DT = deceleration time
dT/dt = rate of increase in temperature over time
D-TGA = complete transposition of the great arteries
DTI = Doppler tissue imaging
$dyne \cdot s \cdot cm^{-5}$ = units of resistance

E = early-diastolic peak velocity
E' = early-diastolic tissue Doppler velocity
ECG = electrocardiogram
echo = echocardiography
EDD = end-diastolic dimension
EDP = end-diastolic pressure
EDV = end-diastolic volume
EF = ejection fraction
endo = endocardium
epi = epicardium
EPSS = E-point septal separation
ESD = end-systolic dimension
ESV = end-systolic volume
ETT = exercise treadmill test

Δf = frequency shift
f = frequency
FL = false lumen
F_n = near field
F_o = resonance frequency
F_s = scattered frequency
FSV = forward stroke volume
F_T = transmitted frequency

HCM = hypertrophic cardiomyopathy
HFpEF = heart failure with preserved ejection fraction
HFrEF = heart failure with reduced ejection fraction
HPRF = high pulse repetition frequency
HR = heart rate
HV = hepatic vein
Hz = Hertz (cycles per second)

I = intensity of ultrasound exposure
IAS = interatrial septum

ICE = intracardiac echocardiography
inf = inferior
IV = intravenous
IVC = inferior vena cava
IVCT = isovolumic contraction time
IVRT = isovolumic relaxation time

LA = left atrium
LAA = left atrial appendage
LAD = left anterior descending coronary artery
LAE = left atrial enlargement
lat = lateral
LCC = left coronary cusp
LMCA = left main coronary artery
LPA = left pulmonary artery
LSPV = left superior pulmonary vein
L-TGA = corrected transposition of the great arteries
LV = left ventricle
LVH = left ventricular hypertrophy
LVID = left ventricular internal dimension
LVOT = left ventricular outflow tract

MAC = mitral annular calcification
MI = myocardial infarction or mechanical index
    (depends on context)
M-mode = motion display (depth versus time)
MR = mitral regurgitation
MRI = magnetic resonance imaging
MS = mitral stenosis
MV = mitral valve
MVA = mitral valve area
MVL = mitral valve leaflet
MVR = mitral valve replacement

NBTE = nonbacterial thrombotic endocarditis
NCC = noncoronary cusp

ΔP = pressure gradient
P = pressure
PA = pulmonary artery
PAP = pulmonary artery pressure
PCI = percutaneous coronary intervention
PDA = patent ductus arteriosus or posterior descending artery (depends on context)
PE = pericardial effusion
PEP = preejection period
PET = positron emission tomography
PFO = patent foramen ovale
PISA = proximal isovelocity surface area
PLAX = parasternal long-axis
PM = papillary muscle
PMVL = posterior mitral valve leaflet
post = posterior (or inferior-lateral) ventricular wall
PR = pulmonic regurgitation
PRF = pulse repetition frequency
PRFR = peak rapid filling rate
PS = pulmonic stenosis

PSAX = parasternal short-axis (view)
PV = pulmonary vein
PVC = premature ventricular contraction
PV_D = pulmonary vein diastolic velocity
PVR = pulmonary vascular resistance
PW = pulsed wave
PWT = posterior wall thickness

Q = volume flow rate
Q_p = pulmonic volume flow rate
Q_s = systemic volume flow rate

r = correlation coefficient
R = ventricular radius
RA = right atrium
RAE = right atrial enlargement
RAO = right anterior oblique
RAP = right atrial pressure
RCA = right coronary artery
RCC = right coronary cusp
R_e = Reynolds number
RF = regurgitant fraction
R_o = radius of microbubble
ROA = regurgitant orifice area
RPA = right pulmonary artery
RSPV = right superior pulmonary vein
RSV = regurgitant stroke volume
RV = right ventricle
RVE = right ventricular enlargement
RVH = right ventricular hypertrophy
RVol = regurgitation volume
RVOT = right ventricular outflow tract

SAM = systolic anterior motion
SC = subcostal
SEE = standard error of the estimate
SPPA = spatial peak pulse average
SPTA = spatial peak temporal average
SSN = suprasternal notch
STE = speckle tracking echocardiography
STEMI = ST-segment elevation myocardial infarction
STJ = sinotubular junction
STVL = septal tricuspid valve leaflet
SV = stroke volume or sample volume (depends on context)
SVC = superior vena cava

$T^{1/2}$ = pressure half-time
TAPSE = tricuspid annular plane systolic excursion
TAVR = transcatheter aortic valve replacement
TD = thermodilution
TEE = transesophageal echocardiography
TGC = time-gain compensation
Th = wall thickness
TL = true lumen
TN = true negatives
TOF = tetralogy of Fallot

TP = true positives
TPV = time to peak velocity
TR = tricuspid regurgitation (jet)
TS = tricuspid stenosis
TSV = total stroke volume
TTE = transthoracic echocardiography
TV = tricuspid valve

V = volume or velocity (depends on context)
VAS = ventriculo-atrial septum
Veg = vegetation
V_{max} = maximum velocity
VSD = ventricular septal defect
VTI = velocity-time integral

Z = acoustic impedance

Symbols	Greek Name	Used for
α	alpha	Frequency
γ	gamma	Viscosity
Δ	delta	Difference
θ	theta	Angle
λ	lambda	Wavelength
μ	mu	Micro-
π	pi	Mathematical constant (approx. 3.14)
ϱ	rho	Tissue density
σ	sigma	Wall stress
τ	tau	Time constant of ventricular relaxation

Units of Measure

Variable	Unit	Definition
Amplitude	dB	Decibels = a logarithmic scale describing the amplitude ("loudness") of the sound wave
Angle	degrees	Degree = (π/180) radians. Example: intercept angle
Area	cm^2	Square centimeters. A 2D measurement (e.g., end-systolic area) or a calculated value (e.g., continuity equation valve area)
Frequency (f)	Hz kHz MHz	Hertz (cycles per second) Kilohertz = 1000 Hz Megahertz = 1,000,000 Hz
Length	cm mm	Centimeter (1/100 m) Millimeter (1/1000 m or 1/10 cm)
Mass	g	Grams (e.g., LV mass)
Pressure	mm Hg	Millimeters of mercury, 1 mm Hg = 1333.2 dyne/cm^2, where dyne measures force in cm $\cdot$ mg $\cdot$ s^{-2}
Resistance	dyne $\cdot$ s $\cdot$ cm^{-5}	Measure of vascular resistance
Time	s ms μs	Second Millisecond (1/1000 s) Microsecond
Ultrasound intensity	W/cm^2 mW/cm^2	Where watt (W) = joule per second and joule = m^2 $\cdot$ kg $\cdot$ s^{-2} (unit of energy)
Velocity (v)	m/s cm/s	Meters per second Centimeters per second
Velocity-time integral (VTI)	cm	Integral of the Doppler velocity curve (cm/s) over time (s), in units of cm
Volume	cm^3 mL L	Cubic centimeters Milliliter, 1 mL = 1 cm^3 Liter = 1000 mL
Volume flow rate (Q)	L/min mL/s	Rate of volume flow across a valve or in cardiac output L/min = liters per minute mL/s = milliliters per second
Wall stress	dyne/cm^2 kdyn/cm^2 kPa	Units of meridional or circumferential wall stress Kilodynes per cm^2 Kilopascals where 1 kPa = 10 kdyn/cm^2

Key Equations

ULTRASOUND PHYSICS	
Frequency	f = cycles/s = Hz
Wavelength	$\lambda = c/f = 1.54/f$ (MHz)
Doppler equation	$v = c \times \Delta f / [2F_T (\cos\Theta)]$
Bernoulli equation	$\Delta P = 4V^2$

LV IMAGING	
Stroke volume	SV = EDV − ESV
Ejection fraction	EF(%) = (SV/EDV) × 100%
Wall stress	σ = PR/2Th

DOPPLER VENTRICULAR FUNCTION	
Stroke volume	SV = CSA × VTI
Rate of pressure rise	dP/dt = 32 mm Hg/time from 1 to 3 m/s of MR CW jet (sec)
Myocardial performance index	MPI = (IVRT + IVCT)/SEP

PULMONARY PRESSURES AND RESISTANCE	
Pulmonary systolic pressure	$PAP_{systolic} = 4(V_{TR})^2 + RAP$
PAP (when PS is present)	$PAP_{systolic} = [4(V_{TR})^2 + RAP] - \Delta P_{RV-PA}$
Mean PA pressure	$PAP_{mean} = Mean \Delta P_{RV-RA} + RAP$
Diastolic PA pressure	$PAP_{diastolic} = 4(V_{PR})^2 + RAP$
Pulmonary vascular resistance	$PVR = 10(V_{TR})/VTI_{RVOT}$

AORTIC STENOSIS	
Maximum pressure gradient (integrate over ejection period for mean gradient)	$\Delta P_{max} = 4(V_{max})^2$
Continuity equation valve area	$AVA(cm^2) = [\pi(LVOT_D/2)^2 \times VTI_{LVOT}]/VTI_{AS\text{-}Jet}$
Simplified continuity equation	$AVA(cm^2) = [\pi(LVOT_D/2)^2 \times V_{LVOT}]/V_{AS\text{-}Jet}$
Velocity ratio	$Velocity\ ratio = V_{LVOT}/V_{AS\text{-}Jet}$

MITRAL STENOSIS	
Pressure half-time valve area	$MVA_{Doppler} = 220/T\frac{1}{2}$

AORTIC REGURGITATION	
Total stroke volume	$TSV = SV_{LVOT} = (CSA_{LVOT} \times VTI_{LVOT})$
Forward stroke volume	$FSV = SV_{MA} = (CSA_{MA} \times VTI_{MA})$
Regurgitant volume	RVol = TSV − FSV
Regurgitant orifice area	$ROA = RSV/VTI_{AR}$

MITRAL REGURGITATION	
Total stroke volume (or 2D or 3D LV stroke volume)	$TSV = SV_{MA} = (CSA_{MA} \times VTI_{MA})$
Forward stroke volume	$FSV = SV_{LVOT} = (CSA_{LVOT} \times VTI_{LVOT})$
Regurgitant volume	RVol = TSV − FSV
Regurgitant orifice area	$ROA = RSV/VTI_{AR}$
PISA method	
Regurgitant flow rate	$R_{FR} = 2\pi r^2 \times V_{aliasing}$
Orifice area (maximum)	$ROA_{max} = R_{FR}/V_{MR}$
Regurgitant volume	$RV = ROA \times VTI_{MR}$

AORTIC DILATION

Predicted sinus diameter
  Children (<18 years): Predicted sinus dimension = 1.02 + (0.98 BSA)
  Adults (18-40 years): Predicted sinus dimension = 0.97 + (1.12 BSA)
  Adults (>40 years): Predicted sinus dimension = 1.92 + (0.74 BSA)
Ratio = Measured maximum diameter/Predicted maximum diameter

PULMONARY (Q_P) TO SYSTEMIC (Q_S) SHUNT RATIO

$$Q_p{:}Q_s = [CSA_{PA} \times VTI_{PA}]/[CSA_{LVOT} \times VTI_{LVOT}]$$

1 Principles of Echocardiographic Image Acquisition and Doppler Analysis

BASIC PRINCIPLES

- Knowledge of basic ultrasound principles is needed for interpretation of images and Doppler data.
- Appropriate adjustment of instrument parameters is needed to obtain diagnostic information.

❖ KEY POINTS

- ❏ The appropriate ultrasound modality (two-dimensional [2D] or three-dimensional [3D] imaging, pulsed Doppler, color Doppler, etc.) is chosen for each type of needed clinical information.
- ❏ Current instrumentation allows modification of many parameters during data acquisition, such as depth, gain, harmonic imaging, wall filters, and so on.
- ❏ Artifacts must be distinguished from anatomic findings on ultrasound images.
- ❏ Accurate Doppler measurements depend on details of both blood flow interrogation and instrument acquisition parameters.

ULTRASOUND WAVES

- Ultrasound waves (Table 1.1) are mechanical vibrations with basic descriptors including:
  - ○ Frequency (cycles per second = Hz, 1000 cycles/second = MHz)
  - ○ Propagation velocity (about 1540 m/s in blood)
  - ○ Wavelength (equal to the propagation velocity divided by frequency)
  - ○ Amplitude (decibels [dBs])
- Ultrasound waves interact with tissues (Table 1.2) in four different ways:
  - ○ Reflection (used to create ultrasound images)
  - ○ Scattering (the basis of Doppler ultrasound)
  - ○ Refraction (used to focus the ultrasound beam)
  - ○ Attenuation (loss of signal strength in the tissue)

❖ KEY POINTS

- ❏ Tissue penetration is greatest with a lower frequency transducer (e.g., 2 to 3 MHz)
- ❏ Image resolution is greatest (about 1 mm) with a higher frequency transducer (e.g., 5 to 7.5 MHz) (Fig. 1.1)
- ❏ Amplitude ("loudness") is described using the logarithmic dB scale; a 6 dB change represents a doubling or halving of signal amplitude.
- ❏ Acoustic impedance depends on tissue density and the propagation velocity of ultrasound in that tissue.
- ❏ Ultrasound reflection occurs at smooth tissue boundaries with different acoustic impedances (such as between blood and myocardium). Reflection is greatest when the ultrasound beam is *perpendicular* to the tissue interface.
- ❏ Ultrasound scattering that occurs with small structures (such as red blood cells) is used to generate Doppler signals. Doppler velocity recordings are most accurate when the ultrasound beam is *parallel* to the blood flow direction.
- ❏ Refraction of ultrasound can result in imaging artifacts due to deflection of the ultrasound beam from a straight path.

TRANSDUCERS

- Ultrasound transducers use a piezoelectric crystal to alternately transmit and receive ultrasound signals (Fig. 1.2).
- Transducers are configured for specific imaging approaches—transthoracic, transesophageal, intracardiac, and intravascular (Table 1.3).

TABLE 1.1   Ultrasound Waves

	Definition	Examples	Clinical Implications
Frequency (*f*)	The number of cycles per second in an ultrasound wave: f = cycles/s = Hz	Transducer frequencies are measured in MHz (1,000,000 cycles/s). Doppler signal frequencies are measured in KHz (1000 cycles/s).	Different transducer frequencies are used for specific clinical applications, because the transmitted frequency affects ultrasound tissue penetration, image resolution, and the Doppler signal.
Velocity of propagation (c)	The speed that ultrasound travels through tissue	The average velocity of ultrasound in soft tissue about 1540 m/s.	The velocity of propagation is similar in different soft tissues (blood, myocardium, liver, fat, etc.) but is much lower in lung and much higher in bone.
Wavelength (λ)	The distance between ultrasound waves: $\lambda = c/f = 1.54/f$ (MHz)	Wavelength is shorter with a higher frequency transducer and longer with a lower frequency transducer.	Image resolution is greatest (about 1 mm) with a shorter wavelength (higher frequency). Depth of tissue penetration is greatest with a longer wavelength (lower frequency).
Amplitude (dB)	Height of the ultrasound wave or "loudness" measured in decibels (dB)	A log scale is used for dB. On the dB scale, 80 dB represents a 10,000-fold and 40 dB indicates a 100-fold increase in amplitude.	A very wide range of amplitudes can be displayed using a gray scale display for both imaging and spectral Doppler.

TABLE 1.2   Ultrasound Tissue Interaction

	Definition	Examples	Clinical Implications
Acoustic impedance (Z)	A characteristic of each tissue defined by tissue density (ρ) and propagation of velocity (c) as: $z = \rho \times c$	Lung has a low density and slow propagation velocity, whereas bone has a high density and fast propagation velocity. Soft tissues have smaller differences in tissue density and acoustic impedance.	Ultrasound is reflected from boundaries between tissues with differences in acoustic impedance (e.g., blood versus myocardium).
Reflection	Return of ultrasound signal to the transducer from a smooth tissue boundary	Reflection is used to generate 2D cardiac images.	Reflection is greatest when the ultrasound beam is perpendicular to the tissue interface.
Scattering	Radiation of ultrasound in multiple directions from a small structure, such as blood cells	The change in frequency of signals scattered from moving blood cells is the basis of Doppler ultrasound.	The amplitude of scattered signals is 100 to 1000 times less than reflected signals.
Refraction	Deflection of ultrasound waves from a straight path due to differences in acoustic impedance	Refraction is used in transducer design to focus the ultrasound beam.	Refraction in tissues results in double image artifacts.
Attenuation	Loss in signal strength due to absorption of ultrasound energy by tissues	Attenuation is frequency dependent with greater attenuation (less penetration) at higher frequencies.	A lower frequency transducer may be needed for apical views or in larger patients on transthoracic imaging.
Resolution	The smallest resolvable distance between two specular reflectors on an ultrasound image	Resolution has three dimensions—along the length of the beam (axial), lateral across the image (azimuthal), and in the elevational plane.	Axial resolution is most precise (as small as 1 mm), so imaging measurements are best made along the length of the ultrasound beam.

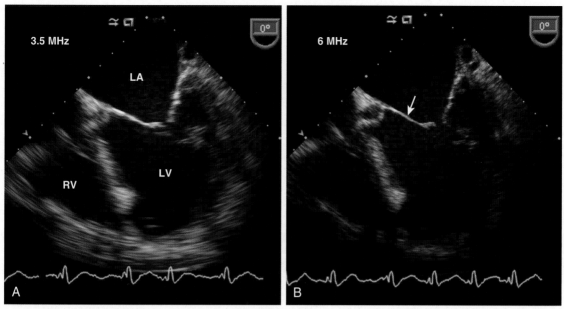

Fig 1.1 The effect of transducer frequency on penetration and resolution. In this transesophageal 4-chamber view recorded at a transmitted frequency of 3.5 MHz (A) and 6 MHz (B), the higher frequency transducer provides better resolution—for example, the mitral leaflets *(arrow)* look thin, but the depth of penetration of the signal is very poor, so the apical half of the LV is not seen. With the lower frequency transducer, improved tissue penetration provides a better image of the LV apex but image resolution is poorer, with the mitral leaflets looking thicker and less well defined.

■ The basic characteristics of a transducer are:
  ○ Transmission frequency (from 2.5 MHz for transthoracic to 20 MHz for intravascular ultrasound)
  ○ Bandwidth (range of frequencies in the transmitted ultrasound pulse)
  ○ Pulse repetition frequency (the number of transmission-receive cycles per second)
  ○ Focal depth (depends on beam shape and focusing)
  ○ Aperture (size of the transducer face or "footprint")
  ○ Power output

❖ **KEY POINTS**

❑ The time delay between transmission of an ultrasound burst and detection of the reflected wave indicates the depth of the tissue reflector.

❑ The pulse repetition frequency is an important factor in image resolution and frame rate.

❑ A shorter transmitted pulse length results in improved depth (or axial) resolution.

❑ A wider bandwidth provides better resolution of structures distant from the transducer.

❑ The shape of the ultrasound beam depends on several complex factors. Each type of transducer focuses the beam at a depth appropriate for the clinical application. Some transducers allow adjustment of focal depth.

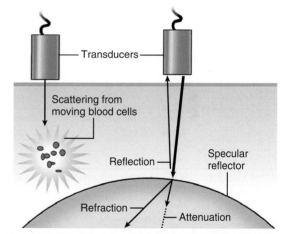

Fig 1.2 Diagram of the interaction between ultrasound and body tissues. Doppler analysis is based on the scattering of ultrasound in all directions from moving blood cells with a resulting change in frequency of the ultrasound received at the transducer. 2D imaging is based on reflection of ultrasound from tissue interfaces (specular reflectors). Attenuation limits the depth of ultrasound penetration. Refraction, a change in direction of the ultrasound wave, results in imaging artifacts. *(From Otto, CM: Textbook of clinical echocardiography, ed 6, Elsevier, 2018, Philadelphia.)*

❑ A smaller aperture is associated with a wider beam width; however, the smaller "footprint" may allow improved angulation of the beam in the intercostal spaces. This is most evident clinically with a dedicated non-imaging continuous-wave (CW) Doppler transducer.

ULTRASOUND IMAGING

Principles

- The basic ultrasound imaging modalities are:
  - M-mode—a graph of depth versus time
  - 2D—a sector scan in a tomographic image plane with real-time motion
  - 3D—a selected cutaway real-time image in a 3D display format or a 3D volume of data (see Chapter 4)
- System controls for 2D imaging typically include:
  - Power output (transmitted ultrasound energy)
  - Gain (amplitude of the received signal)
  - Time gain compensation (differential gain along the ultrasound beam)
  - Depth of the image (affects pulse repetition frequency and frame rate)
  - Gray scale/dynamic range (degree of contrast in the images)

❖ **KEY POINTS**

❏ M-mode recordings allow identification of very rapid intracardiac motion, because the sampling rate is about 1800 times per second compared to a 2D frame rate of 30 frames per second (Fig. 1.3).

TABLE 1.3	Ultrasound Transducers		
	Definition	**Examples**	**Clinical Implications**
Type	Transducer characteristics and configuration Most cardiac transducers use phased array of piezoelectric crystals	Transthoracic (adult and pediatric) Non-imaging CW Doppler 3D echocardiography TEE Intracardiac	Each transducer type is optimized for a specific clinical application. More than one transducer may be needed for a full examination.
Transmission frequency	The central frequency emitted by the transducer	Transducer frequencies vary from 2.5 MHz for transthoracic echo to 20 MHz for intravascular imaging.	A higher frequency transducer provides improved resolution but less penetration. Doppler signals are optimal at a lower transducer frequency than used for imaging.
Power output	The amount of ultrasound energy emitted by the transducer	An increase in transmitted power increases the amplitude of the reflected ultrasound signals.	Excessive power output may result in bioeffects measured by the mechanical and thermal indexes.
Bandwidth	The range of frequencies in the ultrasound pulse	Bandwidth is determined by transducer design.	A wider bandwidth allows improved axial resolution for structures distant from the transducer.
Pulse (or burst) length	The length of the transmitted ultrasound signal	A higher frequency signal can be transmitted in a shorted pulse length compared with a lower frequency signal.	A shorter pulse length improves axial resolution.
Pulse repetition frequency (PRF)	The number of transmission-receive cycles per second	The PRF decreases as imaging (or Doppler) depth increases because of the time needed for the signal to travel from and to the transducer.	Pulse repetition frequency affects image resolution and frame rate (particularly with color Doppler)
Focal depth	Beam shape and focusing are used to optimize ultrasound resolution at a specific distance from the transducer	Structures close to the transducer are best visualized with a short focal depth, distant structures with a long focal depth.	The length and site of a transducer's focal zone is primarily determined by transducer design, but adjustment during the exam may be possible.
Aperture	The surface of the transducer face where ultrasound is transmitted and received	A small non-imaging CW Doppler transducer allows optimal positioning and angulation of the ultrasound beam.	A larger aperture allows a more focused beam. A smaller aperture allows improved transducer angulation on TTE imaging.

❏ Ultrasound imaging resolution is more precise along the length of the ultrasound beam (axial resolution) compared with lateral (side to side) or elevational ("thickness" of the image plane) resolution.

❏ Lateral resolution decreases with increasing distance from the transducer (Fig. 1.4).

❏ Harmonic imaging improves endocardial definition and reduces near-field and side-lobe artifacts (Fig. 1.5).

Imaging Artifacts

■ Common imaging artifacts result from:
  ○ A low signal-to-noise ratio
  ○ Acoustic shadowing
  ○ Reverberations
  ○ Beam width
  ○ Lateral resolution
  ○ Refraction
  ○ Range ambiguity
  ○ Processing

❖ **KEY POINTS**

❏ A shadow occurs distal to a strong ultrasound reflector because the ultrasound wave does not penetrate past the reflector (Fig. 1.6).

❏ Signals originating from the edges of the ultrasound beam or from side lobes can result in imaging or Doppler artifacts.

❏ Deviation of the ultrasound beam from a straight pathway due to refraction in the tissue results in the structure appearing in the incorrect location across the sector scan (Fig. 1.7).

❏ Ultrasound reflected back and forth between two strong reflectors creates a reverberation artifact.

❏ Reflected ultrasound signals received at the transducer are assumed to originate from the preceding transmitted pulse. Signals from very deep structures or signals that have been re-reflected will be displayed at one-half or twice the actual depth of origin.

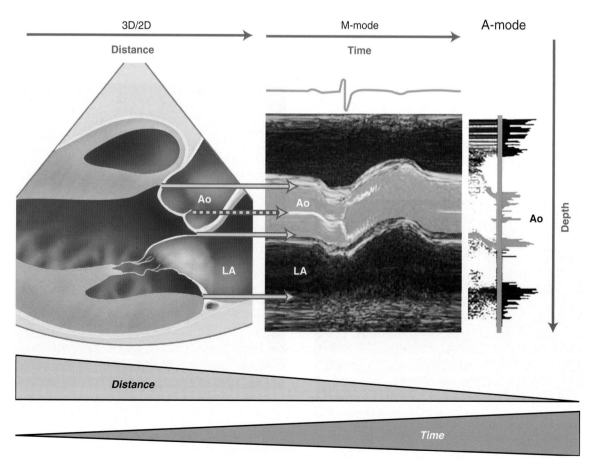

Fig 1.3 3D, 2D, M-mode, and A-mode recordings of aortic valve motion. This illustration shows the relationship between the 3D and 2D long-axis image of the aortic valve *(left)*, which shows distance in both the vertical and horizontal directions, M-mode recording of aortic root *(Ao)*, LA, and aortic valve motion, which shows depth versus time *(middle)* and A-mode recording *(right)*, which shows depth only (with motion seen on the video screen). Spatial relationships are best shown with 3D/2D, but temporal resolution is higher with M-mode and A-mode imaging. *(From Otto, CM: Textbook of clinical echocardiography, ed 6, Elsevier, 2018, Philadelphia.)*

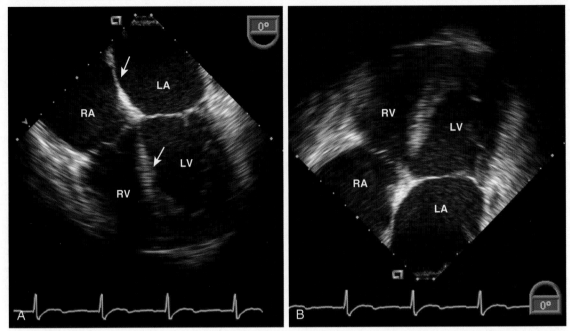

Fig 1.4 **Lateral resolution with ultrasound decreases with the distance of the reflector from the transducer.** (A) In this TEE image oriented with the origin of the ultrasound signal at the top of the image, thin structures close to the transducer, such as the atrial septum *(upper arrow)*, appear as a dot because lateral resolution is optimal at this depth. Reflections from more distant structures, such as the ventricular septum *(lower arrow)*, appear as a broad line due to poor lateral resolution. (B) When the image is oriented with the transducer at the bottom of the image, the effects of depth on lateral resolution are more visually apparent. The standard orientation for echocardiography with the transducer as the top of the image is based on considerations of ultrasound physics, not on cardiac anatomy.

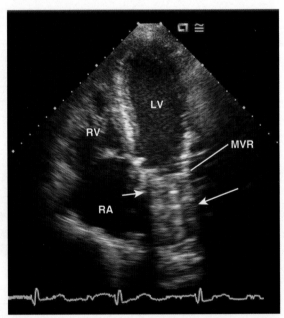

Fig 1.6 **Acoustic shadowing and reverberations.** This apical 4-chamber view in a patient with a mechanical mitral valve replacement *(MVR)* illustrates the shadowing (dark area, *small arrow*) and reverberations (white band of echoes, *large arrow*) that obscure structures (in this case, the left atrium) distal to the valve.

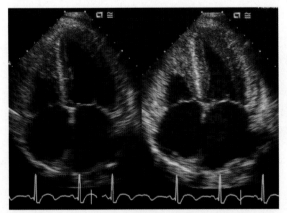

Fig 1.5 **Harmonic imaging compared with fundamental frequency imaging.** Harmonic imaging improves identification of the LV endocardial border, as seen in this apical 4-chamber view recorded with a 4-MHz transducer using *(left)* fundamental frequency imaging and *(right)* harmonic imaging.

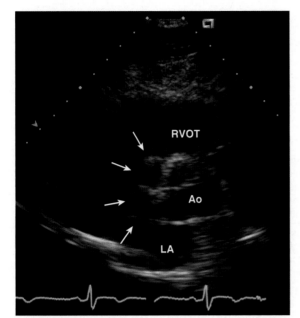

Fig 1.7 **Refraction artifact.** In this parasternal short-axis image of the aortic valve *(Ao)*, a refraction artifact results in the appearance of a "second" aortic valve *(arrows)*, partly overlapping with the actual position of the aortic valve. *RVOT,* Right ventricular outflow tract.

DOPPLER

- Doppler ultrasound is based on the principle that ultrasound backscattered (F_s) from moving red blood cells will appear higher or lower in frequency than the transmitted frequency (F_T) depending on the speed and direction of blood flow (v), the speed of sound in blood (c), and the cosine (cos) of the angle between the ultrasound beam and direction of blood flow (θ). (Table 1.4).
- The Doppler equation is:

$$v = c\,(F_S - F_T)/[2F_T\,(\cos\ \theta)]$$

- Accurate blood flow measurements depend on a parallel intercept angle θ (a cosine of 1.0). between the ultrasound beam and direction of blood flow.
- There are three basic Doppler modalities: pulsed Doppler, color flow imaging, and CW Doppler ultrasound.

❖ KEY POINTS

- ❏ The speed (c) of ultrasound in blood is about 1540 m/s.
- ❏ Blood flow velocity will be underestimated with a nonparallel intercept angle; the error is only 6% with an angle of 20 degrees but increases to 50% at a 60-degree angle.

- ❏ When the ultrasound beam is perpendicular to flow, there is no Doppler shift, and blood flow is not detected, even when present.
- ❏ The standard Doppler velocity display (or spectral recording) shows time on the horizontal axis and velocity on the vertical axis with signal amplitude displayed using a dB gray scale (Fig. 1.8).
- ❏ Standard Doppler instrument controls are:
  - ❏ Power output
  - ❏ Receiver gain (Fig. 1.9)
  - ❏ High-pass ("wall") filters (Fig. 1.10)
  - ❏ Velocity range and baseline shift
  - ❏ Post-processing options

Pulsed Doppler

- Pulsed Doppler allows measurement of blood flow velocity at a specific intracardiac site.
- The depth of interrogation (or sample volume) is determined by the time interval between transmission and sampling of the backscattered signal.
- Signal aliasing limits the maximum velocity measurable with pulsed Doppler.

❖ KEY POINTS

- ❏ A pulse of ultrasound is transmitted and then the backscattered signal is analyzed at a time interval corresponding to the transit time from the depth of interest.
- ❏ The pulsed Doppler interrogation line and sample volume are displayed on the 2D image, with the transducer switched to Doppler only during data recording.
- ❏ Pulse repetition frequency is the number of transmission/receive cycles per second, which is determined by the depth of the sample volume.
- ❏ The maximum frequency detectable with intermittent sampling is one-half the pulse repetition frequency (or Nyquist limit).
- ❏ The direction of blood flow for frequencies in excess of the Nyquist limit is ambiguous, a phenomenon called *signal aliasing* (Fig. 1.11)
- ❏ The effective velocity range for pulsed Doppler can be doubled by moving the baseline to the edge of the spectral display.
- ❏ The sample volume length can be adjusted to localize the signal (short length) or improve signal strength (long length).
- ❏ Pulsed Doppler is used to measure normal intracardiac transvalvular flow velocities.
- ❏ Variations of the pulsed Doppler principle are used to generate color Doppler flow images and tissue Doppler recordings.

TABLE 1.4	Doppler Physics		
	Definition	**Examples**	**Clinical Implications**
Doppler effect	The change in frequency of ultrasound scattered from a moving target: $v = c \times \Delta F / [2F_T (\cos \theta)]$	A higher velocity corresponds to a higher Doppler frequency shift, ranging from 1 to 20 kHz for intracardiac flow velocities.	Ultrasound systems display velocity, which is calculated using the Doppler equation, based on transducer frequency and the Doppler shift, assuming cos θ equals 1.
Intercept angle	The angle (θ) between the direction of blood flow and the ultrasound beam	When the ultrasound beam is parallel to the direction of blood flow (0° or 180°), cos θ is 1 and can be ignored in the Doppler equation.	Velocity is underestimated when the intercept angle is not parallel. This can lead to errors in hemodynamic measurements.
CW Doppler	Continuous ultrasound transmission with reception of Doppler signals from the entire length of the ultrasound beam	CW Doppler allows measurements of high velocity signals but does not localize the depth of origin of the signal.	CW Doppler is used to measure high velocities in valve stenosis and regurgitation.
Pulsed Doppler	Pulsed ultrasound transmission with timing of reception determining depth of the backscattered signal	Pulsed Doppler samples velocities from a specific site but can only measure velocity over a limited range.	Pulsed Doppler is used to record low velocity signals at a specific site, such as LV outflow velocity or LV inflow velocity.
Pulse repetition frequency (PRF)	The number of pulses transmitted per second	PRF is limited by the time needed for ultrasound to reach and return from the depth of interest. PRF determines the maximum velocity that can be unambiguously measured.	The maximum velocity measurable with pulsed Doppler is about 1 m/s at 6 cm depth.
Nyquist limit	The maximum frequency shift (or velocity) measurable with pulsed Doppler equal to ½ PRF	The Nyquist limit is displayed as the top and bottom of the velocity range with the baseline centered.	The greater the depth, the lower the maximum velocity measurable with pulsed Doppler.
Signal aliasing	The phenomenon that the direction of flow for frequency shifts greater than the Nyquist limit cannot be determined	With aliasing of the LV outflow signal, the peak of the velocity curve is "cut off" and appears as flow in the opposite direction.	Aliasing can result in inaccurate velocity measurements if not recognized.
Sample volume	The intracardiac location where the pulsed Doppler signal originated	Sample volume depth is determined by the time interval between transmission and reception. Sample volume length is determined by the duration of the receive cycle.	Sample volume depth and length are adjusted to record the flow of interest.
Spectral analysis	Method used to display Doppler velocity data versus time, with gray scale indicating amplitude	Spectral analysis is used for both pulsed and CW Doppler.	The velocity scale, baseline position, and time scale of the spectral display are adjusted for each Doppler velocity signal.

Color Doppler

- Color Doppler uses the pulsed Doppler principle to generate a 2D image or "map" of blood flow velocity superimposed on the 2D real-time image (Table 1.5).
- Color Doppler signals, like all pulsed Doppler velocity data, are angle dependent and subject to signal aliasing.

- The frame rate for color Doppler imaging depends on:
  - Pulse repetition frequency (depth of color sector)
  - Number of scan lines (width of color sector and scan line density)
  - Number of pulses per scan line (affects accuracy of mean velocity calculation)

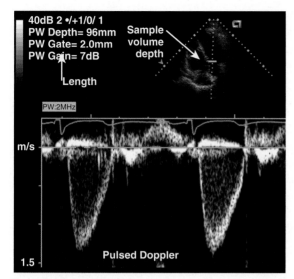

Fig 1.8 Doppler spectral tracing. LV outflow velocity was recorded with pulsed Doppler ultrasound from the apex. The sample volume depth (time for transmission and reception of the signal) is shown on a small 2D image with the length (sampling duration) indicated by the pulsed wave *(PW)* gate size. The spectral tracing shows time *(horizontal axis)*, velocity *(vertical axis)*, and signal strength *(gray scale)*. The baseline has been shifted upward to show the entire velocity curve directed away from the transducer. Some diastolic LV inflow is seen above the baseline, directed toward the transducer.

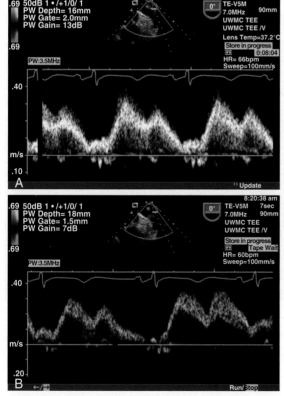

Fig 1.9 Pulsed Doppler gain setting. The effect of Doppler gain settings are shown for a TEE recording of pulmonary vein inflow. Excess noise is eliminated; then the gain is decreased from 13 dB **(A)** to 7 dB **(B)**.

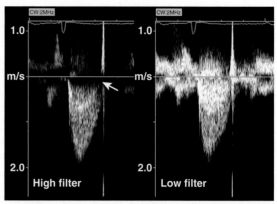

Fig 1.10 Wall filter settings. An aortic outflow signal is recorded with CW Doppler with the high pass ("wall") filter set at a high and low level. With the higher filter, low velocity signals are eliminated as shown by the blank space adjacent to the baseline *(arrow)*. This tracing enhances identification of the maximum velocity and recognition of the valve closing click. At the lower filter setting, the velocity signals extend to the baseline, making measurement of time intervals more accurate, but there also is more low velocity noise in the signal, related to motion of cardiac structures.

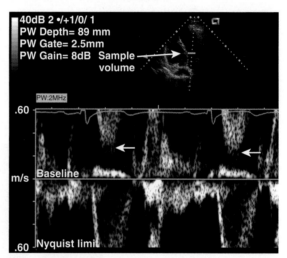

Fig 1.11 Signal aliasing. LV outflow velocity recorded from the apical approach with the sample volume on the LV side of the aortic valve. The spectral tracing is shown in the standard format with the baseline in the center of the scale and the Nyquist limit at the top and bottom of the scale. Signal aliasing is present with the top of the LV outflow signal seen in the reverse channel *(arrows)*. This degree of aliasing is easily resolved by shifting the baseline, as seen in Fig. 1.8. Aliasing with higher velocity flow is best resolved using CW Doppler ultrasound.

❖ KEY POINTS

- Color Doppler is recorded in real time simultaneous with 2D imaging.
- Flow toward the transducer typically is shown in red, with flow directed away from the transducer in blue (Fig. 1.12).
- When velocity exceeds the Nyquist limit, signal aliasing occurs so that faster flows toward the transducer alias from red to blue and vice versa for flow away from the transducer.
- The amount of variation in the velocity signal from each site can be coded on the color scale as variance.

TABLE 1.5	Color Doppler Flow Imaging		
	Definition	**Examples**	**Clinical Implications**
Sampling line	Doppler data is displayed from multiple sampling lines across the 2D image	Instead of sampling backscattered signals from one depth (as in pulsed Doppler), signals from multiple depths along the beam are analyzed.	A greater number of sampling lines results in denser Doppler data but a slower frame rate.
Burst length	The number of ultrasound bursts along each sampling line	Mean velocity is estimated from the average of the backscattered signals from each burst.	A greater number of bursts results in more accurate mean velocity estimates but a slower frame rate.
Sector scan width	The width of the displayed 2D and color image	A greater sector width requires more sampling lines or less dense velocity data.	A narrower sector scan allows a greater sampling line density and faster frame rate.
Sector scan depth	The depth of the displayed color Doppler image	The maximum depth of the sector scan determines PRF (as with pulsed Doppler) and the Nyquist limit.	The minimum depth needed to display the flow of interest provides the optimal color display.
Color scale	Color display of Doppler velocity and flow direction	Most systems use shades of red for flow toward the transducer and blue for flow away from the transducer.	The color scale can be adjusted by shifting the baseline and adjusted the maximum velocity displayed (within the Nyquist limit).
Variance	The degree of variability in the mean velocity estimate at each depth along a sampling line	Variance typically is displayed as a green scale superimposed on the red–blue velocity scale. Variance can be turned on or off.	A variance display highlights flow disturbances and high velocity flow, but even normal flows will be displayed as showing variance if velocity exceeds the Nyquist limit.

PRF, Pulse repetition frequency.

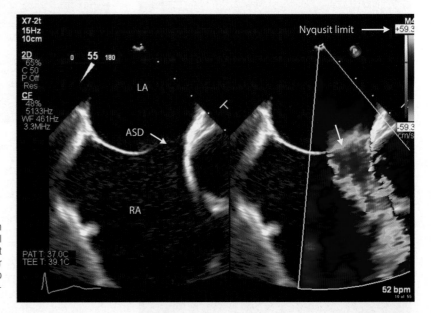

Fig 1.12 **Color Doppler flow mapping.** In this transesophageal view of the interatrial septum, flow across the atrial septal defect *(ASD)* is directed away from the transducer from the *LA* to *RA* but aliases from blue to orange because the velocity exceeds the Nyquist limit of 59 cm/s.

- Variance reflects either signal aliasing (high velocity flow) or the presence of multiple flow velocities or directions (flow disturbance).
- Color Doppler is most useful for visualization of spatial flow patterns; for this purpose, examiner preference determines the most appropriate color scale.
- For color Doppler measurements, such as vena contracta width or proximal isovelocity surface area (PISA) measurements, a color scale without variance is optimal.

❏ The maximum velocity measurable with color Doppler is determined by the Nyquist limit, but the baseline can be shifted or the velocity scale can be reduced.

Continuous-Wave Doppler

- CW Doppler uses two ultrasound crystals to continuously transmit and receive ultrasound signals.
- CW Doppler allows accurate measurement of high flow velocities without signal aliasing.
- Signals from the entire length of the ultrasound beam are included in the spectral CW Doppler recording.

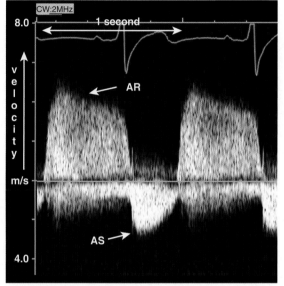

Fig 1.13 **CW Doppler recording.** The spectral recording of antegrade (aortic stenosis, *AS*) and retrograde flow (aortic regurgitation, *AR*) across the aortic valve shows time *(horizontal axis in seconds)*, velocity *(vertical axis in m/s)*, and signal strength *(gray scale)*. High velocity flow can be measured without aliasing using CW Doppler, as shown in the aortic regurgitant velocity over 4 m/s in this example.

❖ KEY POINTS

- ❏ CW Doppler is used to measure high velocity flows, for example, across stenotic and regurgitant valves (Fig. 1.13).
- ❏ The CW Doppler signal is recorded as a spectral tracing with the scale and baseline adjusted as needed to display the signal of interest.
- ❏ CW Doppler can be recorded with a standard transducer with the CW interrogation line shown on the 2D image; however, a dedicated non-imaging CW transducer is optimal due to a higher signal-to-noise ratio and better angulation with a smaller transducer.
- ❏ The lack of range resolution means that the origin of the CW signal must be inferred from:
  - ❏ Characteristics of the signal itself (timing, shape, and associated flow signals)
  - ❏ Associated 2D imaging and pulsed or color Doppler findings
- ❏ Underestimation of blood flow velocity occurs when the CW Doppler beam is not parallel to the flow of interest.

Doppler Artifacts

- Artifacts with pulsed or CW Doppler spectral recordings include:
  - ○ Underestimation of velocity because of a non-parallel intercept angle
  - ○ Signal aliasing (with pulsed Doppler)
  - ○ Range ambiguity
  - ○ Beam width artifacts with superimposition of multiple flow signals
  - ○ Mirror image artifact (Fig. 1.14)
  - ○ Transit time effect
  - ○ Electronic interference

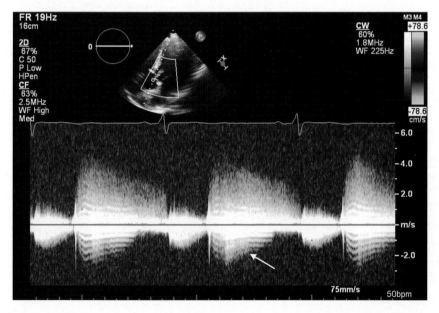

Fig 1.14 **Doppler artifacts.** Appropriate use of instrumentation allows minimization of many ultrasound artifacts. This recording of an aortic regurgitation velocity signal shows marked channel cross-talk (signal below the baseline that does not correlate with an actual intracardiac flow) due to high signal intensity with coarse fluttering of the incompetent valve leaflet. This recording would be improved by a higher wall filter and lower gain setting.

- Artifacts with color Doppler flow imaging (Table 1.6) include:
  - Shadowing resulting in inability to detect flow abnormalities
  - Ghosting from strong reflectors leading to flashes of color across the image plane
  - Gain too low (loss of true signal) or gain too high (speckle pattern across the image)
  - Intercept angle, including absence of detectable flow at a 90° angle
  - Signal aliasing (Fig. 1.15)
  - Electronic interference

❖ **KEY POINTS**

- The potential for underestimation of velocity is the most important clinical limitation of Doppler ultrasound.
- Signal aliasing limits measurement of high velocities with pulsed Doppler and may confuse interpretation of color Doppler images.
- Range ambiguity with CW Doppler is obvious. With pulsed Doppler, range ambiguity occurs when signals from two times, three times or more the sample volume depth return to the transducer during a receive cycle.
- A mirror image artifact is common on spectral tracings and may be reduced by lowering power output and gain.
- As ultrasound propagates through moving blood, there is a slight change in ultrasound frequency, called the *transit time effect*. The transit time effect results in slight blurring of the edge of the CW Doppler spectral display, particularly for high velocity flows.
- Acoustic shadowing can be avoided by using an alternate transducer position; for example, transesophageal imaging of a mitral prosthetic valve.
- Color ghosting is seen in only one or two frames of the cardiac cycle, whereas blood flow signals demonstrate physiologic timing.

BIOEFFECTS AND SAFETY

- A simple measure of ultrasound exposure is the "duty factor," defined as percent of time ultrasound is being transmitted.
- Two types of ultrasound bioeffects are important with diagnostic imaging:
  - Thermal (heating of tissue due to the interaction of ultrasound energy with tissue)
  - Cavitation (the creation or vibration of small gas-filled bodies)
- Ultrasound exposure is measured by the:
  - Thermal index (TI; the ratio of transmitted acoustic power to the power needed to increase temperature by 1°C)
  - Mechanical index (MI; the ratio of peak rarefactional pressure to the square root of transducer frequency)

TABLE 1.6 Ultrasound Terminology: Ultrasound Safety

	Definition	Examples	Clinical Implications
Exposure Intensity (I)	Ultrasound exposure depends on power and area: I = power/area = watt/cm^2	Common measures of intensity are the SPTA or the SPPA.	Transducer output and tissue exposure affect the total ultrasound exposure of the patient.
Thermal bioeffects	Heating of tissue due to absorption of ultrasound energy described by the thermal index (TI)	The degree of tissue heating is affected by tissue density and blood flow. TI is the ratio of transmitted acoustic power to the power needed to increase temperature by 1°C. TI is most important with Doppler and color flow imaging.	Total ultrasound exposure depends on transducer frequency, power output, focus, depth, and exam duration. When the TI exceeds 1, the benefits of the study should be balanced against potential biologic effects.
Cavitation	Creation or vibration of small gas-filled bodies by the ultrasound wave	Mechanical index (MI) is the ratio of peak rarefactional pressure to the square root of the transducer frequency. MI is most important with 2D imaging.	Cavitation or vibration of microbubbles occurs with higher intensity exposure. Power output and exposure time should be monitored.

SPPA, Spatial peak pulse average; *SPTA*, spatial peak temporal average.

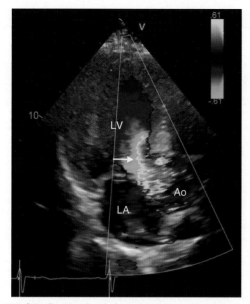

Fig 1.15 **Color Doppler signal aliasing.** In this apical long-axis view, the antegrade flow in the LV outflow tract, away from the transducer, aliases from blue to red because velocity exceeds the Nyquist limit of 61 cm/s. The shape of the aliasing transition across the outflow tract also depends in the exact angle between the ultrasound beam and blood flow stream; a nonparallel intercept angle underestimates velocity, so aliasing occurs closer to the aortic valve even when velocities are uniform across the outflow tract. Ao, Aorta.

❖ **KEY POINTS**

❏ The degree of tissue heating depends on the ultrasound energy imparted to the tissue and on characteristics of the tissue, including tissue density and blood flow.

❏ The total ultrasound exposure depends on transducer frequency, focus, power output, and depth, as well as the duration of the examination.

❏ Cavitation or vibration of microbubbles occurs with higher intensity ultrasound exposure.

❏ When the TI or MI exceeds 1, the benefit of the ultrasound examination should be balanced against potential biologic effects.

❏ Power output and exposure time should be monitored during the echocardiographic examination.

❏ Duty factor ranges from <1% for pulsed Doppler or imaging to 100% for CW Doppler.

THE ECHO EXAM

Basic Principles

Optimization of Echocardiographic Images

Instrument Control	Data Optimization	Clinical Issues
Transducer	• Different transducer types and transmission frequencies are needed for specific clinical applications. • Transmission frequency is adjusted for tissue penetration in each patient and for ultrasound modality (Doppler versus imaging).	• A higher transducer frequency provides improved resolution but less penetration. • A larger aperture provides a more focused beam.
Power output	• Power output reflects the amount of ultrasound energy transmitted to the tissue. • Higher power output results in greater tissue penetration.	• Potential bioeffects must be considered. • Exam time and mechanical and thermal indexes should be monitored.
Imaging mode	• 2D imaging is the clinical standard for most indications. • M-mode provides high time resolution along a single scan line. • 3D imaging provides improved appreciation of spatial relationships.	• Optimal measurement of cardiac chambers and vessels requires a combination of imaging modes.
Transducer position	• Acoustic windows allow ultrasound tissue penetration without intervening lung or bone tissue. • Transthoracic acoustic windows include parasternal, apical subcostal, and suprasternal. • TEE acoustic windows include high esophageal and transgastric.	• Optimal patient positioning is essential for acoustic access to the heart. • Imaging resolution is optimal when the ultrasound beam is reflected perpendicular to the tissue interface. • Doppler signals are optimal with the ultrasound beam is aligned parallel to flow.
Depth	• Depth is adjusted to show the structure of interest. • PRF depends on maximum image depth.	• PRF is higher at shallow depths, which contributes to improved image resolution. • Axial resolution is the same along the entire length of the ultrasound beam. • Lateral and elevations resolution depend on the 3D shape of the ultrasound beam at each depth.
Sector width	• Standard sector width is 60°, but a narrower sector allows a higher scan line density and faster frame rate.	• Sector width should be adjusted as needed to optimize the image. • Too narrow a sector might miss important anatomic or Doppler findings.
Gain	• Overall gain affects the display of the reflected ultrasound signals.	• Excessive gain obscures border identification. • Inadequate gain results failure to display reflections from tissue interfaces.
TGC	• TGC adjusts gain differentially along the length of the ultrasound bean to compensate for the effects of attenuation.	• An appropriate TGC curve results in an image with similar brightness proximally and distally in the sector image.
Grey scale or Dynamic range	• Ultrasound amplitude is displayed using a dB scale in shades of grey.	• The range of displayed amplitudes is adjusted to optimize the image using the dynamic range or compression controls.

Optimization of Echocardiographic Images—Cont'd

Instrument Control	Data Optimization	Clinical Issues
Harmonic imaging	• Harmonic frequencies are proportional to the strength of the fundament frequency but increase with depth of propagation.	• Harmonic imaging improves endocardial definition and decreased near field and side lobe artifacts. • Flat structures, such as valves, appear thicker with harmonic than with fundamental imaging. • Axial resolution is reduced.
Focal depth	• Transducer design parameters that affect focal depth include array pattern, aperture size, and acoustic focusing.	• The ultrasound beam is most focused at the junction between the near zone and far field of the beam pattern. • Transducer design allows a longer focal zone. In some cases, focal zone can be adjusted during the examination.
Zoom mode	• The ultrasound image can be restricted to a smaller depth range and narrow section. The maximum depth still determines PRF, but scan line density and frame rate can be optimized in the region of interest.	• Zoom mode is used to examine areas on interest identified on standard views.
ECG	• The ECG signal is essential for triggering digital cine loop acquisition.	• A noisy signal or low amplitude ECG results in incorrect triggering or inadvertent recording of an incomplete cardiac cycle.

dB, Decibel; *ECG,* electrocardiogram; *PRF,* pulse repetition frequency; *TGC,* time gain compensation.

Optimization of Doppler Recordings

Modality	Data Optimization	Common Artifacts
Pulsed	• 2D guided with "frozen" image • Parallel to flow • Small sample volume • Velocity scale at Nyquist limit • Adjust baseline for aliasing • Use low wall filters • Adjust gain and dynamic range	• Non-parallel angle with underestimation of velocity • Signal aliasing. Nyquist limit = ½ pulse repetition frequency (PRF) • Signal strength/noise
Continuous wave	• Dedicated non-imaging transducer • Parallel to flow • Adjust velocity scale so flow fits and fills displayed range • Use high wall filters • Adjust gain and dynamic range	• Nonparallel angle with underestimation of velocity • Range ambiguity • Beam width • Transit time effect
Color flow	• Use minimal depth and sector width for flow of interest (best frame rate) • Adjust gain just below random noise • Color scale at Nyquist limit • Decrease 2D gain to optimize Doppler signal • 3D color imaging allows better visualization of the size and shape of jet geometry proximal to a restrictive orifice (e.g., valve regurgitation)	• Shadowing • Ghosting • Electronic interference

SELF-ASSESSMENT QUESTIONS

Questions 1-5

Which ultrasound imaging interaction best describes the findings in each of the following images:

    A. Reverberation
    B. Ring-down
    C. Scattering
    D. Refraction
    E. Attenuation

Question 1:

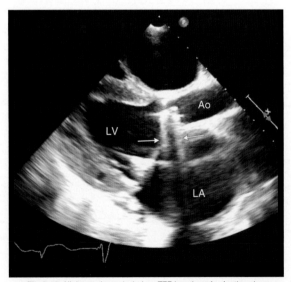

Fig 1.16 Parasternal long-axis view.

Question 2:

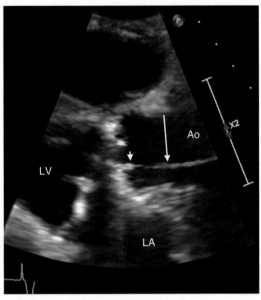

Fig 1.17 High esophageal window, TEE imaging. *Ao,* Aortic valve.

Question 3:

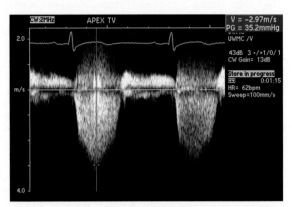

Fig 1.18 Tricuspid regurgitant jet.

Question 4:

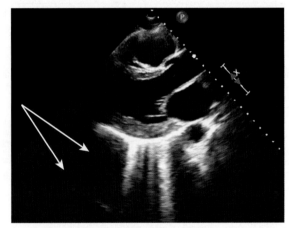

Fig 1.19 Parasternal long-axis view.

Question 5:

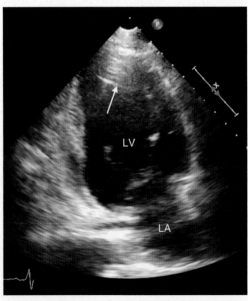

Fig 1.20 Apical 4-chamber view.

Question 6

Which of the following would reduce echocardiographic attenuation of an ultrasound signal?
- **A.** Increase the sector depth
- **B.** Apply water-soluble gel to the transducer
- **C.** Move the transducer laterally over the left lung
- **D.** Decrease the power output
- **E.** Raising the transducer frequency

Question 7

Compared to pulsed-wave Doppler, CW Doppler:
- **A.** Has a duty factor of 1
- **B.** Is more susceptible to nonparallel alignment
- **C.** Has a lower Nyquist limit
- **D.** Has less range ambiguity
- **E.** Has a larger aperture when using a dedicated transducer

Question 8

Which of the following most affects frame rate during color Doppler imaging?
- **A.** Burst length
- **B.** Color scale
- **C.** Electronic interference
- **D.** Variance setting
- **E.** Intercept angle

Question 9

In this TEE color Doppler long axis image of the descending thoracic aorta (Fig. 1.21), the interposed black region between the red and blue color Doppler shift is the result of:
- **A.** Acoustic shadowing
- **B.** Intercept angle
- **C.** Electronic interference
- **D.** Signal aliasing
- **E.** Flow disruption

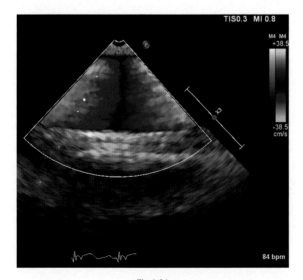

Fig 1.21

Question 10

Which of the following allows measurement of higher velocities with pulsed Doppler ultrasound?
- **A.** Shifting the baseline
- **B.** Decreasing the pulse repetition frequency
- **C.** Increasing depth
- **D.** Decreasing the Nyquist limit

Question 11

The black signal seen on the parasternal long-axis view shown (Fig. 1.22) is best explained by:
- **A.** Acoustic shadowing
- **B.** Intercept angle
- **C.** Electronic interference
- **D.** Reverberations
- **E.** Refraction of the ultrasound beam

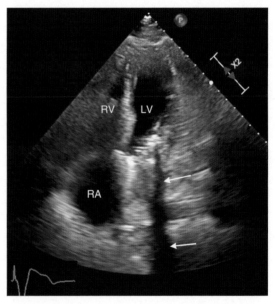

Fig 1.22

Question 12

Which of the following is least affected by increasing width of the 2D scanning sector?
- **A.** Temporal resolution
- **B.** Spatial resolution
- **C.** Axial resolution

Questions 13-17

Select the Doppler modality that offers the best diagnostic data for Questions 13 to 17:

  A. Color Doppler imaging
  B. Pulsed Doppler imaging
  C. CW Doppler imaging

Question 13: Myocardial velocity for evaluation of LV diastolic function

Question 14: Vena contracta for mitral valve regurgitation severity assessment

Question 15: Pulmonary venous flow reversal for mitral regurgitation severity assessment

Question 16: Velocity of the aortic jet in a patient with severe aortic stenosis

Question 17: Tricuspid regurgitation velocity in a patient with pulmonary hypertension

ANSWERS

Answer 1: D

In this parasternal long-axis image of a patient with a bileaflet mechanical aortic valve, strong reflections from one of the valve occludes *(short arrow)* appears as a linear echo in the aorta due to refraction of the strong reflector being displayed as a line across the width of the image *(long arrow)*.

Answer 2: A

This parasternal long axis image of a patient with a bileaflet mechanical aortic valve (and a mitral valve clip) shows reverberations from the aortic valve obscuring the left atrium. Reverberation occurs if strong specular reflectors result in the ultrasound signal going back and forth between the two reflectors before returning to the transducer. The received delayed signal is assigned to expected depth based on the time interval from transmission, leading to display of multiple echodensities in a line distal to the actual structure. In this case, reverberation between the two valve leaflets result in linear artifacts distal to the valve. There also is an acoustic shadow from the mechanical aortic valve between the two reverberation artifacts.

Answer 3: C

Doppler ultrasound sends a signal that is reflected and backscattered off of small structures, such as red blood cells. The reflected backscatter frequencies will be dependent on the speed and direction of blood flow. Based on the Doppler equation, higher Doppler frequency shifts are associated with a higher velocity recording. Peak tricuspid regurgitant jet velocity is the highest recorded velocity from the Doppler envelope. The highest velocity is recorded when the ultrasound beam is parallel with flow.

Answer 4: E

Attenuation describes the loss in ultrasound signal strength due to tissue absorption of ultrasound energy, resulting in poor image quality in the far field. Use of a lower frequency transducer aids tissue penetration, improving image quality, but will relatively lower image resolution in the near field.

Answer 5: B

High amplitude oscillations of the piezoelectric crystal elements may create an acoustic noise artifact, termed *ring-down artifact*, or *near field clutter*, which limits image resolution within 1 to 2 cm of the transducer. This is commonly seen in apical view images of the LV, with an artifact in the LV apex. Multiple views of the LV are needed to correctly identify the artifact.

Answer 6: B

Attenuation is the loss of signal intensity as the ultrasound wave travels through the tissue and back to the transducer. Attenuation is dependent on acoustic properties of the tissue, transducer frequency, acoustic pressure (power), and travel distance. Air produces significant attenuation that is minimized by applying gel to a transducer and avoiding lung tissue. Lowering the transducer frequency improves tissue penetration by increasing the ultrasound wavelength and thus reduces attenuation. Increasing the ultrasound power results in a stronger signal reflected back to the transducer. Increasing sector depth leads to more attenuation by increasing the distance the ultrasound signal travels.

Answer 7: A

The duty factor is the percent of time between ultrasound pulses used for transmitting the ultrasound signal. A CW Doppler continuously sends and receives ultrasound signal and thus has a duty factor of 100% (or 1), whereas a pulsed Doppler typically has a duty factor of 5%. Continuous sampling of the ultrasound signal leads to range ambiguity but allows for measuring higher velocities by eliminating the Nyquist limit. A dedicated CW Doppler transducer has a smaller surface footprint (aperture), allowing for optimal positioning and angulation of the ultrasound beam. All forms of Doppler are equally susceptible to nonparallel alignment, leading to underestimation of frequency shifts.

Answer 8: A

Burst length represents the number of ultrasound bursts transmitted along each sample line in the imaging sector. A higher number of bursts increases the accuracy of mean velocity assessment, but, because of increased data acquisition, results in a slower frame rate. Color scale shows the direction and velocity of flow. Shifting the color scale increases identification of lower velocity flow as long as the maximum velocity is within the Nyquist limit. Beyond the Nyquist limit, there is aliasing of the signal. Electronic interference affects image quality and therefore resolution of velocities within the color sector, but it does not affect frame rate. Variance displays flow turbulence in the color sector and is superimposed on the standard color velocity scale. Although variance can be toggled on/off and affects the display of flow turbulence, the color frame rate is not affected. With Doppler imaging, the signal is optimized when the ultrasound beam is parallel with flow. If flow is perpendicular to the ultrasound beam (90° intercept angle), this is displayed as absence of color, or no detectable flow, but does not affect imaging frame rate.

Answer 9: B

Color Doppler imaging samples blood velocity moving toward (displayed as red) or away (displayed as blue) from the transducer. Maximal velocities are obtained when flow is parallel to the ultrasound beam. In this TEE long-axis view of the descending thoracic aorta, systolic blood flow is from right to left across the image; thus flow toward the transducer on the right is displayed in red and flow away from the transducer is displayed in blue. Flow perpendicular to the transducer, in this case the interposed black region, is recorded as an absent signal. Thus, this black region is due to a perpendicular intercept angle in this image. Acoustic shadowing occurs when a strong specular reflector, such as prosthetic valves or calcium, blocks ultrasound penetration distal to the reflector. Electronic interference is displayed as an overlaying artifact, which is not associated with the image and may extend beyond tissue borders. Signal aliasing results in flow being displayed as if it were due to flow opposite in direction to actual flow. So, flow toward the transducer, by convention shown in red, would be displayed as blue, and vice versa. Signal aliasing often is seen on subcostal images of the proximal abdominal aorta. Disruption of flow would be accompanied by turbulent and disarrayed flow with aliasing of the color Doppler signal at the point of disruption, which is not seen on this image of a normal descending thoracic aorta.

Answer 10: A

To accurately measure the velocity of a sound wave, the signal must be sampled at least twice per wavelength. Aliasing occurs from under-sampling of the backscattered signal, resulting in ambiguity in measuring the Doppler frequency shift with higher frequency shifts appearing as lower velocities in the opposite direction. The maximum pulse repetition frequency, or Nyquist limit, is the sampling rate at a given depth of interrogation for a given transmitted frequency. Thus, the highest velocity measurable without aliasing is limited to one-half of the pulse repetition frequency (Nyquist limit). Decreasing the pulse repetition frequency (and hence Nyquist limit) will decrease the measurable velocity and lead to more aliasing. The pulse repetition frequency decreases with increasing depth as more time is required to transmit and receive the backscattered signals. Shifting the baseline does not change the Nyquist limit but acts as an electronic "cut and paste" moving the signal in the opposite channel to show the physiologic velocity curve, in effect looking like less aliasing in one direction of flow.

Answer 11: A

This 2D image in an apical four-chamber view shows severe mitral leaflet and annular calcification resulting in an acoustic shadow. Calcium is a strong specular reflector, which blocks ultrasound penetration distally. Most of the transmitted ultrasound beam reflects from the calcium back to the transducer. This is shown on the generated image as a bright echodensity at the site of calcium with shadowing of the signal in the distal field. On 2D imaging, a parallel intercept angle between the structure of interest and the ultrasound beam results in image "drop out," as few signals are reflected from the anatomic structure. Electronic interference typically has a geometric pattern and affects the entire 2D image. Reverberations appear as multiple bright echo-densities distal to the anatomic structure, whereas refraction results in the structure of interest appearing lateral to the actual location.

Answer 12: C

With scanned (2D) imaging, the image sector is formed by multiple adjacent scan lines where the transducer sweeps the ultrasound beam across the imaging field. Rapid image processing allows for real-time imaging. Widening the scanning sector allows for improved spatial resolution across the imaging field. Because time is incurred sweeping the ultrasound beam across the imaging field with 2D imaging, temporal resolution is optimal with M-mode imaging, which images only along a single scan line. A wider 2D scanning sector decreases imaging frame rate and decreases temporal resolution. Axial resolution (longitudinal resolution) is resolution in the direction parallel to the ultrasound beam. Because resolution is the same at any point along an ultrasound beam, axial resolution is not affected by scanning sector width.

Answers 13-17

Answer 13: **B**
Answer 14: **A**
Answer 15: **B**
Answer 16: **C**
Answer 17: **C**

CW Doppler imaging allows accurate measurement of high velocity flow without aliasing of the signal. Clinically, CW Doppler is used whenever a high velocity signal is present—for example, with aortic stenosis, tricuspid regurgitation, mitral regurgitation, or a ventricular septal defect. However, with CW Doppler, sampling occurs along the line of interrogation without localization of the point of maximum velocity along that line (lack of range resolution). The origin of the high velocity signal is inferred from imaging data or localized using pulsed Doppler or color flow imaging.

Color Doppler imaging is useful for evaluating the spatial distribution of flow, which is especially helpful in determining the severity and mechanism of regurgitant flow. The width of the color Doppler regurgitant jet, the vena contracta, is a reliable measure of regurgitation severity.

Pulsed-wave Doppler imaging allows spatial localization of a velocity signal but is best used for low velocity signals with a maximum velocity that is below the Nyquist level. Clinical examples of the use of pulsed Doppler include LV inflow across the mitral valve, pulmonary venous flow, and LV outflow velocity proximal to the aortic valve (even when aortic stenosis is present). With velocities that exceed the Nyquist limit, aliasing of the pulsed-wave Doppler signal occurs, which precludes accurate velocity measurements. Conventional Doppler imaging assesses blood flow velocity by measuring signals from moving blood cells. With myocardial tissue Doppler imaging, as is used for LV diastolic function assessment, pulsed Doppler is used to quantify the lower velocity signals of myocardial tissue motion.

2 The Transthoracic Echocardiogram

STEP-BY-STEP APPROACH

Step 1: Clinical Data

- The indication for the study determines the focus of the examination.
- Key clinical history and physical examination findings and results of any previous cardiac imaging studies are noted.

   ❖ KEY POINTS

   - The goal of the echo study is to answer the specific question asked by the referring provider.
   - Blood pressure is recorded at the time of the echo, because many measurements vary with loading conditions.
   - Knowledge of clinical data ensures that the echo study includes all the pertinent images and Doppler data. For example, when a systolic murmur is present, the echo study includes data addressing all the possible causes for this finding.
   - Data from previous imaging studies may identify specific areas of concern, such as a pericardial effusion noted on chest computed tomography (CT) imaging.
   - Detailed information about previous cardiac procedures assists in interpretation of post-operative findings, evaluation of implanted devices (such as prosthetic valves or percutaneous closure devices), and detection of complications.
   - Use of precise anatomic terminology facilitates accurate communication of imaging results (Table 2.1).

Step 2: Patient Positioning

- A steep left lateral position provides acoustic access for parasternal and apical views (Fig. 2.1).

- The subcostal views are obtained when the patient is supine; if needed, the legs are bent to relax the abdominal wall.
- Suprasternal notch views are obtained when the patient is supine with the head turned toward either side.

❖ KEY POINTS

- Images may be improved with suspended respiration, typically at end-expiration but sometimes at other phases of the respiratory cycle.
- An examination bed with an apical cutout allows a steeper left lateral position, often providing improved acoustic access for apical views.
- Imaging can be performed with either hand holding the transducer and with the examiner on either side of the patient. However, imaging from the patient's left side avoids reaching over the patient and is essential for apical views when the patient's girth is larger than the arm span of the examiner.
- Prolonged or repetitive imaging requires the examiner to learn ergonomic approaches to minimize mechanical stress and avoid injury.

Step 3: Instrumentation Principles

- A higher transducer frequency provides improved resolution but less penetration of the ultrasound signal.
- Harmonic imaging is frequently used to improve image quality, particularly recognition of endothelial borders.
- Depth, zoom mode, and sector width are adjusted to optimize the image and frame rate, depending on the structure or flow of interest (Fig. 2.2).
- Gain settings are adjusted to optimize the data recording while avoiding artifacts.

TABLE 2.1	Terminology for Normal Echocardiographic Anatomy
Aorta*	Sinuses of Valsalva Sinotubular junction Coronary ostia Ascending aorta Descending thoracic aorta Proximal abdominal aorta
Aortic valve	Right, left, and non-coronary cusps Nodules of Arantius Lambl excrescence
Mitral valve	Anterior and posterior leaflets Posterior leaflet scallops (lateral, central, medial) Chordae (primary, secondary, tertiary; basal, and marginal) Commissures (medial and lateral)
Left ventricle	Wall segments (see Chapter 8) Septum, free wall Base, apex Medial and lateral papillary muscles
Right ventricle	Inflow segment Moderator band Outflow tract (conus) Supraventricular crest Anterior, posterior, and conus papillary muscles
Tricuspid value	Anterior, septal, and posterior leaflets Chordae Commissures
Right atrium	RA appendage SVC and IVC junctions Valve of IVC (Chiari network) Coronary sinus ostium Crista terminalis Fossa ovalis Patent foramen ovale
Left atrium	LA appendage Superior and inferior left pulmonary veins Superior and inferior right pulmonary veins Ridge at junction of LA appendage and left superior pulmonary vein
Pericardium	Oblique sinus Transverse sinus

IVC, Inferior vena cava; *SVC,* superior vena cava.

*The term *aortic root* is used inconsistently, sometimes meaning the aortic sinuses and sometimes meaning the entire segment of the aorta from the annulus to the arch (including sinuses and ascending aorta).

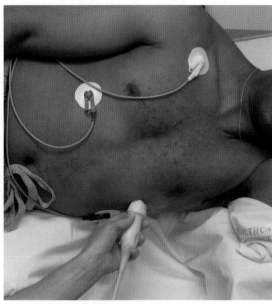

Fig. 2.1 **Patient positioning for transthoracic echocardiography.** The patient is positioned in a steep left lateral decubitus position on an examination bed with a removable section cut out of the mattress to allow placement of the transducer on the apex by the sonographer as shown. Ultrasound gel is used to enhance coupling between the transducer face and the patient's skin. The sonographer sits on an adjustable chair and uses the left hand for scanning and the right hand to adjust the instrument panel. The room is darkened to improve visualization on the ultrasound instrument display screen.

- ❏ With harmonic imaging, flat structures (such as valve leaflets) appear thicker than with fundamental imaging.
- ❏ Frame rate is higher for a shorter depth or a narrower sector; a fast frame rate is especially important with Doppler color flow imaging.
- ❏ Too narrow a sector may miss important anatomic or physiologic findings.
- ❏ Excessive gain results in artifacts with both imaging and Doppler, whereas inadequate gain results in data loss.

Step 4: Data Recording

- ■ Representative digital images from the echo study are saved to document the findings and for later review and measurement.
- ■ Echo images include an electrocardiogram (ECG) tracing for timing purposes.
- ■ A 2-beat cine loop is adequate for sinus rhythm; longer timed cycles are used when atrial fibrillation or other arrhythmia is present.

❖ **KEY POINTS**

- ❏ Two-dimensional (2D) echo images in each view are recorded first with a depth and sector width that encompasses all the structures in the image plane and then at a depth and sector width optimized for the structures of interest (Fig. 2.3).

❖ **KEY POINTS**

- ❏ Although the control panel varies for each instrument, the basic functions are similar for all ultrasound systems.
- ❏ The highest frequency that penetrates adequately to the depth of interest is used for optimal imaging.

Patient information		Power output		Alpha numeric keyboard		Physiologic inputs	
Transducer Selection						ECG size and position	Respiration
TTE 3 MHz	TTE 5 MHz	TEE	CWD				

IMAGING						**DOPPLER**		
M-mode	2D	3D	Harmonic			Pulsed	CW	Color
Depth		TGC		**Common controls** (used for all modalities)		Doppler scale		Baseline
Sector width				Trackball		High pass filter		Color variance
Focal depth						Dynamic range		Color scale
Dynamic range				Gain	Record			
Post-processing				Measurements and calculations		Spectral display sweep speed		Sample volume size

Fig. 2.2 Schematic diagram illustrating the typical features of a simplified echocardiographic instrument panel. Each ultrasound system has a unique instrument panel, ranging from simple to complex, often now integrated into an interactive screen rather than physical buttons. However, the functions controlled by the instrument panel fall into several basic categories as shown schematically here. Understanding the basic principles of ultrasound physics, imaging and Doppler parameters allow the operator to quickly master the interface for any given ultrasound system. Additional options are provided as needed for advanced imaging modalities, such as 3D imaging or speckle tracking strain.

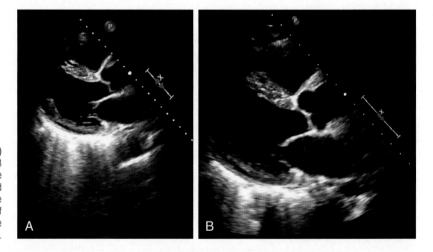

Fig. 2.3 Parasternal long-axis view. (A) Initially images are recorded at a depth of 18 cm to show the structures posterior to the heart *(top)*. **(B)** Next, images are recorded with the depth decreased to 13 cm and the resolution mode used (note that the top of the displayed image now is 2 cm from the skin) to focus on the aortic and mitral valves.

- Additional zoom mode images of normal and abnormal findings are recorded as needed.
- Three-dimensional (3D) imaging is used routinely for measurement of ventricular volumes and as needed for other cardiac structures (see Chapters 4 and 6).
- Spectral pulsed and continuous-wave (CW) Doppler data are recorded with the baseline and velocity range adjusted so that the flow signal fits but fills the vertical axis. The time scale is adjusted to maximize the accuracy of measurements (usually an x-axis of 100 mm/s) (Fig. 2.4).
- Color Doppler is recorded after sector width and depth are adjusted to optimize frame rate and gain is set just below the level that results in background speckle.
- The variance mode on the color scale is preferred by many examiners (including the authors) to enhance recognition of abnormal flows.

- Some normal flows result in a variance display—for example, when left ventricular (LV) outflow velocity exceeds the Nyquist limit and signal aliasing occurs (Fig. 2.5).

Step 5: Examination Sequence

- Subsequent chapters provide details on the elements of the examination for each clinical condition needed for a final diagnosis.
- These examination elements are incorporated into a systemic patient study sequence.

❖ KEY POINTS

- There are several approaches to an examination sequence; any of these are appropriate if a complete systemic examination is performed.
- In some clinical situations, a limited examination may be appropriate, with the study components selected by the referring or performing physician.

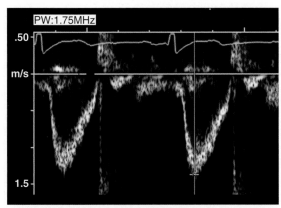

Fig. 2.4 Pulsed Doppler velocity recording. The spectral display of the pulsed wave *(PW)* Doppler signal is shown with the baseline shifted and velocity scale adjusted to avoid aliasing and to use the full vertical axis to improve measurement accuracy; for example, the signal fits but fills the graphical display. The horizontal time scale is 100 mm/s, which is standard for most Doppler recordings.

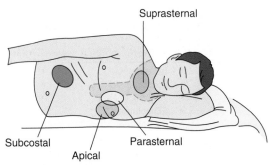

Fig. 2.6 Standard acoustic windows. The positions on the chest wall where ultrasound can reach the cardiac structures without intervening lung or bone include the parasternal, apical, subcostal, and suprasternal notch windows. The parasternal and apical windows typically are optimal with the patient in a steep left lateral position. For the subcostal window, the patient is supine with the knees flexed to relax the abdominal vasculature. For the suprasternal notch window, the patient is supine with the head tilted back and to one side.

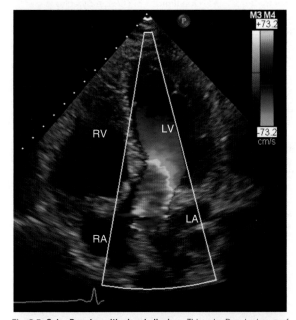

Fig. 2.5 Color Doppler with signal aliasing. This color Doppler image of LV outflow in an anteriorly angulated apical 4-chamber view shows signal aliasing adjacent to the septum in the subaortic region. Although this appearance may be due to an asymmetric flow profile, the effects of intercept angle also may be important. Even if the velocity is identical across the outflow tract, compared with the region along the anterior mitral valve leaflet, the region adjacent to the septum the Doppler beam is more parallel to the flow direction. The higher Doppler shift results in signal aliasing. Aliasing at the aortic valve level is expected because the aortic velocity typically exceeds the Nyquist limit at this depth (0.73 m/s in this example).

❏ The approach suggested here is based on obtaining all data (imaging and Doppler) for each acoustic window (parasternal, apical, subcostal, and suprasternal) before moving to the next acoustic window; this approach minimizes the time needed to reposition the patient between acoustic windows (Fig. 2.6).

❏ Some examiners prefer to obtain all the imaging data and then obtain all the Doppler data; this approach allows the Doppler data recording to be tailored to the imaging findings.

❏ With any approach, the examiner may need to go back to previous acoustic windows at the end of the examination if additional views or measurements are needed based on abnormal findings.

❏ The examination sequence also may need to be modified depending on patient factors (inability to move, bandages, etc.) or the urgency of the examination.

❏ Basic measurements are made as the examination is performed (Table 2.2) or during review of images at completion of the study. Normal values for chamber sizes are provided in Chapter 6 (Tables 6.2 and 6.3) and for the aorta in Chapter 16 (Tables 16.1 and 16.2).

Step 6: Parasternal Window

Long-Axis View

■ Many echocardiographers start with the parasternal long-axis view with:
  ○ Imaging to show the aortic and mitral valves, left atrium, aortic sinuses and ascending aorta, LV basal segments, and the right ventricular (RV) outflow tract
  ○ Color Doppler to screen for aortic and mitral regurgitation
■ Standard measurements include:
  ○ LV end-diastolic and end-systolic diameters; diastolic thickness of the septum and LV inferior-lateral wall just apical from the mitral leaflet tips (Fig. 2.7)
  ○ Aortic diameter at end-diastole (Fig. 2.8)
  ○ Left atrial anterior–posterior dimension
  ○ Vena contracta width for aortic and mitral regurgitation

TABLE 2.2   Basic Echo Imaging Measurements

Cardiac Structure	Basic Measurements	Additional Measurements	Technical Details
Left ventricle	• ED dimension • ES dimension • Wall thickness • ED volume • ES volume • Ejection fraction	• Stroke volume • LV mass • Global longitudinal strain	• 2D imaging is used to ensure measurements are centered and perpendicular to the long axis of the LV. • M-mode provides superior time resolution and more accurate identification of endocardial borders. • LV volumes and ejection fraction are measured by 2D and 3D imaging. • LV volumes and stroke volume often are indexed to body size.
Left atrium	• AP diameter	• LA area • LA volume	• Left atrial anterior–posterior dimension provides a quick screen but may underestimate LA size. • When LA size is important for clinical decision making, measurement of LA volume is helpful.
Right ventricle	• Visual estimate of size • TAPSE	• ED RV outflow tract diameter • ED RV length and diameter	• Quantitation of RV size by echo is challenging due to the complex 3D shape of the chamber. • TAPSE via M-mode is a quantitative measure of RV systolic function.
Right atrium	• Visual estimate of size		• RA size is usually compared to the LA in the apical 4-chamber view.
Aorta	• ED diameter at sinuses	• Maximum diameter indexed to expected dimension • Diameter at multiple sites in aorta	• With 2D echo, inner edge to inner edge measurements are more reproducible. • Measurements are made at end-diastole by convention, but end-systolic measurements also may be helpful.
Pulmonary artery		• Diameter	

AP, Anterior–posterior; *ED,* end-diastole (onset of the QRS); *ES,* end-systole (minimum LV volume); *TAPSE,* tricuspid annular plane systolic excursion.

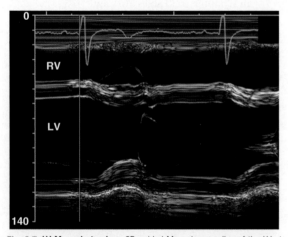

Fig. 2.7 LV M-mode tracing. 2D-guided M-mode recording of the LV at the mitral chordal level. End-diastolic measurements of wall thickness and cavity dimension are made at the onset of the QRS, as shown. End-systolic measurements are made at the maximum posterior motion of the septum (when septal motion is normal) or at minimal LV size. The rapid sampling rate with M-mode allows more accurate identification of the endocardial border, which is distinguished from chordae or trabeculations as being a continuous line in diastole, with the steepest slope during systole.

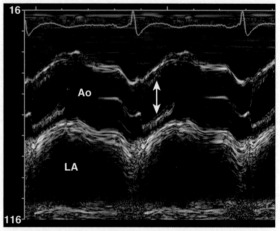

Fig. 2.8 Aortic valve M-mode tracing. 2D guided M-mode recording of the aortic valve *(Ao)* and LA allows measurement of aortic root dimension at end-diastole using a leading-edge to leading-edge approach; the aortic leaflet separation *(arrows);* and the left atrial maximum anterior–posterior dimension in early diastole. The fine fluttering of the aortic valve leaflets is normal.

❖ **KEY POINTS**

◻ Images are initially recorded at a depth that includes the descending thoracic aorta to detect pleural and pericardial effusions.

◻ Next, depth is reduced to the level of the posterior wall for assessment of the size and function of the base of the LV basal segments and the RV outflow tract.

◻ The aortic and mitral valves are examined with zoom mode sweeping through the valve planes from medial to lateral to assess valve anatomy and motion (Fig. 2.9).

◻ M-mode tracings of the mitral valve can aid in timing of leaflet motion, such as systolic anterior motion in hypertrophic cardiomyopathy or posterior buckling in mitral valve prolapse.

◻ Left atrium (LA) anterior–posterior dimension may underestimate LA enlargement; LA volume is measured from apical views.

◻ The aortic sinuses of Valsalva and sinotubular junction are visualized first from the standard window and then with the transducer moved up one or more interspaces to visualize the proximal and mid-ascending aorta (Fig. 2.10).

◻ Color Doppler of aortic and mitral valves is used to screen for valve regurgitation. If more than physiologic regurgitation is present, further evaluation is needed as discussed in Chapter 12.

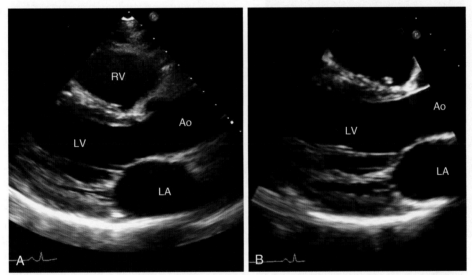

Fig. 2.9 **Mitral valve imaging.** (A) First the mitral valve is examined at a standard depth in the parasternal long-axis view. (B) Then zoom mode (ZOOM) is used to optimize visualization of the aortic and mitral valves. The image plane is angled slightly medial and lateral to encompass the medial and lateral aspects of the valve. Some normal thin mitral chords are well seen in this slightly laterally angulated view, extending from the mitral closure plane to the papillary muscle.

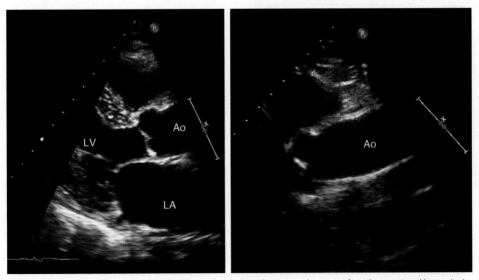

Fig. 2.10 **Ascending aorta.** The ascending aorta is visualized by moving the transducer up an interspace from the parasternal long-axis view. *Ao,* Aorta.

Right Ventricular Inflow View

- From the long-axis view, the image plane is angled medially to show the RV inflow view (Fig. 2.11) with:
  - Imaging of the right atrium (RA), tricuspid valve, and RV
  - Color Doppler evaluation of tricuspid regurgitation (vena contracta width)
  - CW Doppler recording of tricuspid regurgitant (TR) jet velocity
- Standard measurements include:
  - Maximum tricuspid regurgitant velocity (Fig. 2.12)

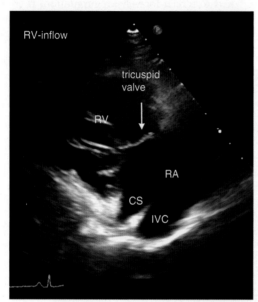

Fig. 2.11 **RV inflow view.** From the parasternal long-axis view, the image plane is angulated medially to visualize the RV inflow view with the RV, RA, coronary sinus *(CS)*, inferior vena cava *(IVC)*, and tricuspid valve.

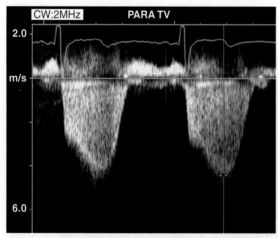

Fig. 2.12 **Tricuspid regurgitant (TR) jet velocity.** The tricuspid regurgitation jet is recorded with CW Doppler from both the parasternal RV inflow view and from the LV apex. Only the highest velocity is reported, in normal sinus rhythm, because the apparent lower velocity signal is due to a nonparallel intercept angle between the ultrasound beam and regurgitant jet. This example shows a high velocity jet consistent with severe pulmonary hypertension. The maximum velocity is measured at the edge of the dense "envelope" of flow, avoiding the faint signals due to gain and transit time effects.

❖ KEY POINTS

- ❏ Slide the transducer apically one interspace if views are not obtained from the standard window.
- ❏ Adjust depth to include the RA, RV, and tricuspid valve.
- ❏ The entrance of the coronary sinus and the inferior vena cava (IVC) into the RA are seen in this view.
- ❏ A small amount of tricuspid regurgitation on color Doppler is seen in most (>80%) normal individuals and sometimes is referred to as *physiologic.*
- ❏ The CW Doppler TR jet is recorded from multiple views; the highest velocity represents the most parallel intercept angle with flow and is used to estimate pulmonary pressure; lower velocity recordings are ignored.

Right Ventricular Outflow View

- From the long-axis view, the image plane is angled laterally to show the RV outflow view (Fig. 2.13) with:
  - Imaging of the RV outflow tract, pulmonic valve, and main pulmonary artery
  - Color Doppler evaluation of pulmonic regurgitation (Fig. 2.14)
  - Pulsed Doppler recording of pulmonary artery flow (Fig. 2.15)
- Standard measurements include:
  - Antegrade velocity in the pulmonary artery

❖ KEY POINTS

- ❏ Slide the transducer cephalad one interspace if views are not obtained from the standard window.
- ❏ Adjust depth to include the RV outflow tract, main pulmonary artery, and pulmonary artery bifurcation.
- ❏ The pulmonic valve often is difficult to visualize in adults, but a small amount of pulmonic regurgitation typically is present with a normally functioning valve.
- ❏ The pulsed Doppler recording of flow in the main pulmonary artery is helpful for assessment of pulmonary pressures and to exclude pulmonic stenosis or a patent ductus arteriosus.

Short-Axis View

- From the long-axis view, the image plane is rotated 90 degrees to show the short-axis plane with:
  - Imaging and color Doppler at the level of the aortic valve to evaluate the aortic, tricuspid, and pulmonic valves (Fig. 2.16)
  - 2D imaging and color Doppler evaluation of the interatrial septum; imaging at the level of the mitral valve for evaluation of mitral leaflet anatomy and motion and LV size and function (Fig. 2.17)
  - Imaging at the mid-papillary muscle level to evaluate global and regional LV size and function (Fig. 2.18)

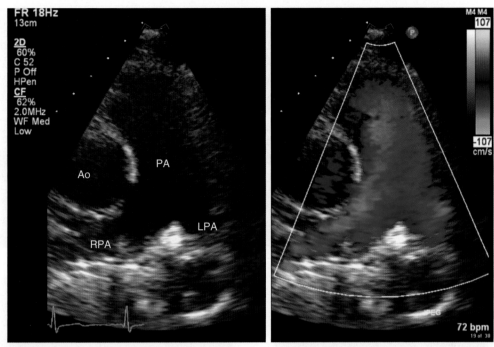

Fig. 2.13 **RV outflow view.** The 2D and color Doppler RV outflow view, obtained by angulating the transducer laterally from the parasternal long-axis view, shows the RV outflow tract, pulmonic valve, main pulmonary artery *(PA)*, and left and right branch pulmonary arteries *(LPA* and *RPA)*. *Ao,* Aorta.

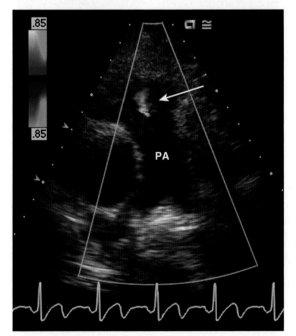

Fig. 2.14 **Color Doppler of pulmonic valve regurgitation.** Color Doppler in a RV outflow view showing a narrow jet of pulmonic regurgitation *(arrow)* in diastole. Mild pulmonic regurgitation is seen in about 80% of normal adults. *PA,* Pulmonary artery.

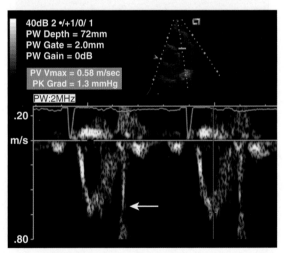

Fig. 2.15 **Pulsed Doppler recording of normal flow in the RV outflow tract.** The pulmonic valve closure click indicates that the sample volume is on the RV side of the valve. Normal flow shows a smooth velocity curve that peaks in mid-systole with a velocity less than 1 m/s.

- Standard measurements include:
  - M-mode or 2D measurements of the aorta, LA, and LV using the combination of long and short-axis view to ensure the dimensions are measured in the minor axis of each chamber or vessel (see Table 2.1)

❖ **KEY POINTS**

- ❏ The aortic and pulmonic valves normally are perpendicular to each other (when the aortic valve is seen in short axis, the pulmonic valve is seen in long axis).
- ❏ Zoom mode is used to identify the number of aortic valve leaflets, taking care to visualize the leaflets in systole.
- ❏ A bicuspid aortic valve is a common abnormality with a prevalence of about 1% of the total

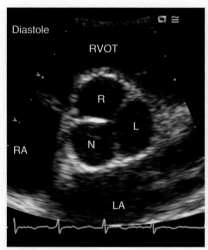
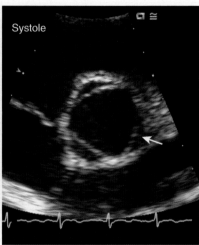

Fig. 2.16 Aortic valve imaging. Parasternal short-axis view of a normal trileaflet aortic valve in diastole *(left)* and in systole *(right)*. The normal positions of the right *(R)*, left *(L)*, and noncoronary *(N)* cusps are seen in diastole. In systole, the open left coronary cusp often is difficult to see *(arrow)*, because the leaflet edge is parallel to the ultrasound beam. However, the three commissures of the open valve are clearly visualized. *RVOT,* Right ventricular outflow tract.

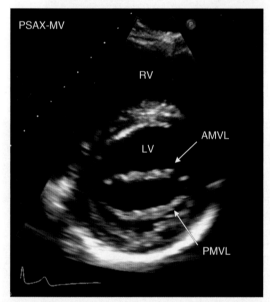
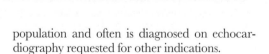

Fig. 2.17 Mitral valve imaging. Parasternal short-axis view of the left ventricle at the level of the mitral valve showing both anterior and posterior valve leaflets. *AMVL,* Anterior mitral valve leaflet; *PMVL,* posterior mitral valve leaflet; *PSAX-MV,* parasternal short-axis–mitral valve.

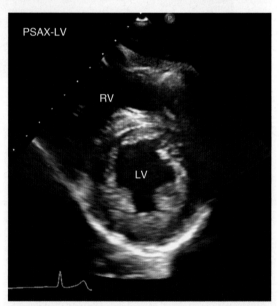

Fig. 2.18 LV short-axis view. Parasternal short-axis *(PSAX)* view of the LV at the papillary muscle level. The LV cavity should appear circular in this view, and an elliptical shape suggests an oblique intercept angle. This view sometimes requires the transducer be moved slightly apically from the short-axis view of the aortic valve, instead of just tilting the transducer toward the apex from a fixed position on the chest wall.

population and often is diagnosed on echocardiography requested for other indications.

- 3D imaging is useful for better definition of aortic or mitral valve anatomy in selected cases.
- The coronary artery ostia may be seen originating in expected positions from the right and left coronary sinuses.
- The atrial septum is seen in the short-axis view at the aortic valve level. Color flow imaging may help detect a patent foramen ovale but must be distinguished from normal flow in the RA (inflow from the superior and IVC and regurgitation across the tricuspid valve), all of which are adjacent to the atrial septum.

- Parasternal views of the LV at the papillary muscle level provide optimal endocardial definition and are used in conjunction with apical views for detection of regional wall motion abnormalities.

Step 7: Apical Window

Imaging Four-Chamber, Two-Chamber, and Long-Axis Views

- The apical window usually corresponds to the point of maximal impulse and is optimized with the patient in a steep left lateral position.

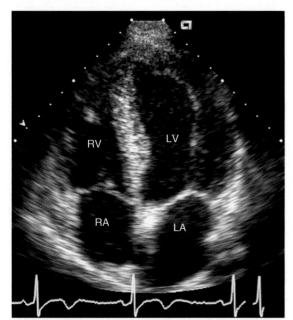

Fig. 2.19 **Apical 4-chamber view.** The transducer is correctly positioned over the LV apex as shown by the longer LV length than width and ellipsoid shape of the chamber. Foreshortening of this view results in a more spherical appearance of the LV. This older adult has both enlargement of atrium and some benign thickening (lipomatous hypertrophy) of the atrial septum. The loss of signal in the mid-segment of the atrial septum is an artifact, because the thin fossa ovalis is parallel to the ultrasound beam at this point resulting in echo "dropout."

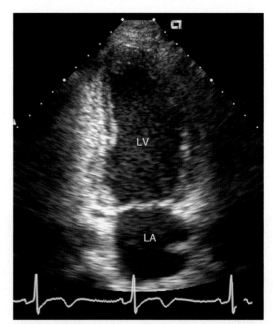

Fig. 2.20 **Apical 2-chamber view.** This view is obtained by rotating the transducer about 60° counterclockwise from the 4-chamber view.

- Images are obtained in 4-chamber (Fig. 2.19), 2-chamber (Fig. 2.20), and long-axis (Fig. 2.21) views to evaluate:
  - 2D images for LV size, wall thickness, global and regional systolic function, and longitudinal strain measurements
  - 3D full volume imaging for measurement of ventricular volumes and ejection fraction
  - RV size, wall thickness, and systolic function
  - Anatomy and motion of the mitral and tricuspid valves
  - LA and RA size and coronary sinus anatomy
  - The amount of pericardial fluid, if present
- Standard measurements include:
  - 2D apical biplane ejection fraction (see Chapter 5)
  - Global longitudinal strain
  - 3D LV ejection fraction
  - Measurement of LA area or volume when clinically indicated (Fig. 2.22)
  - Tricuspid annular plane systolic excursion (TAPSE) and other quantitative measures of RV systolic function (see Chapter 6)

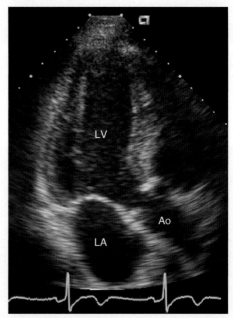

Fig. 2.21 **Apical long-axis view.** This view is obtained by rotating an additional 60° counterclockwise to obtain an image similar to the parasternal long-axis view. *Ao,* Aortic.

❖ **KEY POINTS**

- ❑ The three apical views are at approximately 60 degrees of rotation from each other; however, image planes are based on cardiac anatomy, not external reference points, so that slight adjustment of transducer position and angulation often is needed to optimize the image.
- ❑ Initial views are recorded at the maximum depth to see all the cardiac chambers and surrounding pericardium.

- Evaluation of the LV and RV are based on images with the depth adjusted to just beyond the valve annular plane. The RV is best visualized using zoom mode (Fig. 2.23).
- Left-sided echo contrast should be used to improve identification of LV endocardial borders when needed.
- Visual estimates of LV ejection fraction are appropriate only if quantitative measurements are not possible.
- From the 4-chamber view, the image plane is angled anteriorly to visualize the aortic valve (sometimes called the *5-chamber view*); this view is useful for Doppler recordings, but image quality is suboptimal at the depth of the aortic valve from the apical window (Fig. 2.24).
- The image plane is angled posteriorly to visualize the length of the coronary sinus and its entrance into the RA (Fig. 2.25).
- The LA appendage is not well visualized on transthoracic imaging, and the sensitivity for detection of LA thrombus is low. Transesophageal imaging is needed when atrial thrombus is suspected.
- The descending thoracic aorta is seen in cross section behind the left atrium in the long-axis view and in a longitudinal plane from the 2-chamber view with lateral angulation.

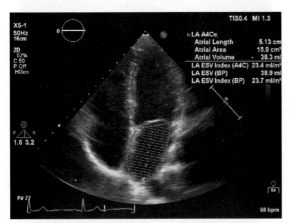

Fig. 2.22 Left atrial volume measurement. Left ventricle volume is measured in the apical 4-chamber view by tracing the inner edge of the atrial border at end-systole. At the mitral annulus, a straight line from leaflet insertion to leaflet insertion is used for this calculation. The area is also traced in the 2-chamber view for a biplane volume calculation.

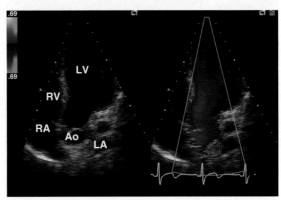

Fig. 2.24 Anteriorly angulated apical 4-chamber view (or 5-chamber view). Anterior angulation from the 4-chamber view allows visualization of the LV outflow tract and an oblique view of the aortic *(Ao)* valve. Laminar flow in the LV outflow tract is demonstrated with color Doppler.

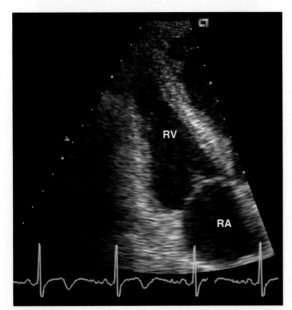

Fig. 2.23 Apical view focusing on the RV. RV size and function are best estimated by centering the RV in the image plane and adjusting depth and zoom appropriately.

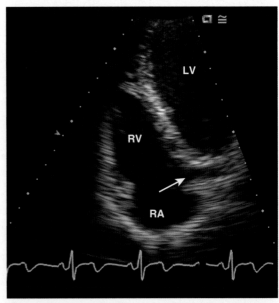

Fig. 2.25 Coronary sinus. The entrance of the coronary sinus *(arrow)* into the RA is visualized by posterior angulation from the apical 4-chamber view.

❑ With active adjustment of the imaging plane, pacemaker leads can be "tracked" visually at the entry into the heart along the course of the lead (RA, RV, coronary sinus).

Doppler Data

■ The apical window provides an intercept angle that is relatively parallel to flow for the aortic, mitral, and tricuspid valves. Standard data recording includes:

   ○ Pulsed Doppler recordings of transmitral flow, pulmonary vein inflow, and LV outflow (Fig. 2.26)

   ○ Color Doppler evaluation of mitral and tricuspid regurgitation

   ○ CW Doppler recordings of mitral, tricuspid, and aortic antegrade flow and regurgitation (Fig. 2.27)

■ Standard measurements include:

   ○ Pulsed Doppler antegrade mitral early (E) diastolic filling and atrial (A) filling velocities

   ○ Pulsed Doppler LV outflow and CW Doppler aortic flow velocities

   ○ Maximum velocity of the TR jet

   ○ Additional measurements as clinically indicated (see specific chapters for each clinical condition)

❖ **KEY POINTS**

❑ Transmitral and pulmonary venous inflow velocities are helpful for evaluation of LV diastolic dysfunction (see Chapter 7). Pulsed Doppler tissue velocities of the myocardial septal or lateral wall also are helpful for evaluation of diastolic function.

❑ There is only a small increase in velocity from the LV outflow tract to the ascending aorta in normal individuals (see Chapter 11).

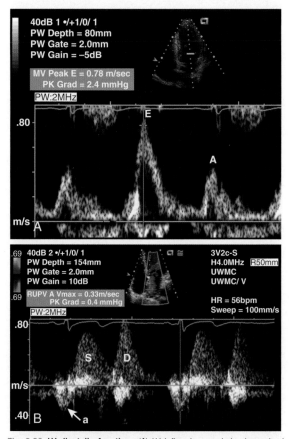

Fig. 2.26 LV diastolic function. (A) LV inflow is recorded using pulsed Doppler with the sample volume positioned at the mitral leaflet tips in diastole. The typical early (E) diastolic filling velocity and atrial (A) velocity are seen. **(B)** Left atrial inflow is recorded with the pulsed Doppler sample volume in the right superior pulmonary vein in an apical 4-chamber view. The normal pattern of systolic (S) and diastolic (D) inflow with a small atrial (a) flow reversal are seen.

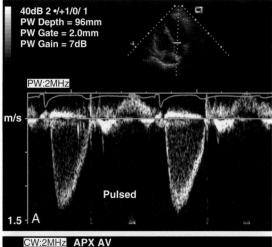

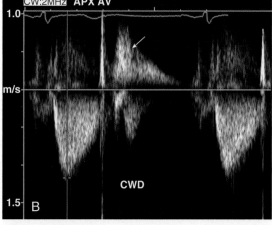

Fig. 2.27 LV outflow. (A) LV outflow is recorded with the Doppler sample volume on the LV side of the aortic valve either in an anteriorly angulated 4-chamber view or in an apical long-axis view. The normal smooth "envelope" of flow with dense signals along the outer edge and few velocity signals within the curve are seen. Again, the baseline and scale are adjusted to prevent aliasing and allow accurate measurements. **(B)** Aortic flow velocity is recorded from an apical approach using CW Doppler (CWD). This velocity tracing includes signals from the entire length of the ultrasound beam so that the velocity curve is filled in by lower velocities proximal to the valve. The aortic closing click is seen. In diastole, the relatively broad CW beam intersects the LV inflow curve (arrow).

- ☐ The CW Doppler recordings of aortic, mitral, and tricuspid regurgitation provide data on the severity of regurgitation (based on the density of the signal) and the transvalvular hemodynamics (based on the shape and density of the time velocity curve).
- ☐ Color flow Doppler from the apical approach is helpful for evaluation of jet direction and for visualization of proximal jet geometry (vena contracta) and the proximal isovelocity surface area (PISA).
- ☐ Apical color Doppler is less helpful for aortic regurgitation, because beam width is greater at the depth of the aortic valve than at the mitral valve.

Step 8: Subcostal Window

- ■ The subcostal window provides:
  - ○ An alternate acoustic window for evaluation of LV and RV systolic function (Fig. 2.28)
  - ○ An optimal angle to evaluate the interatrial septum
  - ○ Estimation of RA pressure based on the size and respiratory variation in the IVC (Fig. 2.29)
  - ○ Pulsed Doppler evaluation of hepatic vein flow (right atrial inflow) and proximal abdominal aortic flow, when clinically indicated (Fig. 2.30)
  - ○ An alternate acoustic window for evaluation of pericardial effusion and detection of abdominal ascites

❖ **KEY POINTS**

- ☐ Estimation of RA pressure is a standard part of the examination used to calculate pulmonary systolic pressure.
- ☐ Atrial septal defects often are best visualized on imaging and with color Doppler using a low Nyquist setting from the subcostal window.
- ☐ Hepatic vein flow patterns are helpful for detection of severe tricuspid regurgitation and for evaluation of pericardial disease.
- ☐ Descending aortic holodiastolic flow reversal is seen with severe aortic regurgitation; persistent holodiastolic antegrade flow is seen with aortic coarctation.

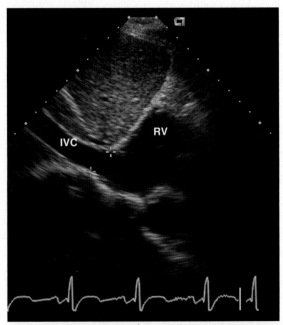

Fig. 2.29 Inferior vena cava (IVC). The IVC is examined from the subcostal view with the size and respiratory variation used to estimate right atrial pressure, as discussed in Chapter 6.

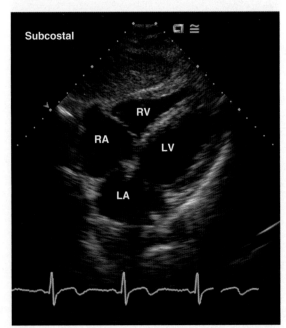

Fig. 2.28 Subcostal 4-chamber view. This view is useful for evaluation of RV and LV function. This view also is best for evaluation of the atrial septum because the ultrasound beam is perpendicular to the septum from this transducer position.

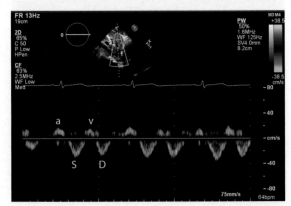

Fig. 2.30 Hepatic vein flow. Pulsed Doppler velocities are recorded from the subcostal view to evaluate right atrial filling when tricuspid regurgitation or pericardial disease is of concern. *a,* Atrial; *D,* diastolic wave; *S,* systolic wave; *v,* ventricular.

Step 9: Suprasternal Window

- The suprasternal window is a standard part of the examination of patients with diseases of the aortic valve or aorta.
- The suprasternal window provides:
  - Images of the aortic arch and proximal descending thoracic aorta (Fig. 2.31)
  - Pulsed and CW Doppler evaluation of descending aortic flow, when clinically indicated (Fig. 2.32)

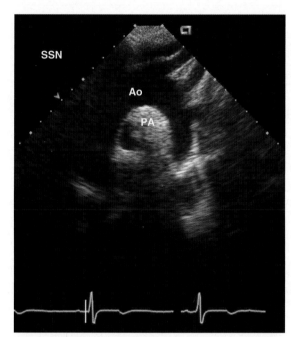

Fig. 2.31 Suprasternal notch *(SSN)* view. This view shows the ascending aorta *(Ao)*, arch, and descending thoracic aorta. A small segment of the right pulmonary artery *(PA)* is seen in cross section.

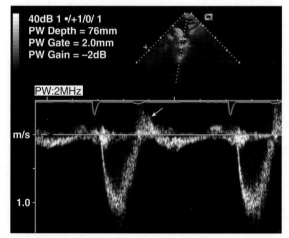

Fig. 2.32 Normal pattern of flow in the descending thoracic aorta. There is antegrade flow in systole, brief diastolic flow reversal as a result of aortic recoil and coronary blood flow, a small amount of antegrade flow in mid-diastole, and slight reversal just before the next cardiac cycle.

- A parallel intercept angle with the aortic velocity in some patients with native or prosthetic aortic valve disease

❖ KEY POINTS

- Aortic disease, such as aortic dissection, may be visualized from this window.
- An increased systolic velocity with persistent antegrade flow ("runoff") in diastole is seen with an aortic coarctation.
- Holodiastolic flow reversal in the descending aorta suggests significant aortic valve regurgitation.

Step 10: The Echo Report

- The echo report consists of four sections:
  - Clinical Data
  - Measurements
  - Echo Findings
  - Conclusions (with recommendations)

❖ KEY POINTS

- The Clinical Data section includes the reason for the study, pertinent history and physical examination findings, cardiac medications, and blood pressure.
- Standard measurements are indicated in the example (Table 2.3) with additional measurements as clinically indicated.
- The Echo Findings section documents what views and flow were recorded and describes any abnormal and key normal findings.
- The Conclusions section indicates the major diagnosis, associated findings, and pertinent negative findings (depending on the indication for the study).
- Image stills taken from the echo study addressing important findings may be incorporated into the final report.
- When clinically appropriate, specific recommendations are made. These include:
  - The clinical significance of the findings
  - Recommendations for cardiology evaluation and periodic follow-up
- Serious unexpected findings are communicated promptly directly to the referring physician.
- When data are not definitive, the findings are described along with a differential diagnosis to explain these findings.
- Additional diagnostic approaches are recommended as appropriate.

TABLE 2.3   Sample Echo Report

Name_____ Date of Study_____
Age: 45 years   Sex: M
Indication: Systolic murmur on auscultation
Cardiac medications: None
Clinical history: Chest pain on exertion, systolic murmur, no prior cardiac procedures
Blood pressure: 118/68 mm Hg   Heart rate: 60 bpm   Rhythm: NSR
Sonographer: BKS   Image quality: Excellent

Measurements

	Dimensions (cm)	Normal Values (Men)
LV chamber		
End-systole	3.2	2.1–4.0 cm
End-diastole	5.4	4.2–5.9 cm
Wall thickness (diastole)	0.8	0.6–1.0 cm
2D ejection fraction	65%	≥55 %
3D ejection fraction	64%	≥55 %
Left atrium	3.6	3.0–4.0 cm
Aortic sinus	2.9	<4.0 (<2.1 cm/m^2)

Doppler Flows

	Regurgitation	Velocity (m/s)	
Aortic valve	None	LV outflow tract	1.0
		Aorta	1.4
Mitral valve	Trace	E	1.0
		A	0.4
Pulmonary valve	Trace		
Tricuspid valve	Mild	TR jet	2.3

		Normal Values
RA pressure estimate (mm Hg)	5	0–5
PA pressure estimate (mm Hg)	26	20–30

Findings

Left ventricle	Wall thickness, internal dimension and systolic function are normal with an estimated ejection fraction of 65%. There are no resting regional wall motion abnormalities.
Left atrium	Size is normal.
Aortic valve	Trileaflet with normal systolic opening and no regurgitation.
Aortic root	Normal dimensions with normal contours of the sinuses of Valsalva.
Mitral valve	Normal anatomy and motion with no stenosis and only physiologic regurgitation.
PA pressures	Estimated pulmonary systolic pressure is normal at 21-26 mm Hg, based on the velocity in the TR jet and the size and respiratory variation of the inferior vena cava.
Right heart	Right ventricular size and systolic function are normal. Tricuspid and pulmonic valves show normal anatomy and Doppler flows. Right atrial size is normal.
Pericardium	No effusion.

Conclusions

1. Normal valve anatomy and function.
2. Normal left ventricle with an estimated ejection fraction of 65%.
3. Normal pulmonary pressures and right heart.

Given these findings, the murmur appreciated on physical examination most likely is a benign flow murmur. Although resting left ventricular regional function is normal, coronary disease cannot be excluded on a resting study. If there is concern that chest pain may be due to coronary disease, a stress study should be considered.
Signed: _____MD

THE ECHO EXAM

A Complete Echo Exam = Core Elements + Additional Components

Diagnostic TTE: Core Elements

Modality	Window	View/Signal	Basic Measurements
Clinical data		Indication for echo Key history and PE findings Previous cardiac imaging data	Blood pressure at time of Echo Exam
2D imaging	Parasternal	Long axis Short-axis aortic valve Short-axis mitral valve Short-axis LV (papillary muscle level) RV inflow	LV end-diastole and end-systole dimensions LV end-diastole wall thickness Aortic end-diastole sinus dimension LA dimension
	Apical	4-chamber Anteriorly angulated 4-chamber 2-chamber Long axis	Visual estimate or biplane ejection fraction
	Subcostal	4-chamber IVC with respiration Proximal abdominal aorta	
	Suprasternal	Aortic arch	
Pulsed Doppler	Parasternal	PA flow	PA velocity
	Apical	LV inflow LV outflow	E velocity A velocity LV outflow velocity
Color flow	Parasternal	Long axis: Aortic and mitral valves Short axis: Aortic and pulmonic valves RV inflow: Tricuspid valve	Color flow to identify regurgitation of all four valves. If more than mild, measure vena contracta
	Apical	4-chamber: Mitral and tricuspid valves Long axis: Aortic and mitral valves	
CW Doppler	Parasternal	Tricuspid valve Pulmonic valve	TR-jet velocity
	Apical	Aortic valve Mitral valve Tricuspid valve	Aortic velocity TR jet (pulmonary pressures)

A-velocity, Late diastolic ventricular filling velocity with atrial contraction; *E-velocity,* early-diastolic peak velocity; *IVC,* Inferior vena cava; *PA,* pulmonary artery; *PE,* pericardial effusion; *TR,* tricuspid regurgitation.

Diagnostic TTE: Additional Components

Abnormality on Core Elements	Additional Echo Exam Components (Chapter)
Reason for Echo	**Additional Components to Address Specific Clinical Question***
Left Ventricle	
Decreased ejection fraction	See Systolic Function (6)
Abnormal LV filling velocities	See Diastolic Function (7)
Regional wall motion abnormality	See Ischemic Heart Disease (8)
Increased wall thickness	See Hypertrophic Cardiomyopathy, Restrictive Cardiomyopathy and Hypertensive Heart Disease (9)
Valves	
Imaging evidence for stenosis or an increased antegrade transvalvular velocity	See Valve Stenosis (11)
Regurgitation greater than mild on color flow imaging or CW Doppler	See Valve Regurgitation (12)
Prosthetic valve	See Prosthetic Valves (13)
Valve mass or suspected endocarditis	See Endocarditis and Masses (14,15)
Right Heart	
Enlarged RV	See Pulmonary Heart Disease and Congenital Heart Disease (9,17)
Elevated TR-jet velocity	See Pulmonary Pressures (6)
Pericardium	
Pericardial effusion	See Pericardial Effusion (10)
Pericardial thickening	See Constrictive Pericarditis (10)
Great Vessels	
Enlarged aorta	See Aortic Disease (16)

TR, Tricuspid regurgitation.

*The echo exam should always include additional components to address the clinical indication. For example, if the indication is "heart failure," additional components to evaluate systolic and diastolic function are needed even if the core elements do not show obvious abnormalities. If the indication is "cardiac source of embolus," the additional components for that diagnosis are needed.

Principles of Doppler Quantitation

Method	Assumptions/Characteristics	Examples of Clinical Applications
Volume flow Stroke volume (SV) = CSA × VTI	• Laminar flow • Flat flow profile • Cross-sectional area (CSA) and velocity time integral (VTI) measured at same site	• Cardiac output • Continuity equation for valve area • Regurgitant volume calculations • Intracardiac shunts, pulmonary to systemic flow ratio
Velocity–pressure relationship $\Delta P = 4v^2$	• Flow limiting orifice • CW Doppler velocity (v) signal recorded parallel to flow	• Stenotic valve gradients • Calculation of pulmonary pressures • LV dP/dt
Spatial flow patterns	• Proximal flow convergence region • Narrow flow stream in orifice (vena contracta) • Downstream flow disturbance	• Detection of valve regurgitation and intracardiac shunts • Level of obstruction • Quantitation of regurgitant severity

SELF-ASSESSMENT QUESTIONS

Question 1

Identify the numbered "spaces" in Fig. 2.33:

1. _____
2. _____
3. _____
4. _____
5. _____

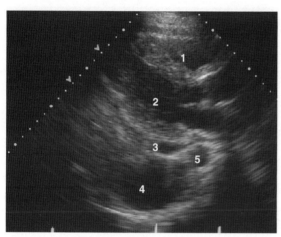

Fig. 2.33

Question 2

From the image presented (Fig. 2.34), identify which echo finding is indicated by the arrow:

A. Eustachian valve
B. Atrial myxoma
C. Crista terminalis
D. Thebesian valve

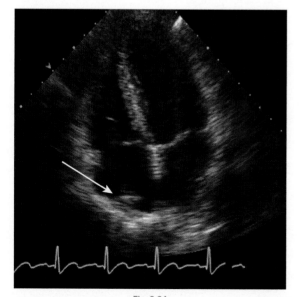

Fig. 2.34

Question 3

The structure identified by the arrow in Fig. 2.35 is which of the following?

A. LV false chord
B. Vegetation
C. Apical thrombus
D. Moderator band

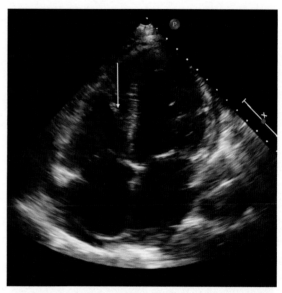

Fig. 2.35

Question 4

A 52-year-old woman underwent echocardiography for atypical chest pains, worse with lying down and after eating. The structure identified by the * in Fig. 2.36 is most likely which of the following?

A. Hiatal hernia
B. Hepatic cyst
C. Aortic aneurysm
D. LA myxoma
E. Dilated coronary sinus

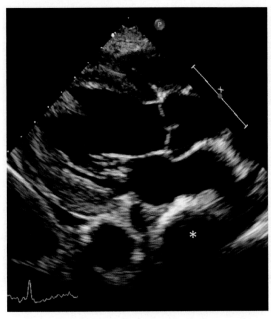

Fig. 2.36

Question 5

In the short-axis view of the mitral valve provided (Fig. 2.37), name the scallops labeled a to f.:

a. _____
b. _____
c. _____
d. _____
e. _____
f. _____

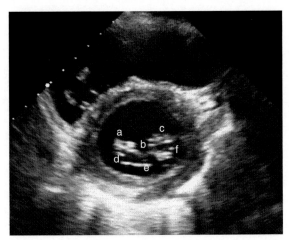

Fig. 2.37

Question 6

This Doppler flow signal (Fig. 2.38) is most consistent with:

A. LV inflow
B. LV outflow
C. Pulmonary vein flow
D. Pulmonary artery flow
E. Descending aorta flow

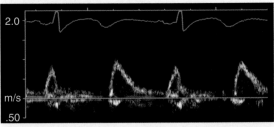

Fig. 2.38

Question 7

Which of the following descriptions would not be a normal flow pattern in a young individual?
A. A LV early inflow velocity higher than a late diastolic peak velocity
B. A RV early inflow velocity higher than a late diastolic peak velocity
C. A negative systolic peak systolic velocity in the pulmonary vein
D. A negative late diastolic peak velocity in the pulmonary vein
E. A negative systolic and diastolic peak velocity in the central hepatic vein

Question 8

This Doppler tracing (Fig. 2.39) is most consistent with:
A. Aortic stenosis
B. Aortic regurgitation
C. Mitral stenosis
D. Mitral regurgitation
E. Tricuspid regurgitation

Question 9

The atrial border tracing for left atrial volume measurement should be traced:
A. In the parasternal long-axis view
B. To include the atrial appendage
C. From the mitral annular plane
D. At end-diastole

Question 10

You are asked to review an echocardiogram of a patient who is a cardiac transplant recipient. Serial echocardiograms in the past document an LV end-diastolic dimension of 4.5 cm. The LV dimension from today's study is provided (Fig. 2.40). The most likely explanation for the change between studies is:
A. Measurement error
B. Interval LV enlargement
C. Physiologic variability
D. Misaligned ultrasound

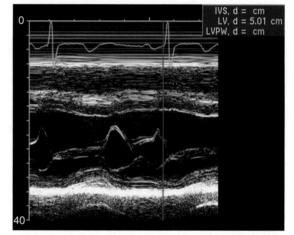

Fig. 2.40

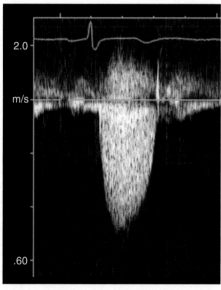

Fig. 2.39

ANSWERS

Answer 1

1. RV
2. LV
3. Pericardial effusion
4. Pleural effusion
5. Descending thoracic aorta

This is a parasternal long-axis view of the heart, set to a depth of over 18 cm. The numbered echolucent space closest to the transducer (1) is the RV, and the adjacent chamber (2) is the LV. This patient has a small pericardial effusion that is circumferential but more prominent posteriorly to the heart (3). The pericardial effusion is easily seen tracking anteriorly to the descending thoracic aorta (5), which is imaged in cross section. There is a small strip of pericardial fluid seen anterior to the RV as well. Posterior to the heart is a large left-sided pleural effusion (4), which is seen tracking posterior to the descending thoracic aorta.

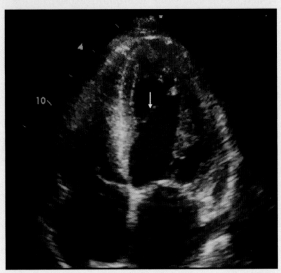

Fig. 2.41

Answer 2: C

The crista terminalis is the embryologic line of union between the trabeculated appendage and the RA. When echo imaging planes go through the mid-portion of the crista terminalis, as is seen in the apical 4-chamber view, a prominent junction line appears as a circular echodensity along the right atrial wall. The Eustachian valve overlies the inferior vena cava (IVC), lies at the junction of the IVC and RA, and is variable in size, length, and prominence in individuals. The function of the Eustachian valve was to direct intra-uterine flow of oxygenated blood from the IVC to the fossa ovalis. An atrial myxoma is a benign cardiac tumor, most commonly seen in the LA, but can also be seen in the RA (≈20% to 30% of cases). Echocardiographic appearance of myxomas is heterogenous, typically a multilobular mass with a pedunculated attachment point on or near the interatrial septum. The thebesian valve is a membranous structure that originates at the superior vena cava, at the orifice of the coronary sinus. It is highly variable in size among individuals and is not commonly seen.

Answer 3: D

The structure is a moderator band, a muscular bundle that carries the right bundle branch of the conduction system. The moderator band, along with the more apically located tricuspid valve and trabeculated apex, helps identify the morphologic RV. The band is in the RV and is generally thicker than an LV false chord (Fig. 2.41, arrow). Apical thrombus and vegetations are more often irregular-shaped masses that form in areas with stagnant or irregular blood flow and have independent motion compared to normal ventricular structures.

Answer 4: A

The structure noted with the * is a hiatal hernia. Extracardiac findings are identified in approximately 5% of echocardiograms and should be noted by the echocardiographer. A hiatal hernia is not uncommon and can produce external compression on the left atrium. A descending aortic aneurysm can have similar appearance, but the circumferential aorta can be seen adjacent to the more irregular-shaped hernia in the figure. If there is an ability to distinguish the structures by 2D and color Doppler, a repeat image after drinking a carbonated beverage can demonstrated opacification of the hiatal hernia. Other extracardiac findings (such as hepatic or renal cysts) can appear as echolucent cystic structures but are more commonly seen in subcostal windows. A LA myxoma is an echodense intracardiac mass more characteristically attached to the interatrial septum. The coronary sinus is seen adjacent to the atrioventricular groove, posterior to the left atrium and anterior to the descending aorta.

Answer 5

The anterior mitral valve leaflet is larger than the posterior leaflet, with the coaptation line between the leaflets showing a semi-circular appearance in short-axis views of the valve. There are three scallops of each valve, numbered 1 through 3. By convention, A1 (answer "c") and P1 (answer "f") coapt and lie along the lateral aspect of the valve. Similarly, A3 (answer "a") and P3 (answer "d") coapt and lie along the medial aspect (closer to the aortic valve). A2 is label "b," and P2 is label "e." It is important to follow anatomical landmarks, because the images appear "flipped" with transesophageal imaging compared to

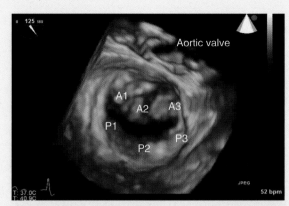

Fig. 2.42

transthoracic imaging, although enface views of the mitral valve by TEE are most commonly obtained via 3D imaging (Fig. 2.42).

Answer 6: A

LV inflow in diastole consists of an early (E) diastolic peak with a second peak occurring with atrial (A) contraction. Pulsed Doppler recording of pulmonary vein flow is low velocity with signals for systole and diastole, as well as slight reversal of flow after atrial contraction. Aortic and pulmonary outflow occur in systole with an ejection curve shape, with a mid-systolic peak for the pulmonary artery and an early systolic peak for aortic flow. Descending aorta flow also occurs in systole, directed away from the transducer.

Answer 7: C

Systolic flow reversal in the pulmonary vein is not a normal finding and is an indication of high left atrial pressure commonly from severe mitral regurgitation. Normal LV and RV filling is characteristic of higher velocity in early diastolic (E wave) than during the atrial kick (A wave) in late diastole. The atrial kick causes a normal reversal of flow in the pulmonary

veins (answer d), resulting in a negative velocity when imaged from a transthoracic apical 4-chamber view. The central hepatic vein is imaged from a subcostal view, and normal central venous flow is away from the transducer (negative velocity) during both ventricular systole (right atrial filling) and diastole (atrium acts as a conduit to RV filling).

Answer 8: A

This is a CW Doppler recording (note velocity scale) showing a systolic flow signal, directed away from the transducer with a maximum velocity of 4.8 m/s. Aortic stenosis is differentiated from mitral regurgitation in the delay after the QRS signal before flow, which corresponds to isovolumic contraction before aortic valve opening. Mitral regurgitation peak velocities may be in this range when recorded from an apical window, reflecting the over 100 mm Hg pressure difference between the LV and LA in systole. If mitral stenosis or aortic regurgitation were present, a typical Doppler signal would be present in diastole. Aortic regurgitation results in a high velocity diastolic flow signal, due to the diastolic pressure difference between the aorta and LV. Tricuspid regurgitation is longer in duration than aortic stenosis (no isovolumic contraction).

Answer 9: C

The left atrial border tracing for volume measurement should be performed from an apical window when the atria are maximally filled, which occurs at end-systole. Measurements should be taken from both the apical 2-chamber (Fig. 2.43A) and the apical 4-chamber (Fig. 2.43B) views.

Care should be taken that images are optimized and not foreshortened so that volumes are not underestimated. The border tracing should follow the blood-tissue border of the LA and a horizontal line across the mitral annulus. The atrial area between

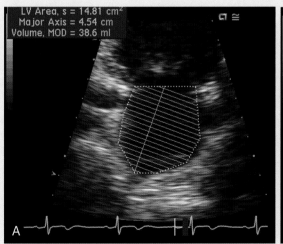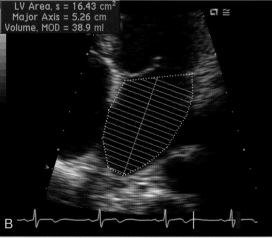

Fig. 2.43

the mitral annular plane and the mitral leaflet coaptation point should be excluded. The left atrial appendage and the pulmonary vein ostia should also be excluded from the atrial area measurement. If either the 2-chamber or 4-chamber view is suboptimal, then a single apical view measurement can be used twice in the left atrial volume calculation. The parasternal long-axis view is useful to provide an anterior–posterior left atrial dimension, but, because it is a single linear measurement of the atria, may underestimate overall left atrial size. Border tracings from the parasternal long-axis view would be inaccurate as this view does not allow for full visualization of the atria.

Answer 10: D

The LV end-diastolic dimension is measured at 5.0 cm on the provided M-mode tracing. This is 0.5 cm larger than previous measurements, which is greater than expected for physiologic variability with changes in loading conditions. Interval change from the prior study or measurement variability should be considered, but only once proper alignment of the M-mode ultrasound beam is ensured. 2D-guided M-mode allows for spatial alignment of the M-mode ultrasound beam to ensure cardiac dimension measurements that are perpendicular to the endocardial border. Misaligned M-mode tracings lead to oblique images of the LV and overestimation of cardiac dimensions. The dimension was measured correctly from the M-mode image, but the beam itself is misaligned. In this patient, a 2D image shows

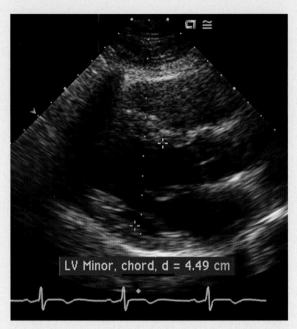

LV Minor, chord, d = 4.49 cm

Fig. 2.44

misalignment of the M-mode beam (dashed line), demonstrating the end-diastolic dimension (cross marks) is actually unchanged from previous studies, at 4.5 cm (Fig. 2.44)

Although 2D imaging improves spatial resolution, M-mode has significantly improved temporal resolution, which may allow for better visualization of the blood-tissue border if image quality is suboptimal.

3 Transesophageal Echocardiography

STEP-BY-STEP APPROACH

Step 1: Clinical Data

- In addition to the indication for the study and the cardiac history, clinical data establishing the safety of the transesophageal echocardiography (TEE) procedure are needed.
- The risk of the TEE procedure is related to both moderate sedation and esophageal intubation.
- Informed consent is obtained before the procedure.

❖ **KEY POINTS**

- ❑ Informed consent includes a description of the procedure with explanation of the expected benefits and potential risks.
- ❑ Complications serious enough to interrupt the procedure occur in less than 1% of cases, and the reported mortality rate is less than 1 in 10,000.
- ❑ Significant esophageal disease, excessive bleeding risk, and tenuous respiratory status are contraindications to TEE.
- ❑ The risk of hemodynamic compromise and respiratory depression are assessed using standard pre-anesthesia protocols and risk levels.
- ❑ Risk is higher in patients with impaired respiratory status or a history of sleep apnea.
- ❑ Patients typically have no oral intake for at least 6 hours before the procedure, except in emergencies.
- ❑ In anticoagulated patients, the level of anticoagulation is checked before the TEE to ensure it is in the therapeutic range.

Step 2: TEE Protocol

- The moderate sedation standards at each institution apply to TEE procedures.

- Typically, these include having a credentialed health care provider monitor level of consciousness, blood pressure, electrocardiogram, and arterial oxygen saturation.
- Oral suction is used to clear secretions and maintain an open airway.
- The study is optimally performed with a physician to manipulate the probe and direct the examination, a cardiac sonographer to optimize image quality and record data, and a nurse to monitor the patient.

❖ **KEY POINTS**

- ❑ Adequate local anesthesia of the pharynx improves patient comfort and tolerance.
- ❑ The specific choice and dose of pharmacologic agents for sedation are based on institutional protocols.
- ❑ Endocarditis prophylaxis is not routinely recommended for TEE.
- ❑ The TEE probe is inserted via a bite block using ultrasound gel for lubrication and to provide acoustic coupling between the ultrasound transducer and the wall of the esophagus.
- ❑ The TEE probe is advanced and diagnostic images are obtained in standard image planes by turning the probe and rotating the image plane (Fig. 3.1).
- ❑ All health care providers involved in the procedure use universal precautions to prevent exposure to body fluids.

Step 3: Basic Examination Principles

- Although the TEE study is directed toward answering the clinical question, a complete systemic examination is recorded unless precluded by the clinical situation.

- Standard tomographic planes are used to evaluate cardiac chambers and valves with side-by-side, simultaneous display of orthogonal imaging planes (90° offset) when needed.
- The structure or flow of interest is centered in the image plane with depth and sector width adjusted to optimize image quality.
- Three-dimensional (3D) imaging using real-time zoom mode and acquisition of full volume 3D datasets is used for measurement of left ventricular (LV) volumes and ejection fraction and for visualization of mitral valve anatomy.
- Additional 3D imaging is based on the clinical diagnosis and two-dimensional (2D) imaging findings.

❖ KEY POINTS

- In stable patients, a complete TEE examination is recommended with recording of all standard image planes and Doppler flows.
- In unstable patients, the examination should focus on the key diagnostic issues first, with additional recordings as tolerance and time allow.
- Each cardiac structure is evaluated in at least two orthogonal views or, ideally, using a rotational scan of the structure.
- The structure of interest is centered in the image plane with transducer frequency, depth, and zoom adjusted to optimize visualization.
- With color Doppler, frame rate is optimized by decreasing depth and sector width to focus on the flow of interest.
- Only one to two beats of each view are recorded so that the examiner can move quickly through the examination sequence. The total intubation time for a complete TEE ranges from less than 10 minutes for a relatively normal study to up to 30 minutes for complex examinations.

Step 4: Imaging Sequence

- The basic imaging sequence suggested in the Echo Exam Basic Transesophageal Echocardiography Exam Sequence table at the end of this chapter is organized by probe position, because this is the most efficient approach to examination in most cases.
- The imaging sequence is adjusted to focus on the key issues in unstable patients.
- This step-by-step approach describes the evaluation of each anatomic structure. This evaluation often is incorporated into the standard exam sequence shown in the Echo Exam table.

❖ KEY POINTS

- The probe position is constrained by the position of the esophagus so that optimal views are not always possible.
- The terms *advance* and *withdraw* refer to the vertical motion of the probe in the esophagus and stomach (Fig. 3.2).
- The term *turn* refers to manual rotation of the entire probe toward the patient's right or left side.
- The terms *flexion* and *extension* refer to motion of the tip of the probe in a plane parallel to the long-axis of the probe, controlled by a large dial at the base of the probe (Figs. 3.3 and 3.4).
- The term *rotation* refers to the electronic movement of the image plane in a circular fashion, controlled by a button on the probe and displayed as an angle on the image (Fig. 3.5).

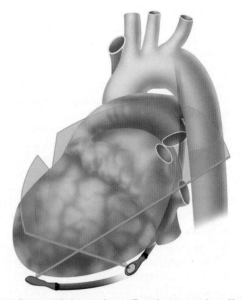

Fig. 3.2 Transgastric image planes. From the transgastric position, the probe is positioned near the gastroesophageal junction to obtain a short-axis view of the LV or is advanced into the stomach to obtain an "apical" view. Transgastric apical images may show a foreshortened LV because the true LV apex often does not lie on the diaphragm. *(From Otto, CM: Textbook of clinical echocardiography, ed 6, Philadelphia, 2018, Elsevier.)*

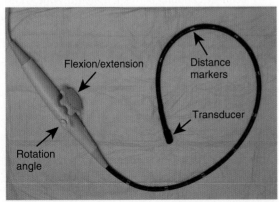

Fig. 3.1 TEE probe. The transesophageal multiplane transducer is at the tip of a steerable probe. The probe motion is controlled by the dials, with the rotational angle of the image plane adjusted with a button.

❑ The exact degree of rotation needed for a specific view varies from patient to patient, depending on the relationship between the heart and esophagus. The values given here are a starting point; image planes are adjusted based on cardiac anatomy, not specific rotation angles.

❑ If a specific view or flow is difficult to obtain, continue with the examination and return to this view later in the study.

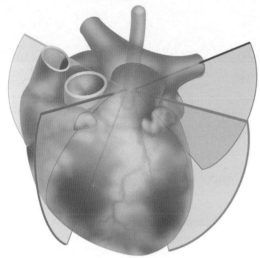

Fig. 3.3 **Turning the TEE probe.** From a mid-esophageal position, turning the image plane from left to right provides images of the left pulmonary veins *(purple)*, aorta and LV *(blue)*, RV *(green)*, and RA with superior and inferior vena cava (SVC and IVC) *(yellow)*. *(From Otto, CM: Textbook of clinical echocardiography, ed 6, Philadelphia, 2018, Elsevier.)*

❑ The specific views and flows recorded depend on the clinical indication and the findings of the study.

❑ Although modification of the exam sequence often is necessary, the examiner should quickly review a checklist of the recorded data before removing the probe to ensure a complete exam.

Step 5: Left Ventricle

■ The LV is evaluated in the mid-esophageal 4-chamber, 2-chamber, and long-axis views.

■ A 3D full-volume image dataset of the LV is obtained from a mid-TEE position for measurement of LV volumes and ejection fraction.

■ Additional views of the LV include the transgastric short-axis view and the transgastric apical view.

❖ **KEY POINTS**

❑ The starting point for a TEE is a 4-chamber view recorded from a mid-esophageal position (0° rotation) at maximum depth to show the entire LV. Typically the probe is extended to include as much of the apex as possible (Fig. 3.6).

❑ With the probe centered behind the left atrium (LA) and the LV apex in the center of the image, the image plane is rotated to about 60° to obtain a 2-chamber view and then rotated further to about 120° for a long-axis view, followed by a multi-beat full volume 3D acquisition.

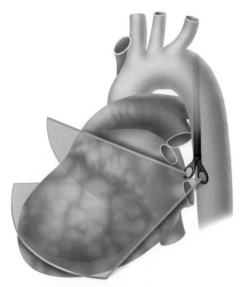

Fig. 3.4 **TEE probe angulation.** From a mid-esophageal position with the probe at 0° rotation, the transducer tip is extended to obtain a 4-chamber view or flexed for a short-axis view of the left atrial appendage. *(From Otto, CM: Textbook of clinical echocardiography, ed 6, Philadelphia, 2018, Elsevier.)*

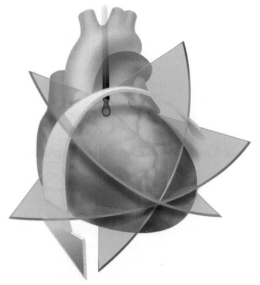

Fig. 3.5 **TEE image plane rotation.** Rotation of the image plane starting from the 4-chamber view, with the LV apex centered in the image, allows a 2-chamber view (see Fig. 3.6) at approximately 60° rotation and a long-axis view at approximately 120° rotation. Slight repositioning and angulation of the transducer may be needed as the image plane is rotated to ensure inclusion of the LV apex in the image. *(From Otto, CM: Textbook of clinical echocardiography, ed 6, Philadelphia, 2018, Elsevier.)*

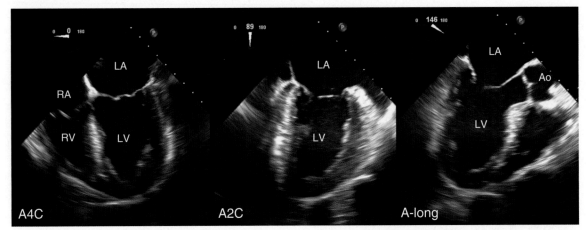

Fig. 3.6 TEE views of the LV. With the LV apex centered in the image plane at 0°, the apical 4-chamber *(A4C)* view is obtained. When the angle is adjusted to about 60°, an apical 2-chamber *(A2C)* view is obtained showing the anterior and inferior LV walls. With further rotation of the image plane, typically to about 120°, an apical long-axis view *(A-long)* is obtained with the aortic valve and ascending aorta *(Ao)* and the inferior-lateral (posterior) and anterior septal walls of the LV. These views are oriented by the cardiac anatomy, not a specific rotation angle. In this patient, obtaining a long-axis view with the ascending aorta and LV correctly aligned required rotation of the image plane to 146°.

❑ The transducer position, angulation, and exact degree of rotation are adjusted to optimize each view.
❑ Regional ventricular function is evaluated as follows:
  ❑ Lateral wall and inferior septum in the 4-chamber view
  ❑ Anterior and inferior walls in the 2-chamber view
  ❑ Anterior septum and the inferior-lateral (or posterior) wall in the long-axis view
❑ Quantitative ejection fraction measurements are made using the 3D full-volume acquisition with automated border detection or the 2D biplane approach with tracing of endocardial borders at end-diastole and end-systole in 4-chamber and 2-chamber views (Fig. 3.7).
❑ An apical LV thrombus may be missed, because the apex is in the far field of the TEE image; transthoracic imaging is more sensitive for detection of apical thrombus.

Step 6: Left Atrium and Atrial Septum

■ The body of the LA is evaluated in the midesophageal 4-chamber, 2-chamber, and long-axis views.
■ The LA appendage is imaged in at least two orthogonal planes at 0° and 90° using the biplane mode or rotating between image planes.
■ 3D imaging of the LA appendage is helpful in selected cases for thrombus detection or procedural planning.
■ The pulmonary veins are identified using 2D and color Doppler imaging most easily in the 0° image plane, although views at 90° also may be helpful.

❖ **KEY POINTS**

❑ Images of the LA are recorded at a shallow depth to focus on the structure of interest.
❑ The atrial septum is best examined by centering the septum in the image plane in the 4-chamber view and then slowly rotating the image plane, keeping the septum centered, from 0° to 120° (Fig. 3.8). A 3D volumetric image also can be recorded.
❑ The atrial appendage is imaged using a high frequency transducer, zoom mode, and a narrow sector to improve image resolution (Fig. 3.9). Simultaneous biplane imaging of the LA appendage or sequential images in a rotational scan are recommended for detection of LA appendage thrombus.
❑ Flow in the atrial appendage is recorded with a pulsed Doppler sample volume about 1 cm from the mouth of the appendage (Figs. 3.10 and 3.11).
❑ The pulmonary veins are most easily identified using color Doppler with the aliasing velocity decreased to about 20 to 30 cm/s.
❑ The left superior pulmonary vein (LSPV) is located adjacent to the atrial appendage and enters the atrium in an oblique anterior to posterior direction.
❑ The left inferior pulmonary vein, seen by advancing the probe a few centimeters, enters the atrium in a left lateral to medial direction (Fig. 3.12).
❑ The right pulmonary veins are imaged in the 0° plane by turning the probe toward the patient's right side.
❑ The superior vein enters the atrium in an anterior–posterior direction; the inferior vein is seen by advancing the probe and enters in a right lateral to medial direction (Fig. 3.13).

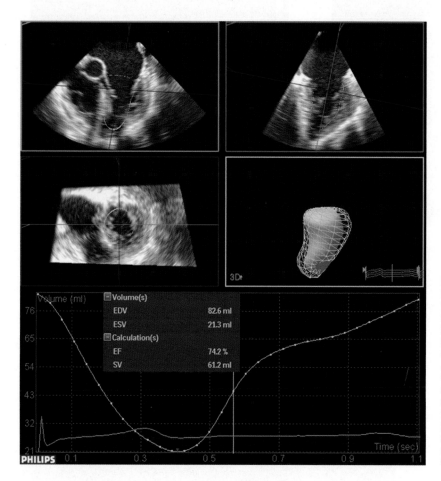

Fig. 3.7 3D LV volume measurement. Ejection fraction measured with TEE 3D imaging. A full volume dataset is acquired from a high TEE position with the volume including the entire LV chamber. Automatic borders are reviewed and edited as needed, in 4-chamber *(upper left)*, 2-chamber *(upper right)*, and short-axis *(lower left)* views. A reconstruction 3D LV volume is shown *(lower right)* with a wire frame for end-diastole and a moving yellow surface for each frame over the cardiac cycle. A graph of LV volume versus time is shown at the bottom. Separate lines also can be displayed for each myocardial segment to evaluate regional function.

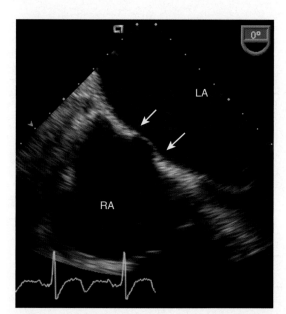

Fig. 3.8 Atrial septum. The atrial septum is examined by centering the septum in the image plane at 0° rotation and then slowly rotating the image plane to 120°. The thin fossa ovalis *(between arrows)* is clearly seen on this image.

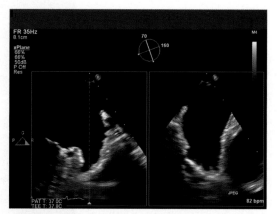

Fig. 3.9 LA appendage. Two views of the LA appendage at about 70° and 160° rotation are obtained simultaneously using biplane imaging. The typical crescent shape of the appendage is seen, and the normal ridge is seen between the LA appendage and left superior pulmonary view.

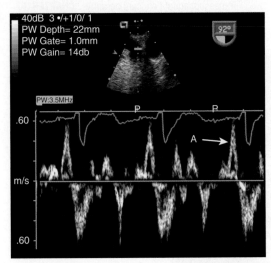

Fig. 3.10 **Sinus rhythm.** Doppler flow patterns in the atrial appendage are recorded with the sample volume in the appendage about 1 cm from the entrance into the LA. In this patient in sinus rhythm, the normal antegrade flow, with a velocity greater than 0.4 m/s after the p-wave, is seen *(arrow)*.

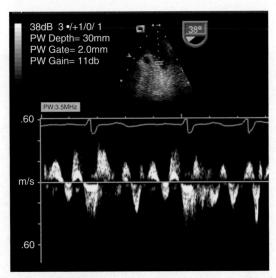

Fig. 3.11 **Atrial fibrillation.** Atrial appendage flow in a patient in atrial fibrillation shows a rapid, irregular low velocity flow pattern.

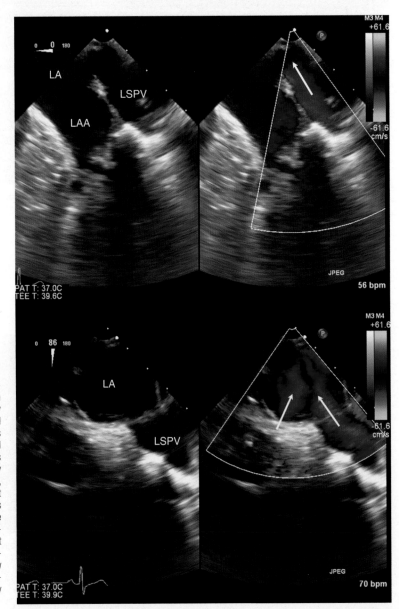

Fig. 3.12 **Left pulmonary veins.** From the standard 4-chamber view at 0° *(top)*, the left atrium appendage *(LAA)* and left superior pulmonary vein *(LSPV)*, with flow into the LA, are visualized by moving the transducer up in the esophagus and flexing the probe tip. There often is a normal prominent ridge, seen as a rounded mass in this view, between the atrial appendage and pulmonary vein. With rotation of the image plane to about 90°, with the transducer turned toward the patient's left side, both left pulmonary veins are visualized. In this image, superior structures are to the right of the image and inferior structures to the left. The left inferior pulmonary vein is not clearly seen because it enters the atrium at a perpendicular angle to the ultrasound beam, but color Doppler shows the inflow signal *(arrows)*. The LSPV enters with the flow direction parallel to the ultrasound beam and is easily seen with both 2D and color Doppler imaging.

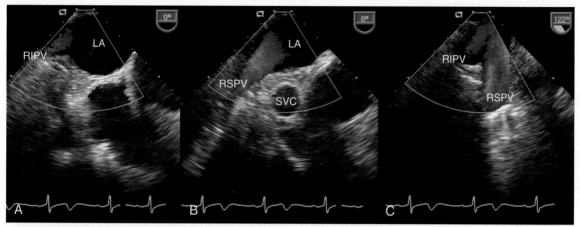

Fig. 3.13 **Right pulmonary veins.** The right pulmonary veins are identified in the 0° image plane by turning the transducer toward the patient's right side. **(A)** The right inferior pulmonary vein is seen with color Doppler entering the LA at a relatively perpendicular angle to the ultrasound beam. **(B)** The probe is withdrawn 1 to 2 cm to visualize the right superior pulmonary vein, which enters the atrium relatively parallel to the ultrasound beam direction. **(C)** The right pulmonary veins also can be imaged in the orthogonal plane by rotating the image plane to a longitudinal view, with the right superior pulmonary vein on the right and the inferior pulmonary vein on the left. *RIPV,* Right inferior pulmonary vein; *RSPV,* right superior pulmonary vein; *SVC,* superior vena cava.

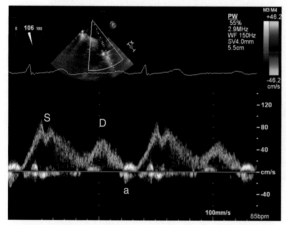

Fig. 3.14 **Pulmonary vein flow.** Pulsed Doppler tracing of normal flow in the left superior pulmonary vein (LSPV) shows systolic *(S)* and diastolic *(D)* inflow with a small reversal of flow with atrial *(a)* contraction.

- ❏ Pulmonary vein flow is recorded with pulsed Doppler in one or more pulmonary veins, depending on the clinical indication for the study (Fig. 3.14).
- ❏ An orthogonal view at 90° also may be helpful, turning the probe rightward for the right pulmonary veins and leftward for the left pulmonary veins (see Figs. 3.12 and 3.13).

Step 7: Mitral Valve

- The mitral valve is evaluated starting in the 4-chamber view and then rotating the image plane slowly to 120° (long-axis view), keeping the valve centered in the image.
- Additional views of the mitral valve include the transgastric short-axis and 2-chamber view.
- 3D imaging of the mitral valve is recommended in most patients, particularly for myxomatous mitral

valve disease, other leaflet abnormalities, or annular dilation.

- TEE provides optimal evaluation of mitral regurgitant severity, allowing a parallel angle between the flow direction and ultrasound beam for continuous-wave (CW) Doppler, excellent visualization of the jet origin and direction, and accurate measurement of vena contracta width and proximal isovelocity surface area (PISA) radius.

❖ KEY POINTS

- ❏ The image depth is adjusted to just fit the mitral valve on the image. Transducer frequency, harmonic imaging, and gain are adjusted to improve the image (Fig. 3.15).
- ❏ The mitral valve is first evaluated with 2D imaging alone to focus on the details of valve anatomy.
- ❏ 3D real-time zoom and full volumes imaging are recommended when the valve is abnormal (Fig. 3.16).
- ❏ A second rotational scan is performed using color Doppler to evaluate for mitral regurgitation. Regurgitation is evaluated based on measurement of the vena contracta, evaluation of pulmonary venous flow pattern, the CW Doppler signal, and quantitative parameters, as discussed in Chapter 12 (Fig. 3.17).
- ❏ Simultaneous split screen 2D and color imaging shortens the exam time, but eccentric jets might be missed due to the narrower sector width compared to full screen imaging.
- ❏ The transgastric view of the mitral valve offers improved visualization of the subvalvular apparatus, although concurrent evaluation by transthoracic imaging also may be needed.

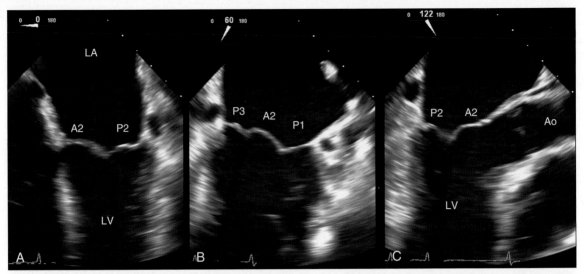

Fig. 3.15 Mitral valve. (A) The mitral valve is imaged starting at 0° rotation with the valve centered in the image plane and the depth adjusted to focus on the valve. The image plane is then slowly rotated, keeping the mitral valve centered, to examine the entire valve apparatus. (B) At about 60° rotation (2-chamber image plane), the lateral *(P1)* and medial *(P3)* scallops of the posterior mitral leaflet and the central segment of the anterior leaflet are typically seen. (C) In the long-axis view at about 120° rotation, the central segment of the anterior leaflet and the *P2* segment of the posterior leaflet are seen. *Ao,* Ascending aorta.

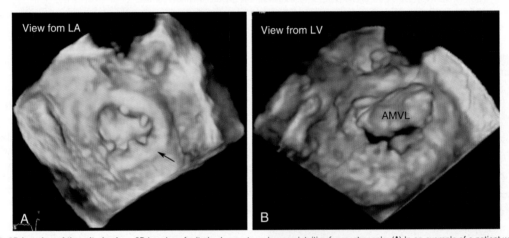

Fig. 3.16 3D imaging of the mitral valve. 3D imaging of mitral valve anatomy is more intuitive for most people. (A) In an example of a patient with a prior surgical valve repair, the image with the viewer looking at the left atrial side of the valve (the surgical view) shows a mitral annular ring *(arrow)* with the leaflets closed in systole. The aortic valve is at the top of the image. (B) A view from the LV side in diastole show a prominent anterior mitral valve leaflet *(AMVL)* with the mitral orifice in black under the open leaflet.

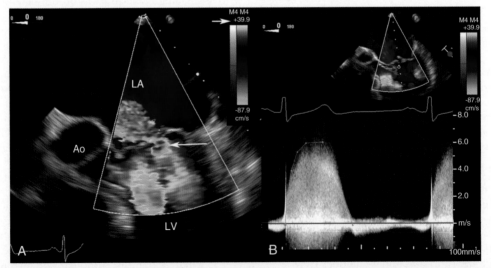

Fig. 3.17 Mitral regurgitation. (A) Color Doppler is used to identify the presence of mitral regurgitation (MR) and to evaluate severity based on vena contracta width and by the proximal isovelocity surface area *(long arrow)* approach with the aliasing velocity set to 30-40 cm/s in the direction of flow *(short arrow)* (see Chapter 12). (B) The density and shape CW Doppler velocity curve also are useful for confirming the identity and evaluating severity of regurgitation. The peak velocity and velocity time integral of the MR curve are measured *(green line)* for calculation of regurgitant orifice area (ROA) and regurgitant volume.

Step 8: Aortic Valve and Ascending Aorta

- The aortic valve and proximal ascending aorta are evaluated in standard long- and short-axis views.
- Aortic regurgitation is evaluated by color Doppler in mid-esophageal views.

❖ KEY POINTS

- ❑ The aortic valve is best seen in the long-axis view (at about 120°) and in a short-axis view of the valve (at about 30° to 50° rotation), using a shallow-depth, high frequency transducer, zoom mode, and narrow 2D sector (Figs. 3.18 and 3.19).
- ❑ From the standard long-axis view, the TEE probe is turned rightward and leftward to see the medial and lateral aspects of the valve. The probe also is withdrawn higher in the esophagus to see as much of the ascending aorta as possible.
- ❑ From the short-axis view, the probe is slowly advanced and withdrawn to visualize the areas immediately inferior and superior to the valve plane.
- ❑ 3D full-volume acquisition improves diagnosis of a bicuspid valve (Fig. 3.20).
- ❑ Aortic regurgitation can be evaluated by color Doppler, with measurement of vena contracta, although precise quantitation of regurgitant severity may be difficult on TEE, because the Doppler beam cannot be aligned parallel to flow (Fig. 3.21).

- ❑ CW Doppler of the aortic regurgitant jet sometimes can be recorded from a transgastric apical view, but underestimation of velocity is likely because of a nonparallel intercept angle between the ultrasound beam and regurgitant jet (Fig. 3.22).
- ❑ Transthoracic imaging often provides more precise quantitation of regurgitant severity.

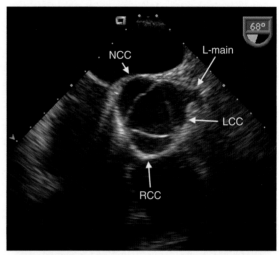

Fig. 3.19 Aortic valve short-axis view. This view is obtained by centering the valve in the long-axis image and then rotating the image plane to about 45°. This zoomed image shows the right coronary cusp *(RCC)*, left coronary cusp *(LCC)*, and noncoronary cusp *(NCC)* in systole. The left main *(L-main)* coronary artery is also seen.

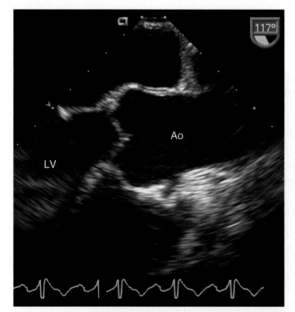

Fig. 3.18 Aortic valve long-axis view. This view typically is obtained at about 120° rotation. The exact rotation angle needed varies between patients; the image plane is adjusted to the standard image plane based on anatomy, not a specific rotation angle. Note that the right coronary ostium is seen in this view. *Ao,* Aortic valve.

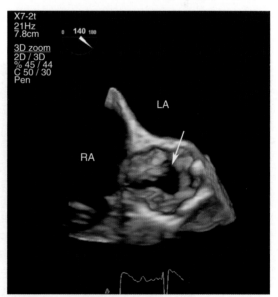

Fig. 3.20 3D imaging of the aortic valve. Using 3D TEE imaging, the aortic valve can be viewed from the perspective of the aorta, looking "down" on the valve, similar to a short-axis view. In this mid-systolic imaging, moderately restricted opening of a trileaflet valve is seen due to calcific aortic stenosis.

Step 9: Coronary Arteries

- The left main coronary artery is easily seen in the short-axis view of the aorta valve (see Fig. 3.19).
- The right coronary artery may be seen in a long-axis view of the ascending aorta or in the short-axis view of the aortic valve, but it can be identified in only about 20% of cases (see Fig. 3.18).

❖ KEY POINTS

- ❏ The left main coronary is slightly superior to the aortic valve plane.
- ❏ Visualization of the coronary ostium is enhanced by using a high frequency transducer and zoom mode.
- ❏ The bifurcation of the left main into the left anterior descending and circumflex coronaries is frequently visualized, but the more distal vessels are not seen in most patients.
- ❏ Identification of the coronary ostium is most important in adolescents and young adults with exertional symptoms and in patients with prior aortic root surgery with coronary reimplantation (Fig. 3.23).

Step 10: Right Ventricle and Tricuspid Valve

- The right ventricle (RV) and tricuspid valve are evaluated in the mid-esophageal 4-chamber and RV inflow views (Fig. 3.24).
- Additional views of the RV and tricuspid valve include the transgastric short-axis view and RV inflow views.

❖ KEY POINTS

- ❏ In the initial TEE 4-chamber images, RV size and systolic function are evaluated.

- ❏ The RV also is seen in the short-axis view, starting at the aortic valve level and slowly advancing the transducer to see the tricuspid valve and RV.
- ❏ From the transgastric short-axis view, the image plane is rotated to 90° and the probe is turned rightward to obtain a view of the right atrium (RA), tricuspid valve, and RV, similar to a transthoracic RV inflow view (Fig. 3.25).

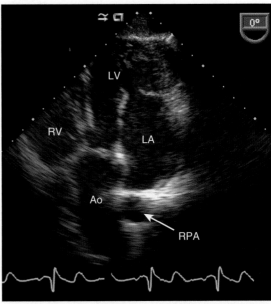

Fig. 3.22 **Transgastric apical view.** From a deep transgastric position, an anteriorly angulated 4-chamber view is obtained by flexion of the probe tip. This image plane does not pass through the true LV apex, with obvious foreshortening of the LV in this image. The ascending aorta *(Ao)* and right pulmonary artery *(RPA)* are seen.

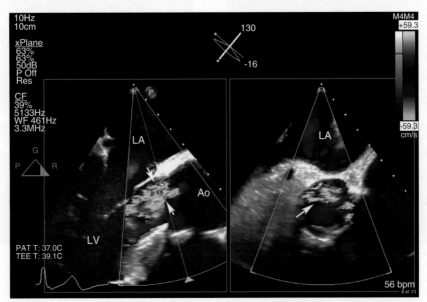

Fig. 3.21 **Aortic regurgitation.** Color Doppler in simultaneous long- *(left)* and short-axis *(right)* images allows detection of aortic regurgitation. Regurgitant severity is evaluated by measurement of vena contracta width in the long-axis view and the size of the regurgitant signal compared to outflow tract area in the short-axis view. This example shows a wide jet with a vena contract width of 9 mm, consistent with severe regurgitation.

- Tricuspid valve anatomy and motion and color Doppler tricuspid regurgitation are evaluated in each of these views.
- A CW Doppler recording of tricuspid regurgitant jet velocity may be obtained from the esophageal 4-chamber or short-axis view, although underestimation of velocity because of a poor intercept angle is possible.

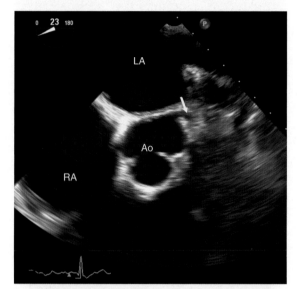

Fig. 3.23 **Left main coronary artery.** The left coronary artery is seen by moving the image plane slightly superior to the aortic valve short-axis image plane. The left main coronary artery *(arrow)* ostium is seen originating from the aorta just superior to the aortic valve. *Ao,* Ascending aorta.

Step 11: Right Atrium

- The RA is evaluated in the mid-esophageal 4-chamber view and in the 90° view of the RA (Fig. 3.26).
- Additional views of the RA include a low atrial view, at the level of the coronary sinus, and the transgastric 2-chamber view of the right side of the heart.

❖ **KEY POINTS**

- The RA is visualized by rotating the image plane to 90° and turning the probe rightward to obtain a longitudinal view of the RA, including the entrances of the superior and inferior vena cava (IVC).
- The trabeculated RA appendage may be seen adjacent to the entry of the superior vena cava into the atrium.
- The IVC can be evaluated by advancing the probe slowly toward the gastroesophageal junction.
- The central hepatic vein enters the IVC at a perpendicular angle, allowing Doppler recording of hepatic vein flow when indicated.
- From the standard 4-chamber plane at 0° the probe is advanced to obtain a low atrial view and the junction of the coronary sinus with the RA. The size and flow characteristics of the coronary sinus can be evaluated in this view when needed.

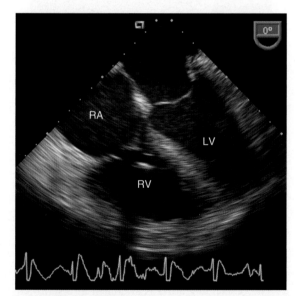

Fig. 3.24 **TEE view of RV.** The RV is seen in the 4-chamber view, but it often is helpful to turn the transducer toward the RV to focus on RV size and systolic function. This patient has moderate RV dilation and systolic dysfunction. Rotation of the image plane allows evaluation of the RV outflow tract in the short-axis view at the aortic valve level.

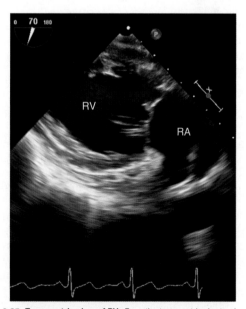

Fig. 3.25 **Transgastric view of RV.** From the transgastric short-axis view, the image plane is rotated to between 60° and 90°. From the 2-chamber view of the LV, the probe is turned toward the patient's right side to obtain this view of the RA, tricuspid valve, and RV.

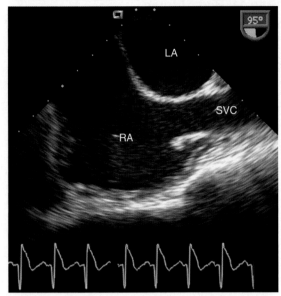

Fig. 3.26 **Bicaval view.** A long-axis view of the RA is obtained with the image plane rotated to 90° and the transducer turned toward the patient's right side. The superior vena cava *(SVC)* enters the atrium near the trabeculated atrial appendage. When the transducer is advanced in the esophagus, the entrance of the inferior vena cava (IVC) into the atrium also may be seen in this view.

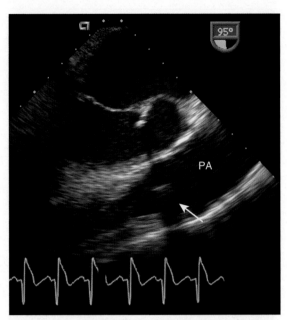

Fig. 3.27 **Pulmonic valve.** With the transducer in the high esophageal position, the pulmonary artery *(PA)* is seen with the image plane rotated to 90° and the transducer turned slightly toward the patient's left side. The anteriorly located pulmonic valve *(arrow)* is relatively distant from the transducer, so image quality often is suboptimal.

Step 12: Pulmonic Valve and Pulmonary Artery

■ The pulmonic valve and pulmonary artery are visualized in a high esophageal view in the 0° image plane or in a 90° image plane with the transducer turned toward the left (RV outflow view) (Fig. 3.27).

■ Images of the pulmonic valve may be suboptimal because the valve is in the far field of the image, and it may be obscured by the air-filled bronchus at this level of the esophagus.

❖ **KEY POINTS**

❏ The pulmonic valve also may be visualized in the transgastric short-axis view.

❏ Doppler flow in the pulmonary artery can be recorded from the high esophageal position.

❏ Evaluation of pulmonic regurgitation with color Doppler is performed in the RV outflow view. However, transthoracic imaging of the pulmonic valve often provides more accurate data.

❏ The pulmonary artery bifurcation and proximal right and left pulmonary arteries may be seen in a high esophageal view, but visualization of more distal pulmonary arteries is rarely possible (Fig. 3.28).

❏ Cardiac magnetic resonance imaging provides an alternate approach to evaluation of the pulmonic valve and pulmonary artery.

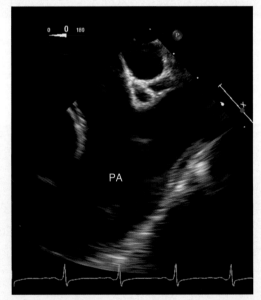

Fig. 3.28 **Pulmonary artery.** The main pulmonary artery *(PA)* and pulmonary artery bifurcation seen in a very high transesophageal view. This probe position may not be well tolerated in some patients, and this image cannot be obtained in all patients.

Step 13: Descending Aorta and Aortic Arch

■ The descending aorta is evaluated in a short-axis view, starting at the transgastric level, by turning the probe leftward to identify the vessel and then slowly withdrawing the probe to visualize each segment of the descending thoracic aorta (Fig. 3.29).

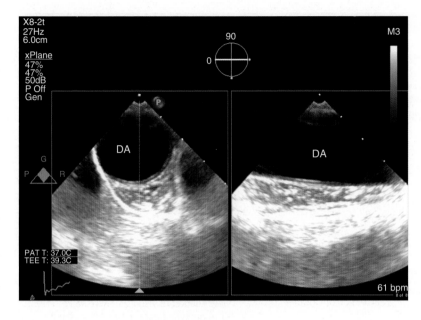

Fig. 3.29 **Descending aorta.** TEE biplane imaging of the descending aorta *(DA)* with the transducer turned toward the patient's left side. In the cross-sectional view on the left, the vertical line indicates the position of the image plane for the long-axis view on the right.

■ Once the probe reaches the level of the aortic arch, the image plane is turned rightward and the probe extended to visualize the arch and ascending aorta.

❖ KEY POINTS

❏ Between the segment of the ascending aorta visualized in the high esophageal long-axis view and the aortic arch, there is a segment of the ascending aorta that may be missed on TEE imaging.

❏ In addition to short-axis images of the descending aorta, the longitudinal view may be simultaneously obtained by biplane or the short-axis image plane may be rotated to 90° to provide a longitudinal view of the extent of disease. However, the short-axis view should always be used to ensure that the medial and lateral aspects of the aorta are examined, which would be missed in a single longitudinal image plane.

❏ Normal structures adjacent to the aorta (connective tissue, lymph nodes) should not be mistaken for pathologic aortic conditions.

Step 14: The TEE Report

■ The TEE report provides a systematic summary of the findings arranged by anatomic structure.

■ The study includes the diagnostic implications of the findings, notes any limitations of the study, and suggests further evaluation as appropriate.

❖ KEY POINTS

❏ The TEE report includes evaluation of:
  ❏ LV size and function
  ❏ RV size and function
  ❏ LA and atrial appendage anatomy and evidence for thrombus
  ❏ Anatomy of the interatrial septum and location of the four pulmonary veins
  ❏ Aortic, mitral, tricuspid, and pulmonic valve anatomy and function
  ❏ Abnormalities of the ascending aorta, descending aorta, or aortic arch
  ❏ Presence (or absence) or a pericardial effusion

❏ Integration of the data to provide a specific diagnosis (such as, "These findings are diagnostic for endocarditis.") is provided whenever possible.

❏ Any unresolved clinical issues and areas of uncertainty are identified, and specific approaches to resolving these issues are recommended.

❏ The TEE report also includes the details of the procedure, including informed consent, patient monitoring, medications, and any procedural complications.

THE ECHO EXAM

Basic Transesophageal Echocardiography Exam Sequence

Probe Position	View	Typical Rotation Angle	Modality	Focus On
Mid-esophageal *Set depth to include LV apex*	4-chamber	0°	2D and color Doppler	• LV size, global and regional function • In 4-chamber view, angulate anteriorly to see aortic valve • Aortic and mitral valve anatomy, motion and flow patterns • RV size and systolic function • LA and RA size • Pericardial effusion
	2-chamber	60°	2D and color Doppler	
	Long axis	120°	2D and color Doppler	
	3D volume	—	Full volume capture (4 beat)	• 3D LV for calculation of volumes and EF
Mid-esophageal *↓ depth and center mitral valve images*	4-chamber	0°	2D and color Doppler	• Mitral valve anatomy and motion • Mitral regurgitation • Split screen 2D/color unless wider field of view needed to visualize entire valve • PISA and vena contracta if MR present
	2-chamber	60°	2D and color Doppler	
	Long axis	120°	2D and color Doppler	
	3D volume	—	Real-time zoom mode and full volume capture (4 beat)	• Mitral valve anatomy and motion from LA and LV views
	Doppler	—	Pulsed and CW Doppler	• Pulsed Doppler LV inflow if needed for diastolic function • CW Doppler of MS or MR jet if more than mild
Mid-upper esophageal *Center aortic valve images*	Long axis	120°	2D and color Doppler	• Aortic valve • Split screen 2D/color unless wider field of view needed to visualize entire valve
	Long axis	120°	2D, biplane imaging and color Doppler	• Aorta, start with aortic valve centered then withdraw transducer slightly to visualize ascending aorta • Right coronary artery ostium may be visualized
	Short axis	30-50°	2D and color Doppler	• Aortic valve • Split screen 2D/color unless wider field of view needed to visualize entire valve • Withdraw probe slightly to see left main coronary artery ostium • 3D imaging of aortic valve if number of leaflets not well seen
Mid-esophageal *Move probe to center LAA*	Depth to show LAA	2D scan from 0 to 90°	2D (resolution mode, 7 MHz transducer)	• LA appendage
	Depth to show LAA	Biplane imaging	2D (resolution mode, 7 MHz transducer)	• LA appendage
	Doppler	—	Pulsed Doppler	• Flow signal recoded with sample volume about 1 cm into LA appendage
Mid-upper esophageal	Left pulmonary veins	0° or 90°	2D and color Doppler	• At 0° turn probe leftward and angulate to see LSPV • Advance probe to see inferior vein • Use of color with low aliasing velocity aids identification of veins • Also can be seen in 90° view

Probe Position	View	Typical Rotation Angle	Modality	Focus On
	Right pulmonary veins	0° or 90°	2D and color Doppler	• At 0° turn probe rightward and angulate to see right superior pulmonary vein • Advance probe to see inferior vein • Use of color with low aliasing velocity aids identification of veins • Also can be seen in 90° view
	Doppler	—	Pulsed Doppler	• Record pulmonary vein flow in one or more pulmonary veins
Mid-esophageal *Turn rightward to center atrial septum*	Rotational scan	0° → 90°	2D and color Doppler	• Atrial septum • Split screen 2D/color unless wider field of view needed to visualize entire atrial septum • Biplane imaging is an alternative option • 3D imaging if ASD present with real-time zoom and full volume for measurement of ASD size
	SVC/IVC view	90°	2D and color Doppler	• RA and atrial appendage • SVC and IVC
Mid-esophageal *Turn rightward to visualize right heart*	4-chamber	0°	2D and color Doppler	• RV • RA • Tricuspid valve
	Short axis RV	60°	2D and color Doppler	• Tricuspid valve
	RV outflow	90°	2D and color Doppler	• Pulmonic valve and pulmonary artery
Transgastric	Short-axis	0°	2D or biplane imaging	• LV wall motion, wall thickness, chamber dimensions • RV size and function
	Long-axis	90°	2D or biplane imaging	• LV and mitral valve • Turn medially to image RV and tricuspid valve
	Right heart	90°	2D	• Turn medially to image RV and tricuspid valve
Transgastric apical	4-chamber	0°	2D, color and CW Doppler	• Useful for antegrade aortic flow but may still be nonparallel intercept angle
Transgastric to upper esophageal	Descending thoracic aorta	0°	2D or biplane imaging	• Image aorta from the diaphragm to aortic arch
		90°	Color, pulsed and CW Doppler	• Doppler evaluation of aorta if 2D imaging suggests dissection • CW Doppler for diastolic flow reversal if AR present
	Arch and ascending aorta	0°	2D	• When TEE probe reaches proximal descending thoracic aorta, turn rightward to see arch and ascending aorta
		90°	2D	

AR, Aortic regurgitation; *ASD,* atrial septal defect; *EF,* ejection fraction; *LAA,* left atrium appendage; *LSPV,* left superior pulmonary vein; *MR,* mitral regurgitation; *MS,* mitral stenosis; *PISA,* proximal isovelocity surface area.

SELF-ASSESSMENT QUESTIONS

Question 1

The following Doppler tracing (Fig. 3.30) was acquired on TEE imaging. This signal is most consistent with:
- **A.** Aortic stenosis
- **B.** Aortic regurgitation
- **C.** Mitral stenosis
- **D.** Mitral regurgitation
- **E.** Tricuspid regurgitation

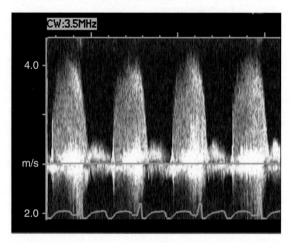

Fig. 3.30

Question 2

You are asked to quantitate mitral regurgitation severity in a patient with mitral valve prolapse, and the following color Doppler image is obtained (Fig. 3.31). To complete your evaluation, based on the image provided, you recommend:
- **A.** Record mitral inflow Doppler signal
- **B.** Color Doppler interrogation of pulmonary veins
- **C.** Adjust color Doppler baseline
- **D.** Measure medial to lateral diameter of isovelocity hemisphere

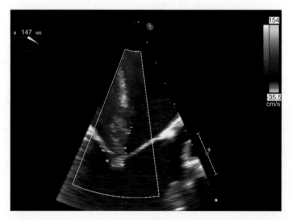

Fig. 3.31

Question 3

In the image provided, name the labeled structures (Fig. 3.32).
- **a.** _____
- **b.** _____
- **c.** _____
- **d.** _____
- **e.** _____

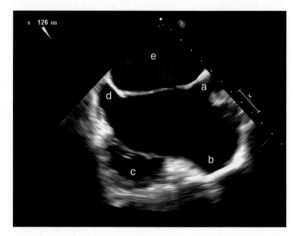

Fig. 3.32

Question 4

From the following view, identify the structures labeled *a* to *e*. (Fig. 3.33):
- **a.** _____
- **b.** _____
- **c.** _____
- **d.** _____
- **e.** _____

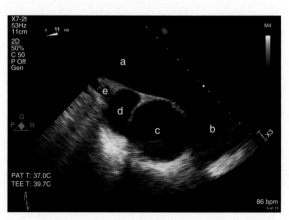

Fig. 3.33

Question 5

You are asked to evaluate a patient with a history of a bioprosthetic aortic valve and suspected aortic regurgitation. The following image is obtained from a mid-esophageal long-axis view at 130° (Fig. 3.34).

Which additional imaging view of the aortic valve would aid in visualizing the regurgitant jet?
- **A.** High-esophageal short-axis view
- **B.** Transgastric long-axis view
- **C.** Mid-esophageal 4-chamber view
- **D.** Deep gastric short-axis view

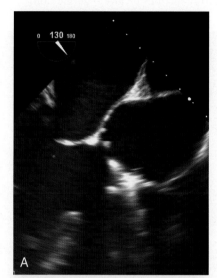

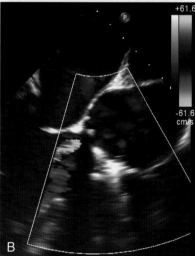

Fig. 3.34

Question 6

A TEE is ordered in a patient in whom a type A aortic dissection is suspected. Imaging of the distal ascending aorta is hindered by:
- **A.** Ultrasound attenuation in the far-field
- **B.** Interposition of trachea
- **C.** Ring-down, or near field clutter artifact
- **D.** Anatomic constraint of esophagus for the TEE probe

Question 7

You are called urgently to the operating room to aid cardiovascular imaging in a patient after coronary bypass grafting surgery who has just been taken off the cardiopulmonary bypass pump. The anesthesiologist has noted new ST segment elevation on the electrocardiogram monitor. You note heterogeneity in wall motion in the indicated area (arrows, Fig. 3.35) and conclude:
- **A.** Left anterior descending artery distribution ischemia
- **B.** Cardiogenic shock and global myocardial ischemia
- **C.** Left circumflex artery distribution ischemia
- **D.** Right coronary artery distribution ischemia

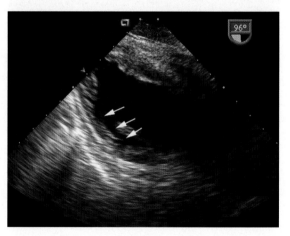

Fig. 3.35

Question 8

A TEE is performed to evaluate for endocarditis. After recording the transgastric view, the probe is withdrawn back into the esophagus. In this position, there is resistance to further withdrawal of the probe. The next best step would be to:
- **A.** Withdraw the probe
- **B.** Retroflex the probe
- **C.** Rotate the probe
- **D.** Advance the probe

Question 9

A 66-year-old man presents with dyspnea. Electrocardiography demonstrates newly diagnosed atrial fibrillation, and a TEE is ordered to evaluate for left atrial appendage thrombus before direct current cardioversion (Fig. 3.36). What abnormality is identified in the left atrial appendage?

A. Reverberation artifact
B. Left atrial appendage thrombus
C. Atrial appendage trabeculation
D. Spontaneous echo contrast

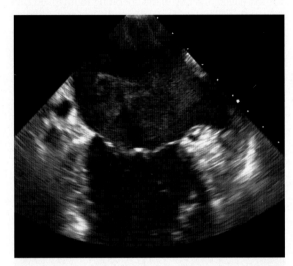

Fig. 3.36

Question 10

A male with previous mitral valve replacement underwent transesophageal echocardiogram for shortness of breath. 3D full volume color Doppler from a slightly rotated surgeon's atrial view was obtained (Fig. 3.37). The finding (arrow) is best described as which of the following.

A. Aortic regurgitation
B. Lateral paravalvular regurgitation
C. Medial paravalvular regurgitation
D. Prosthetic mitral stenosis
E. Prosthetic mitral valve regurgitation

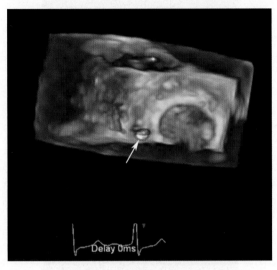

Fig. 3.37

ANSWERS

Answer 1: B

This is a CW Doppler tracing (note velocity scale) with a maximum velocity about 4 m/s and with flow occurring in diastole, directed toward the transducer, consistent with aortic regurgitation. Aortic stenosis, mitral regurgitation, and tricuspid regurgitation might have a similar velocity, but all occur in systole. Mitral stenosis would be a lower velocity diastolic signal, usually directed away from the transducer from a mid-TEE 4-chamber view. The tracing was obtained in a patient with a bicuspid aortic valve where the aortic regurgitant jet was directly posteriorly (Fig. 3.38).

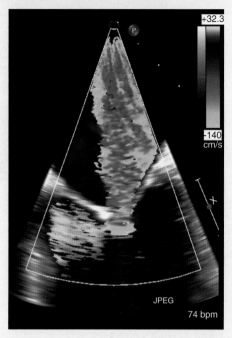

Fig. 3.39

(parallel to valve plane) diameter of the hemisphere. The ROA is then calculated using the velocity time integral from the regurgitant jet. To make this measurement, a spectral Doppler tracing of the mitral regurgitant signal (not the mitral inflow Doppler signal) is needed. A semi-quantitative evaluation of regurgitation severity is a demonstration of systolic flow reversal in the pulmonary veins. This requires spectral Doppler imaging, not color Doppler interrogation of pulmonary venous flow.

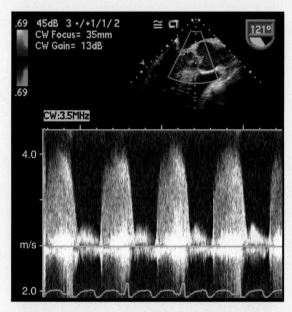

Fig. 3.38

Answer 2: C

Assessment of mitral regurgitation severity requires visualization of the regurgitant jet from multiple views. Quantitation of severity may include calculation of the regurgitant orifice area (ROA) using the proximal isovelocity surface area (PISA) measurement. To do this, the color Doppler baseline should be moved in the direction of flow. In this example, the baseline was moved opposite to regurgitant flow (an error), seen in the upper right indicator with the baseline moved downward. Once a clear isovelocity hemisphere is identified, the PISA radius should be measured and the aliasing velocity recorded (Fig. 3.39).

The PISA radius is the distance from the hemisphere edge to the valve plane, not the medial to lateral

Answer 3

    a. Superior vena cava (SVC)
    b. Right atrial appendage
    c. Right ventricle
    d. Inferior vena cava (IVC)
    e. Left atrium

This image is taken from the mid-esophageal window slightly rotated from a bicaval view. The indicator in the upper left hand portion of the image shows it is recorded from 126°. The inter-atrial septum bisects the image. Above the inter-atrial septum is the left atrium (e). Entering the right atrium from the right side of the image is the SVC (a), and the IVC (d). At the lower right side of the image, the right atrial appendage (b) is seen. At the lower left side of the image, the tricuspid valve is seen, adjacent to the right ventricle (c). Additional imaging from this patient revealed a small secundum atrial septal defect (Fig. 3.40).

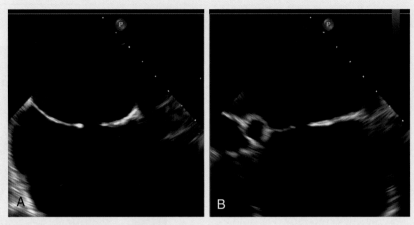

Fig. 3.40

Answer 4

a. Right pulmonary artery
b. Main pulmonary artery
c. Ascending aorta
d. Superior vena cava
e. Right superior pulmonary vein

Fig. 3.33 shows a mid- to upper-esophageal short-axis view of the ascending aorta (c). In the image, other great vessels can be identified with bifurcation of the main pulmonary artery (b) into the right pulmonary artery (a). Turning the probe to the left (counterclockwise) may show the left pulmonary artery, but this is frequently obstructed by interference from the trachea. Doppler assessment of the pulmonary artery may be useful form this view. Short-axis views of the superior vena cava (d) and right superior pulmonary vein (e) are also seen. This view may not be obtainable in all patients or be poorly tolerated if the probe is too high in the esophagus. Color Doppler can demonstrate flow to help identify the structures as vessels.

Answer 5: B

Fig. 3.34 shows the aortic valve in long axis. There is significant acoustic shadowing from the valve occluders of the left ventricular outflow tract (LVOT), and the regurgitant jet is not clearly seen. Transgastric views allow visualization of the valve prosthesis from a vantage point apical to the LVOT. A gastric long-axis view (120°) would be needed to image the regurgitant jet in the LVOT (Fig. 3.41). In the image below, turbulent flow in the LVOT is seen with color Doppler imaging just below the mitral valve (right side of image). From this view, the regurgitant jet is also aligned parallel to flow for Doppler interrogation.

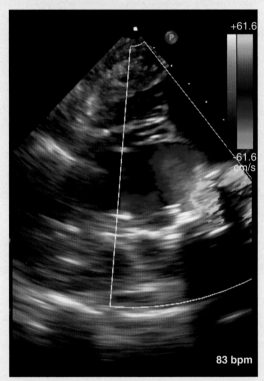

Fig. 3.41

Answer 6: B

The trachea at the level of the distal ascending aorta anatomically lies between the esophagus and the aorta. Near-field clutter artifacts and ultrasound attenuation are not prominent factors hindering imaging of the aorta. There is no anatomic constraint in the esophagus to view the aorta, which does lie in the imaging sector; rather, imaging of this portion of the aorta is obscured due to poor ultrasound penetration through tracheal air.

Answer 7: A

The image is taken from a long-axis gastric view of the LV. In this view, the inferior wall is closer to the transducer and the anterior wall is in the far field. New wall motion abnormalities in the anterior wall are consistent with a left anterior descending artery coronary distribution.

Answer 8: D

In the transgastric view, optimization of the short-axis view of the LV typically involves flexion of the transducer for superior angulation of the probe tip. Once completed, flexion of the probe tip should be relaxed before withdrawal back into the esophagus; otherwise, the tip may be withdrawn in the fully flexed/folded position. In this probe position, withdrawing, retroflexing, or rotating the probe further may perforate the esophagus. The esophagus is too narrow to correct a folded probe within the esophagus. The probe should be readvanced to the stomach where the tip can be relaxed. If a folded TEE probe is suspected, chest radiography may be used to confirm the suspicion before further probe manipulation.

Answer 9: B

In patients with atrial fibrillation undergoing evaluation for direct current (DC) cardioversion who have not been on chronic anticoagulation, TEE is needed to visualize the left atrial appendage. The appendage should be visualized from several views. This image was taken from the 90° mid-esophageal view. The atrial appendage thrombus is seen in the mid-right hand part of the image, with a globular echodensity filling the distal half of the appendage. Spontaneous echo contrast appears as a mobile, swirling signal, and suggests decreased blood velocity or stasis of flow, which has not consolidated into frank thrombus. In Fig. 3.36, spontaneous echo contrast is seen in the mid-portion of the LA, just above the mitral valve, but not in the appendage. Often, spontaneous echo contrast does coexist with a true appendage thrombus. Atrial trabeculations are atrial muscle seen in cross section, commonly seen protruding along the lateral wall of the appendage. Because trabeculations are contiguous with the atrial wall, contractile motion of the trabeculations should be seen with atrial activity. Spontaneous echo contrast appears as swirling echodensity within the body of the appendage and is consistent with low-velocity flow. A reverberation artifact from the ridge between the appendage and the left upper pulmonary vein are common and often difficult to differentiate from a thrombus. Artifact is more likely if the abnormality cannot be demonstrated from multiple image planes.

Answer 10: B

The image demonstrates a lateral paravalvular leak occurring outside of the prosthetic mitral valve suture ring and not within the prosthetic valve leaflets (answer E). Flow through the aortic valve is seen at the 11 o'clock position but would not be consistent with regurgitation (answer A) during ventricular systole that can be seen by electrocardiogram (ECG) and closed mitral valve leaflets. Similarly the flow would not be consistent with mitral stenosis (answer D) given the flow is outside the suture ring and during systole. The orientation in this view would be lateral for the flow on the left side from this 3D view near the left atrial appendage (Fig. 3.42).

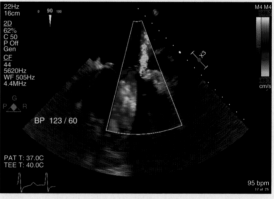

Fig. 3.42

4 Specialized Echocardiography Applications

STRESS ECHOCARDIOGRAPHY

- Stress echocardiography uses echo imaging concurrently with increases in myocardial work, achieved either with an exercise protocol or pharmacologic agent. Stress echo is useful for diagnosis and management of patients with:
  - Coronary artery disease (see Chapter 8)
  - Aortic valve stenosis (see Chapter 11)
  - Mitral valve stenosis or regurgitation (see Chapters 11 and 12)
  - Hypertrophic cardiomyopathy (see Chapter 9)
  The specific stress modality depends on the clinical diagnosis and type of information needed for decision making (Table 4.1).

THREE-DIMENSIONAL ECHOCARDIOGRAPHY

Image Acquisition and Display

- Three-dimensional (3D) echocardiographic image formats include (Table 4.2):
  - *Real-time narrow sector 3D imaging:* Beat-by-beat view with a wider image plane than standard two-dimensional (2D) imaging
  - *Real-time 3D-zoom volume rendered images:* Full-volume acquisition rotated to show a perspective-type image from different points of view
  - *Full-volume gated acquisition volume rendered images:* Multiple-beat full-volume, rotated and cropped to show the structures of interest
  - *Simultaneous multiplane mode:* Simultaneous display of two 2D image planes
  - *3D color Doppler imaging:* Real-time or full-volume color Doppler data acquisition
- 3D echocardiography facilitates recognition of complex intracardiac spatial relationships.

❖ KEY POINTS

- ❏ Real-time narrow sector 3D imaging provides a beat-by-beat image similar to a 2D image but with a thicker image plane.
- ❏ Real-time 3D-zoom volume rendered images show a full-volume image rotated to show the structure of interest in real time (Fig. 4.1).
- ❏ Full-volume gated acquisition volumes are used for quantitative analysis with the ability to examine the 3D image volume in any tomographic plane, typically with three orthogonal planes used to select the optimal site for measurement (Fig. 4.2).
- ❏ Image resolution decreases with acquisition of larger 3D data volumes but is improved by acquiring multiple smaller data volumes across the sector and integrating the volumes ("stitching") to form one larger volume.
- ❏ The simultaneous multiplane mode allows display of two or more 2D image planes in real-time (Fig. 4.3).
- ❏ 3D color Doppler imaging allows acquisition of a 3D volume of Doppler data at a slower frame rate than 2D imaging.

Examination Protocol

- A systematic protocol for 3D imaging ensures a complete examination (Table 4.3).
- Typically, 2D images are optimized before transitioning to the 3D mode.
- A full-volume acquisition of the left ventricle (LV) allows quantitation of LV volumes, ejection fraction, and regional wall motion.
  - Standard orientation of 3D-zoom real-time images for evaluation of valve anatomy facilitate recognition of anatomic abnormalities.

TABLE 4.1	Clinical Applications of Stress Echocardiography		
Clinical Indication	**Stress Modality**	**Protocol**	**Interpretation**
Detection or evaluation of coronary artery disease	Exercise	• Maximum treadmill exercise provides highest workload with image acquired immediately after exercise; or • Supine bicycle exercise (allows continuous imaging). • Compare rest and stress cine loop images of the LV in standard views.	• Normal wall motion at rest and a regional wall motion abnormality with stress indicates ischemia. • Abnormal regional wall motion at rest that persists with stress indicates prior infarction.
	Pharmacologic	• Dobutamine is infused beginning at low dose (5 or 10 μg/kg/min), increasing by 10 μg/kg/min every 3 minutes to a maximum dose of 40 μg/kg/min or target heart rate of 85% maximum predicted. • Atropine may also be used to achieve target heart rate. • Comparison of rest versus peak stress cine loop images of the LV in standard views.	• Normal wall motion at rest and a regional wall motion abnormality with stress indicate ischemia. • Abnormal regional wall motion at rest that persists with stress indicates prior infarction.
Myocardial viability	Dobutamine stress	• Dobutamine is infused beginning at low dose (5 μg/kg/min) and increasing to 10 μg/kg/min. • The stress test may be continued to evaluate for ischemia as above. • Images of the LV in cine loop format at baseline and low-dose dobutamine (increase in contractility with no change in heart rate) are compared.	• Viability is diagnosed when an area of hypokinesis or akinesis at rest shows improved wall motion at low-dose dobutamine. • If wall motion again worsens at higher dobutamine doses, ischemia also is present (the biphasic response to stress).
Postcardiac transplant myocardial ischemia	Dobutamine stress	• Use standard dobutamine stress echo protocol. • Compare rest versus peak stress cine loop images of the LV in standard views.	• A new wall motion abnormality with stress is consistent with inducible ischemia. • Balanced ischemia (equal involvement of all major coronary arteries) or small-vessel disease may be missed on stress echocardiography.
Low output aortic stenosis (AS)	Dobutamine stress	• Measure stroke volume and ejection fraction as dobutamine is increased from 0 to 20 μg/kg/min in 5 μg/kg/min increments. • Measure AS velocity, mean gradient, and valve area at each stress level. • Stop for symptoms or when a hemodynamic endpoint is reached.	• Severe AS is present if aortic velocity increases to at least 4 m/s and valve area remains less than 1 cm^2. • Failure of stroke volume or EF to increase by at least 20% is termed "lack of contractile reserve" and connotes a poor clinical outcome.
Mitral valve disease	Exercise stress	• Measure TR jet velocity at baseline and at peak exercise stress on maximum treadmill testing or with supine bicycle exercise. • The transmitral pulsed or CW Doppler velocity curve also may be evaluated at rest and with exercise. • MR may be evaluated using CW and color Doppler (optional).	• The primary goal is to assess peak PA pressure with exercise (and change from baseline), calculated from the TR jet velocity. • With MS, the transmitral velocity and mean gradient will increase as expected for the increase in flow rate; this measurement is rarely diagnostically useful. • With primary MR, severity may increase with exercise (e.g., with mitral prolapse), but quantitation at peak exercise is challenging. The change in PA pressure is a surrogate for the increase in regurgitation.

Continued

TABLE 4.1	Clinical Applications of Stress Echocardiography—cont'd		
Hypertrophic cardiomyopathy (HCM)	Exercise stress	• Supine bicycle stress is preferred for evaluation of HCM, because it allows data recording at each stress level. • LV outflow velocity is recorded with pulsed and CW Doppler at baseline and with stress. • MR also is evaluated with CW and color Doppler.	• Latent LV outflow obstruction is present when the resting subaortic gradient is <30 mm Hg but increases to >30 mm Hg with stress. • Separating the LV outflow signal from the higher-velocity MR signal can be challenging in some cases. • Useful features in identifying the origin of the Doppler signal are timing of flow onset relative to the QRS signal, shape of the velocity curve, delineation of a smooth dark edge to the velocity curve, and recordings showing separate LV outflow and MR CW Doppler flow curves.

EF, Ejection fraction; *MR,* mitral regurgitation; *MS,* mitral stenosis; *PA,* pulmonary artery; *TR,* tricuspid regurgitation.

TABLE 4.2	3D Imaging Modalities	
	Advantages	**Limitations**
Real-time 3D mode—narrow section, volume-rendered images	• Rapid acquisition, familiar image planes • Image can be rotated, helpful with complex cardiac anatomy	Narrow sector; entire structure does not fit in imaging plane.
Real-time "zoom" volume-rendered cropped images	• Shows anatomy in "surgical" views • Enlarged 3D image of structure of interest	A wider field of view decreases spatial and temporal resolution.
Full-volume gated acquisition for volume-rendered cropped images	• High spatial resolution • High temporal resolution • Quantitation of LV volumes and ejection fraction • Provides 3D LV shape and dyssynchrony	May be difficult to optimize image quality for all structures in the field of view. "Stitch" artifacts occur because of patient and respiratory motion.
Full-volume gated acquisition for multiple 2D tomographic slices	• Accurate measurements of cardiac dimensions • More objective and less operator-dependent than standard 2D imaging • Visualization of all myocardial segments simultaneously	Endocardial definition may be suboptimal depending on transducer position.
Simultaneous multiplane 2D imaging	• Simultaneous images in two defined planes • Highest spatial resolution • Highest temporal resolution	Only two planes visualized.
3D color Doppler	• Visualization of 3D geometry of vena contracta and proximal isovelocity surface area for regurgitant lesions • Location of paravalvular prosthetic leaks and intracardiac shunts	Slow frame rate with low temporal resolution.

○ The orientation of the aortic valve on 3D imaging is with the right coronary cusp located inferiorly when viewed from either the aortic or LV side of the valve.

○ The orientation of the mitral valve is with the anterior mitral leaflet at the top of the image when viewed from the LV or left atrium (LA) side of the valve.

○ The interatrial septum is shown with the right upper pulmonary vein at 1 o'clock when viewed from the LA side. From the right atrium (RA) side, the superior vena cava is at the 11 o'clock position.

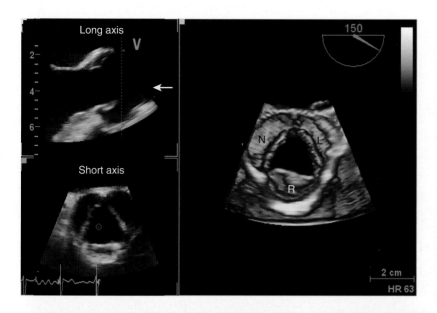

Fig. 4.1 **3D zoom of the aortic valve.** On TEE imaging, a 3D real-time zoom image of the aortic valve is obtained with the long- and short-axis 2D views and the 3D view from the aortic side of the leaflet showing the right *(R)*, left *(L)*, and noncoronary *(N)* leaflets.

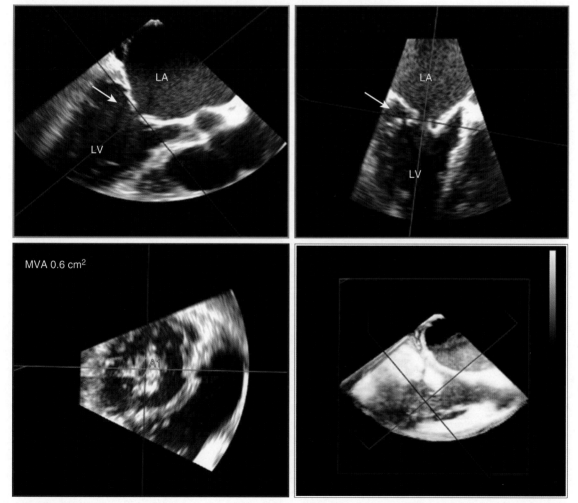

Fig. 4.2 **3D measurement of mitral valve area.** A full-volume 3D acquisition *(lower right)* is used for quantitative measurements. The 4-chamber *(upper left)* and 2-chamber *(upper right)* image planes are used to align the image planes in two orthogonal views to obtain a short-axis view of the mitral valve area *(MVA)* at the leaflet tips *(lower left)*. The colored lines in each view correspond to the image plane shown in each colored box. The position of the short-axis MVA view *(blue box)* is adjusted by moving the blue line in the 4-chamber and 2-chamber views until the correct position and alignment is achieved. This patient has severe mitral stenosis with a valve area of 0.6 cm^2.

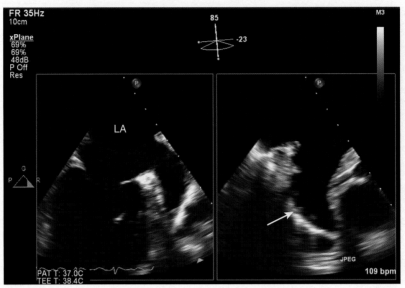

Fig. 4.3 Biplane imaging. Simultaneous imaging of the left atrial appendage using biplane imaging allows evaluation for atrial thrombus. Normal pectinate muscles in the appendage are seen *(arrow)*.

TABLE 4.3	EAE/ASE Recommendations for a Systematic 3D Study		
	TTE Image Acquisition	**TEE Image Acquisition**	**Sequence for TEE Full-Volume Image Orientation (see Fig. 4.7)**
Aortic valve	PLAX with and without color, narrow angle and zoomed	60° mid-esophageal short-axis with and without color, zoomed or full-volume 120° mid-esophageal long-axis with and without color, zoomed or full-volume	2D views at 60° and 120° with aortic valve centered in acquisition boxes Live 3D to optimize gain Full-volume acquisition, and then rotated 90° clockwise around *y*-axis
Mitral valve	PLAX with and without color, narrow angle and zoomed A4C with and without color, narrow angle and zoomed	0-120° mid-esophageal with and without color, zoomed	2D views at 90° and 120° with mitral valve centered in acquisition boxes Full-volume acquisition, rotated 90° counterclockwise around *x*-axis and then 90° counterclockwise in plane so that aortic valve is superior
LV	A4C, narrow and wide angle	0-120° mid-esophageal view including entire LV, full-volume	Full-volume acquisition for quantitation of LV volumes, ejection fraction, and regional wall motion Data displayed as a moving 3D surface-rendered image with color coding and as a time graph
RV	A4C with image tilted to put RV in center of image	0-120° mid-esophageal view, tilted to put RV in center of image, full-volume	
Atrial septum	A4C, narrow angle and zoomed	0° with probe rotated toward atrial septum, zoomed or full-volume	
Pulmonic valve	RV outflow view with and without color, narrow angle and zoomed	90° high-esophageal view with and without color, zoomed 120° mid-esophageal three-chamber view with and without color, zoomed	2D high-esophageal view at 0° with pulmonic valve centered in acquisition box Full-volume acquisition, rotated 90° counterclockwise around *x*-axis, then rotate in plane 180° counterclockwise so that anterior leaflet is superior

TABLE 4.3	EAE/ASE Recommendations for a Systematic 3D Study—cont'd		
	TTE Image Acquisition	**TEE Image Acquisition**	**Sequence for TEE Full-Volume Image Orientation (see Fig. 4.7)**
Tricuspid valve	A4C with and without color, narrow angle and zoomed RV inflow view with and without color, narrow angle and zoomed	0-30°mid-esophageal four-chamber view with and without color, zoomed 40° transgastric view with anteflexion with or without color, zoomed	TTE* 2D views in off-axis A4C view with tricuspid valve centered in acquisition boxes Full-volume acquisition, rotated 90° counterclockwise around x-axis and then rotate 45° in plane so that septal leaflet is in 6 o'clock position

A4C, Apical four-chamber view; narrow angle, real-time volume rendered tomographic imaging in standard image planes; *ASE,* American Society of Echocardiography; *ESE,* European Association of Echocardiography; *PLAX,* parasternal long-axis view; *SAX,* short-axis view; zoomed, real-time volume rendered 3D imaging rotated to intracardiac views.

*3D images of the tricuspid valve are best obtained from transthoracic, not TEE, imaging.

Summarized from Lang RM, Badano LP, Tsang W, et al: EAE/ASE recommendations for image acquisition and display using three-dimensional echocardiography. *J Am Soc Echocardiogr* 25(1):3-46, 2012.

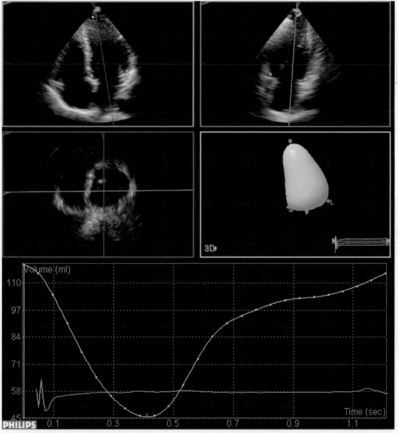

Fig. 4.4 **3D LV volume measurement.** A full-volume acquisition of the LV from a TTE apical window is used. Standard image planes in 4-chamber *(upper left)*, 2-chamber *(upper right)*, and short-axis *(lower left)* views allow review and editing of automated border detection. The reconstruction 3D LV volume is shown in the lower right panel. Data for the entire cardiac cycle are shown as beating images, and a graph of LV volume versus time is shown at the bottom for one cardiac cycle. End-diastole volume is at the left of the graph (119 mL) with end-systolic volume (46) at the nadir of the volume curve. Stroke volume is 119–46 = 73 mL. Ejection fraction is 73/119 = 61%.

Quantitation From 3D Datasets

- LV volumes, ejection fraction, and regional wall motion are measured with 3D imaging.
  - A full-volume acquisition that includes the entire LV is obtained.
  - Endocardial borders are automatically identified with manual adjustment as needed by the echocardiographer (Fig. 4.4).
  - A moving 3D surface rendered image is provided with color coding for regional systolic function (Fig. 4.5).

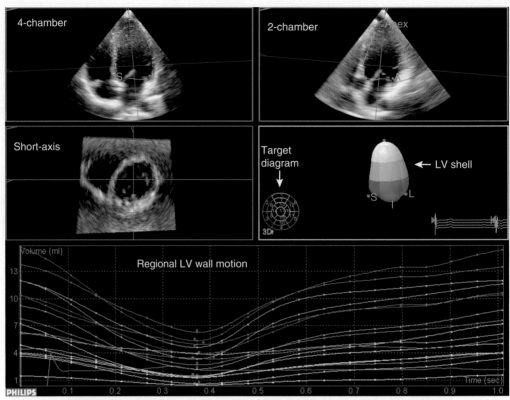

Fig. 4.5 **3D analysis of regional ventricular function.** Regional wall motion is displayed as a beating 3D heart and as a graph of volume versus time with color coding for each myocardial segment with images in the same orientation as Fig. 4.4.

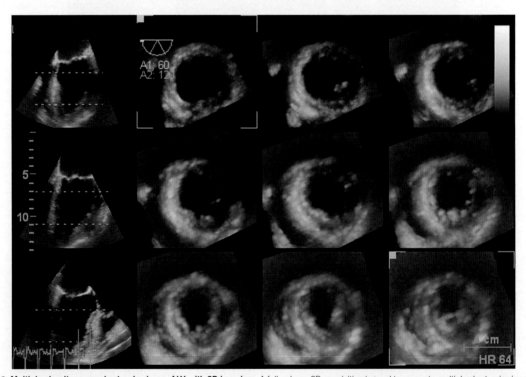

Fig. 4.6 **Multiple simultaneous short-axis views of LV with 3D imaging.** A full-volume 3D acquisition is used to generate multiple short-axis views of the LV for evaluation of regional function.

- A graphical display of motion versus time allows evaluation of regional function and strain.
- Multiple short-axis views of the LV can be displayed simultaneously to enhance diagnosis of the presence and extent of regional wall motion abnormalities (Fig. 4.6).
- Measurements of complex valve anatomy are made from full-volume 3D data acquisition.
- A full-volume 3D dataset is acquired with several cardiac cycles "stitched" together to form the full image of the aortic or mitral valve.
- Stitch artifact is avoided by having the patient stay still and suspend respiration; data acquisition should be repeated if a discontinuity between image segments is present.
- For measurement of mitral orifice area with rheumatic mitral stenosis, x, y, and z image planes are aligned to obtain an image plane at the minimum orifice, which is then traced at the white–black interface.
- Aortic valve and LV outflow measurements also can be made with this approach.

CLINICAL UTILITY

- Routine use of 3D imaging is recommended for:
  - Quantitation of LV volumes and ejection fraction
  - Evaluation of mitral valve anatomy (valve area in mitral stenosis)
  - Guidance of transcatheter procedures
- 3D imaging also is useful for:
  - Evaluation of mitral valve anatomy before and after mitral valve repair in patients with mitral regurgitation
  - Visualization of the size and shape of atrial septal defects in patients undergoing transcatheter closure (Table 4.4)

TABLE 4.4	Clinical Applications of 3D Echocardiography	
Application	**3D Approach**	**Comments**
LV function	• Surface-rendered LV volumes, ejection fraction and regional wall motion derived from a gated full-volume 3D acquisition	• 3D echo underestimates LV volumes compared to CMR data. • Trabeculae and papillary muscles are included in the LV chamber.
RV function	• Volume-rendered images allow visualization of entire RV. • Surface-rendered images may allow measurement of volumes and ejection fraction.	• 3D measurement of RV volumes and ejection fraction requires further validation but is a promising approach.
Mitral valve	• Volume-rendered images show mitral valve anatomy en face from the LA or LV side of the valve. • Accurate measurement of valve area in mitral stenosis using 3D-guided 2D image planes. • Annular shape and dimensions from volumetric images. • 3D color Doppler shows jet origin and direction.	• 3D TEE is recommended for guidance of interventional mitral valve procedures. • 3D TTE or TEE is recommended for clinical evaluation of mitral valve pathology.
Aortic valve and sinuses	• Volume-rendered images obtained from TTE parasternal or TEE high-esophageal views provide optimal spatial resolution. • Planimetry of aortic valve area is possible on 2D images derived from the 3D full-volume data set. • 3D images demonstrate the oval shape of the aortic annulus.	• 3D imaging may be helpful in determining the mechanism of aortic regurgitation and defining the number of valve leaflets. • 3D imaging is recommended for guidance of transcatheter aortic valve implantation.
Pulmonic valve and pulmonary artery	• The pulmonic valve can be imaged using biplane or real-time 3D imaging.	• Routine 3D pulmonic valve imaging is not recommended.
Tricuspid valve	• 3D volume-rendered images of the tricuspid valve are acquired in a similar fashion to those for the mitral valve.	• 3D views of the tricuspid valve may be helpful in determining the mechanism of valve regurgitation.
LA and RA	• 3D volume-rendered images of the atrial septum are helpful for defining the location, size, and shape of atrial septal defects and for guiding transcatheter closure procedures.	• 3D imaging may improve assessment of LA volume but is not a routine measurement.
LA appendage	• 3D volume-rendered images are helpful in guiding transcatheter LA appendage closure.	• Biplane imaging of the LA appendage is useful in evaluating for LA thrombus.

Continued

TABLE 4.4	Clinical Applications of 3D Echocardiography—cont'd	
Application	**3D Approach**	**Comments**
3D stress echocardiography	• 3D imaging provides simultaneous evaluation of wall motion in all myocardial segments, improved visualization of the LV apex, and rapid image acquisition at peak stress.	• Disadvantages of 3D stress imaging include lower frame rates and spatial resolution compared to 2D imaging. • Not all 3D systems allow side by side review of rest and stress images.

CMR, cardiac magnetic resonance.
Data from Lang RM, Badano LP, Tsang W, et al: EAE/ASE recommendations for image acquisition and display using three-dimensional echocardiography. *J Am Soc Echocardiogr* 25(1):3-46, 2012.

Limitations

- Current ultrasound systems display 3D images on a 2D screen.
- Spatial and temporal resolutions are lower than for 2D imaging.
- Imaging artifacts (shadowing, reverberations, ultrasound drop-out, etc.) seen on 2D imaging also affect 3D imaging.
- 3D volume stitching artifact is more prominent when acquiring data subvolumes during arrhythmia, such as atrial fibrillation.

MYOCARDIAL MECHANICS

Basic Principles

- LV function is incompletely described by simple measures, such as ejection fraction or diastolic filling patterns.
- Myocardial strain, strain rate, and measures of synchrony attempt to provide an integrated, precise description of ventricular contraction and relaxation.

❖ **KEY POINTS**

- ❑ LV contraction occurs simultaneously in the longitudinal, radial, and circumferential directions.
- ❑ Rotation is the circular motion of the LV myocardium around its long axis, measured in degrees.
- ❑ The LV apex and base rotate in opposite directions during contraction; the absolute difference in rotation between the apex and base is "twist," and the gradient in rotation angle from base to apex is "torsion."

Tissue Doppler Velocities

- Tissue Doppler measures the velocity of myocardial motion, displayed as a velocity curve for a single point or as a color display across the 2D image plane.
- Tissue Doppler velocities are measured relative to the position of the transducer, like all Doppler signals, so that accurate measurements depend on a parallel alignment between the Doppler beam and direction of motion.

❖ **KEY POINTS**

- ❑ Recording tissue Doppler velocity at a single location, for example, adjacent to the mitral annulus for evaluation of diastolic function, provides a standard velocity versus time spectral display output.
- ❑ Tissue Doppler velocities also can be displayed for multiple points across the 2D image using a color display, analogous to color Doppler flow mapping for blood flow velocities.
- ❑ Tissue Doppler signals are high amplitude and low velocity. Recording requires adjusting the instrument settings with:
  - ❑ A low velocity range (usually ± 0.2 m/s)
  - ❑ Very low gain and wall filter settings
- ❑ Tissue Doppler velocity is recorded in the apical 4-chamber view with a 2-mm sample volume positioned in the septal myocardium about 1 cm apical from the mitral annulus. The lateral annulus can be used if septal motion is abnormal.
- ❑ The normal tissue Doppler velocity curve shows an early diastolic velocity (E′) toward the apex, followed by a late diastolic velocity (A′) reflecting atrial filling. In systole (S), the myocardial velocity is directed away from the apex with the velocity reflecting LV systolic function (Fig. 4.7).

Strain and Strain Rate

- Strain rate (SR) is the rate of change in myocardial length, normalized for the original length calculated from the difference in velocities at two myocardial sites (V_1 and V_2), and divided by the distance (D) between them (units are s^{-1}).

$$SR = (V_2 - V_1)/D \qquad (4.1)$$

- Strain is a measure of deformation of a material, defined as the difference between the original length (L_0) and final length (L), expressed as a percent (units are a dimensionless percent) of the original length:

$$Strain = [(L - L_0)/L_0 \times 100\% \qquad (4.2)$$

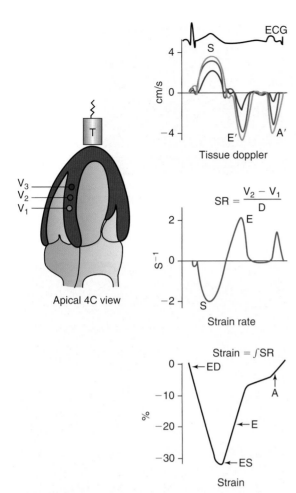

$$SR = \frac{V_2 - V_1}{D}$$

$$Strain = \int SR$$

Fig. 4.7 **Schematic diagram of the derivation of strain rate and strain from myocardial tissue velocities.** From the apical view at least three Doppler sample volumes are positioned in the myocardium about 12 mm apart. The three graphs on the right show one cardiac cycle, matched for timing as shown by the electrocardiogram *(ECG)* at the top. The tissue Doppler tracings show mean velocity versus time with the line colors corresponding to each sample volume position. Strain rate *(SR)* is calculated for each time point at the change in velocity *(V)* between each two-sample volume positions, divided by the distance *(D)* between them. Strain is determined by integration of the strain rate to generate a curve similar to a LV volume curve with a rapid decrease in strain during ejection *(ED to ES)* and a rapid increase in strain in early diastole *(E)* with another increase in late diastole after atrial contraction *(A).*

❖ **KEY POINTS**

❑ Myocardial shortening (systole) is a negative strain rate. Lengthening (diastole) is a positive strain rate. Thus the strain rate curve looks like a mirror image of a tissue Doppler velocity curve (see Fig. 4.7).

   ❑ With Doppler tissue velocity data, strain is calculated by integrating the strain rate curve over time.

   ❑ With speckle-tracking echocardiography (STE), strain is measured directly from the change in distance between two points in the myocardium.

❑ Global longitudinal strain (GLS) is a measure of LV systolic function with a normal peak GLS of about −20% (normal range of −16% to −22%) and is relatively insensitive to changes in loading conditions.

❑ Strain is analogous to ejection fraction (change in length versus volume over time), and the strain curve is similar in shape to a ventricular volume curve.

❑ Regional LV function can be evaluated using strain rate or strain imaging, as well as global LV systolic function.

❑ Speckle-tracking GLS is preferred over tissue Doppler velocity derived GLS, because it is more reproducible and is not angle dependent.

Speckle Tracking Strain Imaging

■ Speckle tracking uses small reflectors in the myocardium to track motion, allowing calculation of LV strain.

■ Unlike tissue Doppler, speckle-tracking strain is not dependent on the angle between the ultrasound beam and direction of motion.

❖ **KEY POINTS**

❑ Speckle tracking provides a direct measure of strain defined as the change in length of myocardium relative to the original length.

❑ Speckle tracking is displayed as a 2D color-coded image, alongside a graphic display of strain for different myocardial segments (Fig. 4.8).

❑ Longitudinal strain can be measured from apical views, circumferential strain from short-axis views, and radial strain from various 2D views.

Dyssynchrony, Twist, and Torsion

Dyssynchrony is defined as spatial variation in the timing of LV contraction, most often seen in patients with a low ejection fraction or regional wall motion abnormalities.

■ Dyssynchrony is qualitatively easily appreciated on 2D imaging; various quantitative measures have been proposed, but there is little data on clinical utility.

❖ **KEY POINTS**

❑ One measure of dyssynchrony is a difference >130 ms in septal to posterior wall delay, defined as the interval between the QRS and the maximum inward motion of the myocardium. This measure is affected by other factors that alter septal motion.

❑ Interventricular dyssynchrony is reflected by a >40 ms difference between the LV and right ventricle (RV) preejection periods (time from QRS to antegrade aortic or pulmonic flow).

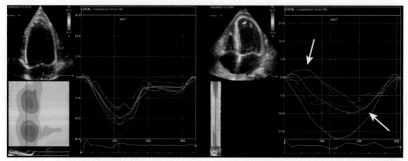

Fig. 4.8 Speckle-tracking echocardiography (STE) showing long-axis strains. The left panel shows the typical strain pattern from a normal LV. The right panel shows recordings from a patient with an anterior myocardial infarction. In the apical LV segments *(arrows)*, there is lengthening during early systole, and there is postsystolic shortening.

❑ Tissue Doppler allows 2D display of dyssynchrony and measurement for multiple myocardial segments. Dyssynchrony is present when there is a difference of at least 65 ms in the tissue Doppler S-wave peaks between opposing LV walls in apical 4-chamber or long-axis views.

CONTRAST ECHOCARDIOGRAPHY

■ Intravenous injection of microbubbles to opacify the cardiac chambers or evaluate myocardial perfusion is called *contrast echocardiography.*

■ Agitated saline contrast opacifies the right heart and is used for detection of right to left intracardiac shunting based on the appearance of contrast in the left heart.

■ Smaller microbubbles (1 to 5 μm diameter) transverse the pulmonary vasculature, allowing left heart chamber and myocardial opacification.

❖ **KEY POINTS**

❑ The most common use of right-sided contrast is to detect a patent foramen ovale, either on transthoracic or transesophageal imaging (Fig. 4.9).

❑ Left heart contrast typically is used to enhance LV endocardial border detection when transthoracic image quality is suboptimal (Fig. 4.10).

❑ In patients with LV thrombus or mass, use of left heart contrast outlines the intra-chamber mass, which does not fill with contrast (negative filling defect).

❑ Instrument settings to optimize left heart contrast images include:

  ❑ A decrease in power output (to a mechanical index of about 0.5)

  ❑ A lower transducer frequency

  ❑ An increase in overall gain and dynamic range

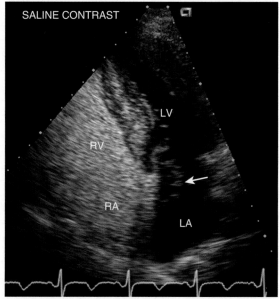

Fig. 4.9 Right heart saline contrast. Intravenous injection of agitated saline provides opacification of the right heart chambers. A small amount of contrast is seen in the LA *(arrow)* consistent with the presence of patent foramen ovale.

  ❑ Focal depth at the mid- or near-field of the image

❑ When microbubble density is too high, excessive apical contrast results in shadowing of the rest of the ventricle (Fig. 4.11A).

❑ A low microbubble density or high mechanical index results in a swirling appearance with inadequate LV opacification (see Fig. 4.11B).

❑ Left-sided contrast is contraindicated in patients with:

  ❑ A significant right-to-left shunt or a bidirectional shunt

  ❑ Hypersensitivity to echo contrast

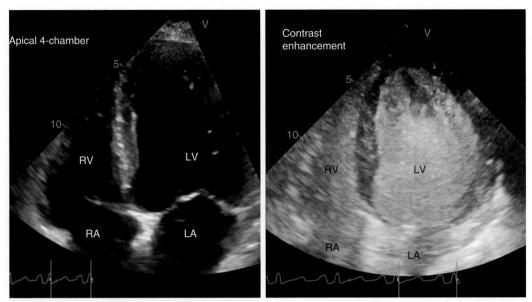

Fig. 4.10 **Left heart contrast.** In this patient with suboptimal endocardial definition in the apical 4-chamber view *(left)*, intravenous injection of a left heart contrast agent opacifies the LV, providing improved endocardial definition for better evaluation of LV regional and overall systolic function *(right)*.

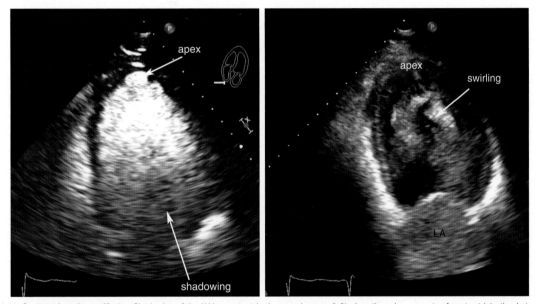

Fig. 4.11 **Contrast imaging artifacts.** Shadowing of the LV by contrast in the apex is seen *(left)* when the volume or rate of contrast injection is too high. Swirling of ventricular contrast *(right)* with poor definition of the endocardium is seen when the volume of contrast is too low or when the mechanical index is too high, which results in destruction of microbubbles.

❑ Caution is needed (with blood pressure, arterial oxygen saturation, and electrocardiogram [ECG] monitoring) in patients with:
  ❑ Pulmonary hypertension or
  ❑ Unstable cardiopulmonary conditions
❑ Assessment of myocardial perfusion by contrast echocardiography is not widely used for clinical diagnosis, although there is ongoing development of this approach.

INTRACARDIAC ECHOCARDIOGRAPHY

■ Intracardiac echocardiography (ICE) is performed in the cardiac catheterization or electrophysiology laboratory using a small high frequency transducer (5 to 10 MHz) on the tip of a catheter.
■ ICE imaging is used to guide percutaneous interventions and complex electrophysiology procedures.

❖ **KEY POINTS**

❏ ICE typically is performed by the physician performing the invasive procedure.

❏ Manipulation of the transducer-tipped catheter requires considerable experience in intracardiac procedures.

❏ Images are obtained primarily from the RA, allowing evaluation of the:
  ❏ Interatrial septum
  ❏ LA, atrial appendage, and pulmonary veins
  ❏ Mitral valve and base of the LV
  ❏ Tricuspid valve and RV (Fig. 4.12)

❏ ICE is used to guide procedures including:
  ❏ Atrial septal defect closure
  ❏ Patent foramen ovale closure
  ❏ Arrhythmia ablation procedures
  ❏ Other complex percutaneous procedures

❏ Some procedures (such as balloon mitral valvuloplasty) can be monitored by intracardiac, transesophageal, or transthoracic imaging.

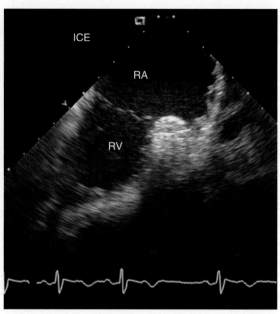

Fig. 4.12 **Intracardiac echocardiography (ICE).** The catheter-tip transducer is located in the RA with visualization of the trabeculated RA appendage, tricuspid valve, and RV.

THE ECHO EXAM SPECIALIZED ECHO APPLICATIONS

Modality	Instrumentation	Clinical utility	Special training
3D echo	Volume-rendered images Surface-rendered LV volumes Simultaneous 2D images	• LV volumes, EF, and regional wall motion • Mitral valve anatomy • Procedural guidance	• Image acquisition and analysis
Tissue Doppler strain rate and strain	Tissue Doppler and 2D imaging are used to measure strain rate: $SR = (V_2 - V_1) / D$	• Strain rate is a measure of ventricular contractility. • Strain rate is integrated to determine strain, a measure of regional myocardial function.	• Data acquisition and analysis • Clinical interpretation of data
Myocardial speckle tracking	Strain is measured directly from the motion of myocardial speckles as: $[(L - L_0) / L_0] \times 100\%$	• Myocardial speckle tracking is angle independent. • Analysis can be performed after image acquisition.	• Data acquisition and analysis • Clinical interpretation of data
Myocardial dyssynchrony	Multiple 2D pulsed Doppler and tissue Doppler methods	• The degree of dyssynchrony is altered in various disease states.	• Data acquisition and analysis • Clinical interpretation of data
Contrast echo	Microbubbles for right or left heart contrast	• Detection of patent foramen ovale • LV endocardial definition	• Intravenous administration of contrast agents • Knowledge of potential risks
Intracardiac echo (ICE)	5-10 MHz catheter-like intracardiac probe	• Interventional procedures (ASD closure) • EP procedures	• Invasive cardiology training and experience
Point-of-care ultrasound study (POCUS) (see Chapter 5)	Small, inexpensive ultrasound instruments	• Bedside evaluation by physician for pericardial effusion, LV global function, and LV regional function	• At least Level 1 echo training
Procedural Guidance (see Chapter 18)	Complete TEE and/or TTE ultrasound system	• Intraoperative evaluation of structural heart disease immediately before and after the procedure • Procedural guidance of transcatheter procedures for structural heart disease	• Echocardiography training (often performed by cardiac anesthesiologists)

ASD, Atrial septal defect; *EF*, ejection fraction; *EP*, electrophysiology.

SELF-ASSESSMENT QUESTIONS

Question 1

Exercise echocardiography is a reasonable consideration in patients with:
- **A.** Previous myocardial infarction
- **B.** Symptomatic aortic stenosis
- **C.** Acute aortic dissection
- **D.** Severe systemic hypertension

Question 2

A 54-year-old woman presents with complaints of episodic dyspnea, which can occur both at rest or on exertion but is not reliably provoked. She has no cardiovascular risk factors. TTE demonstrates an ejection fraction of 64%, and a global longitudinal strain (GLS) of −23% (Fig. 4.13). Based on the speckle tracking echocardiographic image and strain data provided, what additional testing would likely be most useful in evaluating her symptoms?
- **A.** Septal myocardial tissue Doppler velocity
- **B.** Pulmonary function testing
- **C.** Measure 3D systolic and diastolic LV volumes
- **D.** Coronary angiography

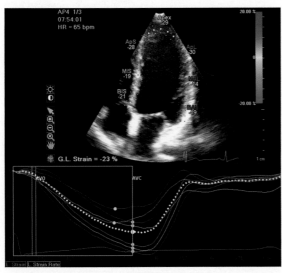

Fig. 4.13

Question 3

Which of the following would aid in improving echocardiographic image quality when using microbubble transpulmonary contrast?
- **A.** Concentrate microbubble solution
- **B.** Set focus depth in near field
- **C.** Decrease transmit frequency
- **D.** Increase mechanical index

Question 4

Which of the following will improve the frame rate of a 3D echocardiography image?
- **A.** Changing from a real-time narrow zoom to single-beat, full-volume acquisition
- **B.** Using 3D color flow Doppler imaging
- **C.** Increasing from a single-beat to a four-beat volume acquisition
- **D.** Extending the elevation width of a 3D-zoom image
- **E.** Displaying the 3D image using multiple 2D tomographic planes

Question 5

TTE was requested in a 57-year-old man with a stroke to evaluate for a patent foramen ovale. Agitated saline contrast was injected via a right antecubital vein at rest and again following Valsalva maneuver for a total of six injections. Several microbubbles were first seen in the LA eight cardiac cycles after injection. These data are most consistent with:
- **A.** Persistent left superior vena cava
- **B.** Patent foramen ovale
- **C.** Transpulmonary passage of contrast
- **D.** Nondiagnostic study

Question 6

A 62-year-old man is referred for cardiac stress testing for symptoms of intermittent chest discomfort when he lifts or carries heavy loads. His past medical history includes tobacco use and treated hypertension. His baseline ECG shows normal sinus rhythm with criteria for LV hypertrophy.

The most appropriate test to obtain would be:
- **A.** Treadmill ECG stress test
- **B.** Exercise stress echocardiogram
- **C.** Dobutamine stress echocardiogram
- **D.** Cardiopulmonary exercise stress test

Question 7

Which of the following statements best describes speckle tracking echocardiographic imaging?
- **A.** Measures low-level myocardial velocities
- **B.** Dependent on angle of interrogation
- **C.** Measures absolute change in length of myocardium
- **D.** Simultaneous measurement across image plane

Question 8

A 58-year-old male patient presents for follow-up after a recent transmural myocardial infarction. TTE was obtained. Because of poor endocardial definition, transpulmonary microbubble contrast was used, and the following apical long-axis view image was obtained (Fig. 4.14). Based on the image provided, you conclude that the infarct involved:

A. Left anterior descending artery distribution
B. Right coronary artery distribution
C. Left circumflex coronary artery distribution
D. Septal perforator distribution

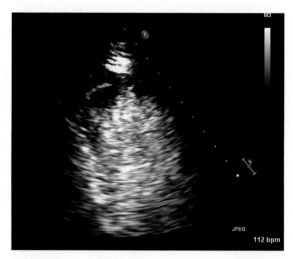

Fig. 4.14

Question 9

List the units of measure for strain, strain rate, speckle tracking, and tissue Doppler.

Question 10

A transthoracic study was obtained in a 41-year-old patient with a history of recurrent dizziness (Fig. 4.15). The image is most consistent with:

A. Perimembranous ventricular septal defect
B. Anomalous coronary artery
C. Secundum atrial septal defect
D. Anomalous pulmonary return
E. No intracardiac shunt

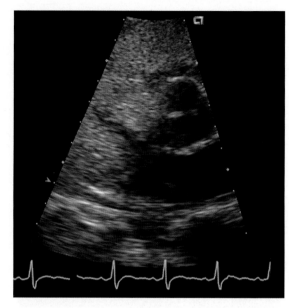

Fig. 4.15

Question 11

Echocardiography in a 56-year-old man with progressive shortness of breath showed a low voltage ECG, severe LV hypertrophy, and a dilated LA. Speckle-tracking global longitudinal strain was performed (Fig. 4.16). The most likely diagnosis is:

   A. Normal LV systolic function
   B. Normal LV diastolic function
   C. Coronary artery disease
   D. Apical hypertrophic cardiomyopathy
   E. Amyloid heart disease

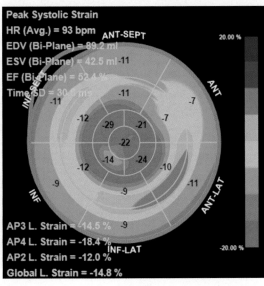

Fig. 4.16

Question 12

A 72-year-old male with a dilated cardiomyopathy underwent echocardiography for evaluated of LV function. Contrast echocardiography was requested to evaluate for LV thrombus and wall motion assessment. Based on review of images from a previous echocardiographic study (Fig. 4.17), which of the following is most accurate?

   A. The mechanical index was set too high, resulting in failure of LV opacification due to destruction of transpulmonary contrast microbubbles.
   B. The sonographer should alert the physician to the presence of interatrial shunting before requesting an order for transpulmonary contrast.
   C. A larger-bore intravenous line was needed for adequate contrast opacification.
   D. The sonographer should proceed with the left heart contrast study with routine patient discharge immediately after the procedure.

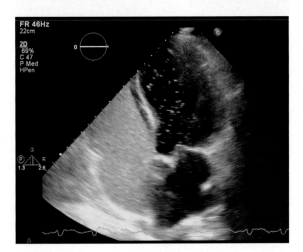

Fig. 4.17

ANSWERS

Answer 1: A

In patients with a recent myocardial infarction who did not undergo angiography, a submaximal stress test is appropriate 3 to 6 days after the initial event, because it provides valuable prognostic information by risk-stratifying patients on the basis of exercise tolerance and residual ischemia. Echocardiographic imaging also allows localization of the culprit vessel and the size of the ischemic territory at risk. Exercise echocardiography should not be done within 72 hours of an acute myocardial infarction in the absence of revascularization, because it may provoke an arrhythmic event. Other contraindications to exercise testing include patients with uncontrolled arrhythmias, severe symptomatic aortic stenosis, and acute aortic dissection. In patients with severe systemic hypertension (systolic blood pressure >200 mm Hg), blood pressure should be controlled, if necessary with medications, before stress testing.

Answer 2: B

Of the options listed, pulmonary function testing would be most likely to provide an etiology of the patient's dyspnea. Left atrial size is small, arguing against high left atrial pressures and diastolic dysfunction. Therefore answer A, septal myocardial tissue Doppler velocity, which is used to calculate E:e′ ratio, would be less helpful. Coronary angiography should only be performed if there is high clinical suspicion for coronary artery disease. In this case, the patient has a paucity of cardiovascular risk factors, and her symptoms are not classic for myocardial ischemia. Global longitudinal strain is a representative aggregate of longitudinal strain from several myocardial segments, represented in the lower left-hand side of Fig. 4.13 as G.L. Strain. Longitudinal strain is the relative motion toward the transducer, and a negative value in excess of −17% is consistent with normal systolic function. Each of the separate segments is color coded, with that color-coded line plotted below the 2D imaging along the time dimension. Although measurement of 3D LV volumes would allow calculation of the ejection fraction (EF), we are already told this patient's EF is normal (64%), and the image shows all segments contracting synchronously, which suggests normal regional wall motion. In contrast, a 2-chamber image taken from a different patient (Fig. 4.18) shows LV chamber dilation, dyssynchronous motion of the myocardial segments, and a global longitudinal strain of −4%.

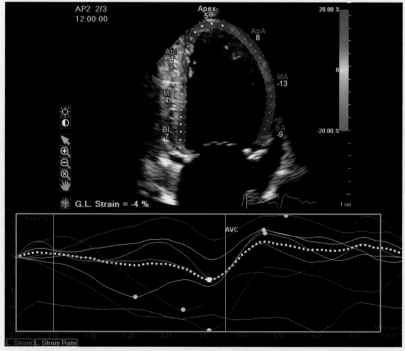

Fig. 4.18

Answer 3: C

Blood and microbubbles have different densities. The relative change in density causes a change in acoustic impedance that reflects transmitted ultrasound waves back to the transducer. However, microbubbles also are destroyed by strong ultrasound signals. Ultrasound machine settings, which improve image quality during microbubble contrast by preserving bubble integrity, include decreasing acoustic power both by decreasing the mechanical index (power output) and decreasing ultrasound transmit frequency. Image quality is also improved by increasing the focal depth from the transducer but not to the point where attenuation occurs; usually microbubble imaging is optimal with the focal depth set in the mid-field. If ultrasound microbubble density is too high, as would occur with concentrating the microbubble solution, then most of the ultrasound is reflected back to the transducer with shadowing of distal structures.

Answer 4: C

Temporal resolution with low frame rates is an inherent problem in 3D echocardiography. The most common method to improve frame rates in by using a multibeat acquisition that images narrower subvolumes that are "stitched" together to form the desired pyramidal volume. This method can be used to improve temporal resolution but can produce stitching artifacts due to an irregular rhythms or translational movement of the structure of interest or probe. Other methods to improve temporal resolution involve narrowing the sector or pyramidal size. Answer A and D would increase pyramidal volume and thus decrease frame rates. Color Doppler (answer B), similar to 2D imaging, reduces temporal resolution. Multiple display options are available for 3D imaging, including volume rendering, surface rendering, and multiple tomographic slices. However, the display option (answer E) does not affect temporal resolution.

Answer 5: C

This was an adequate, diagnostic agitated saline contrast study. A total of six injections were performed, both at rest and following a Valsalva maneuver. Following release of the Valsalva maneuver, there is a transient increase in right atrial pressure relative to left atrial pressure, which would increase the likelihood of transient right to left shunting. Several injections (>5) are typically needed to ensure that interatrial shunting, if present, is identified. Although microbubbles are seen in the LA, this occurred after eight cardiac cycles. This suggests transpulmonary transit of microbubbles rather than intracardiac shunting. A persistent left superior vena cava can also be identified with an agitated saline contrast study, where saline is injected into the left antecubital vein and bubbles are seen opacifying the enlarged coronary sinus (transported via the persistent left superior vena cava) before opacifying the RA.

Answer 6: B

This patient has several cardiovascular risk factors and has exertional chest discomfort so that further evaluation for coronary artery disease is indicated. The most appropriate next test is exercise stress echocardiography, because the patient is ambulatory and his symptoms are provoked by exercise. Echocardiographic imaging allows detection of ischemic myocardium based on the presence of a regional wall motion abnormality with stress but not at rest. Exercise stress testing is preferred over pharmacologic (dobutamine) stress testing when it can be performed, because additional data are obtained on exercise tolerance and the workload required for symptom provocation. A treadmill ECG test would not be helpful, because this patient has an abnormal baseline ECG, which increases the likelihood of a false-positive study when the ECG alone is used to detect ischemia. A cardiopulmonary stress test concurrently measures oxygen consumption with the stress test but is not typically used in conjunction with imaging for ischemia. Cardiopulmonary exercise testing is most useful to separate the pulmonary from cardiac component of exercise limitation in patients with symptoms of unclear etiology, to objectively measure exercise capacity in patient with chronic heart failure or congenital heart disease, and to measure exercise tolerance during cardiopulmonary rehabilitation.

Answer 7: D

Myocardial strain and strain rate provide data on ventricular contraction and relaxation. Echocardiographic measurement of myocardial strain may be obtained by either tissue myocardial Doppler imaging or speckle tracking strain imaging. Tissue myocardial Doppler imaging tracks low level myocardial velocities; as such, it is subject to the inherent features of Doppler imaging, and is dependent on the angle of interrogation between the transducer and myocardial motion. Speckle tracking utilizes reflections from bright echogenic spots (natural acoustic markers) in the myocardium as they move throughout the cardiac cycle. Speckle tracking provides a direct measure of the change in length of the speckle relative to the original length. This relative (not absolute) measure is displayed, often with color mapping, of the multiple, simultaneous measurements, which are taken across an image plane.

Answer 8: A

The image is taken from the apical long-axis view. The LV outflow tract is to the right of the image. In this view, the anterior septum is shown on the right and the inferolateral wall is shown on the left of the image. Microbubble transpulmonary contrast opacifies the endocardial border of the LV. There is thinning of the LV apex, with a large echolucent filling defect in the apex, consistent with an apical thrombus. In patients with poor imaging, qualitulmonary contrast is commonly needed to better evaluate regional wall motion. Often, it is difficult to exclude an apical thrombus due to artifact (near field clutter) or poor image quality. In these cases, transpulmonary contrast will not penetrate the thrombus, and a negative filling defect is seen. This distribution of wall motion abnormality is most consistent with a left anterior descending distribution with transmural infarction involving the entire apex.

Answer 9

Strain rate is the rate of change in myocardial length, normalized for the original length. Strain rate is calculated from the difference in velocities at two myocardial sites (V_1, V_2) divided by the distance between them; the units are $(m/s)/m$. Thus, strain rate simplifies to $1/s$ or s^{-1}.

Strain is a measure of myocardial deformation. Strain of a myocardial segment is defined as the difference between baseline myocardial length (L_0) and final contraction length (L), relative to the original length, or $(L - L_0)/L_0$. The length units in the numerator and denominator cancel each other so that strain measurements are dimensionless. In clinical practice, strain is typically expressed as a percentage.

Speckle tracking follows the motion of small reflectors in the myocardium, allowing calculation of LV strain at multiple sites, and is usually displayed as a 2D color-coded image. Because it measures strain, speckle tracking is also dimensionless.

Tissue Doppler measures velocity of myocardial motion; velocity is lower than the velocity of blood flow but is still typically reported in units of either meters/second or centimeters/second.

Answer 10: C

Fig. 4.15 is an image from an agitated saline contrast study, taken from the parasternal short-axis view. The aortic valve is in the center of the image, the LA is in the lower right section of the image, and the RA and RV are seen opacified by saline contrast. There is a dark, negative washout of contrast that originates at the interatrial septum and goes toward the RA. This finding is consistent with flow of noncontrast blood from left to right across an intracardiac shunt, at the interatrial septum. If left atrial pressure is significantly higher than right atrial pressure, then right to left shunting will not occur following agitated saline contrast injection. Anomalous takeoff of the coronary arteries is not diagnosed with an agitated saline contrast study. Anomalous pulmonary vein return would return oxygenated blood from the pulmonary circulation back to the right heart, but would not insert at the interatrial septum, so that neither a positive or negative contrast jet would be seen. A perimembranous ventricular septal defect (VSD) would not be seen in this view, but could also cause a negative washout of contrast if present (would be seen best from a parasternal long-axis view or apical 4-chamber view).

Answer 11: E

The patient has features of cardiac amyloidosis, including unexplained LV hypertrophy, low-voltage electrocardiogram (ECG), and a reduced global longitudinal strain (GLS) with apical sparing pattern as demonstrated on the bullseye peak systolic strain display. The work-up of infiltrative disease and amyloid should be sought and screening for amyloid protein by serum protein electrophoresis is warranted. The patient does not have normal systolic function (answer A). Although the ejection fraction is minimally reduced, it is only one measure of systolic function. Another measure of systolic myocardial mechanics, the GLS, is below the normal range (-16% to -22%) in this patient. The GLS in this example is demonstrating peak systolic strain values and is not a diastolic parameter (answer B). Furthermore, the LV hypertrophy and left atrial dilation makes it unlikely to have normal diastolic function. The patient has reduced longitudinal strain values in the basal and mid-wall segments with apical sparing, which would not be consistent with a coronary distribution (answer C). The patient is less likely to have hypertrophic cardiomyopathy (answer D) given a low voltage ECG. Apical hypertrophic cardiomyopathy more commonly has large voltages with deep t-wave inversions and does not show normal apical strain.

Answer 12: B

Fig. 4.17 shows an agitated saline contrast study that is positive for a significant number of microbubbles crossing into the LA and LV, indicating a right-to-left intracardiac shunt. Although a high mechanical index can destroy microbubbles producing a swirling artifact when using transpulmonary contrast (answer A), the image shows excellent opacification of the RV on the agitated saline study. A larger IV catheter (answer C) is not needed, because there is an adequate opacification of the RV. The use of left-sided echo contrast requires a physician's order to decide the necessity of contrast administration in the clinical setting and generally is contraindicated in patients with an intracardiac shunt. High-risk patients who do receive contrast injections should have blood pressure and electrocardiographic monitoring for 30 minutes after the study, because rare cardiovascular complications have been reported, rather than being discharged home immediately after the study (answer D).

5 | Clinical Indications and Quality Assurance

BASIC PRINCIPLES

- The value of echocardiography for a specific diagnosis depends on the reliability of the echocardiographic data and integration with other clinical information.
- The framework for echocardiographic data acquisition and reporting is a structured diagnostic approach to the question posed by the requesting physician.

❖ KEY POINTS

- ❑ The echocardiographic study seeks to provide the appropriate data for clinical decision making depending on the patient's symptoms, signs, and known diagnoses.
- ❑ The list of possible diagnoses that might explain the clinical findings, called the *differential diagnosis*, is mentally constructed at the beginning of the echocardiographic study.
- ❑ As the study proceeds, some diagnoses are excluded, whereas others may be suggested by specific findings.
- ❑ Pertinent positive data include abnormal echocardiographic findings.
- ❑ Pertinent negative data include normal echocardiographic findings that help narrow the differential diagnosis.

Understand the Reliability of Echocardiography for the Specific Diagnosis

- The accuracy of echocardiography describes the agreement between an echocardiographic measurement or diagnosis and an external reference standard, such as another imaging approach or clinical outcomes (Fig. 5.1).

- The precision of an echocardiographic measurement is affected by variability in recording, measuring, and interpreting the echocardiographic data.
- Expertise in image acquisition and interpretation affect the reliability of echocardiographic data.

❖ KEY POINTS

- ❑ *Sensitivity* is the percent of patients with the diagnosis correctly identified by echocardiography.
- ❑ *Specificity* is the percent of patients without the diagnosis correctly identified by echocardiography.
- ❑ *Positive predictive value* is the percent of patients with a positive echocardiogram who actually have the diagnosis.
- ❑ *Negative predictive value* is the percent of patients with a negative echocardiogram who do not actually have the diagnosis.
- ❑ *Accuracy* indicates what proportion of all studies indicated a correct diagnosis.
- ❑ The positive and negative predictive value of a test depends on the prevalence of disease in addition to sensitivity and specificity.
- ❑ Each laboratory should periodically review the reproducibility of the echocardiographic measurements.
- ❑ The effect of variability is minimized when images from sequential studies are compared side by side.

Integrate the Clinical Data and the Echocardiographic Findings (Fig. 5.2)

- The likelihood ratio indicates the probability of disease in a patient with a positive or negative echocardiographic finding; a positive likelihood ratio greater than 10 or a negative likelihood ratio less than 0.1 indicates an excellent diagnostic test.

- Pre- and posttest probability estimates integrate the likelihood of disease before the echocardiogram is performed with the echocardiographic results.
- The threshold approach to clinical decision making indicates that diagnostic testing (such as, echocardiography) is most helpful in patients where the results will change either one of the following:
  ○ Treatment strategy
  ○ Diagnostic strategy

❖ **KEY POINTS**

- The positive likelihood ratio is calculated as the true positive rate divided by the false-positive rate. The negative likelihood ratio is the false-negative rate divided by the true-negative rate.
- The pretest probability of disease is the probability of disease before echocardiography is done—for example, consideration of cardiac risk factors and symptoms in a patient scheduled for stress echocardiography provides an estimate of the probability of coronary artery disease.

- Echocardiography is most helpful when the pretest likelihood of disease is intermediate and echocardiography has a high accuracy for the diagnosis.
- When the pretest likelihood of disease is very low, an abnormal echocardiographic finding often is a false-positive result.
- Conversely, when the pretest likelihood of disease is very high, the failure to demonstrate the disease on echocardiography often is a false negative.
- With the threshold approach, the upper threshold is the point where the risk of the test is higher than the risk of treating the patient; for example, additional diagnostic testing should not delay surgical intervention for an acute ascending aortic dissection.
- The lower threshold for transthoracic echocardiography (TTE) occurs only with a very low probability of disease; the major potential adverse effect is a false-positive result leading to further inappropriate testing or therapy.

Recommend Additional Diagnostic Testing as Appropriate

- The interpretation of the echocardiogram lists the pertinent positive and negative findings along with any confirmed diagnoses.
- The differential diagnosis of equivocal findings is indicated and appropriate additional diagnostic testing is recommended when the echocardiographic results are not diagnostic.

❖ **KEY POINTS**

- Echocardiography provides qualitative and quantitative information on cardiac structure and function and often provides a definitive diagnosis.
- Positive findings are more helpful than negative findings; for example, a dissection flap seen on TTE is diagnostic for a dissection, but its absence does not exclude this possibility.

ECHO	Disease	
	Present	Absent
Positive	True positives	False positives
Negative	False negatives	True negatives

→ Positive predictive value
→ Negative predictive value

↓ Sensitivity   ↓ Specificity

$$\text{Accuracy} = \frac{\text{TP} + \text{TN}}{\text{All tests}}$$

Fig. 5.1 **Accuracy of a diagnostic test.** Sensitivity and specificity in comparison with positive and negative predictive value. Predictive values depend on the prevalence of disease in the population. *TN,* True negatives; *TP,* true positives.

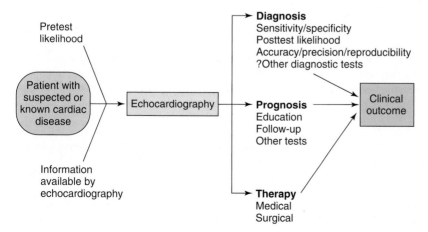

Pretest likelihood

Patient with suspected or known cardiac disease → Echocardiography

Information available by echocardiography

Diagnosis
Sensitivity/specificity
Posttest likelihood
Accuracy/precision/reproducibility
?Other diagnostic tests

Prognosis
Education
Follow-up
Other tests

Therapy
Medical
Surgical

→ Clinical outcome

Fig. 5.2 **Flow chart illustrating the impact of echocardiographic results on diagnosis, prognosis, and therapy.** The effects of echocardiography on clinical outcome are the best measure of the usefulness of the test result.

- A noncardiac cause for symptoms is likely when the appropriate echocardiographic study is normal. For example, normal resting echo in a patient with a systolic murmur is consistent with a benign flow murmur. A normal stress echo in a patient with chest pain indicates that coronary disease is not a likely cause of symptoms.
- The echocardiographer often needs to assist in choosing the optimal diagnostic approach (e.g., TTE or transesophageal echocardiography [TEE], stress echocardiography, contrast study) based on the indication for the study.
- Additional diagnostic studies, with either another echocardiographic modality or an alternate imaging approach, are recommended after review of the echocardiographic exam.

DIAGNOSTIC THINKING FOR THE ECHOCARDIOGRAPHER

- The echocardiographer needs:
  - Clinical data to estimate the pretest likelihood of disease before starting the exam
  - An understanding of pertinent positive and negative findings for each clinical indication
  - Knowledge of the reliability of echocardiography for each diagnosis
  - The ability to integrate the echocardiographic findings with the clinical data
- The "Echo Exam" section summarizes the approach by anatomic diagnosis.
- Examples of the approach to common clinical indications for echocardiography are discussed in the next section.

ECHOCARDIOGRAPHY FOR COMMON SIGNS AND SYMPTOMS

Murmur

- The echocardiographic differential diagnosis for a murmur is based on an anatomic approach with evaluation of all four valves and a search for an intracardiac shunt (Fig. 5.3).
- Many patients referred to echocardiography for a murmur on auscultation have no significant structural heart disease. In this setting, the physical exam finding is most likely a benign flow murmur.

❖ **KEY POINTS**

- The echocardiography request form may not specify the type of murmur (e.g., systolic or diastolic), so a systemic echocardiographic exam is essential.
- Normal physiologic regurgitation rarely accounts for an audible murmur.

- The most common pathologic causes for a murmur in adults are aortic valve stenosis and mitral valve regurgitation.
- Murmurs typically are due to high-velocity intracardiac flows (e.g., aortic stenosis or mitral regurgitation), because low-velocity flows (e.g., tricuspid regurgitation with normal pulmonary pressures) are not usually audible with a stethoscope.
- Conditions that cause increased cardiac output (e.g., anemia or pregnancy) may cause a murmur due to high velocity transvalvular flow in patients with otherwise anatomically normal valves.
- Congenital heart disease may first be diagnosed in an adult based on finding a murmur. In patients with an atrial septal defect, the murmur is due to increased pulmonary blood flow volume, not to flow across the atrial septum.

Chest Pain

- The echocardiographic differential diagnosis for chest pain is based on the major clinical diagnoses that are of immediate clinical concern (Fig. 5.4).
- When the echocardiogram does not establish a diagnosis, further evaluation may be needed emergently.

❖ **KEY POINTS**

- Acute chest pain is a medical emergency, because the differential diagnosis includes acute coronary syndromes and aortic dissection, both of which require immediate treatment.
- An abnormal echocardiographic finding (such as anterior wall hypokinesis) may prompt further diagnostic and therapeutic interventions (such as coronary angiography).
- An acute pulmonary embolism, if large enough, may show signs of right heart strain and increased pulmonary pressures. A smaller pulmonary embolism may have no significant findings on echocardiography.
- Even when the transthoracic echocardiogram is normal, further evaluation may be needed—for example, TEE or chest computed tomography (CT) in a patient with suspected aortic dissection.
- Normal resting wall motion does not exclude the possibility of significant coronary artery disease. Wall motion is abnormal only after infarction or with ongoing myocardial ischemia.
- The presence of a pericardial effusion is consistent with pericarditis, although not all patients with pericarditis have an effusion.
- In a patient with aortic dissection, pericardial fluid may be due to rupture of the aorta into the pericardial space.
- With significant left ventricle (LV) outflow obstruction, the increase in LV myocardial wall stress and oxygen demand results in angina-type chest pain.

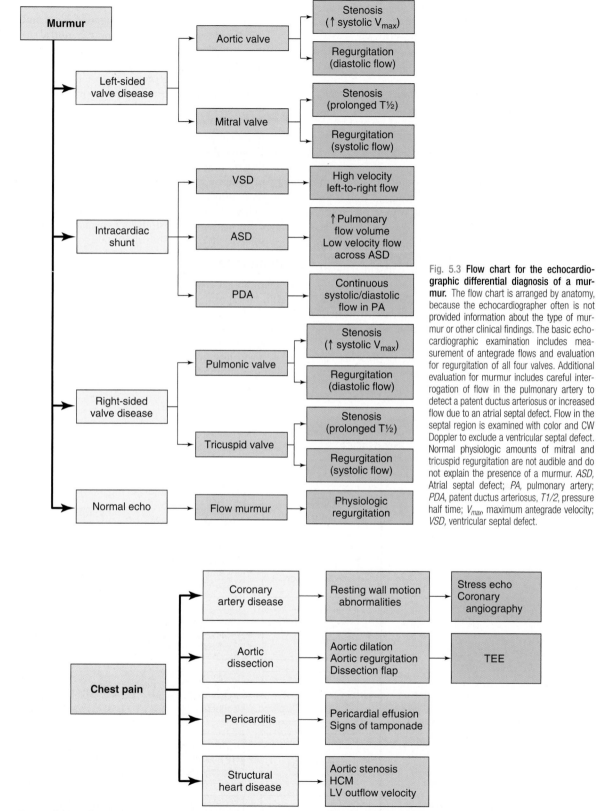

Fig. 5.3 Flow chart for the echocardiographic differential diagnosis of a murmur. The flow chart is arranged by anatomy, because the echocardiographer often is not provided information about the type of murmur or other clinical findings. The basic echocardiographic examination includes measurement of antegrade flows and evaluation for regurgitation of all four valves. Additional evaluation for murmur includes careful interrogation of flow in the pulmonary artery to detect a patent ductus arteriosus or increased flow due to an atrial septal defect. Flow in the septal region is examined with color and CW Doppler to exclude a ventricular septal defect. Normal physiologic amounts of mitral and tricuspid regurgitation are not audible and do not explain the presence of a murmur. *ASD*, Atrial septal defect; *PA*, pulmonary artery; *PDA*, patent ductus arteriosus; *T1/2*, pressure half time; V_{max}, maximum antegrade velocity; *VSD*, ventricular septal defect.

Fig. 5.4 Echocardiographic approach to evaluation of chest pain. The primary goal in the acute setting is to exclude life-threatening conditions, such as an acute coronary syndrome or acute aortic dissection. With both acute and chronic chest pain, further diagnostic evaluation often is needed. *HCM,* Hypertrophic cardiomyopathy.

Heart Failure or Dyspnea

- Symptoms of dyspnea, edema, and decreased exercise tolerance are nonspecific, with a wide differential diagnosis that includes cardiac and noncardiac conditions.

- Heart failure, defined as the inability of the heart to supply adequate blood flow at a normal filling pressure, is the clinical consequent of several types of heart disease (Fig. 5.5).

❖ **KEY POINTS**

- ❏ Heart failure may be due to systolic dysfunction (called heart failure with reduced ejection fraction [HFrEF]) or may occur with a preserved ejection fraction (HFpEF).
- ❏ HFrEF may be due to a cardiomyopathy, coronary disease with prior infarction, long-standing valvular heart disease, or congenital heart disease.
- ❏ HFpEF, associated with diastolic dysfunction, is seen with hypertensive heart disease, hypertrophic cardiomyopathy, and infiltrative myocardial disease.
- ❏ Constrictive pericarditis often presents as right heart failure, with ascites and peripheral edema.

- ❏ Heart failure occurs in patients with valvular heart disease, even when LV function is normal, due to obstruction of blood flow (e.g., mitral stenosis) or elevated pulmonary diastolic pressure (e.g., mitral regurgitation).
- ❏ Pulmonary hypertension due to left heart disease, pulmonary vascular disease, or underlying lung disease leads to right heart failure with a dilated hypokinetic right ventricle (RV), sometimes called *cor pulmonale.*
- ❏ Heart failure in patients with congenital heart disease may be due to ventricular dysfunction, obstructive or regurgitant lesions, or intracardiac shunts.
- ❏ When heart failure is present with a normal echocardiographic study, noncardiac causes for the patient's symptoms should be considered.

Palpitations

- Palpitations are the patient's awareness of a forceful, rapid, or irregular heart rhythm.
- The primary approach to evaluation of palpitations includes resting and ambulatory electrocardiogram (ECG) monitoring.
- Echocardiography allows evaluation of any underlying anatomic abnormalities associated with the cardiac arrhythmia.

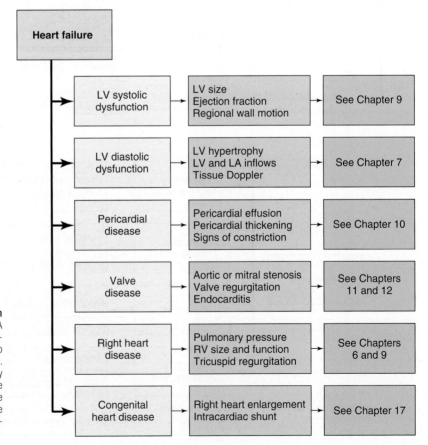

Fig. 5.5 Echocardiographic approach to patients referred for heart failure. A systemic echocardiographic study will include the 2D views and Doppler flows to identify each of these possible diagnoses. In addition, the sonographer should mentally "check off" each of these conditions as the exam progresses to ensure that the entire differential diagnosis is considered. If the echocardiographic study is normal, a noncardiac cause of symptoms is likely.

- Echocardiography typically is normal in patients with a supraventricular arrhythmia and no prior cardiac history.
- Conditions associated with supraventricular arrhythmias include:
  - Ebstein anomaly in patients with preexcitation syndromes
  - Prior surgery for congenital heart disease
- Atrial fibrillation often is associated with hypertensive heart disease, mitral valve disease, and LV systolic dysfunction.
- The prevalence of atrial fibrillation increases with age (present in about 4% of people older than 60 years of age).
- Left atrium (LA) thrombi are associated with atrial fibrillation but are not reliably visualized on TTE; TEE imaging is more accurate for diagnosis of atrial thrombi.
- Echocardiography often is abnormal in patients with ventricular arrhythmias. Quantitative evaluation of LV systolic function is particularly important in these patients.
- Diseases that affect the RV (such as RV dysplasia) also may present with palpitations.

Embolic Event

- An intracardiac thrombus or mass may result in a systemic embolic event.
- Aortic atheroma is present in 20% of patients with an embolic event.
- The presence of a patent foramen ovale or atrial septal aneurysm is associated with an increased prevalence of systemic embolic events in younger adults (<60 years old).

❖ KEY POINTS

- A systematic transthoracic examination is the first step in evaluation for a potential cardiac source of embolus, but TEE is a more sensitive diagnostic approach.
- Conditions associated with systemic embolic events include:
  - Atrial fibrillation
  - LA thrombus
  - Prosthetic heart valves
  - Valvular vegetations (bacterial or nonbacterial thrombotic endocarditis)
  - Patent foramen ovale
  - Aortic atheroma
  - LV thrombus (e.g., after anterior myocardial infarction)
  - Left-sided cardiac tumors (atrial myxoma, valve fibroelastoma)

- In patients with a systemic embolic event, a cardiac source must be presumed to the cause when there is atrial fibrillation, a prosthetic valve, an intracardiac thrombus, or a tumor.
- Other common potential causes of embolic events include patent foramen ovale in patients under age 60 years and aortic atheroma.
- Diagnosis of a patent foramen ovale is based on demonstration of right to left shunting at rest or after Valsalva maneuver, following right heart agitated saline contrast. TEE is more sensitive than TTE for detection of a patent foramen ovale, which is present in about 30% of normal individuals.

Fever/Bacteremia

- Echocardiography is the primary approach to diagnosis of endocarditis in patients with bacteremia (Fig. 5.6).
- In most patients, TTE is the initial approach, but TEE is more sensitive for detection of valvular vegetations.
- Complications of endocarditis (e.g., abscess, fistula) are best evaluated by TEE.
- Patients with an intracardiac device (pacer, defibrillator, or chronic indwelling intravascular line, such as a hemodialysis catheter) should undergo echocardiography to exclude a lead infection.

❖ KEY POINTS

- Detection of valvular vegetations is a major criterion for diagnosis of endocarditis.
- Specificity of TTE for detection of a vegetation is high (i.e., the finding of a vegetation is diagnostic) but sensitivity is low; therefore failure to demonstrate vegetations does not rule out the diagnosis.
- When bacteremia or other clinical signs of endocarditis are present, TEE is appropriate unless the likelihood of endocarditis is very low and image quality is high on transthoracic imaging.
- Both TTE and TEE are appropriate with suspected prosthetic valve endocarditis, because posterior structures are shadowed by the prosthetic valve on transthoracic imaging, whereas anterior structures are shadowed on TEE imaging.
- Detection of vegetations is enhanced by scanning across the valve, using multiple images planes and using nonstandard views, on both TTE and TEE imaging.

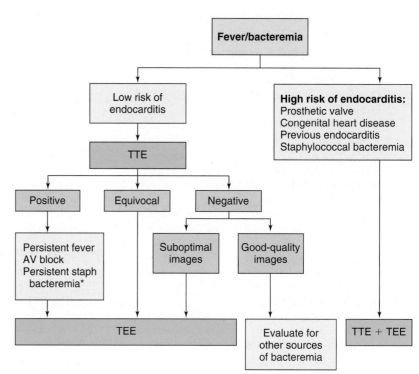

Fig. 5.6 Flow chart for a suggested approach to evaluation of patients with fever and/or bacteremia who are referred for echocardiography. *AV,* Atrioventricular.

*Or other signs of paravalvular abscess or persistent infection.

THE ECHO EXAM

Indications for Transthoracic Echocardiography

Clinical Diagnosis	Key Echo Findings	Limitations of Echo	Alternate Approaches
Valvular Heart Disease			
Valve stenosis	Cause of stenosis, valve anatomy Transvalvular ΔP, valve area Chamber enlargement and hypertrophy LV and RV systolic function Associated valvular regurgitation	Possible underestimation of stenosis severity Possible coexisting coronary artery disease	Cardiac cath CMR
Valve regurgitation	Mechanism and cause of regurgitation Severity of regurgitation Chamber enlargement LV and RV systolic function PA pressure estimate	TEE indicated for evaluation of mitral regurgitant severity and valve anatomy (especially before MV repair)	Cardiac cath CMR
Prosthetic valve function	Evidence for stenosis Detection of regurgitation Chamber enlargement Ventricular function PA pressure estimate	TTE is limited by shadowing and reverberations. TEE is needed for suspected prosthetic MR due to "masking" of the LA on TTE.	Cardiac cath Fluoroscopy
Endocarditis	Detection of vegetations (TTE sensitivity 70%–85%) Presence and degree of valve dysfunction Chamber enlargement and function Detection of abscess Possible prognostic implications	TEE more sensitive for detection of vegetations (>90%) A definite diagnosis of endocarditis also depends on bacteriologic criteria TEE more sensitive for abscess detection	Blood cultures and clinical findings also are diagnostic criteria for endocarditis.
Coronary Artery Disease			

Acute myocardial infarction	Segmental wall motion abnormality reflects "myocardium at risk"
	Global LV function (EF)
	Complications:
	  Acute MR vs. VSD
	  Pericarditis
	  LV thrombus, aneurysm, or rupture
	  RV infarct
		Coronary artery anatomy itself not directly visualized	Coronary angio (cath or CT)
			Radionuclide or PET imaging

Angina	Global and segmental LV systolic function Exclude other causes of angina (e.g., AS, HCM)	Resting wall motion may be normal despite significant CAD Stress echo needed to induce ischemia and wall motion abnormality	Coronary angio (cath or CT) Radionuclide or PET imaging ETT

Indications for Transthoracic Echocardiography

Clinical Diagnosis	Key Echo Findings	Limitations of Echo	Alternate Approaches
Pre-revascularization/post-revascularization	Assess wall thickening and endocardial motion at baseline Improvement in segmental function postprocedure	Dobutamine stress and/or contrast echo needed to detect viable but nonfunctioning myocardium	CMR Coronary angio (cath or CT) Radionuclide or PET imaging Contrast echocardiography
End-stage ischemic disease	Overall LV systolic function (EF) PA pressures Associated MR LV thrombus RV systolic function		Coronary angio (cath or CT) Radionuclide or PET imaging CMR for myocardial viability
Cardiomyopathy			
Dilated	Chamber dilation (all four) LV and RV systolic function (qualitative and EF) Coexisting atrioventricular valve regurgitation PA systolic pressure LV thrombus	Indirect measures of LV-EDP Accurate EF may be difficult if image quality is poor	CMR for LV size, function and myocardial fibrosis LV angiography with left and right heart hemodynamics
Restrictive	LV wall thickness LV systolic function LV diastolic function PA systolic pressure	Must be distinguished from constrictive pericarditis	Cardiac cath with direct, simultaneous RV and LV pressure measurement after volume loading CMR
Hypertrophic	Pattern and extent of LV hypertrophy Dynamic LVOT obstruction (imaging and Doppler) Coexisting MR Diastolic LV dysfunction	Exercise echo needed to detect inducible LVOT obstruction	CMR Strain and strain rate imaging
Hypertension			
	LV hypertrophy LV diastolic dysfunction LV systolic function Aortic valve sclerosis, MAC	Diastolic dysfunction precedes systolic dysfunction, but detection is challenging because of impact of age and other factors.	Speckle tracking strain and strain rate imaging LV twist and torsion
Pericardial Disease			
	Pericardial thickening Detection, size, and location of PE 2D signs of tamponade physiology Doppler signs of tamponade physiology	Diagnosis of tamponade is a hemodynamic and clinical diagnosis. Constrictive pericarditis is a difficult diagnosis. Not all patients with pericarditis have an effusion.	Intracardiac pressure measurements for tamponade or constriction CMR or CT to detect pericardial thickening
Aortic Disease			
Aortic dilation	Cause of aortic dilation Accurate aortic diameter measurements Anatomy of sinuses of Valsalva (especially Marfan syndrome) Associated aortic regurgitation	The ascending aorta is only partially visualized on TTE in most patients.	CT, CMR, TEE

Indications for Transthoracic Echocardiography

Clinical Diagnosis	Key Echo Findings	Limitations of Echo	Alternate Approaches
Aortic dissection	2D images of ascending aorta, aortic arch, descending thoracic, and proximal abdominal aorta Imaging of dissection "flap" Associated aortic regurgitation Ventricular function	TEE more sensitive (97%) and specific (100%) Cannot assess distal vascular beds	Aortography CT CMR TEE
Cardiac Masses			
LV thrombus	High sensitivity and specificity for diagnosis of LV thrombus Suspect with apical wall motion abnormality or diffuse LV systolic dysfunction	Technical artifacts can be misleading. 5-MHz or higher frequency transducer and angulated apical views needed.	LV thrombus may not be recognized on radionuclide or contrast angiography.
LA thrombus	Low sensitivity for detection of LA thrombus, although specificity is high Suspect with LA enlargement, MV disease	TEE is needed to detect LA thrombus reliability.	TEE
Cardiac tumors	Size, location, and physiologic consequences of tumor mass	Extracardiac involvement not well seen Cannot distinguish benign from malignant or tumor from thrombus	TEE CT CMR Intracardiac echo
Pulmonary Hypertension			
	PA pressure estimate Evidence of left-sided heart disease to account for increased PA pressures RV size and systolic function (cor pulmonale) Associated TR	Indirect PA pressure measurement Difficult to determine pulmonary vascular resistance accurately	Cardiac cath
Congenital Heart Disease			
	Detection and assessment of anatomic abnormalities Quantitation of physiologic abnormalities Chamber enlargement Ventricular function	No direct intracardiac pressure measurements Complicated anatomy may be difficult to evaluate if image quality is poor (TEE helpful)	CMR with 3D reconstruction Cardiac cath TEE 3D Echo

AS, Aortic stenosis; *CAD,* coronary artery disease; *CMR,* cardiac magnetic resonance imaging; *CT,* computed tomography; *EDP,* end-diastolic pressure; *EF,* ejection fraction; *ETT,* exercise treadmill test; *HCM,* hypertrophic cardiomyopathy; *LVOT,* left ventricular outflow tract; *MAC,* mitral annular calcification; *MR,* mitral regurgitation; *MV,* mitral valve; *PA,* pulmonary artery; *PE,* pericardial effusion; *PET,* positron emission tomography; *VSD,* ventricular septal defect.

SELF-ASSESSMENT QUESTIONS

Select the best diagnostic modality option available for the clinical scenario presented in questions 1 to 14 from the following list:

A. Transthoracic echocardiography (TTE)
B. Dobutamine stress echocardiography (DSE)
C. Transesophageal echocardiography (TEE)
D. Intracardiac echocardiography (ICE)
E. Exercise stress echocardiography (ESE)
F. Saline contrast echocardiography
G. Left-sided contrast echocardiography
H. No further diagnostic testing needed.

Question 1

A 26-year-old man with a history of prior endocarditis and bioprosthetic aortic valve replacement due to intravenous drug use presents with fever and bacteremia. Electrocardiogram (ECG) demonstrates a prolonged PR interval compared to previous ECGs.

Question 2

A 47-year-old woman undergoing percutaneous closure of an atrial septal defect with minimal conscious sedation.

Question 3

A 40-year-old man with known hypertrophic cardiomyopathy presents with several episodes of exertional presyncope. A TTE performed 1 month ago demonstrated a LV outflow tract velocity of 1.8 m/s following Valsalva maneuver with a maximal, diastolic septal wall thickness of 18 mm.

Question 4

A 17-year-old asymptomatic male undergoing a sports physical in preparation for participation on an intramural school sports team presents for evaluation. He had received a screening ECG and was noted to have prominent voltage in the precordial leads (S wave in V3 = 25 mm).

Question 5

A 76-year-old man presents to the emergency department following a syncopal episode. His medical history includes hypertension, advanced chronic kidney disease, and dyslipidemia. During his evaluation, he has ongoing, severe precordial chest pain that radiates to his midscapular region. Blood pressure in his right arm is 160/80 mm Hg, and in his left arm it is 140/96 mm Hg. A 12-lead ECG performed in the emergency room (ER) shows sinus rhythm at 120 bpm. There are no ischemic changes on the ECG tracings, and blood work obtained is unrevealing. Chest radiography shows a wide mediastinum.

Question 6

A 50-year-old woman had undergone cardiac transplantation 8 years ago for nonischemic cardiomyopathy. Two years ago, she had developed exertional dyspnea, and diagnostic evaluation at that time identified mild to moderate range transplant vasculopathy. The patient was treated medically with resolution of symptoms. She is currently asymptomatic and presents for routine clinical evaluation.

Question 7

A 60-year-old man presents for annual follow-up of mitral valve prolapse and moderate-severe mitral regurgitation. He exercises regularly, with lap swimming several times per week; LV size and systolic function are normal, and estimated pulmonary systolic pressure is 30 mm Hg.

Question 8

A 43-year-old woman presents with dyspnea. Her medical history includes breast cancer, and she has completed several rounds of chemotherapy and radiation treatment. A 12-lead ECG shows sinus tachycardia with a ventricular rate of 125 bpm; there is low voltage throughout the precordial leads.

Question 9

A 91-year-old woman presents for routine clinical evaluation. She has no known cardiac history. Her medical history includes only mild hypertension. On physical examination, there is an early peaking systolic murmur heard at the upper right sternal border, which does not radiate. The other heart sounds are normal.

Question 10

A 49-year-old woman with symptomatic rheumatic mitral stenosis undergoing evaluation for percutaneous mitral valvotomy.

Question 11

A 65-year-old man with type 2 diabetes mellitus undergoing preoperative evaluation for bilateral femoral artery bypass surgery.

Question 12

A 58-year-old smoker with chronic obstructive pulmonary disease and dilated cardiomyopathy due to ischemic heart disease presents with new onset, right-sided weakness, splenic infarct, and ischemic toe digits.

Question 13

A 50-year-old woman with a mechanical mitral valve replacement for rheumatic stenosis 12 years ago presents for routine clinical evaluation. She exercises regularly, walking daily. She was last seen in follow-up 3 years ago and had an unremarkable transthoracic echocardiogram at that time. She has had no complaints since her last visit.

Question 14

A 62-year-old man presents to the emergency room with left-sided weakness. The patient recalls similar symptoms 2 months prior, which resolved on their own. Past medical history includes coronary artery disease with a history of a prior coronary stent in the right coronary artery following a myocardial infarction 8 months ago. TTE at that time showed preserved systolic function with EF 58% and only mild hypokinesis of the inferior wall. No other abnormalities.

ANSWERS

Answer 1: C

Clinical suspicion for endocarditis is high in this patient with bacteremia, and additional diagnostic testing is indicated. The presence of atrioventricular nodal block raises concern for a paravalvular abscess with intramyocardial extension affecting conduction pathways. TTE imaging is inadequate for definitive evaluation of paravalvular abscess, particularly in a patient with a prosthetic aortic valve, because reverberations and acoustic shadowing from the prosthetic valve may obscure or limit visualization of a paravalvular abscess. An aortic paravalvular abscess may extend into the septum, affecting the conduction system, but may also extend into the posterior aortic annulus, adjacent to the anterior mitral valve leaflet. With TEE imaging, there is no interposed ribs/lung tissue between the transducer and the heart, so image quality is improved and posterior cardiac structures are better visualized compared with TTE imaging.

Answer 2: D

Intraprocedural echocardiography (ICE) is commonly utilized in procedural-based echocardiographic studies to aid in real-time catheter and device placement during the procedure. In this case, ICE assists in quantifying the size, location, and number of defects. ICE imaging also allows for Doppler assessment of interatrial flow and adequacy of surround rims for device deployment. Visualization of cardiac structures during a procedure may also be obtained with TEE, typically performed by cardiac anesthesiologists trained in periprocedural TEE imaging. However, continuous imaging with TEE during a procedure necessitates intubation and ventilator support to minimize patient discomfort with prolonged TEE probe placement during a procedure. TTE is difficult to perform concurrently with procedures due to interference of transducer placement with the sterile field.

Answer 3: E

This patient presents with presyncope and further diagnostic testing is indicated. Repeat TTE is unlikely to demonstrate a significant interval change compared to a prior study only 1 month before. Patients with hypertrophic cardiomyopathy may develop LV outflow tract obstruction, which is only manifest with physical activity. If there is concurrent systolic anterior motion of the mitral valve with physical activity, LV outflow obstruction may be exacerbated. Provoked LVOT gradients reflect true peak stress gradients when measured in real time. Exercise may be performed using a standard treadmill protocol or with a supine bicycle. With treadmill exercise, echocardiographic data are recorded at baseline and immediately after exercise. Bicycle stress ergometry allows continuous echocardiographic images, because the patient lies recumbent and, with some systems, an integrated stress bed can be maneuvered to allow for optimal patient positioning. TEE imaging is not optimal for patients with hypertrophic cardiomyopathy, because TEE is a resting study, and the LVOT jet is difficult to align in a parallel manner with the transducer due to the physical constraints of the esophagus.

Answer 4: A

This patient's abnormal baseline ECG is consistent with LV hypertrophy.

Patients with hypertrophic cardiomyopathy who participate in competitive sports are at increased risk of sudden cardiac death. Therefore this patient warrants additional evaluation. TTE allows for visualization of cardiac size and function, including myocardial thickness. Competitive athletes may have concentric hypertrophy (not hypertrophic cardiomyopathy) that regresses with abstinence from participation in sports; in cases where a diagnosis of hypertrophic cardiomyopathy is equivocal, additional imaging modalities (such as cardiac magnetic resonance imaging) that allow for a more detailed evaluation of the morphologic, functional, and tissue abnormalities associated with hypertrophic cardiomyopathy (HCM) myocardial fibrosis and scarring may be needed.

Answer 5: C

This patient has complaints of severe, ongoing chest discomfort. He also had a syncopal event, but a 12-lead ECG performed during active pain does not show evidence of myocardial ischemia. However, he has unequal blood pressures in his arms, and his chest radiograph shows an enlarged aorta. This clinical presentation is most consistent with an acute aortic dissection. Computed tomography (CT) imaging with contrast is the first diagnostic test at most centers but might best be avoided in this patient with chronic renal disease. TEE allows for visualization of the proximal ascending aorta, aortic arch, and proximal descending thoracic aorta. Only a small portion of the distal ascending is not well seen due to the overlying trachea where air obscures ultrasound penetration. TEE also allows for visualization of cardiac function to evaluate regional wall motion. Transthoracic imaging allows visualization of myocardial function, but visualization of the ascending aorta is not optimal, particularly for definitive evaluation for aortic dissection. If aortic dissection is suspected, other tomographic imaging modalities, such as cardiac computed tomography (CT) or magnetic resonance imaging, would allow evaluation of the aorta. Stress echocardiography could be considered if acute ischemia is excluded by laboratory work-up but the pain is ongoing, once other severe causes of acute chest pain are excluded.

Answer 6: B

TTE allows for resting evaluation of cardiac structures and function. This patient has a history of known transplant vasculopathy. Screening for transplant vasculopathy requires cardiac stress testing. Dobutamine stress testing is the procedure of choice for noninvasive evaluation for transplant vasculopathy given that the autonomic response to exercise is not intact in the denervated, transplanted heart. Treadmill stress echocardiography would provide a reasonable option if the study indication was to assess patient exercise tolerance. In order to ensure adequate achievement of maximal cardiac workload, pharmacologic testing is typically needed. During dobutamine stress echocardiography (DSE) testing, most patients achieve the target heart rate. Like the sympathetic response to exercise, denervated hearts will not have a predictable response to parasympathetic stimulation; therefore response to atropine is typically variable to nonexistent.

Answer 7: C

In patients with chronic mitral regurgitation due to mitral valve prolapse, elective surgical mitral valve repair may be considered even in the absence of symptoms or LV dysfunction if (1) quantitative measures confirm severe regurgitation and (2) valve anatomy is amenable to repair with a high likelihood of a successful procedure. Valve reparability is best evaluated by 3D TEE with full volume imaging to show the location and extent of leaflet prolapse, identify any flail segments, and measure annular size.

Answer 8: A

This patient's clinical history and current presentation are concerning for cardiac tamponade. TTE is diagnostic for pericardial effusion. Cardiac tamponade is a clinical diagnosis that incorporates the clinical presentation, physical examination, and echocardiography findings. Patients with hemodynamically significant effusions are typically symptomatic, with relative hypotension, tachycardia, and significantly increased central venous pressure. This is evident on TTE with a large pericardial effusion with evidence of right-sided chamber collapse; there is respiratory variation in mitral and tricuspid inflow, and plethora of the inferior vena cava (indicating increased central venous pressure).

Answer 9: H

This patient has cardiac murmur heard best over the aortic region. The characteristics of the murmur are benign, early peaking with a normal second heart sound and are consistent with aortic sclerosis. Increased antegrade flow over the cardiac valves increases turbulent flow and commonly produces a benign systolic flow murmur. In an asymptomatic patient, no further diagnostic testing is indicated. In patients with significant stenosis, aortic valve replacement is not recommended for asymptomatic patients.

Answer 10: C

Patients with symptomatic rheumatic mitral stenosis are candidates for percutaneous mitral valvotomy. Before the procedure, TEE is indicated to evaluate for mitral regurgitation and left atrial thrombus. There is an increased likelihood of success with favorable valve anatomy (less leaflet calcification, less leaflet thickening, and less involvement of the subvalvular apparatus). Valvotomy may significantly increase regurgitation, particularly if the valve leaflets are thickened or calcified and leaflet tearing occurs during the procedure. Also, during the procedure, the catheter is in the LA, where a LA thrombus may dislodge if present. Therefore transcatheter valvotomy is contraindicated if there is greater than moderate regurgitation or a LA thrombus at baseline. TTE may be adequate to evaluate mitral regurgitation severity but is not adequate to exclude LA appendage thrombus. Intracardiac echocardiography (ICE) may be used intraprocedurally during the valvuloplasty, but the TEE is first indicated to determine if the patient is a candidate for the procedure.

Answer 11: B

Preoperative evaluation for patients with significant cardiovascular risk factors typically includes provocative stress testing to identify myocardial ischemia. Resting studies (such as TTE or TEE) do not provide evaluation of the cardiac response to stress, as would potentially be encountered intraoperatively. An exercise stress study (treadmill or bicycle stress) is preferred over pharmacologic testing when possible as it provides an evaluation of the cardiac response to physiologic stress. However, given that the patient in this case scenario is undergoing preoperative evaluation for bilateral lower peripheral artery disease, it is unlikely that the workload achieved would be adequate to provide a maximal stress study.

Answer 12: G

This patient presents with signs of cardioembolism in a dilated cardiomyopathy. Thorough evaluation starts with TTE. However, evaluation of LV thrombus can be limited from near-field clutter artifact and suboptimal visualization in patients with poor acoustic apical windows from lung disease. Contrast echocardiography is the modality of choice to improve imaging and identification of the true apex in evaluation of LV thrombus. Although TEE can overcome suboptimal chest wall imaging, identification of the true apex is frequently limited due to confined placement of the transducer in the esophagus. TEE could be warranted to evaluate the left atrial appendage after thrombus is excluded by contrast echocardiography.

Answer 13: H

This patient has had a postoperative TTE that documents normal prosthetic valve function, and she is currently asymptomatic. Routine surveillance echocardiography is not recommended in asymptomatic patients with mechanical prostheses. Patients with bioprosthetic valve prostheses should undergo surveillance TTE 8 to 10 years after placement to exclude valve degeneration and dysfunction. If the patient develops cardiopulmonary symptoms, signs of systemic infection, or clinical suspicion for valve dysfunction, TTE is typically initially obtained. However, because of acoustic shadowing of the prosthesis with limited or no penetration of ultrasound through

prosthetic material, TEE imaging is often also needed to more completely evaluate valve function, particularly with mitral mechanical prostheses, where acoustic shadowing of the LA limits evaluation of the atrial side of the valve.

Answer 14: F

This patient is presenting with neurologic complaints that are recurrent. TTE performed 8 months prior to his current presentation demonstrated relative preservation of LV systolic function with ejection fraction 58%, and only mild hypokinesis of the inferior wall. Agitated saline contrast echocardiography is not a routine component of standard transthoracic imaging protocols. In this case, facilitate diagnosis of a patent foramen ovale, if present. A diagnosis may alter treatment strategies given that these are recurrent symptoms.

Left and Right Ventricular Systolic Function

LEFT VENTRICULAR SYSTOLIC FUNCTION

Step 1: Measure Left Ventricular Size

Left Ventricular Chamber Dimensions

■ Two-dimensional (2D) measurement of left ventricular (LV) minor axis internal dimensions or 2D guided M-mode measurement of LV minor axis internal dimensions at end-diastole and end-systole

❖ KEY POINTS

❑ LV internal dimensions are measured from the parasternal window, because the ultrasound beam is perpendicular to the blood-myocardial interface, providing high axial resolution (Fig. 6.1).

❑ The parasternal long-axis view allows verification that measurements are perpendicular to the long axis of the LV. An oblique angle may not be recognized in short-axis views.

❑ 2D imaging in long- and short-axis views is used to ensure the dimension is measured in the minor axis of the ventricle, and not at an oblique angle, which would overestimate size (Fig. 6.2).

❑ The rapid sampling rate of M-mode (compared with the slow frame rate of 2D imaging) provides more accurate identification of the endocardial borders (Fig. 6.3).

❑ End-diastole measurements are made at the onset of the QRS complex; end-systole measurements are made at the minimum chamber size, just before aortic valve closure.

❑ Measurements are made from the leading edge of the septal endocardial to the leading edge of the posterior LV wall.

❑ The posterior LV wall is identified on M-mode as the steepest, most continuous line. Identification of the endocardial border on 2D images is less reliable.

❑ Measurements of LV internal dimensions and wall thickness are made at the level of the mitral valve chords just apical to the mitral leaflet tips.

2D and 3D Left Ventricular Chamber Volumes

■ LV volumes are more accurate measures of chamber size than linear dimensions; three-dimensional (3D) measured LV volumes are more accurate than 2D calculations of volume. (Table 6.1)

■ 2D echo measures of LV volumes are based on tracing endocardial borders in apical 4-chamber and 2-chamber views at end-diastole and end-systole, with volumes calculated using the biplane method of disks (Fig. 6.4).

■ 3D LV volumes are calculated using semiautomated endocardial border tracing with a full 3D reconstruction of the LV at end-diastole and end-systole (Fig. 6.5). LV end-diastolic volume and end-systolic volume are indexed by dividing by body surface area (Table 6.2 and 6.3).

❖ KEY POINTS

❑ Care is needed to obtain images from a true apical position; use of a steep left lateral decubitus position with an apical cutout in the stretcher allows optimal transducer positioning.

❑ Depth is adjusted so the mitral annulus just fits on the image; gain and processing curves are adjusted to optimize endocardial definition.

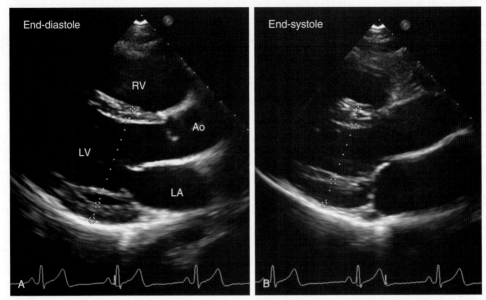

Fig. 6.1 **2D measurement of LV size.** Parasternal long-axis view showing 2D measurement of LV internal dimension at end-diastole (onset of the QRS) from the septal endocardium to the posterior wall endocardium at the level of the mitral valve chords and myocardial thickness at end-diastole and end-systole. This minor axis dimension is measured perpendicular to the long axis of the LV. *Ao,* Aorta.

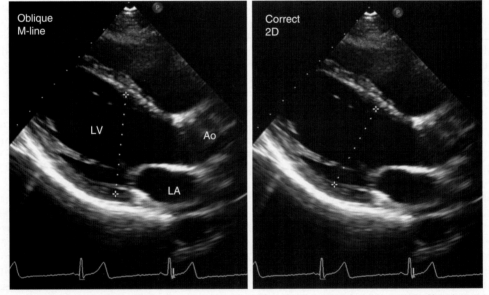

Fig. 6.2 **Oblique LV dimension measurements.** Parasternal long-axis view *(left)* showing that a line oriented to match the M-mode measurement of LV dimensions from this transducer position along the *dotted line,* would overestimate ventricular size, because the sample line is oblique compared to the correct minor axis dimension, shown on the *right. Ao,* Aorta.

❏ Left-sided echo contrast enhances recognition of endocardial borders when image quality is poor.

❏ End-diastolic tracings are made at the onset of the QRS (first frame on digital cine loop); end-systole is defined as minimal LV volume and is identified visually by frame-by-frame viewing of the images (Fig. 6.6).

❏ Volumes are more reflective of the degree of LV dilation than linear dimensions.

❏ The most common limitation of this approach is a foreshortened apical view, resulting in underestimation of ventricular volumes; 3D imaging helps avoid underestimation of LV volumes (Fig. 6.7).

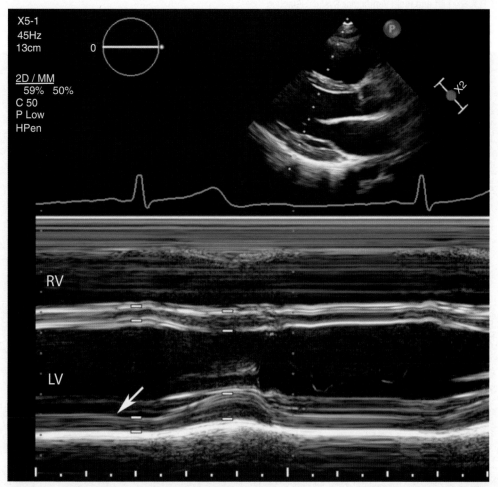

Fig. 6.3 **M-mode LV dimensions.** When the M-mode bean can be aligned perpendicular to the long axis of the LV, based on 2D long- and short-axis views, the advantage of the M-mode recording is a high temporal sampling rate. The rapid motion of the septal and posterior wall endocardium allows precise measurements. The endocardium *(arrow)* typically is the most continuous line with the steepest slope in systole. Measurement of the end-systolic wall thickness and internal dimension (maximal posterior motion of the septum, or minimal LV dimension) is shown by the *horizontal lines*.

	TABLE 6.1	2D and 3D Echocardiographic Measurement of LV Volumes and Ejection Fraction	
	2D	**3D**
Window	Apical • Patient in steep left lateral position • Apical cutout in exam stretcher • Avoid apical foreshortening	Apical • Patient in steep left lateral position • Apical cutout in exam stretcher • Adjust transducer position to ensure inclusion of entire LV
Image acquisition	4-chamber and 2-chamber views • Adjust depth to mitral annulus level. • Adjust gain, time-gain compensation, harmonic imaging, and other instrument parameters to optimize endocardial definition. • Left-sided contrast enhances endocardial border identification when image quality is suboptimal.	Apical volumetric acquisition • Full-volume gated acquisition • Use 2D images for initial positioning and adjusting gain. • Use split screen display of orthogonal views to optimize acquisition. • Breath hold during acquisition to minimize stitch artifacts. • Left-sided contrast enhances endocardial border identification when image quality is suboptimal.
Endocardial borders	Manual tracing at end-diastole and end-systole • End-diastole defined as onset of QRS • End-systole defined as minimal LV volume Trace borders at time of image acquisition and adjust, if needed, on final review.	Semiautomated endocardial border detection • Exclude papillary muscles and trabeculations from LV chamber. • Review and adjust borders after acquisition.
Volume calculations	• Apical biplane formula	• Surface rendered LV volumes

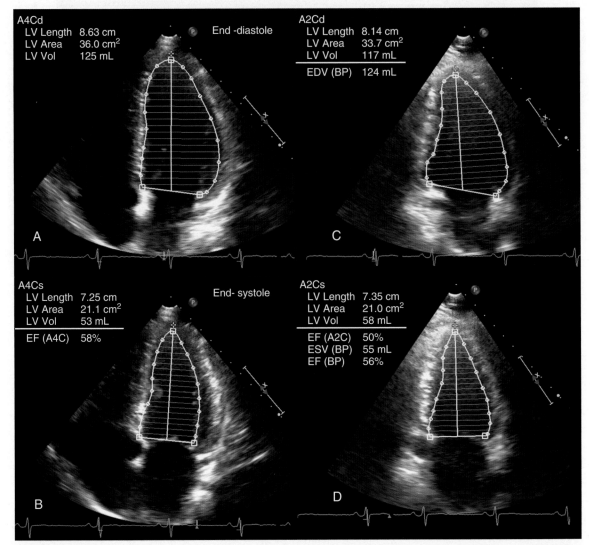

Fig. 6.4 2D LV volumes. LV volumes and ejection fraction (EF) are calculated based on tracing endocardial borders at end-diastole (A and C) and end-systole (B and D) in both apical 4-chamber (A and B) and apical 2-chamber views (C and D). Identification of endocardial borders is optimized by playing the cine loop to show endocardial motion.

- Body surface area may not be the ideal measure but is widely used clinically to index volumes for body size.

Left Ventricular Wall Thickness and Mass

- 2D or 2D-guided M-mode measurement of LV septal and posterior wall thickness at end-diastole are usually are sufficient for clinical care.
- LV mass and wall stress can be calculated from 2D images, if needed.

❖ KEY POINTS

- LV wall thickness is measured from the parasternal window, because the ultrasound beam is perpendicular to the blood-myocardial interface, providing high axial resolution.

- The rapid sampling rate of M-mode (compared with the slow frame rate of 2D imaging) provides more accurate identification of the endocardial borders.
- Wall thickness of both the septum and posterior wall is measured at the level of the mitral valve chordae at end-diastole.
- The septal wall thickness measurement does not include trabeculations on the right ventricular (RV) side of the septum and does not mistake the midseptal stripe for the right-sided endocardium.
- The posterior LV wall thickness is measured from the endocardium to the posterior epicardium.
- LV mass is calculated from endocardial and epicardial border tracing in a short-axis view at the papillary muscle level and measurement of LV length.

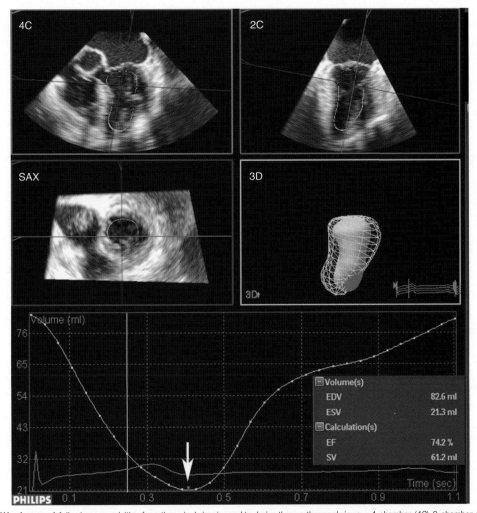

Fig. 6.5 3D LV volumes. A full volume acquisition from the apical view is used to derive three orthogonal views—4-chamber *(4C)*, 2-chamber *(2C)*, and short axis *(SAX)* using the *red, green,* and *blue* image planes as defined by the boxes and lines. After the user selects annular and apical points at end-systole and end-diastole, endocardial borders are detected (which can be edited as needed) to generate a 3D volume reconstruction. A graph of the 3D-derived LV volume over the time frame of one cardiac cycle is shown, with end-systole indicated by the *arrow.*

Step 2: Evaluate Left Ventricular Systolic Performance

2D and 3D Ejection Fraction

- LV ejection fraction is an essential part of the echo examination and should be measured by 2D or 3D methods whenever possible.
- LV ejection fraction is measured from 2D images using the apical biplane method with tracing of endocardial borders at end-diastole and end-systole in apical 4- and 2-chamber views (see Figs. 6.6 and 6.7). However, 3D measurement of LV ejection fraction is recommended when possible.
- If the ejection fraction cannot be measured due to poor endocardial definition, a visual estimate may be reported.

❖ **KEY POINTS**

- LV ejection fraction (EF) is calculated from end-diastolic volume (EDV) and end-systolic volume (ESV) as:

$$EF = [(EDV - ESV)/EDV] \times 100 \qquad (6.1)$$

- When image quality is suboptimal, left-sided contrast may enhance identification of endocardial borders (Fig. 6.8).
- When quantitation of ejection fraction is not needed or is limited by image quality, LV ejection fraction is visually estimated based on parasternal short axis and apical 4-chamber, 2-chamber, and long-axis views.

TABLE 6.2 Reference Values for Echocardiographic Chamber Quantification

Chamber	Measurement	Normal Range (Women)	Normal Range (Men)	Units
Left Ventricle				
	Diastolic diameter	3.8-5.2	4.2-5.8	cm
	Systolic diameter	2.2-3.5	2.5-4.0	cm
	2D diastolic volume	46-106	62-150	mL
	(indexed to BSA)	*29-61*	*34-74*	*mL/m²*
	2D systolic volume	14-42	21-61	mL
	(indexed to BSA)	*8-24*	*11-31*	*mL/m²*
	Ejection fraction	54-74	52-72	%
	Septal wall thickness	0.6-0.9	0.6-1.0	cm
	Posterior wall thickness	0.6-0.9	0.6-1.0	cm
	LV mass (2D method)	66-150	96-200	g
	(indexed to BSA)	*44-88*	*50-102*	*g/m²*
	Relative wall thickness	0.22-0.42	0.24-0.42	
Left Atrium				
	AP diameter	2.7-3.8	3.0-4.0	cm
	(indexed to BSA)	*1.5-2.3*	*1.5-2.3*	*cm/m²*
	LA volume	22-52	18-52	mL
	(indexed to BSA)	*16-34*	*16-34*	*mL/m²*
Right Atrium				
	RA major dimension	1.9-3.1	1.8-3.0	cm
	RA minor dimension	1.3-2.5	1.3-2.5	cm
	2D echo RA volume	9-33	11-39	mL/m²
Right Ventricle		**Normal Range (Women and Men)**		
	RV basal diameter	2.5-4.1		cm
	RV subcostal wall thickness	1.1-0.5		cm
	RVOT proximal diameter	2.1-3.5		cm
	RVOT distal diameter	1.7-2.7		cm
	Fractional area change	35-63		%
	Tricuspid annular excursion (TAPSE)	1.7-3.1		cm

AP, Anterior–posterior; *BSA,* body surface area; *EF,* ejection fraction *RVOT,* RV outflow tract.
Data from Lang RM, Badano LP, Mor-Avi V, et al: Recommendations for cardiac chamber quantification by echocardiography in adults: an update from the American Society of Echocardiography and the European Association of Cardiovascular Imaging, *J Am Soc Echocardiogr* 28(1):1-39.e14, 2015.

TABLE 6.3 Normal Ranges and Severity Partition Cutoff Values for 2D E-Derived LV Ejection Fraction and LA Volume

	Male				Female			
	Normal Range	Mildly Abnormal	Moderately Abnormal	Severely Abnormal	Normal Range	Mildly Abnormal	Moderately Abnormal	Severely Abnormal
LV EF (%)	52-72	41-51	30-40	<30	54-74	41-53	30-40	<30
Maximum LA volume/BSA (mL/m²)	16-34	35-41	42-48	>48	16-34	35-41	42-48	>48

BSA, Body surface area; *EF,* ejection fraction.
From Lang RM, Badano LP, Mor-Avi V, et al: Recommendations for cardiac chamber quantification by echocardiography in adults: an update from the American Society of Echocardiography and the European Association of Cardiovascular Imaging, *J Am Soc Echocardiogr* 28(1):1-39.e14, Table 4, 2015.

- A visual estimate is reported using a descriptive scale as follows:
  - Normal (EF ≥55%)
  - Mildly reduced (EF 45% to 54%)
  - Moderately reduced (EF 30% to 44%)
  - Severely reduced (EF <30%)

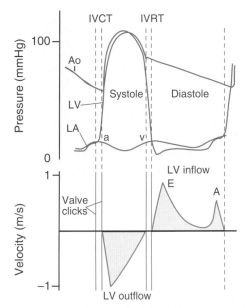

Fig. 6.6 **The cardiac cycle.** LV, aortic *(Ao)*, and LA pressures are shown with the corresponding Doppler LV outflow and inflow velocity curves. The isovolumic contraction time *(IVCT)* represents the time between mitral valve closure and aortic valve opening, while the isovolumic relaxation time *(IVRT)* represents the time between Ao valve closure and mitral valve opening.

Stroke Volume and Cardiac Output

- Stroke volume calculations are increasingly routine, particularly when ventricular function is abnormal and when valve stenosis, valve regurgitation, or an intracardiac shunt is present.
- Stroke volume (SV in cm^3 or mL) is the product of the cross-sectional area (CSA) of flow (in cm^2) multiplied by the velocity-time integral (VTI in cm) of flow at that site (Fig. 6.9):

$$SV = CSA \times VTI \qquad (6.2)$$

- Stroke volume can be calculated at any site where diameter and velocity can be measured but most often is measured in the LV outflow tract (LVOT), just proximal to the aortic valve.
- Cardiac output (CO in L/min) is stroke volume (mL) times heart rate (beats/min), divided by 1000 mL/L:

$$CO = [SV\,(mL) \times heart\,rate\,(beats/m\,in)]\,/1000\,mL/L$$
$$= L/min \qquad (6.3)$$

❖ KEY POINTS

- LVOT diameter (D) is measured from a parasternal long-axis view in mid-systole, from inner edge to inner edge, immediately adjacent to the base of the aortic valve leaflets (Fig. 6.10A).
- CSA is calculated as the area of a circle:

$$CSA = \pi(radius)^2 = 3.14(D/2)^2 \qquad (6.4)$$

- LV outflow velocity is recorded using pulsed Doppler, with a 2- to 3-mm sample volume length, from the apical window with the sample volume just proximal to the aortic valve (see Fig. 6.10B).

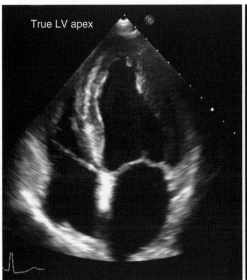
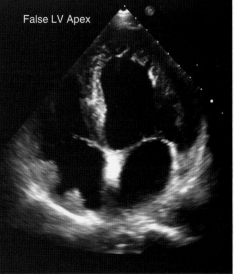

Fig. 6.7 **Apical foreshortening.** When the transducer is on the true apex of the LV, the chamber is ellipsoid *(left)* compared with a foreshortened view *(right)* where the ventricle appears more spherical with a false apex. LV volumes will be underestimated in a foreshortened view, and apical wall motion abnormalities may be missed. This potential error is avoided by moving the transducer down an interspace and laterally to the true apex.

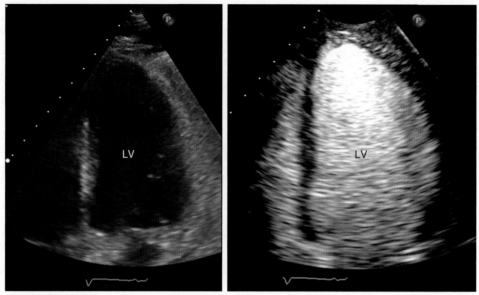

Fig. 6.8 Contrast enhancement. When endocardial borders are poorly seen *(left)*, left-sided contrast *(right)* improves visualization of the LV chamber and allows more accurate measurement of LV volumes.

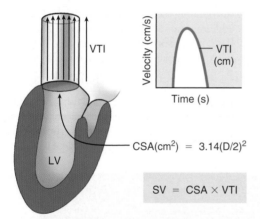

Fig. 6.9 Doppler stroke volume (SV) calculation. The cross-sectional area *(CSA)* of flow is calculated as a circle based on a 2D echo diameter (D) measurement. The length of the cylinder of blood ejected through this CSA on a single beat is the velocity-time integral *(VTI)* of the Doppler curve. Stroke volume *(SV)* then is calculated as CSA × VTI.

$$CSA(cm^2) = 3.14(D/2)^2$$

$$SV = CSA \times VTI$$

- ❑ A visible aortic valve closing click on the Doppler tracing ensures correct sample volume placement.
- ❑ The modal velocity (darkest part of the velocity curve) is traced to obtain the velocity time integral.
- ❑ The velocity time integral represents the "stroke distance" or the length of the cylinder of blood ejected by the LV on each beat.
- ❑ A similar approach can be used to calculate stroke volume across the mitral annulus or the pulmonic valve.
- ❑ In adults, normal stroke volume is about 80 mL, and normal cardiac output is about 6 L/min.
- ❑ Stroke volume and cardiac output are indexed to body surface area. A normal stroke volume index is >35 mL/m².

Global Longitudinal Strain

- ■ Strain is a measure of myocardial shortening that reflects LV systolic performance (Fig. 6.11).
- ■ Speckle tracking strain allows measurement of longitudinal strain in apical 4-chamber, 2-chamber, and long-axis views.
- ■ Global longitudinal strain is measured from all three apical views and displayed as a color-coded chart, a graph of strain over the cardiac cycle and as a single negative number.

❖ KEY POINTS

- ❑ Normal global longitudinal strain is about −20% with smaller negative numbers reflecting impaired ventricular function.
- ❑ Strain is more sensitive than ejection fraction for detection of early myocardial dysfunction.
- ❑ Strain is less dependent on loading conditions compared with ejection fraction.
- ❑ Strain algorithms vary from system to system, so serial studies should use the same equipment and software.

Step 3: Assess Regional Ventricular Function

- ■ Regional (or segmental) ventricular function is evaluated as detailed in Chapter 8.
- ■ Wall motion and thickening for each myocardial segment is graded as normal, hypokinetic, akinetic, or dyskinetic.
- ■ Any areas of thinning and increased echogenicity (consistent with scar) are noted (Fig. 6.12).
- ■ Regional variation in strain also can be used to evaluate segmental wall function.

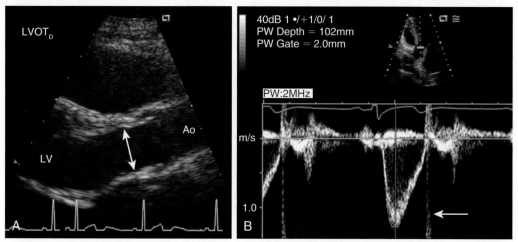

Fig. 6.10 LV outflow tract diameter (LVOT$_D$) and flow. (A) Diameter is measured in a parasternal long-axis view (for axial resolution) in mid-systole using zoom mode. The diameter is measured at the base of the open aortic valve leaflets from the inner edge of the septal endocardium to the inner edge of the anterior mitral leaflet, as shown. (B) The LV outflow velocity curve is recorded from the apical window, so the ultrasound beam is parallel to the direction of flow, with the 2- to 3-mm sample volume on the LV side of the valve. Appropriate positioning is confirmed by the presence of an aortic valve closing click *(arrow)* and no opening click. The Doppler curve should show a narrow band of velocities with a clearly defined peak. The velocity-time integral (VTI) is measured by tracing the modal velocity of the systolic flow signal. *Ao,* Aorta.

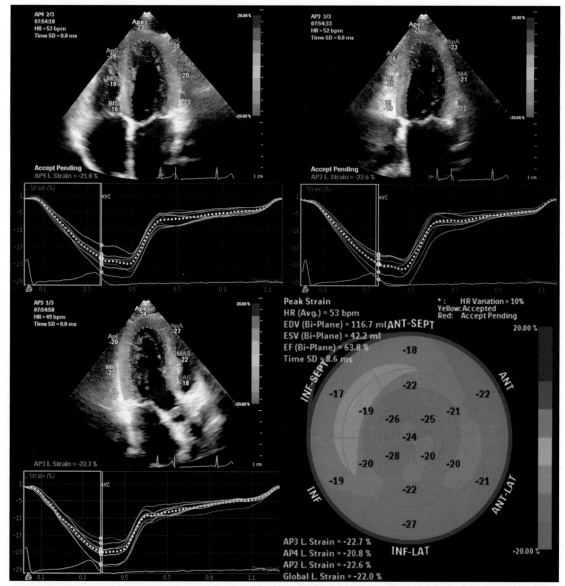

Fig. 6.11 Global longitudinal strain. Longitudinal strain is measured with speckle tracking in apical 4-chamber (AP4, *upper left*), 2-chamber (AP2, *upper right*), and long-axis (AP3, *lower left*) images. Global longitudinal strain (Global L Strain) is shown in the target diagram *(lower right),* measuring −22% in this normal individual. Measurements also include heart rate (HR), end-diastolic volume (EDV), end-systolic volume (ESV), and ejection fraction (EF).

❖ **KEY POINTS**

❑ The presence of wall motion abnormalities in a pattern corresponding to coronary artery perfusion suggests ischemic cardiac disease.

❑ In a short-axis view, the inferior wall may normally flatten along the diaphragm in diastole (with normal systolic motion); this normal pattern should not be mistaken as a wall motion abnormality.

❑ Optimal endocardial definition is needed to evaluate regional function; contrast should be used if needed.

❑ Wall thickening, as well as endocardial motion, should be evaluated for each myocardial segment.

❑ Strain diagrams show regional variation in an easily understood display format.

Step 4: Consider Other Measures of Left Ventricular Systolic Function

Ejection Acceleration Times

■ Normal ventricular function is reflected in a short isovolumic contraction time, rapid acceleration of blood flow in early systole, and a short time from onset to peak flow velocity.

■ A higher ratio of pre-ejection to ejection time indicates ventricular systolic dysfunction.

Left Ventricular *dP/dt*

■ The rate of rise of ventricle pressure, or change in pressure *(dP)* over time *(dt)*, is a load-independent measure of ventricular function.

■ LV *dP/dt* can be calculated from the rise in velocity of the mitral regurgitant-jet (Fig. 6.13).

■ This measurement is useful in selected patients with evidence of ventricular dysfunction or with significant mitral regurgitation.

❖ **KEY POINTS**

❑ The time interval *(dt)* between the points on the mitral regurgitant velocity curve at 1 and 3 m/s is measured in seconds (Fig. 6.14).

❑ The pressure difference *(dP)* between 1 and 3 m/s, calculated using the Bernoulli equation, is:

$$dP = 4(3)^2 - 4(1)^2 = 32 \text{ mm Hg}$$

❑ Thus, *dP/dt* is 32 mm Hg divided by the time interval in seconds.

❑ A normal *dP/dt* is more than 1000 mm Hg/s.

Other Measures

■ Other signs of LV systolic function that are not independently diagnostic may aid in recognition of abnormal function and prompt quantitative evaluation of ventricular function.

■ These findings include increased E-point septal separation, decreased aortic root anterior–posterior motion, and decreased mitral annular apical motion.

❖ **KEY POINTS**

❑ The distance between the most anterior motion of the mitral leaflet and the most posterior motion of the septum normally is only 0 to 5 mm. An increased mitral E-point to septal

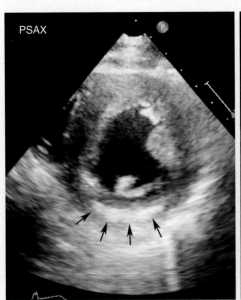
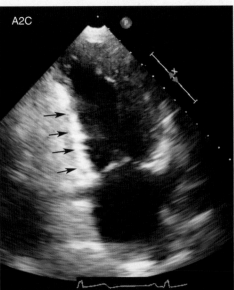

Fig. 6.12 Regional wall motion abnormality. In these parasternal short axis *(left)* and apical 2-chamber *(right)* views, the basal 2/3 of the inferior wall is thin, bright, and akinetic, consistent with a previous inferior myocardial infarction.

separation occurs with LV dilation or systolic dysfunction, aortic regurgitation, or mitral stenosis. This finding is best appreciated on M-mode tracings (Fig. 6.15).

❑ The movement of the aortic root in an anterior-posterior direction on M-mode reflects the filling and emptying of the left atrium (LA), which is confined between the aortic root and spine. A decrease in atrial filling/emptying (e.g., with a low forward stroke volume) results in decreased motion of the aortic root (Fig. 6.16).

❑ Ventricular contraction occurs along the long axis of the ventricle, in addition to circumferential shortening. The mitral annulus moves apically with longitudinal contraction of the LV, with the magnitude of motion reflecting

ventricular function. Reduced apical motion of the annulus (<8 mm) indicates an ejection fraction less than 50% (see Fig. 6.11).

RIGHT VENTRICULAR SYSTOLIC FUNCTION

Step 1: Evaluate Right Ventricular Chamber Size and Wall Thickness

■ RV size and wall thickness are evaluated from multiple views, including parasternal short-axis and RV inflow views, apical 4-chamber view, and subcostal 4-chamber view (Fig. 6.17).

■ RV size is graded qualitatively based on the relative size of the RV and LV:

  ○ Normal (RV < LV, with RV apex more basal than LV apex)

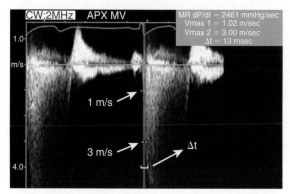

Fig. 6.13 **Mitral regurgitation (MR) for measurement of LV *dP/dt*.** The rate of rise of LV pressure in early systole is calculated by measuring the time integral between 1 and 3 m/s on the mitral regurgitant Doppler velocity curve. This time (t) in seconds is divided by the pressure difference corresponding to a change in velocity from 1 to 3 m/s (32 mm Hg). In this example, the *dP/dt* is 32 mm Hg divided by 0.013 s (13 ms), which equals 2461 mm Hg/s.

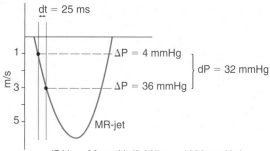

Fig. 6.14 **Schematic diagram showing measurement of *dP/dt* from the mitral regurgitation velocity curve.** The points where the velocity reaches 1 m/s and 3 m/s are identified and the time interval *(dt)* between these two points is measured as shown. The pressure difference *(dP)* between 1 m/s (4 mm Hg) and 3 m/s (36 mm Hg) is 32 mm Hg, so *dP/dt* is calculated as shown. *MR*, Mitral regurgitation.

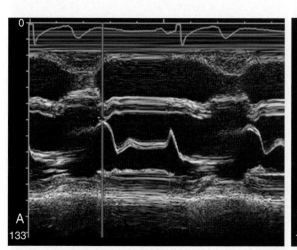

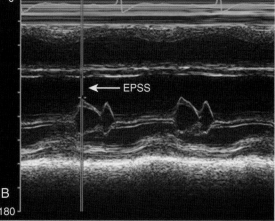

Fig. 6.15 **E-point septal separation *(EPSS).*** The vertical distance between the maximum anterior motion of the mitral leaflet *(E-point)* and the maximum posterior motion of the septum reflects LV size and systolic function. The normal EPSS is less than 5 mm. A larger separation indicates LV dilation or systolic dysfunction. The EPSS also is increased with aortic regurgitation due to impingement of the regurgitant jet on the anterior mitral leaflet and with mitral stenosis, due to restricted motion of the mitral leaflet. Examples of a normal **(A)** and increased **(B)** E-point separation (due to a low LV ejection fraction [EF]) are shown.

- ○ Mildly enlarged (enlarged but RV < LV)
- ○ Moderately enlarged (RV = LV)
- ○ Severely enlarged (RV > LV)
- ■ Quantitative end-diastolic measurements of RV size include (Fig. 6.18):
  - ○ Basal dimension measures at the annulus in the apical 4-chamber view (see Table 6.2)
  - ○ Outflow tract distal diameter measured in the parasternal short-axis view
  - ○ Outflow track proximal diameter measured in the parasternal long-axis view

- ■ RV wall thickness is evaluated qualitatively, or free wall thickness can be measured on the subcostal view.

❖ **KEY POINTS**

- ❏ The best views for evaluation of RV size are an apical 4-chamber view tilted toward the RV and a subcostal 4-chamber view.
- ❏ RV size may be overestimated if the apical view is foreshortened, if the transducer is medial to the LV apex, or if the free wall of the RV is not well visualized.

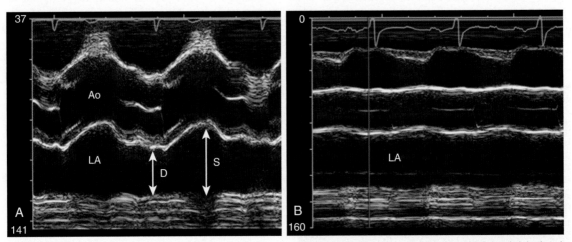

Fig. 6.16 Aortic (Ao) root motion. LA filling in systole results in anterior motion of the Ao root, because LA expansion is constrained posteriorly by the spine. An example of normal Ao root motion on M-mode in a patient with normal LA filling and emptying and a normal cardiac output (CO) **(A)** is compared with the reduced Ao root motion seen in a patient with severe LV dysfunction **(B)** and reduced LA filling and emptying. Conversely, Ao root motion may be increased when significant mitral regurgitation is present. *D,* Diastole; *S,* systole.

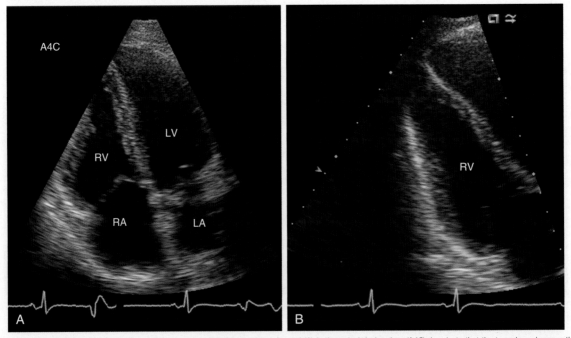

Fig. 6.17 Imaging the RV. Evaluation of RV size and systolic function is performed **(A)** in the apical 4-chamber *(A4C)* view (note that the transducer is correctly located over the LV apex) and **(B)** in a zoom view with the transducer tilted toward the RV.

❏ The subcostal view provides the most reliable estimate of RV size, because the ultrasound beam is perpendicular to the RV free wall and ventricular septum.

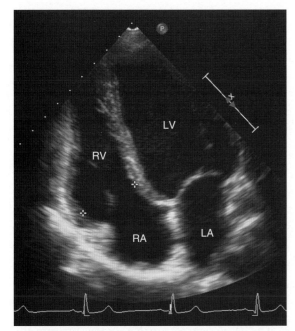

Fig. 6.18 RV dimension measurements. In an apical 4-chamber view, RV diameter is measured at end-diastole from the septum to the free wall at the base of the chamber, as shown by the markers.

❏ RV hypertrophy is seen when the RV free wall is more than 5 mm or when the RV wall appears as thick as the LV wall (Fig. 6.19).

Step 2: Examine the Pattern of Ventricular Septal Motion

■ Ventricular septal motion is evaluated in 2D parasternal long- and short-axis images.

■ M-mode evaluation of ventricular septal motion may be helpful in some cases.

❖ **KEY POINTS**

❏ With RV volume overload, the ventricular septum is flattened in diastole, but in systole the LV assumes the normal circular configuration (Fig. 6.20).

❏ With RV pressure overload, the ventricular septum remains flattened or reversed in systole so that the LV assumes a D shape in the short-axis view (Fig. 6.21).

❏ The pattern of ventricular septum motion is also altered by conduction abnormalities, previous cardiac surgery, and pericardial disease.

Step 3: Measure Right Ventricular Systolic Contraction

■ RV systolic function is assessed from multiple views, including parasternal short-axis and RV inflow views, the apical 4-chamber view, and the subcostal 4-chamber view.

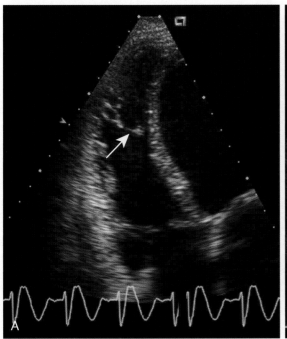

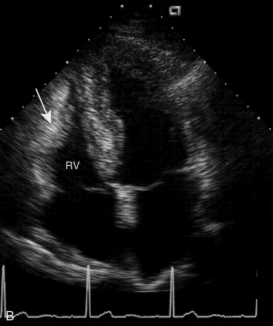

Fig. 6.19 RV wall thickness. The RV free wall normally is thinner than the LV wall, although prominent trabeculations and the moderator band *(arrow)* may be appreciated, as seen in a patient with mild RV dilation **(A)**. An increased thickness of the RV free wall **(B)** is seen in a patient with pulmonary hypertension.

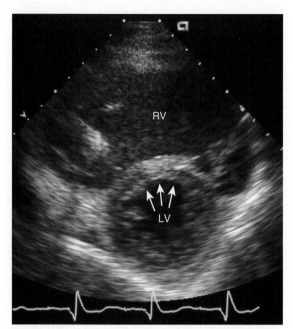

Fig. 6.20 **RV volume overload.** With RV volume overload, the RV is enlarged and septal motion is flat in diastole. However, in systole (shown here), the contour of the septum is normal, with a circular shape of the LV in short axis.

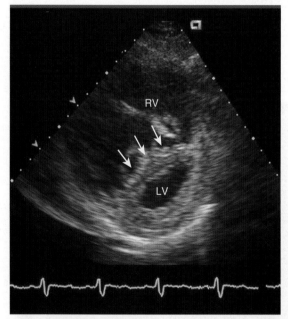

Fig. 6.21 **RV pressure overload.** In contrast to volume overload, RV pressure overload results in septal flattening in both diastole and in systole, as seen on this end-systolic image.

- RV systolic function is graded qualitatively as normal, mildly, moderately, or severely reduced.
- The tricuspid annular plane systolic excursion (TAPSE) toward the apex from end-diastole to end-systole provides a useful measure of longitudinal RV contraction.

- Other measures of RV systolic function include the fractional area change, the tissue Doppler peak systolic velocity at the annulus, and the pulsed or tissue Doppler myocardial performance index.

❖ **KEY POINTS**

- ❏ The best views for evaluation of RV systolic function are an apical 4-chamber view tilted toward the RV and a subcostal 4-chamber view.
- ❏ RV systolic function can be graded in comparison to LV systolic function.
- ❏ If LV systolic function is reduced and the RV looks similar to the LV, the degree of dysfunction is similar.
- ❏ TAPSE is calculated using an M-mode beam from the apex aligned through the tricuspid annulus (normal ≥1.7 cm) (Fig. 6.22).
- ❏ The tricuspid annular tissue Doppler systolic velocity is also recorded from the apical window (Fig. 6.23).

Step 4: Estimate Pulmonary Systolic Pressure

- Noninvasive calculation of pulmonary systolic pressures is possible in more than 80% of transthoracic echocardiograms.
- The RV to right atrium (RA) systolic pressure gradient is calculated from the maximum velocity in the tricuspid regurgitant (TR) jet using the Bernoulli equation (Fig. 6.24).

$$\Delta P_{RV-RA} = 4(V_{TRpeak})^2 \qquad (6.5)$$

- Right atrial pressure, estimated from the size and respiratory variation in the inferior vena cava (IVC), is added to this pressure gradient to determine RV systolic pressure (Table 6.4).

❖ **KEY POINTS**

- ❏ In the absence of pulmonic valve stenosis, RV and pulmonary systolic pressures are the same (Table 6.5).
- ❏ When pulmonic stenosis is present, pulmonary systolic pressure is calculated by subtracting the RV-to-pulmonary artery gradient from the estimated RV systolic pressure.
- ❏ A diligent search for the highest tricuspid regurgitant jet velocity includes continuous-wave (CW) Doppler recording from parasternal and apical views. The highest signal obtained is the most parallel to jet direction.
- ❏ Signal strength may be enhanced by repositioning the patient or having the patient hold their breath at end expiration or in mid-inspiration.
- ❏ The Doppler scale, gain, and wall filters are adjusted to show a gray-scale spectrum with a dense outer edge and smooth systolic curve (Fig. 6.25).

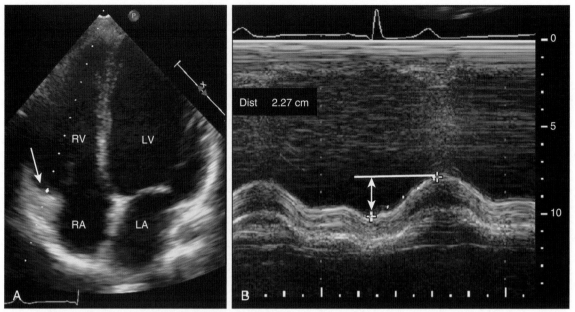

Fig. 6.22 Tricuspid annular plane systolic excursion (TAPSE). (A) In an apical 4-chamber view with the transducer moved over the RV apex, an M-line is positioned through the lateral tricuspid annulus. (B) The vertical distance between the position of the annulus at end-diastole and end-systole (e.g., the motion of the annulus toward the apex in systole) is measured from the M-mode tracing.

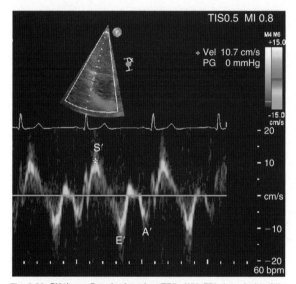

Fig. 6.23 RV tissue Doppler imaging (TDI). With TDI, the velocity of the tricuspid annulus is recorded showing the expected systolic (S′) and diastolic (E′ and A′) tissue velocities, similar to the LV TDI recordings. The peak S′ velocity reflects RV longitudinal shortening.

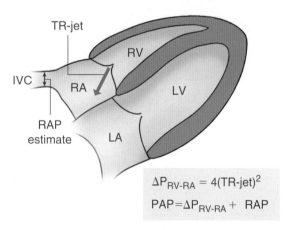

$$\Delta P_{RV\text{-}RA} = 4(TR\text{-jet})^2$$

$$PAP = \Delta P_{RV\text{-}RA} + RAP$$

Fig. 6.24 Estimation of pulmonary artery pressure. The velocity in the tricuspid regurgitant (TR) jet is used to calculate the RV to RA systolic pressure difference, which then is added to an estimate of right atrial pressure *(RAP),* based on the size and respiratory variation in inferior vena cava *(IVC)* diameter. *PAP,* Pulmonary artery pressure.

Step 5: Consider the Cause of an Elevated Pulmonary Systolic Pressure

- Pulmonary hypertension may be due to left-sided heart disease, resulting in an elevated LA pressure and consequent increase in pulmonary pressure.
- Pulmonary hypertension also may be due to a pulmonary arterial disease, lung disease, or pulmonary embolism, or may be due to multiple factors with a systemic disease.

❑ Estimation of RA pressure from the respiratory variation in the inferior vena cava is only useful in spontaneously breathing patients. In ventilated patients, a measured central venous pressure is used or an estimated range of pulmonary pressures is provided (Fig. 6.26).

TABLE 6.4   Estimation of Right Atrial Pressure

| Inferior Vena Cava Diameter* | Change with Sniff | RA Pressure Estimate | |
		Range Estimate‡	ASE Guidelines§
Normal (≤2.1 cm)	Decrease >50%	0-5 mm Hg	3 mm Hg
Normal (≤2.1 cm)	Decrease ≤50%	5-10 mm Hg	8 mm Hg†
Dilated (>2.1 cm)	Decrease >50%	10-15 mm Hg	
Dilated (>2.1 cm)	Decrease ≤50%	15-20 mm Hg	15 mm Hg

*Inferior vena cava (IVC) diameter is measured just proximal to entrance of hepatic veins in a subcostal view. Changes in IVC diameter during the respiratory cycle are not reliable indicators of RA pressure in patients on mechanical ventilation.

†For intermediate values, the RA pressure estimate should be lowered or increased depending on the absence or presence of other signs of elevated RA pressures, including restrictive right-sided diastolic filling pattern, tricuspid E/E' >6, diastolic flow predominance in the hepatic veins (systolic filling fraction <55%), and dilated RA with bulging of the septum toward the LA.

‡Integrated from multiple sources including: Brennan JM, Blair JE, Goonewardena S, et al: Reappraisal of the use of inferior vena cava for estimating right atrial pressure, *J Am Soc Echocardiogr* 20:857-861, 2007; Kircher BH, Himelmann RB, Schiller NG: Noninvasive estimation of right atrial pressure from the inspiratory collapse of the inferior vena cava, *Am J Cardiol* 66:493, 1990; Lang RM, Bierig M, Devereux RB, et al: Recommendations for chamber quantification: a report from the American Society of Echocardiography's Guidelines and Standards Committee and the Chamber Quantification Writing Group, developed in conjunction with the European Association of Echocardiography, a branch of the European Society of Cardiology, *J Am Soc Echocardiogr* 18:1440, 2005.

§Rudksi LG, Lai, WW, Afilalo J, et al: Guidelines for the echocardiographic assessment of the right heart in adults: a report from the American Society of Echocardiography endorsed by the European Association of Echocardiography, a registered branch of the European Society of Cardiology, and the Canadian Society of Echocardiography, *J Am Soc Echocardiogr* 23:685-713, 2010.

TABLE 6.5   Doppler Echo Methods for Estimation of Right Heart Pressures

	Method	Advantages	Potential Limitations
Systolic PA pressure	TR jet: $PAP_{systolic} = 4(V_{TR})^2 + RAP$	• Accurate • Measurable in a high percentage of patients overall (90%)	• Underestimation because of nonparallel intercept angle or inadequate signal strength • Overestimation because of measurement outside well-defined spectral envelope or misidentification of jet signal • Presence of pulmonic stenosis where RV pressure is greater than PA pressure • RA pressure estimate needed
Diastolic PA pressure	PR end-diastolic velocity: $PAP_{diastolic} = 4(V_{PR})^2 + RAP$	• Reflects pulmonary diastolic pressure • Adequate signal in 85% of patients	• Nonparallel intercept angle between jet and ultrasound beam • RA pressure estimate needed
Mean PA pressure	TR jet tracing for mean RV to RA pressure gradient plus RA pressure estimate	• Mean PA pressure is more accurate for identification of pulmonary hypertension	• Nonparallel intercept angle between jet and ultrasound beam • Inadequate signal in some patients
	Pulmonary artery acceleration time	• Readily measured in nearly all patients, including patients with chronic lung disease • Estimates *mean* PA pressure	• Skewed flow profile in pulmonary artery • Measurement variability
RA pressure	IVC diameter and change with respiration or sniff	• Obtainable from subcostal window in most patients • Reliably identifies normal versus severely elevated RA pressure	• IVC collapse not accurate for RA pressure estimates in patients on mechanical ventilation • Less reliable for intermediate values of RA pressure

IVC, Inferior vena cava; *PA*, pulmonary artery; *PAP*, pulmonary artery pressure; *TR*, tricuspid regurgitation.

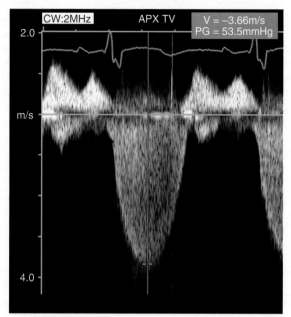

Fig. 6.25 **Tricuspid regurgitant (TR) jet recorded with CW Doppler.** The velocity curve shows a smooth contour with a dark edge and a well-defined peak velocity. Although these characteristics are consistent with a high signal-to-noise ratio, they do not exclude the possibility of underestimation of velocity due to a nonparallel intercept angle between the flow direction and Doppler beam.

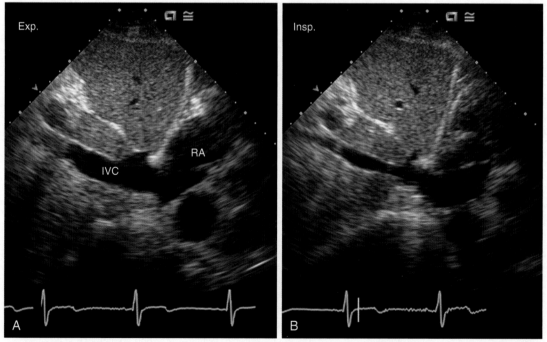

Fig. 6.26 **Estimation of RA pressure.** Zoom views of the inferior vena cava *(IVC)* from the subcostal window are used to visualize the size of the IVC at the caval-RA junction during expiration (1.8 cm in this case) and the change in size during inspiration or with a sniff (>50% in this case), indicating a RA pressure of 0 to 5 mm Hg (see Table 6.4).

❖ KEY POINTS

- ❏ The definition of pulmonary arterial hypertension is a mean pulmonary artery pressure of more than 25 mm Hg at rest with a pulmonary capillary wedge pressure of less than 15 mm Hg.
- ❏ In patients with left-sided heart disease, typically both LA and pulmonary pressures are elevated.
- ❏ If pulmonary systolic pressure is elevated and there is no obvious left-sided heart disease, careful evaluation of LV diastolic function is appropriate.
- ❏ An elevation in pulmonary pressure greater than expected for the degree of left heart disease suggests primary pulmonary vascular disease or lung disease.

Ventricular Systolic Function

	TTE	TEE
LV size and wall thickness	• Linear LV internal dimensions and wall thickness • LV volumes calculated from apical biplane method • 3D volumes when possible	• Linear dimensions can be measured on transgastric short-axis views. • LV volumes can be calculated by the 2D biplane method or by 3D volumes.
LV ejection fraction	• 3D EF when possible • 2D biplane method using 4-chamber and 2-chamber views, taking care to image from tip of LV apex	• 3D volumes and EF recommended on all TEE studies.
LV regional wall motion	• Apical 4-chamber, 2-chamber, and long-axis views plus parasternal long- and short-axis views	• TEE 4-chamber, 2-chamber, and long-axis views plus TG short-axis view. • Apical wall motion may be difficult to assess.
Doppler cardiac output	• LVOT and transmitral flows from apical approach • PA flow from parasternal views	• Transmitral flow in 4-chamber view • PA flow from high TEE view • LVOT flow sometimes obtained from TG long-axis view, but intercept angle may be nonparallel
Speckle tracking strain imaging	• Global longitudinal strain measured from apical views	• Global longitudinal strain measurements supplement 2D and 3D imaging
LV dP/dt	• CW Doppler mitral regurgitant jet	• CW Doppler mitral regurgitant jet
RV size and systolic function	• Apical and subcostal 4-chamber views plus parasternal long- and short-axis views • TAPSE	• TEE 4-chamber view plus transgastric short-axis and RV-inflow views
PA pressure estimates	• TR jet recorded from parasternal and apical views with dedicated CW Doppler transducer	• TR jet may be recorded on TEE 4-chamber or short-axis views, but underestimation is possible due to a nonparallel intercept angle.

CO, Cardiac output; *EF,* ejection fraction; *LVOT,* left ventricular outflow tract; *PA,* pulmonary artery; *TAPSE,* tricuspid annular plane systolic excursion; *TG,* transgastric; *TR,* tricuspid regurgitation.

Technical Details in Evaluation of Ventricular Systolic Function

Parameter	Modality	View	Recording	Measurements
Ejection fraction	3D or 2D	Apical 4-chamber and 2-chamber	Adjust depth, optimize endocardial definition, harmonic imaging, contrast if needed	Careful tracing of endocardial borders at end-diastole and end-systole in both views
Global longitudinal strain	Speckle-tracking strain	Apical 4-chamber, 2-chamber, and long-axis views	Adjust depth, optimize myocardial tracking, record each view and composite data	Global longitudinal strain measurement if myocardial tracking is accurate, regional ventricular function and synchrony
dP/dt	CW Doppler	MR jet, usually from apex	Patient positioning and transducer angulation to obtain highest velocity MR jet, decrease velocity scale, increase sweep speed	Time interval between 1 m/s and 3 m/s on Doppler MR velocity curve
PA pressures	CW Doppler	Parasternal and apical	Patient positioning and transducer angulation to obtain highest-velocity TR jet	Estimate of RA pressure from size and appearance of IVC
Cardiac output	2D and pulsed Doppler	Parasternal LVOT diameter	Ultrasound beam perpendicular to LVOT with depth decreased and gain adjusted to see mid-systolic diameter	LVOT diameter from inner edge to inner edge in mid-systole, adjacent and parallel to aortic valve
		Apical LVOT VTI	LVOT velocity from anterior angulated apical 4-chamber view with sample volume just on LV side of aortic valve	Trace modal velocity of LVOT spectral Doppler envelope

CO, Cardiac output; *EF,* ejection fraction; *IVC,* inferior vena cava; *LVOT,* left ventricular outflow tract; *MR,* mitral regurgitation; *PA,* pulmonary artery; *TR,* tricuspid regurgitation; *VTI,* velocity time integral.

SELF-ASSESSMENT QUESTIONS

Question 1

Calculate LV stroke volume, cardiac output, fractional shortening, and ejection fraction in the following patient:

Heart rate	64 bpm
LV end-diastolic dimension	5.3 cm
LV end-systolic dimension	3.8 cm
3D LV end-systolic volume	50 mL
3D LV end-diastolic volume	122 mL
LV outlfow tract diameter	2.4 cm
LV outlfow tract velocity time integral	15 cm

Question 2

A transthoracic study is obtained in a patient with a history of non-Hodgkin lymphoma who presents with decreased exercise tolerance (Fig. 6.27). The image is most consistent with:

  A. Pericardial effusion
  B. Dilated cardiomyopathy
  C. Pericardial constriction
  D. Restrictive cardiomyopathy

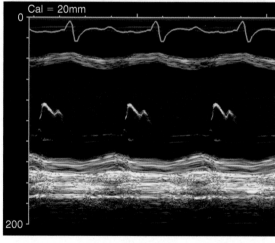

Fig. 6.27

Question 3

In a patient with this tissue Doppler imaging of the tricuspid annulus (Fig. 6.28), which of the following additional findings is most likely?

  A. Tricuspid annular plane systolic excursion measuring 13 mm
  B. Pulsed Doppler myocardial (Tei) performance index measuring 0.35
  C. Fractional area change measuring 50%
  D. RV ejection fraction measuring 48%

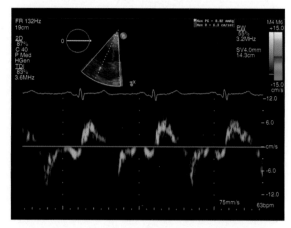

Fig. 6.28

Question 4

A 27-year-old female with shortness of breath underwent echocardiography. Which of the following diagnoses is most consistent with the short-axis views in diastole (Fig. 6.29) and systole?

  A. Left bundle branch block
  B. Mitral stenosis
  C. Primary pulmonary hypertension
  D. Secundum atrial septal defect
  E. Ventricular septal defect

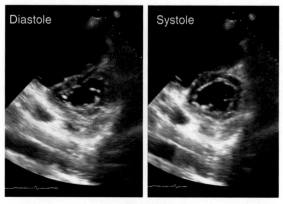

Fig. 6.29

Question 5

A 56-year-old male patient presents with progressive dyspnea. Echocardiography is ordered, and the apical biplane LV tracings provide an LV end-systolic volume of 100 mL and an LV end-diastolic volume of 222 mL. 3D imaging was obtained (Fig. 6.30).

Compared with the 2D method, this 3D assessment of LV size and function shows:

A. A higher ejection fraction
B. The effect of geometric assumptions
C. A smaller stroke volume
D. Less foreshortened image planes
E. Improved endocardial border definition

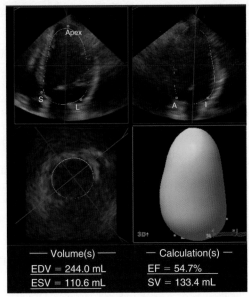

— Volume(s) —	— Calculation(s) —
EDV = 244.0 mL	EF = 54.7%
ESV = 110.6 mL	SV = 133.4 mL

Fig. 6.30

Question 6

An image from a transthoracic echocardiographic study is shown (Fig. 6.31). Based on the image provided, you conclude:

A. RV systolic pressure is 50 mm Hg
B. Pulmonary arterial diastolic pressure is 50 mm Hg
C. RV diastolic pressure is 31 mm Hg
D. Pulmonary arterial systolic pressure is 31 mm Hg

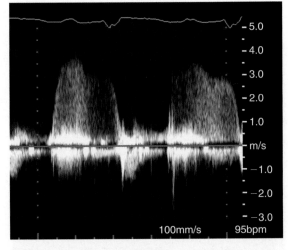

Fig. 6.31

Question 7

A 45-year-old male with carcinoid syndrome underwent transthoracic echocardiography (Fig. 6.32). Imaging includes (A) an apical view of the RV, (B) color Doppler in systole of tricuspid regurgitation, (C) CW Doppler recording of tricuspid regurgitation, and (D) subcostal inferior vena cava (IVC) measurements during deep inspiration. Based on the obtained Doppler and 2D data you conclude:

A. LV size and systolic function are normal.
B. Pulmonary pressures are severely elevated.
C. Tricuspid regurgitation is mild in severity.
D. Right atrial pressure (RAP) is normal.
E. RV dilation is present.

Question 8

A 30-year-old man with dilated cardiomyopathy presents with decompensated heart failure and volume overload. He is referred for echocardiography. Which of the following echocardiographic findings is most likely present?

A. Mitral *dP/dt* 600 mm Hg/s
B. Tricuspid regurgitant peak velocity 2.1 m/s
C. Global longitudinal strain of −22%
D. LV end-diastolic indexed volume 70 mL/m²

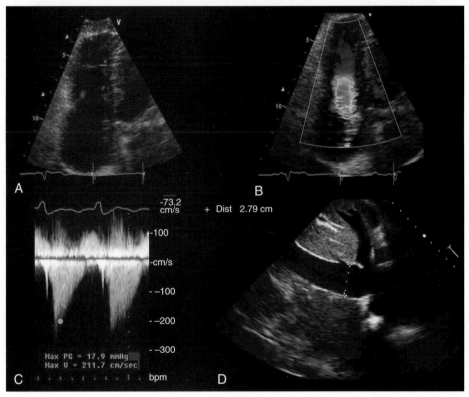

Fig. 6.32

Question 9

Based on the longitudinal strain from the bulls-eye plot (Fig. 6.33), which of the following statements are most likely?

A. The patient has a dilated cardiomyopathy with reduced global systolic function.

B. The patient had a myocardial infraction involving the posterior descending coronary.

C. The patient has a left bundle branch block.

D. The patient has normal myocardial function.

Question 10

Which of the following factors is most likely to result in overestimation of global LV systolic in this patient (see Fig. 6.33)?

A. Apical foreshortening on 3D imaging

B. Geometric assumptions in calculation of 2D biplane ejection fraction

C. Suboptimal alignment of the transducer beam for speckle tracking strain imaging

D. M-mode measurement of endocardial fractional shortening

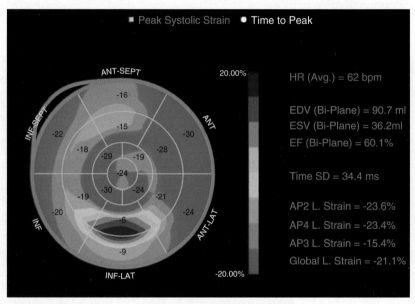

Fig. 6.33

Question 11

Which of the following *least* affects septal myocardial motion?

A. Restrictive cardiomyopathy

B. Pericardial constriction

C. Coronary artery bypass graft surgery

D. Paced ventricular rhythm

E. Primary pulmonary hypertension

ANSWERS

Answer 1:

The stroke volume (SV) is the volume of blood ejected from the LV during systole. SV is calculated as the product of the velocity time integral and cross-sectional area (CSA) at the point of interrogation and at the same point in the cardiac cycle. In this case, SV across the left ventricular outflow tract (LVOT) in systole can be calculated as:

$$CSA_{LVOT} \times VTI_{LVOT}$$

A circular orifice is assumed for the LVOT. Therefore, for this patient, this calculation is:

$$\pi \, (radius_{LVOT})^2 \times VTI_{LVOT} \text{ or}$$
$$\pi \, (2.4/2)^2 \times 15 = 68 \text{ mL}$$

Using the 3D volumes, SV also can be calculated as:

$$LVEDV - LVESV \text{ or}$$
$$122 \text{ mL} - 50 \text{ mL} = 72 \text{ mL}$$

Cardiac output (CO) is the product of SV and heart rate. In this patient,

$$CO = SV \times \text{heart rate} =$$
$$68 \text{ mL} \times 64 \text{ bpm}/(1000 \text{ mL/L}) = 4.4 \text{ L/min}$$

The fractional shortening is measured from the parasternal long-axis LV end-diastolic dimension (EDD) and end-systolic dimension (ESD) dimensions as

$$(EDD - ESD)/EDD =$$
$$(5.3 - 3.8)/5.3 = 0.28 \text{ or } 28\%$$

which is in the normal range. The ejection fraction (EF) is more commonly reported than the fractional shortening and is the relative change in LV end-diastolic volume (EDV) and end-systolic volume (ESV). This is measured as

$$(EDV - ESV)/EDV =$$
$$(122 - 50)/122 \times 100\% = 59\%$$

Answer 2: B

This is an M-mode tracing from the parasternal long-axis view of the heart. LV chamber size is severely dilated with the marks on the vertical axis, each representing 2 cm. The tracing is taken at the mitral valve leaflet tips (seen along the midportion of the image). The end-diastolic dimension is ≈9 cm and the end systolic dimension is ≈7 cm. There is a large separation between the anterior mitral valve leaflet and the anteroseptum (increased E-point septal separation) consistent with severe LV enlargement. A pericardial effusion is not seen. Septal and posterior wall motion is synchronous throughout the cardiac cycle, not consistent with either myocardial restriction or pericardial constriction.

Answer 3: A

Fig. 6.28 demonstrates a reduced apical motion velocity during systole (S′) of only 6 cm/s; a normal S′ would be at least 10 cm/s. Impaired RV systolic function based on S′ would most likely correlate with a reduced tricuspid annular plane systolic excursion (TAPSE) of 13 mm (normal ≥17 mm). The other measures of RV function (answers B through D) are normal values and would be less likely to be associated with impaired RV systolic function. The myocardial performance index is a global measure of RV performance based on the ratio of non-ejection to ejection work of the heart using either pulsed wave spectral Doppler (normal values ≤0.4) or tissue Doppler imaging (normal ≤0.55). A fractional area change is based on the systolic and diastolic area change from a focused apical 4-chamber view and would account for abnormalities in RV free wall motion (normal ≥40%). The non-uniform shape of the RV requires 3D evaluation with either 3D echocardiography or more often cardiac magnetic resonance imaging. The low end for a normal RV ejection fraction (EF) is lower than the LV at approximately 45%.

Answer 4: D

Parasternal short axis views at the level of the mitral valve are consistent with abnormal septal motion from RV volume overload. During diastolic filling (see Fig. 6.29), there is a flattened D-shape septum due to the RV enlargement. The abnormal curvature normalizes in systole (see Fig. 6.29) consistent with a ventricular volume overload condition (such as atrial septal defect). Abnormal septal motion from a left bundle branch block is characterized as dyssynchronous brisk septal motion during early systole. Paradoxical early diastolic motion can be seen with mitral stenosis, but the mitral valve is widely open without any commissural fusion during diastole. RV pressure overload conditions (such as primary pulmonary hypertension and ventricular septal defects) have characteristic paradoxical septal motion in both diastole and systole.

Answer 5: D

Apical biplane calculation of LV ejection fraction (EF) utilizes geometric assumptions for ventricular chamber shape. Tracings are taken at end-diastole and end-systole in the apical 4-chamber and 2-chamber views. 3D imaging does not utilize geometric assumptions, but rather includes the entire LV in the pyramidal dataset. The asymmetric, "true" endocardial border is generally larger than the estimated LV chamber size obtained by standard 2D imaging. Because the entire LV is imaged in 3D, image planes can be adjusted to ensure that the LV apex is included, and images are not foreshortened (as can happen with 2D imaging). Foreshortening of the LV excludes the apex from volume measurements, decreases measured LV volumes, and often erroneously raises EF calculations. However, the imaging frame rate in acquiring a pyramidal data set is lower, and endocardial border definition is not as optimal for 3D imaging relative to standard 2D imaging relative to imaging. In this example, the end-diastolic volume (EDV) and end-systolic volume (ESV) were both higher than the volumes derived from the apical biplane method. However, the relative increase in LV volumes is proportional, such that the calculated EF is the same. For the 2D derived volumes, EF was (222 mL − 100 mL)/222 mL, or 55%, the same as was calculated using the 3D volumes. The stroke volume (SV) for the 3D images was 244 mL − 110 mL = 114 mL, and for the 2D volumes 122 mL. The incremental difference in stroke volume is relatively comparable.

Answer 6: C

This is a CW Doppler tracing in the RV outflow tract, recording pulmonary regurgitant flow. Assuming there is no obstruction of flow across the pulmonic valve, the regurgitant velocity reflects the pulmonary artery to RV diastolic pressure gradient. RV diastolic pressure can be estimated from the end-diastolic velocity utilizing the Bernoulli equation. In this case, the end-diastolic velocity is 2.8 m/s, which correlates with a RV end diastolic pressure of 31 mm Hg. Pulmonary arterial diastolic pressure could then be estimated by adding the central venous pressure estimate. This is obtained by evaluating inferior vena cava (IVC) diameter from the subcostal view and determining whether there is inspiratory collapse. Analogous to this is estimation of RV systolic pressure utilizing the peak tricuspid regurgitant (TR) jet velocity.

Answer 7: E

Fig. 6.32 shows at least moderate RV dilation based on the diameter of the RV at the annulus and an RV apex extending to LV apex. The LV is not visualized so that no conclusions about LV size or systolic function can be made from these images. RA pressure is severely elevated, because there is plethora of the inferior vena cava with distension at 2.8 cm during inspiration, indicating RA pressure is at least 15 mm Hg. Color Doppler shows a very wide vena contracta of the tricuspid regurgitant (TR) jet, consistent with severe (or "wide open") tricuspid regurgitation, which is confirmed by the equal density of forward and reverse flow across the tricuspid valve on the CW Doppler tracing. The triangular-shaped CW Doppler systolic signal is consistent with a high RA pressure, and the low velocity is consistent with a low pressure difference between the RV and RA in systole. Although there is some concern that ignoring effects of acceleration might result in underestimation

of the RV to RA pressure difference by the simplified Bernoulli equation, in clinical practice this effect is small, so it is unlikely that this patient has severe pulmonary hypertension. Direct pressure measurement by catheterization is appropriate when there is concern that pressures may be underestimated by echocardiography.

Answer 8: A

In patients with LV systolic dysfunction, decreased LV contractility results in a reduced rate of pressure rise in early systole, as reflected in the rate of rise in the velocity in the mitral regurgitant jet. A normal rate of rise in pressure (dP/dt) derived from the mitral regurgitant jet is >1000 mm Hg/s. In this patient, a reduced dP/dt is expected. A peak tricuspid regurgitant (TR) jet velocity of 2.1 m/s, utilizing the Bernoulli equation provides a RV systolic pressure of 17 mm Hg (RVSP = 4 $[V_{TR\text{-}jet}]^2$), which is not consistent with decompensated heart failure. With a dilated cardiomyopathy, a reduced LV global longitudinal strain and reduced ejection fraction are expected. An LV global longitudinal strain of −22% is normal. An LV end-diastolic indexed volume of 70 mL/m^2 is normal. LV volumes are indexed to body surface area. For both women and men, a value of ≈75 mL/m^2 is consistent with only mild LV dilation, and a volume over 100 mL/m^2 is consistent with severe LV dilation.

Answer 9: B

Fig. 6.33 provides assessment of global and regional LV systolic function using a 17-segment model. There is reduced regional segmental longitudinal strain in the inferolateral wall consistent with a previous posterior myocardial infarction. The average global longitudinal strain (normal ≥20%) and ejection fraction (EF) are normal; a dilated cardiomyopathy would more likely have reduced measured of global systolic function (answer A) and less likely isolated regional abnormality. Abnormal strain during systole with a left bundle branch (answer C) would demonstrate early preejection and midsystolic shortening of the septal wall but not reduced strain only of the inferolateral wall. Although global measures of function are in the normal range, the regional wall strain abnormalities is not normal (answer D).

Answer 10: B

The speckle-tracking strain imaging bullet diagrams shows severe hypokinesis of the inferolateral wall (in blue). Calculation of 2D bi-plane ejection fraction (EF) is based on tracing endocardial border in the apical 4-chamber and 2-chamber views, which do not include the inferior-lateral (e.g., posterior) wall, thus it does not account for the patient's regional myocardial dysfunction, with overestimation of EF. A more accurate EF would be obtained using 3D echocardiography that would not rely on the geometric assumption of the bi-plane method and is more likely to avoid foreshortening of the apex compared to 2D imaging (answer A). Unlike assessment with Doppler, speckle tracking (answer C) is less dependent on the intercept angle between the ultrasound beam and target, instead relying on tacking motion of unique echo signal patterns (speckles) over the cardiac cycle. The M-mode endocardial fractional shortening (answer D) is based on a single dimension change in size, measured from the septum to inferior-lateral wall, and thus would underestimate global systolic function of this patient.

Answer 11: A

Restrictive cardiomyopathy is most commonly due to an underlying infiltrative process. This process most commonly affects diastolic function, with relative preservation of systolic function. Systolic function is typically synchronous, unless the infiltrative process has affected the electrical conduction pathways. In pericardial constriction, there is a fixed space for cardiac motion. As a consequence, there is often respiratory dependent shifting of septal motion from right to left with transient increases in preload, as occurs with inspiration. Ventricular conduction abnormalities (LBBB, RBBB, or ventricular pacing) alter the sequence of ventricular contraction. Initial activation with an RV apical lead will lead to dyssynchronous contraction of the RV free wall relative to the septum and LV. Cardiac surgery involving the septum can also lead to alteration in the ventricular activation sequence. Pressure overload of the RV, as occurs with severe pulmonary hypertension, results in septal flattening; there is a leftward septal shift throughout the cardiac cycle.

7 Ventricular Diastolic Filling and Function

BASIC PRINCIPLES

- Diastolic dysfunction often occurs in association with abnormal imaging findings (e.g., left ventricular (LV) hypertrophy or impaired systolic function).
- Diastolic dysfunction may be the earliest sign of cardiac disease, often with Doppler findings antedating clinical or imaging signs of dysfunction.
- Chronic elevation of LV diastolic pressure often leads to left atrium (LA) enlargement, a key element in evaluation of LV diastolic dysfunction.

STEP-BY-STEP APPROACH

Step 1: Measure Left Ventricular Inflow Velocities

- LV inflow velocities are recorded at the mitral leaflet tips and at the mitral annulus (Fig. 7.1).
- Standard measurements are E velocity and deceleration time, and A velocity and duration (Fig. 7.2).
- The normal pattern of a higher E than A velocity is reversed with impaired early diastolic relaxation, but the pattern may be "pseudo-normalized" with more severe diastolic dysfunction.

❖ KEY POINTS

- ❑ LV inflow velocities are recorded at the mitral leaflet tips (highest velocity signal) in the apical 4-chamber view using pulsed Doppler with a sample volume of 2.0 to 2.5 mm in length.
- ❑ The Doppler scale, baseline, and gain are adjusted to show a clear velocity curve.
- ❑ Low wall filter settings allow accurate measurements that require identification of where the velocity signal intersects the baseline (Fig. 7.3).
- ❑ Recordings at the leaflet tips are used to measure E and A velocity and deceleration slope. Recordings at the annulus are used to measure A duration.

- ❑ A transient decrease in preload may unmask an impaired relaxation filling pattern in patients with superimposed elevated filling pressures. This is shown by recording LV inflow at the mitral leaflet tips while the patient performs a Valsalva maneuver.

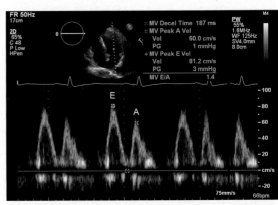

Fig. 7.1 **Normal LV inflow pattern.** LV inflow velocities were recorded using pulsed Doppler with the sample volume at the mitral leaflet tips. *A,* Atrial; *E,* early.

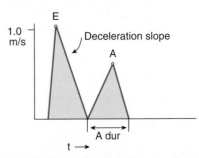

Fig. 7.2 **Schematic diagram showing basic measurements from the LV inflow curve.** The early *(E)* diastolic peak velocity, the velocity after atrial *(A)* contraction, the early diastolic deceleration slope, and the duration of the A velocity *(from the recording at the annulus)*

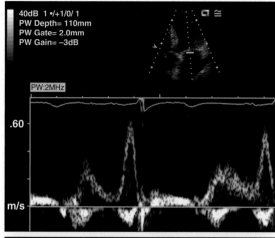

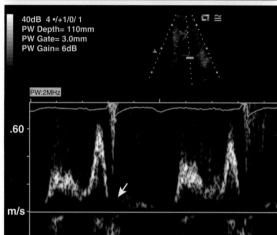

Fig. 7.3 Effect of wall filter settings. Example of LV inflow recorded at the annulus with the wall filters set at a low level (level is set at 1) to allow accurate timing measurements *(top)*. When the wall filter is inappropriately high (level is set at 4), the intersection of the Doppler signal with the baseline is no longer seen, making accurate measurement difficult *(bottom)*.

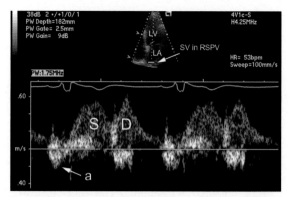

Fig. 7.4 Normal pulmonary vein flow pattern. LA inflow is recorded with the pulsed Doppler sample volume positioned in the right superior pulmonary vein (RSPV) from an apical 4-chamber approach. With atrial contraction, there is a small atrial reversal velocity *(a)*, with a normal pattern of systolic *(S)* and diastolic *(D)* inflow into the atrium.

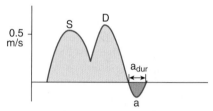

Fig. 7.5 Schematic of measurements for pulmonary vein flow. Typical measurements included the atrial *(a)* reversal peak and duration and peak systolic *(S)* and diastolic *(D)* filling velocities.

Step 2: Record Left Atrial Inflow

- LA inflow velocities are recorded in the right superior pulmonary vein from an apical 4-chamber view on transthoracic echocardiography (TTE) or in any pulmonary vein on transesophageal echocardiography (TEE) (Fig. 7.4).
- Standard measurements are peak systolic velocity, peak diastolic velocity, and the atrial velocity peak and duration (a_{dur}) (Fig. 7.5).
- A PV_a greater than 0.35 m/s and an a_{dur} 20 ms longer than transmitral A duration indicate an elevated LV end-diastolic pressure.

❖ **KEY POINTS**

- ❏ LA inflow velocities from the transthoracic approach may be difficult to record due to poor signal strength at the depth of the pulmonary vein.
- ❏ Color flow imaging may be helpful in locating the pulmonary vein and optimizing sample

volume position. The 2- to 3-mm length sample volume should be at least 1 cm into the pulmonary vein (Fig. 7.6).

- ❏ The Doppler scale, baseline, and gain are adjusted to show a clear spectral signal.
- ❏ Low wall filter settings allow accurate measurements that require identification of where the velocity signal intersects the baseline.

Step 3: Record Tissue Doppler at the Mitral Annulus

- Tissue Doppler myocardial velocities are recorded adjacent to the mitral annulus from a TTE apical approach (Fig. 7.7).
- Standard measurements are the early myocardial velocity (E′) and atrial myocardial velocity (A′) (Fig. 7.8).
- An E′/A′ ratio more than 1.0 is normal, with a reduced ratio indicating impaired early diastolic relaxation.
- A ratio of the transmitral E velocity to the tissue Doppler E′ velocity greater than 15 predicts an LV end-diastolic pressure more than 15 mm Hg.

❖ **KEY POINTS**

- ❏ In the apical 4-chamber view, a small (2 mm) sample volume is positioned in the myocardium about 1 cm from the mitral annulus. The tissue Doppler instrument settings include a velocity scale of about 0.2 m/s, low gain settings, low velocity scale, and low wall filters.

❑ Tissue Doppler recordings at the septal side of the annulus are more reproducible than signals from the lateral wall.

❑ The E′ and A′ velocities are less dependent on preload than the transmitral flow velocities.

Step 4: Measure the Isovolumic Relaxation Time

■ Pulsed Doppler is used to show the time interval between aortic valve closure and mitral valve opening (the isovolumic relaxation time [IVRT]) (Fig. 7.9).

■ The IVRT normally 50 to 100 ms, is prolonged with impaired relaxation but is shortened with severe diastolic dysfunction and reduced compliance (Fig. 7.10).

❖ **KEY POINTS**

❑ In an anteriorly angulated 4-chamber view, a 2- to 3-mm sample volume is positioned midway between aortic and mitral valves to show both LV ejection and LV filling velocity curves.

❑ The wall filters are set at a low level to identify the end of aortic outflow and onset of mitral inflow at their intersection with the baseline.

❑ The time interval is measured in milliseconds (ms).

Step 5: Consider Other Useful Measurements

■ The diastolic slope of the apical color M-mode recording of LV inflow (the propagation velocity)

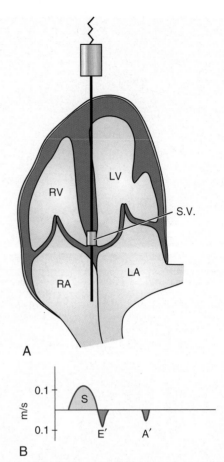

A

B

Fig. 7.7 **Schematic diagram of tissue Doppler measurements.** (A) In the apical 4-chamber view, the sample volume *(SV)* is placed about 1 cm apical to the medial mitral annulus. (B) The typical early *(E′)* and late *(A′)* tissue Doppler velocities are seen in diastole directed away from the transducer (as the ventricle fills). In systole, there is a velocity component toward the transducer corresponding to systolic contraction of the ventricle.

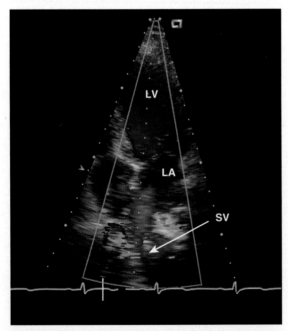

Fig. 7.6 **Identification of the right superior pulmonary vein from the transthoracic apical 4-chamber view.** Color Doppler imaging aids in positioning the pulsed Doppler sample volume *(SV, arrow)* about 1 cm into the pulmonary vein for optimal data quality.

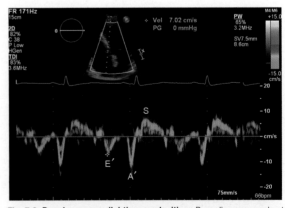

Fig. 7.8 **Doppler myocardial tissue velocities.** Recordings are made at the septal side of the mitral annulus using a small sample volume, with the velocity scale reduced (note that the velocity range is only 0.2 m/s), the wall filters at a low level (setting = 1), and the gain reduced to a very low level (setting = −17 dB) *A′*, Diastolic late velocity; *E′*, diastolic early velocity; *S*, systolic velocity.

reflects the rate of LV diastolic relaxation (Fig. 7.11).

- The rate of decline in velocity of the mitral regurgitant jet at end-systole reflects the early diastolic rate of decline in LV pressure (Fig. 7.12).

❖ KEY POINTS

- ❏ Propagation velocity is measured from an apical view using a narrow sector, a depth that just includes the mitral annulus, with the aliasing velocity set to 0.5 to 0.7 m/s, at a fast (100 to 200 mm/s) sweep speed.
- ❏ The early diastolic $-dP/dt$ is measured from the mitral regurgitant continuous-wave (CW) Doppler curve by measuring the time interval between 3 and 1 m/s and dividing by 32 mm Hg (analogous to measurement of $+dP/dt$ from the early systolic part of the mitral regurgitant velocity curve).

Step 6: Integrate the Data (Table 7.1)

- ■ Measurement of LA size (diameter and/or indexed volume) is useful in the assessment of diastolic function. Chronically elevated LV filling pressure leads to increased LA chamber size.
- ■ Based on integration of data from LA size, LV filling velocities, LA filling velocities, tissue Doppler, and IVRT, diastolic dysfunction can be detected and graded (Fig. 7.13).

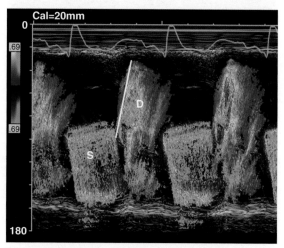

Fig. 7.11 Color M-mode propagation velocity. LV inflow is recorded from an apical view using a color Doppler M-mode beam aligned along the center of the mitral annulus. Thus, the vertical axis is distance from the LA (at about 160 mm depth on the scale) to the apex (at the top of the scale) with the horizontal axis indicating time, using an electrocardiogram for timing of the cardiac cycle. Flow toward the transducer in diastole (D) represents LV filling with the slope of the edge of this signal (line) reflecting the velocity of the movement of blood from the annulus to the apex. S, Systole.

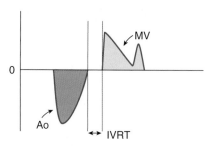

Fig. 7.9 Isovolumic relaxation time (IVRT). This time interval is measured from aortic valve (Ao) closure to mitral valve (MV) opening on the Doppler tracing, corresponding to the phase of the cardiac cycle where LV pressure is rapidly declining, but LV volume is constant.

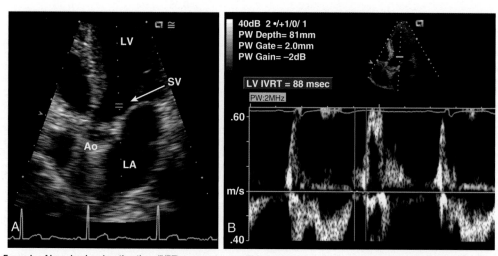

Fig. 7.10 Example of isovolumic relaxation time (IVRT) measurement. (A) In an apical 4-chamber view angulated anteriorly to include the aortic valve, a pulsed Doppler sample volume is positioned on the LV side of the anterior mitral leaflet in systole (to record LV outflow) and on the atrial side in diastole (to record LV inflow). **(B)** The time interval between the end of aortic antegrade flow and the onset of diastolic inflow across the mitral valve is measured. The scale and wall filters have been adjusted to optimize identification of the onset and end of flow, at their intersection with the baseline. A rapid sweep speed (100 mm/s) is used to improve the accuracy of the measurement. In this patient, the IVRT is normal at 88 ms (normal 50 to 100 ms) sample volume. SV, Sample volume.

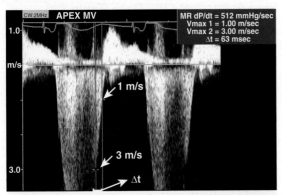

Fig. 7.12 Rate of decline in LV pressure (or negative dP/dt). This measurement can be made from the mitral regurgitant jet velocity as velocity decelerates, analogous to measurement of positive dP/dt from the rate of acceleration in velocity. The pressure difference between 1 and 3 m/s (32 mm Hg) is divided by the time interval (in seconds) measured between these points on the velocity curve at 1 and 3 m/s to give the –dP/dt in mm Hg/s.

- The clinical interpretation of the data also takes several other factors into consideration, including mitral regurgitation, LV systolic function, LV wall thickness, and clinical signs and symptoms.

NORMAL DIASTOLIC FUNCTION (FIG. 7.14)

Characteristic Features

- Normal LA size.
- Transmitral E/A velocity ratio between 1 and 2.
- E deceleration time 150 to 200 ms.
- Tissue Doppler E′/A′ ratio of 1 to 2.
- Pulmonary vein systolic to diastolic flow ratio of 1 or more.
- Pulmonary vein a-velocity less than 0.35 m/s and duration less than 20 ms longer than transmitral A duration.

TABLE 7.1   Classification of Diastolic Dysfunction*

	Normal	Mild (Grade I)	Moderate (Grade II)	Severe† (Grade III)
Pathophysiology		↓ Relaxation Normal LV EDP	↓ Relaxation and ↑ LV EDP	↓ Compliance and ↑↑ LV EDP
E/A ratio¶	≥0.8	<0.8	>0.8 to <2.0§	≥2.0
Valsalva ΔE/A		<0.5	≥0.5	≥0.5
DT (ms)	150-200	>200	150-200	<150
E′ velocity (cm/s)	≥10	<8	<8	<5
E/E′ ratio	≤10	≤10	10-14	>14
IVRT (ms)	50-100	≥100	60-100	≤60
PV S/D	≅1	S > D	S < D	S << D
PVₐ (m/s)	<0.35	<0.35‡	≥0.35	≥0.35
aₐᵤᵣ-Aₐᵤᵣ (ms)	<20	<20‡	≥30	≥30
LA volume index	<34 mL/m²	Mildly enlarged	Moderately enlarged	Severely enlarged

A, Late diastolic ventricular filling velocity with atrial contraction; a_{dur}, duration of pulmonary vein atrial reversal; A_{dur}, duration of transmitral atrial flow signal; *DT*, deceleration time; *E*, early-diastolic peak velocity; *E′*, early-diastolic tissue Doppler velocity; *EDP*, end-diastolic pressure; *IVRT*, isovolumic relaxation time; *PV*, pulmonary vein; PV_a, pulmonary vein atrial reversal.

Data from Nagueh SF et al: Recommendations for the evaluation of left ventricular diastolic function by echocardiography: An update from the American Society of Echocardiography and the European Association of Cardiovascular Imaging, *J Am Soc Echocardiogr* 29(4):277-314, 2016; Rakowki H et al: Canadian consensus recommendations for the measurement and reporting of diastolic dysfunction by echocardiography: from the Investigators of Consensus on Diastolic Dysfunction by Echocardiography, *J Am Soc Echocadiogr* 9(5):736-760, 1996; Yamada H et al: Prevalence of left ventricular diastolic dysfunction by Doppler echocardiography: Clinical application of the Canadian consensus guidelines, *J Am Soc Echocardiogr* 15(10):1238-1244, 2002; Redfield et al: Burden of systolic and diastolic ventricular dysfunction in the community: appreciating the scope of the heart failure epidemic, *JAMA* 289(2):194-202, 2003; Lester et al: Unlocking the mysteries of diastolic function: deciphering the Rosetta Stone 10 years later, *J Am Coll Cardiol* 51(7):679-689, 2008.

*Key measures highlighted.

†An additional grade of irreversible severe dysfunction is characterized by the absence of a decrease in E velocity with the strain phase of the Valsalva maneuver.

‡Pulmonary vein a duration and velocity may be increased if filling pressures are elevated.

§E/A with Valsalva is <1.

¶Only the highlighted rows are included in the ASE Guidelines plus consideration of tricuspid regurgitant jet velocity. In the absence of other causes for elevated pulmonary pressures, a tricuspid regurgitation (TR) velocity over 2.8 m/s is consistent with moderate to severe LV diastolic dysfunction.

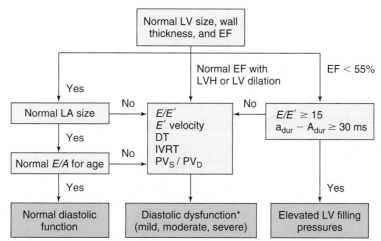

Fig. 7.13 **Suggested algorithm for evaluation of diastolic dysfunction on routine clinical studies.** When LV size, wall thickness, and ejection fraction *(EF)* are normal, further evaluation of diastolic function is needed only if there is left atrial enlargement or an abnormal E/A ratio for age. In patients with ventricular hypertrophy or dilation with a normal EF, diastolic function should be fully evaluated, particularly if there is a clinical concern that diastolic dysfunction may account for symptoms. When the EF is reduced, the first step is to evaluate for elevated filling pressures. If simple criteria for elevated filling pressures are not present, a more complete evaluation of diastolic function is appropriate. *IVRT,* Isovolumic relaxation time; *LVH,* left ventricular hypertrophy. *(From Otto, CM: Textbook of clinical echocardiography, ed 6, Philadelphia, 2018, Elsevier.)*

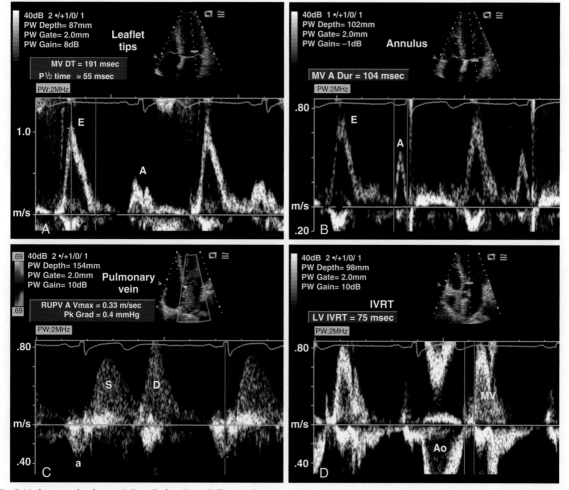

Fig. 7.14 **An example of normal diastolic function.** (A) The LV inflow curve at the mitral leaflet tips shows a normal E and A velocity with a deceleration time of 191 ms. (B) Inflow recorded at the annulus shows the duration of the atrial flow curve (104 ms) is the same as the duration of atrial reversal in the pulmonary vein recording. (C) The pulmonary vein flow also shows normal systolic and diastolic inflow signals. (D) The isovolumic relaxation time (IVRT) is normal at 75 ms. *Ao,* Aorta; *MV,* mitral valve.

Diastolic Filling Versus Diastolic Function

- At a higher heart rate (shorter diastolic filling time), the A velocity may be increased, because it is superimposed on the E deceleration slope (Fig. 7.15).
- The transmitral E/A ratio decreases with age, reversing at about age 50 years. Similarly, the pulmonary vein diastolic flow declines, so the systolic to diastolic ratio increases with age.
- A higher preload increases the transmitral E velocity; hypovolemia results in a lower velocity—with Valsalva maneuver, E velocity falls transiently due to reduced venous return (Fig. 7.16).
- Increased transmitral volume flow due to mitral regurgitation increases the transmitral E velocity.
- Atrial contractile function affects LV filling, LA filling, and tissue Doppler signals (Fig. 7.17).

MILD DIASTOLIC DYSFUNCTION (IMPAIRED RELAXATION) (FIG. 7.18)

- Increased LA diameter and volume are typical.
- Impaired relaxation with reduced early diastolic filling is typical of mild diastolic dysfunction.
- Common causes of diastolic dysfunction include hypertensive heart disease, ischemic disease, or an early infiltrative cardiomyopathy.
- The decreased rate of early diastolic filling is associated with a reduced E velocity (reduced E/A ratio), a reduced E′/A′ ratio on tissue Doppler, reduced pulmonary vein diastolic flow, and a prolonged IVRT.
- LV filling pressure may be normal with mild diastolic dysfunction, so pulmonary vein atrial velocity and duration often are normal.

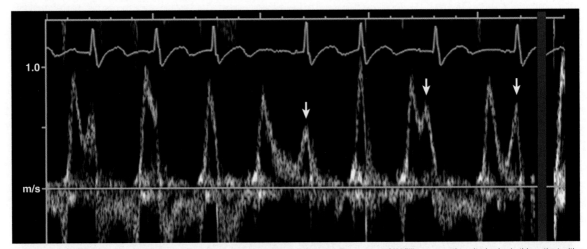

Fig. 7.15 **Diastolic filling pattern changes with changes in the duration of diastole.** The pattern of LV filling across the mitral valve in this patient with a variable R-R interval shows an E/A ratio greater than 1 on the longer R-R interval. However, the A velocities *(arrows)* are higher when superimposed on the E deceleration slope on the shorter R-R intervals. There is fusion of the E and A velocities on the shortest diastolic intervals.

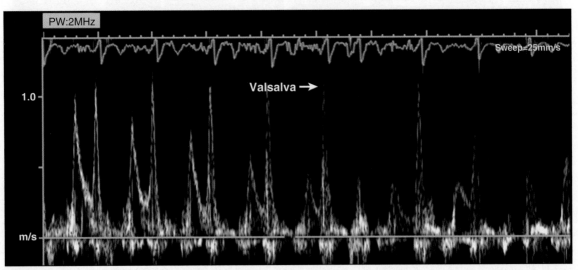

Fig. 7.16 **Diastolic filling pattern changes with changes in preload.** LV inflow recorded at a slow sweep speed during the Valsalva maneuver shows a gradual reduction in E velocity, due to a relative decrease in LV preload, but no change in A velocity. Thus, E/A ratio is dependent on preload.

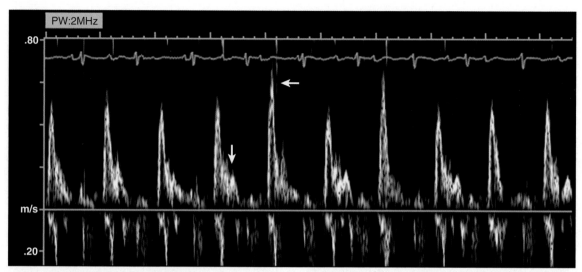

Fig. 7.17 Effect of PR interval on diastolic filling patterns. In this patient with third-degree atrioventricular (AV) block, the height of the E velocity varies with the timing of atrial contraction. When atrial contraction occurs in mid to late diastole, a separate A velocity is seen *(vertical arrow)*, but when atrial contraction occurs in early diastole, a higher (summated) E velocity is seen *(horizontal arrow)*.

MODERATE DIASTOLIC DYSFUNCTION (PSEUDO-NORMALIZATION) (FIG. 7.19)

- LV relaxation is impaired and LV filling pressures are elevated with moderate diastolic dysfunction.
- Typical causes of moderate diastolic dysfunction include dilated, hypertrophic, or restrictive cardiomyopathy.
- In addition to the findings seen with mild diastolic dysfunction, there is evidence for elevated filling pressures, including a higher pulmonary vein a-velocity peak (>0.35 m/s) and duration, an increased E/E′ ratio (>15), and a shorted E velocity deceleration time.
- The LV filling velocity waveform shows an apparently normal E/A ratio of 1 to 2 (pseudo-normal) that is distinguished from a true normal by the tissue Doppler showing an E′/A′ less than 1 and a shortened E velocity deceleration time.
- The change in the transmitral flow pattern with Valsalva maneuver also can be used to identify a pseudo-normal transmitral flow pattern; the E velocity decreases with pseudo-normalization.

SEVERE DIASTOLIC DYSFUNCTION (DECREASED COMPLIANCE) (FIG. 7.20)

- Severe diastolic dysfunction is characterized by decreased compliance, in addition to impaired relaxation, an enlarged LA, and an elevated filling pressure.
- Decreased compliance means there is a greater increase in LV pressure for a given increase in LV volume compared with a normal ventricle.

- Although the E/A ratio is more than 2 and the E′/A′ ratio is more than 1, severe diastolic dysfunction is differentiated from normal by the higher E/A ratio, shorter IVRT, decreased deceleration time (<150 ms), blunted pulmonary vein systolic flow, and increased pulmonary a-wave velocity and duration.
- The E′ velocity is very low (<5 cm/s) with severe diastolic dysfunction.

LEFT ATRIAL PRESSURE ESTIMATES

- Exact measurement of LA (or LV filling) pressure is not possible with echocardiography, but there are several parameters that suggest significant elevation of LA pressures:
  - ○ Pulmonary vein atrial reversal velocity (PVa) more than 0.35 m/s (Fig. 7.21)
  - ○ Pulmonary vein atrial reversal duration (adur) at least 20 ms longer than transmitral A duration (Adur) recorded at the mitral annulus
  - ○ Ratio of transmitral E velocity to myocardial tissue E′ velocity more than 15 (Fig. 7.22)
  - ○ Pulmonary venous diastolic flow deceleration time less than 175 ms
  - ○ E velocity deceleration time less than 150 ms
  - ○ E/A ratio more than 2
- When more than one parameter is consistent with elevated LA pressure, the diagnosis is more certain.
- In patients with atrial fibrillation, parameters of diastolic function that do not rely on atrial contraction may be helpful, including deceleration time, the E/E′ ratio, and the IVRT.

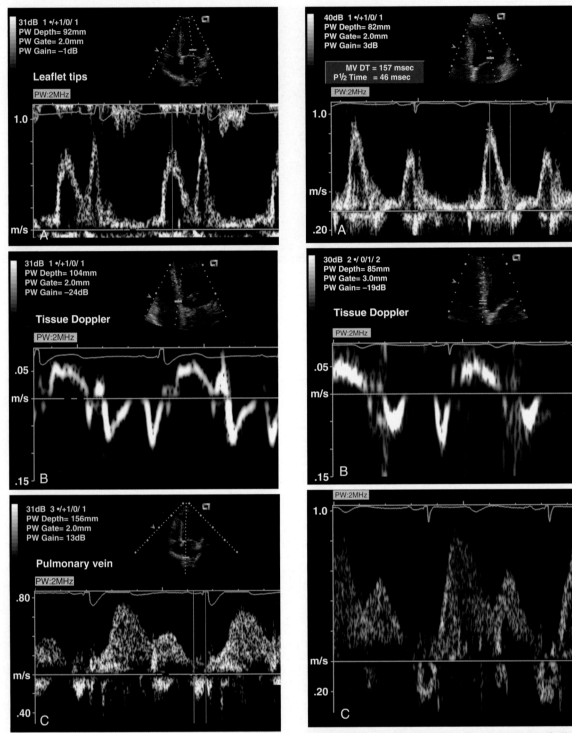

Fig. 7.18 **Example of mild diastolic dysfunction with impaired early diastolic relaxation.** Characteristic findings are an E/A ratio less than 1 on the LV inflow curve (A), a tissue Doppler early to late diastolic velocity ratio less than 1 (B), and a pulmonary vein flow curve with a reduced diastolic inflow curve but a relatively normal atrial reversal velocity and duration (C).

Fig. 7.19 **Moderate diastolic dysfunction (pseudo-normalization).** Characteristic findings include a mitral inflow curve with an E/A velocity between 1 and 2 but a relatively steep deceleration time (157 ms) (A), and a tissue Doppler E′/A′ less than 1 (B). Typically, the pulmonary vein flow signal shows greater systolic than diastolic flow and a prolonged duration and increased velocity of the atrial reversal. However, in this case, the pulmonary venous flow signal (C) does not show these features, suggesting the degree of diastolic function falls between mild-moderate and moderate (pseudonormal) as shown in the classification in the Echo Exam section.

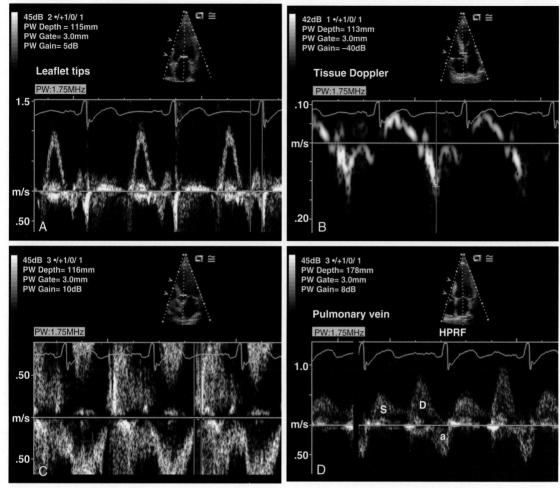

Fig. 7.20 Severe diastolic dysfunction. Characteristic findings include an LV inflow curve with an E/A >2 and a short deceleration time **(A)**, a tissue Doppler E′/A′ more than 1 **(B)**, a short isovolumic relaxation time (IVRT) **(C)**, and reduced systolic flow compared with diastolic flow in the pulmonary vein with a pulmonary vein a-reversal that is prolonged (>20 ms longer than transmitral A duration) and increased in velocity (≥0.35 m/s) **(D)**.

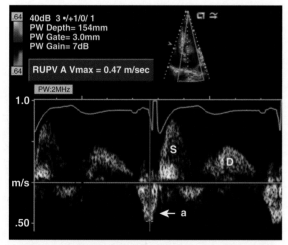

Fig. 7.21 Pulmonary vein recording in a patient with hypertrophic cardiomyopathy and severe diastolic dysfunction. The atrial reversal duration is prolonged with an elevated velocity of 0.47 m/s, suggesting markedly elevated LV filling pressures. *a,* Atrial; *D,* diastole; *S,* systole.

- With mitral valve stenosis or regurgitation, evaluation of LV diastolic function and LA pressure are problematic, because transmitral filling reflects mitral valve hemodynamics, rather than LV diastolic function.

Patterns of diastolic inflow are summarized in Fig. 7.23 for patients with mild, moderate, and severe diastolic dysfunction in comparison to normal filling patterns.

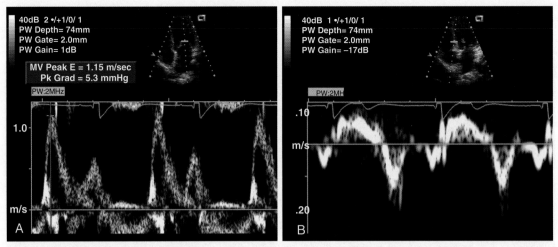

Fig. 7.22 E/E′ as a marker of an elevated LV filling pressure. The ratio of the transmitral E velocity to myocardial tissue Doppler velocity is higher when filling pressures are elevated with a ratio more than 15, indicating a significant elevation. In this example, the ratio is 1.15:0.15 = 7.7, suggesting normal filling pressures.

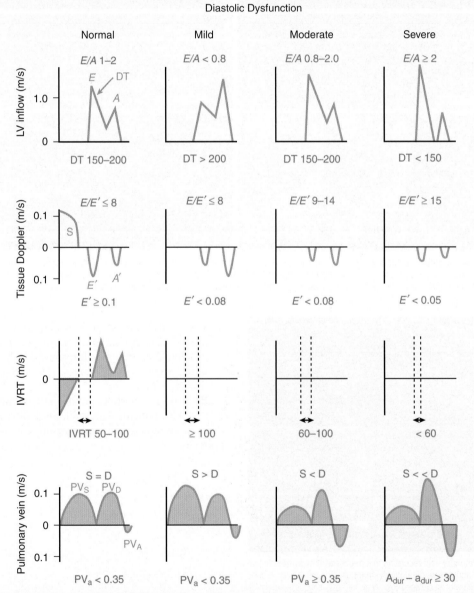

Fig. 7.23 Diagram comparing typical Doppler findings in patients with normal, mild, moderate, and severe diastolic dysfunction. The top row shows LV inflow with early *(E)* and atrial *(A)* phases of diastolic filling. The second row shows tissue Doppler recorded at the septal side of the mitral annulus with the myocardial early *(E′)* and atrial *(A′)* velocities and the expected ratio of E/E′. The third row shows the isovolumic relaxation time *(IVRT)*. The bottom row shows the pulmonary vein *(PV)* inflow pattern with systolic *(S)* and diastolic *(D)* antegrade flow and the pulmonary vein atrial *(PVa)* reversal of flow. *(From Otto, CM: Textbook of clinical echocardiography, ed 6, Philadelphia, 2018, Elsevier.)*

THE ECHO EXAM

Echocardiographic Techniques in Assessment of Diastolic Function

	Clinical Utility	Technical Points	Limitations
Mitral inflow	• Assess LV compliance, relaxation, filling pressures • Short DT associated with poor prognosis • Best used with combined systolic and diastolic heart failure	• Sample volume 1-3 mm, filter at 200 Hz, sweep speed 50-100 mm/s • Measure E- and A-waves, DT, IVRT • A_{dur} measured at mitral annulus	• Preload dependent • E/A ratio can be pseudo-normalized
Pulmonary vein flow	• Assess LV compliance, relaxation, filling pressures • Blunted S and D velocities associated with poor prognosis • Best used with combined systolic and diastolic heart failure • PV_a used to assess pseudo-normalization	• Sample volume 2-3 mm, placed 1-2 cm into the PV, filter at 200 Hz, sweep speed 50-100 mm/s • Measure S, D, and PV_a waves	• Relatively preload independent • Technically difficult to obtain in all patients • Blunted S/D from other conditions including atrial fibrillation and mitral regurgitation
Tissue Doppler imaging	• Assess LV compliance, relaxation, filling pressures • E/E′ ≥15 associated with elevated filling pressures • Best used with primary diastolic heart failure	• Sample volume 2-4 mm at mitral annulus, filter at 200 Hz, sweep speed 50-100 mm/s • Measure S′, E′, and A′ waves	• Relatively preload independent • Angle and translation dependent • Different velocities at annuli (lateral > medial)
Color M-mode	• Assess LV compliance, relaxation, filling pressures • E/V_p >1.5 associated with elevated filling pressures • Best used with primary diastolic heart failure	• Slope of flow propagation (first aliasing velocity) for 4 cm into LV • 2D depth reduced to 16 cm • Move baseline to set color aliasing velocity about 40 cm/s • M-mode sweep recorded at 100 mm/s • Measure V_p slope	• Relatively preload independent • Technically difficult to obtain in all patients • Influenced by LV geometry
Strain imaging	• High time resolution of deformation (sampling rates >200/min) • Allows assessment of regional diastolic deformation	• Global measures include peak early and late diastolic strain rates and time to early peak strain rate	• Circumferential strain should be measured in addition to radial and longitudinal strain • Diastolic strain rate measurements are complex and not yet clinically validated.

A-wave, Filling wave due to atrial contraction; A_{dur}, atrial duration; *D,* diastolic flow; *DT,* deceleration time; *E,* early diastolic filling velocity; *IVRT,* isovolumic relaxation time; *PV,* pulmonary vein; PV_a, pulmonary vein atrial reversal; *S,* systolic flow; V_p, velocity of propagation.

SELF-ASSESSMENT QUESTIONS

Question 1

This mitral inflow signal was recorded in a 72-year-old man with hypertension and aortic stenosis (Fig. 7.24). Which of the following statements about diastolic function is the most likely explanation for this flow pattern?

A. Diastolic function cannot be evaluated due to bradycardia.

B. Diastolic function is normal for age.

C. Mild diastolic dysfunction is present.

D. Moderate diastolic dysfunction is present.

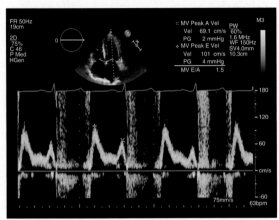

Fig. 7.24

Question 2

A patient is referred for echocardiography and the following image is obtained (Fig 7.25). Progression in the Doppler signal across several cardiac cycles is accounted for by:

A. Shifts in transducer position

B. Change in LV loading

C. Doppler signal optimization

D. Underlying atrial fibrillation

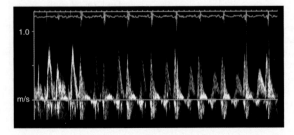

Fig. 7.25

Question 3

Which of the following, if present, least affects echocardiographic Doppler assessment of LV diastolic function?

A. Atrial fibrillation

B. Mitral regurgitation

C. Pulmonary hypertension

D. Mitral stenosis

Question 4

A myocardial tissue Doppler image taken from the septal mitral annulus in an apical 4-chamber view is shown in Fig. 7.26. Identify the labeled velocity peaks with the correct cardiac measurement.

1. Late diastolic velocity (A′)

2. Early diastolic velocity (E′)

3. Isovolumic contraction velocity

4. Isovolumic relaxation velocity

5. Systolic ejection velocity (S′)

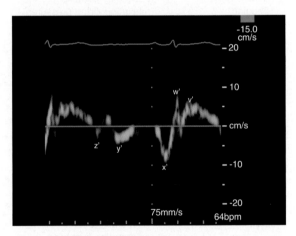

Fig. 7.26

Question 5

This pulmonary vein flow (Fig. 7.27) signal (recorded on TEE imaging) is most consistent with which of the following:
A. Normal diastolic function
B. Severe mitral regurgitation
C. Atrial flutter
D. Diastolic dysfunction

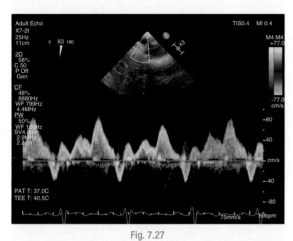

Fig. 7.27

Question 6

What feature of the color Doppler M-mode tracing (as shown in Fig. 7.28) is most useful for LV diastolic assessment?
A. Signal duration
B. Maximal signal distance from mitral valve
C. Slope of signal from mitral valve opening
D. Signal intensity

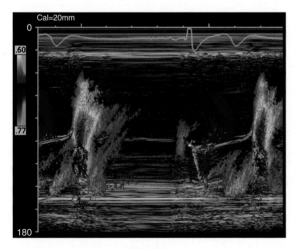

Fig. 7.28

Question 7

Based on the mitral inflow pulsed wave and CW Doppler across the mitral valve (Fig. 7.29), which of the following statements about diastolic function is most accurate?
A. There is normal diastolic function.
B. There is pseudonormalization of mitral inflow velocity.
C. Diastolic function assessment is limited by arrhythmia.
D. Diastolic function is limited by severe mitral regurgitation.

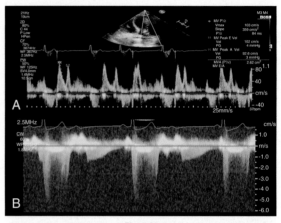

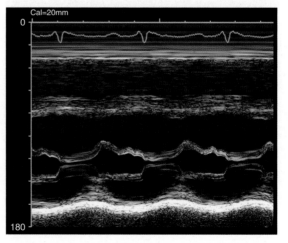

Fig. 7.29

Question 8

Review the M-mode image shown in Fig. 7.30. Which feature of the image is most helpful in evaluating LV diastolic pressure?
A. Late diastole mitral valve motion
B. Peak early mitral valve diastolic displacement
C. Duration diastolic leaflet excursion
D. E-point septal separation

Fig. 7.30

Question 9

Indicate the position for sample volume acquisition for each of the following echocardiographic measures of LV diastolic function (some of the indices may require data from more than one position) (Fig. 7.31):

1. Isovolumic relaxation time (IVRT)
2. E/A ratio
3. $-dP/dt$ calculation
4. E/E′ ratio
5. E-wave deceleration time
6. Mitral A-wave duration
7. Left atrial inflow velocity

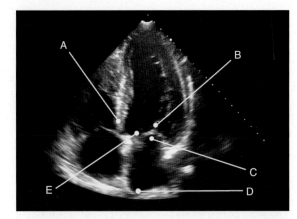

Fig. 7.31

Questions 10-11

Match the images shown in Fig. 7.32 and Fig. 7.33 with the most likely diagnosis:

A. Normal diastolic function
B. Impaired LV relaxation
C. Pseudonormal (moderate diastolic dysfunction)
D. Restrictive LV filling

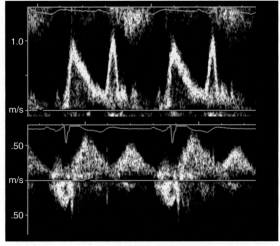

Fig. 7.33 Question 11

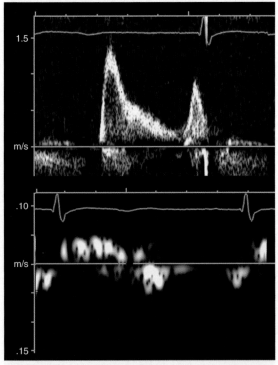

Fig. 7.32 Question 10

ANSWERS

Answer 1: D

The mitral inflow pattern is not consistent with the patient's age, because most patients over age 50 years have impaired relaxation with an E/A ratio <1.0. Given hypertension and aortic stenosis, LV hypertrophy with impaired diastolic relaxation or mild LV diastolic dysfunction might be expected but also would result in an E/A ratio <1.0. Instead, mitral inflow shows an E/A ratio >1.5 and a steep early diastolic deceleration slope, which is suggestive of pseudonormal LV filling consistent with moderate diastolic dysfunction. Additional findings that could confirm this diagnosis include a low tissue Doppler E' velocity, an E/E' ratio of 9 to 14, and a reduced pulmonary vein systolic velocity. An additional interesting finding in Fig. 7.24 is persistent antegrade flow during diastasis (also called an L-wave) that exceeds 20 cm/s, which is due to prominent pulmonary venous flow into the LA in diastole. L-waves may be seen with significant bradycardia and normal diastolic function, but the heart rate is normal at 63 beats per minute, suggesting the L-wave is due to a high diastolic pulmonary venous flow signal. Other echocardiographic features supportive of pseudonormalization include LV hypertrophy and left atrial dilation, which can be visually appreciated in the apical 4-chamber view.

Answer 2: B

This is a pulsed wave Doppler tracing taken at the level of the mitral valve leaflet tips from an apical view. The first two beats show an early (E) wave in diastole that is higher velocity than the late (A) wave velocity. At the third cardiac cycle, the patient performed a Valsalva maneuver, transiently decreasing LV preload, which reduced volume of transmitral flow in early diastole, resulting in a relatively larger contribution of atrial contraction to LV filling. With relaxation of Valsalva, the transmitral filling pattern returned to baseline (not shown). The transducer remained fixed, recording mitral inflow for the duration of the Doppler tracing. The rhythm is not paced nor is it atrial fibrillation, with atrial contraction evidenced by the A-wave throughout the sample. The Doppler signal quality is reasonable, with no changes in recording parameters during the recording.

Answer 3: C

Diastolic dysfunction with either impaired LV relaxation or decreased ventricular compliance impedes LV filling, leading to increased left atrial pressure. Doppler evaluation of diastolic function includes evaluation of transmitral filling (early [E] and late [A] diastolic filling), as well as tissue myocardial velocities in the myocardial wall (E' and A', respectively), measured 1 cm apically from the mitral valve annulus. Although increased LA pressure may lead to pulmonary hypertension, particularly with superimposed intravascular volume overload, the reverse is not true; pulmonary hypertension does not cause LV diastolic dysfunction. Cardiac abnormalities that affect LA pressure and/or the transmitral gradient will affect diastolic function assessment. For mitral regurgitation, increased transmitral volume flow results in an increased transmitral E-velocity, limiting Doppler-derived diastolic function assessment using the E/A ratio alone. For mitral stenosis, the increased pressure gradient at the valve level is directly due to inflow obstruction. Atrial fibrillation results in loss of the atrial contribution to diastolic filling and absence of the A-wave. However, in patients with atrial fibrillation, the transmitral E to myocardial velocity (E') ratio (E:E' ratio) remains a reasonable gauge of LA pressure.

Answer 4:

1. x'
2. y'
3. w'
4. z'
5. v'

Standard clinical measurements for diastolic function include the early-diastolic filling velocity (E') and atrial contraction filling velocity (A'). Systolic velocity (S') may be measured to evaluate systolic function, more commonly in the right ventricle (see Chapter 6). It is important to distinguish the isovolumic relaxation velocity from early diastolic velocity. Isovolumic relaxation has a brisk negative velocity near end-systole with a terminal positive velocity consistent with mild post-systolic shortening. Similarly, there is a normal brief velocity spike during isovolumic contraction before mitral valve closure. Sometimes, as seen here, there is a slight negative velocity component at the end of the isovolumic contraction prior to peak systolic ejection velocity.

Answer 5: D

The pulmonary vein flow is most consistent with diastolic dysfunction. There is a lower peak systolic velocity compared to the peak diastolic velocity. There is an elevated atrial reversal velocity of 40 cm/s. In normal diastolic function with normal left atrial filling pressure, peak systolic flow velocities are higher than peak diastolic velocity. The biphasic systolic flow velocity waves should not be confused with variable atrial flutter waves. TEE imaging can detect biphasic peak systolic flows (S1, S2) in many patients during normal sinus rhythm. The S1 component is from normal atrial relaxation and a second peak from systolic displacement of the mitral valve annulus toward the cardiac apex. Severe mitral regurgitation is more often associated with systolic flow reversal or severe blunting of left atrial systolic filling during normal sinus rhythm.

Answer 6: C

This is a color Doppler M-mode tracing of transmitral flow along the center of the mitral annulus taken from an apical view. With the mitral valve open in diastole, flow toward the transducer is recorded. The slope of the color Doppler signal from the point of valve opening (color propagation velocity [Vp]) reflects the velocity of LV inflow from the mitral valve plane to the apex. A steep slope is consistent with normal diastolic function and a flatter slope suggests higher LV diastolic pressure. The maximal signal distance from mitral valve is the distance where LV inflow velocities were detected. Increased turbulent flow could increase the maximal signal distance from mitral valve detected. The color signal duration corresponds to the time of flow in diastole and the signal intensity reflects the turbulence of flow within the jet; both are not measures of LV diastolic function.

Answer 7: C

The patient has an abnormal cardiac rhythm due to heart block. This irregular bradycardia alters interpretation of the early (E-wave) and atrial (A-wave) LV filling pattern, limiting diastolic classification. Alterations in LV diastolic filling from cardiac rhythm variation and mitral valve disorders limit echocardiographic interpretation of diastolic function. Heart block results in the variable LV filling patterns as the timing of atrial contraction occurs at different points in diastole, sometimes summated with the E-velocity. The patient does not have severe systolic mitral regurgitation based on the intensity of CW Doppler in systole. However, there is diastolic mitral regurgitant flow with atrioventricular dissociation from the heart block.

Answer 8: A

This is an M-mode tracing taken from the parasternal long-axis view at the mitral valve leaflet tips. In the mid-portion of the image, the anterior and posterior mitral valve leaflets are seen opening during diastole. Early diastolic motion of the anterior mitral valve leaflet is concurrent with early LV filling. Mid-diastolic anterior motion of the leaflet is concurrent with atrial contraction and later diastolic filling. Just before systole, there is a very late anterior displacement, or "bump" in the motion of the anterior mitral valve leaflet (Fig. 7.34). This "B-bump" is indicative of an elevated LV end-diastolic pressure. Peak early mitral valve diastolic anterior displacement and E-point septal separation are a reflection of LV chamber size. With dilated cardiomyopathy, apical tethering of the mitral valve leaflet tips may hinder leaflet excursion and increase the distance between the anterior

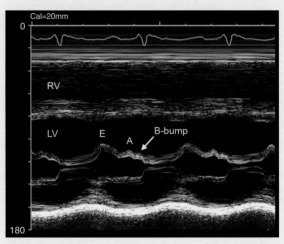

Fig. 7.34

mitral valve leaflet and the interventricular septum. In dilated cardiomyopathy, diastolic function is not normal. LV diastolic pressure may not be significantly elevated if volume status is euvolemic. The duration diastolic leaflet excursion reflects the time in the cardiac cycle spent in diastole and is not reflective of LV diastolic function.

Answer 9

1. Isovolumic relaxation time (E)
2. E/A ratio (B)
3. $-dP/dt$ calculation (C)
4. E/E′ ratio (A, B)
5. E-wave deceleration time (B)
6. Mitral A-wave duration (C)
7. Left atrial inflow velocity (D)

IVRT is recorded from an anteriorly angulated apical 4-chamber view midway between the aortic and mitral valves and is the time duration between aortic valve closure and mitral valve opening. IVRT is prolonged in patients with impaired LV relaxation and is shortened (<50 ms) in patients with decreased LV compliance. LV inflow velocities are recorded at the point where inflow occurs, the mitral leaflet tips, and the mitral annulus. At the mitral valve tips, the highest, or peak, velocity signal for both the E and A waves are measured, and the E/A ratio can be calculated. An E:A ratio less than 1 indicates impaired LV relaxation. An E:A ratio greater than 1 may indicate either normal diastolic function or decreased passive LV compliance, and additional data are needed. The early E-wave deceleration time is also measured from tracings taken at the mitral valve tips, and it is prolonged in patients with impaired LV relaxation and shortened (<150 ms) in patients with decreased LV compliance. The mitral inflow atrial A-wave duration is obtained from the mitral annular position and is compared to left atrial inflow a-wave duration (pulmonary venous flow), whereas pulmonary venous a-wave velocities less than 0.35 m/s are consistent with normal left atrial pressure. The −dP/dt is calculated from the deceleration slope of the CW mitral regurgitant jet, analogous to the dP/dt calculation for assessment of LV systolic function. The CW is aligned along the mitral inflow. Tissue Doppler myocardial velocity samples from the septum (E′ velocity) and the mitral E wave velocity recorded at the tips are a reflection of left atrial pressure, with an E:E′ ratio over 15 consistent with increased left atrial pressure.

Answer 10: A

The left portion of the image (see Fig. 7.32) is of mitral inflow at the level of the mitral valve tips. The sample is E-wave dominant with an E/A ratio greater than 1. The peak E-wave velocity is ≈1 m/s. The middle portion of the image is a tissue Doppler sample from the septum. The peak e′ wave velocity is ≈0.12 m/s. The E/E′ ratio is 8, consistent with normal left atrial pressure. The pulmonary venous atrial wave is not well seen, but pulmonary vein (right panel) systolic and diastolic inflows are about equal, which is normal. The findings in sum support a diagnosis of normal diastolic function.

Answer 11: D

This LV inflow Doppler recording shows an apparently normal E/A velocity ratio of ≈1.8. However, E-wave deceleration slope is steep, consistent with rapid equalization of transmitral pressure gradient during mitral valve opening. The septal myocardial tissue velocity, E′, is markedly reduced at 0.05 cm/s, indicating decreased myocardial motion. The E/E′ ratio of 28 is consistent with severely increased left atrial pressure. Overall these findings are consistent with restrictive LV diastolic function.

Answer 12: B

The LV mitral inflow Doppler signal shows slight reversal of the peak E/A velocities. The E-wave deceleration slope is prolonged, consistent with impaired LV relaxation. The pulmonary vein signal shows the systolic wave is dominant and the pulmonary atrial reversal wave is prolonged with a high peak velocity (≈0.4 m/s), implying increased LA pressure.

8 Coronary Artery Disease

REVIEW OF CORONARY ANATOMY AND LEFT VENTRICULAR WALL SEGMENTS

- Evaluation of coronary disease by echocardiography (echo) is based on visualization of endocardial motion and wall thickening.
- To describe regional myocardial function, the left ventricle (LV) is divided into segments that correspond to the coronary artery blood supply (Fig. 8.1).
- Myocardial infarction results in thinning and akinesis of the affected regions. With myocardial ischemia, wall motion may be normal at rest.
- The ostia of the right and left main coronary arteries often can be identified, but direct visualization of distal coronary anatomy by echo is limited (Figs. 8.2 and 8.3)

❖ KEY POINTS

- ❏ The ventricle is divided into basal, midventricular, and apical segments, plus the tip of the apex.
- ❏ A distal coronary stenosis results in apical abnormalities; a midcoronary lesion results in midventricular and apical wall motion changes; and proximal coronary disease results in abnormalities that extend from the base to the apex.
- ❏ In the short-axis plane, the LV is divided into six segments: anterior, anterior-lateral, inferior-lateral, inferior, inferior-septal, and anterior-septal.
- ❏ The left anterior descending coronary supplies the entire anterior wall, and anterior septum and typically extends to supply the apical segment of the inferior septum and the tip of the apex.
- ❏ The right coronary artery supplies the basal and midventricular segments of the inferior septum and the entire inferior wall and sometimes supplies the inferior-lateral wall.
- ❏ The circumflex coronary artery supplies the entire anterior-lateral and inferior-lateral walls.

STEP-BY-STEP APPROACH

Stress Echocardiography

Basic Principles

- LV global and regional function is normal at rest, even when significant coronary artery disease is present.
- With an increase in myocardial oxygen demand, myocardial ischemia is evidenced by reversible regional hypokinesis or akinesis.
- The basis of a stress echo is a comparison of images of the LV acquired at rest and after induction of

Echo Views for Wall Motion

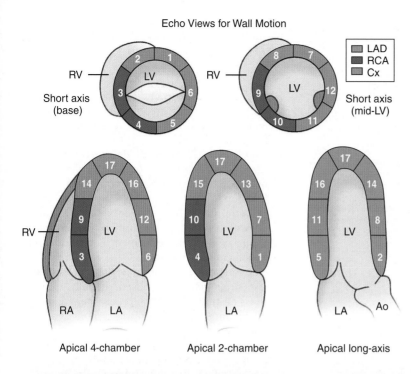

Fig. 8.1 **Echocardiographic views for wall motion evaluation.** In the short-axis view, at the base and midventricular levels, the LV is divided into the anterior *(1, 7),* anterior-septal *(2, 8),* inferior septal *(3, 9),* inferior *(4, 10),* inferolateral *(5, 11),* and anterolateral *(6, 12)* segments. In the apical region, there are four segments: anterior *(13),* septal *(14),* inferior *(15),* and lateral *(16),* plus the tip of the apex *(17).* The territory of the left anterior descending (LAD) artery is indicated in *green,* the right coronary artery (RCA) in *red,* and the left circumflex (Cx) coronary artery in *yellow.*

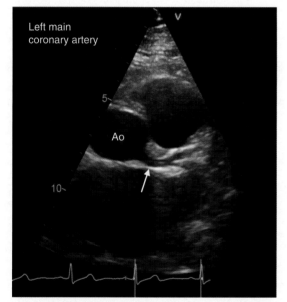

Fig. 8.2 **Left main coronary artery.** The left main coronary artery *(arrow)* is visualized on TTE arising from the aorta *(Ao)* anterior to the LA in a transthoracic parasternal short-axis view just above the aortic valve plane.

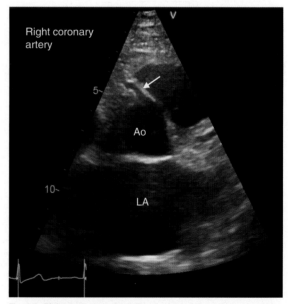

Fig. 8.3 **Right coronary artery.** The right coronary artery *(arrow)* is seen in a transthoracic parasternal short-axis view arising from the aorta *(Ao)* by slight adjustment of the image plane.

myocardial ischemia, either with exercise or pharmacologic intervention (Figs. 8.4 and 8.5).

❖ KEY POINTS

❑ The accuracy of a stress echo correlates with the stress load achieved. Typically, the goal is a peak heart rate at least 85% of the patient's maximum predicted heart rate.

❑ Comparison of resting and stress images is facilitated by acquiring images in a cine loop format, gated from the onset of the QRS to include the same number of frames for each image.

❑ Because ischemia may be induced with the stress protocol, appropriate medical supervision and monitoring is essential for patient safety and to promptly treat any complications of the procedure.

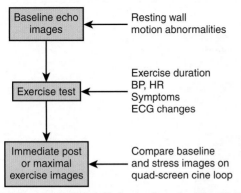

Fig. 8.4 **Flow chart of treadmill stress echocardiography.** *BP,* Blood pressure; *ECG,* electrocardiogram; *HR,* heart rate. (From Otto, CM: *Textbook of clinical echocardiography,* ed 6, Philadelphia, 2018, Elsevier.)

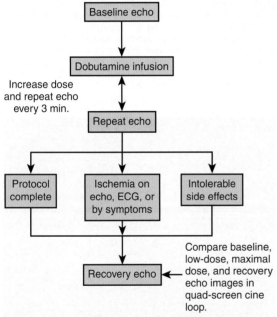

Fig. 8.5 **Flow chart of the protocol for dobutamine stress echocardiography.** (From Otto, CM: *Textbook of clinical echocardiography,* ed 6, Philadelphia, 2018, Elsevier.)

Step 1: Prepare for the Stress Echo

- The patient is instructed not to take beta-blocking medications the day before and day of the stress test.
- The reason for the stress study and the patient history is reviewed, followed by a directed physical examination.
- Informed consent is obtained for either an exercise or pharmacologic stress echo.
- Patient monitoring includes continuous 12-lead electrocardiogram (ECG) monitoring (with a recording at each stress stage) and intermittent blood pressure measurement under the supervision of a qualified medical professional, in a procedure room with resuscitation equipment and medications readily available.

- When needed, an intravenous (IV) line is placed for infusion of dobutamine and/or use of contrast echo.

❖ **KEY POINTS**

- Any potential contraindications or risk factors for the stress study are identified and discussed with the referring health care provider before beginning the test.
- The risks and benefits of the stress echo study are discussed with the patient, in the context of the patient's medical history and cardiac function.
- Because the cardiac sonographer's attention is focused on image acquisition, patient monitoring typically is performed by an additional health care professional.
- The rationale for a pharmacologic versus exercise stress echo is reviewed. Usually, exercise stress is preferred because of the additional information gained regarding hemodynamics and symptoms.
- A pharmacologic (usually dobutamine) stress echo is preferred in patients unable to walk on a treadmill or use a supine bicycle due to orthopedic or vascular problems and in some specific patient subgroups, such as those who have undergone heart transplantation.

Step 2: Evaluate Regional and Global Left Ventricular Systolic Function at Rest

- LV global and regional function is evaluated in parasternal long- and short-axis views and in apical 4-chamber, 2-chamber, and long-axis views (Fig. 8.6).
- The function for each myocardial segment is graded as hyperdynamic, normal, hypokinetic, akinetic, or dyskinetic based on the degree of endocardial motion and wall thickening (Table 8.1).
- Overall LV ejection fraction is visually estimated or (preferably) measured using the apical biplane approach.

❖ **KEY POINTS**

- The four standard views (with the long-axis in apical or parasternal, whichever is best) are recorded in cine loop format. A beat with clear definition of endocardial borders and optimal image plane alignment chosen for each view.
- Three-dimensional (3D) imaging may be used for simultaneous visualization in multiple views when image quality allows.
- Depth is reduced to maximize LV image size, including the mitral annulus but not the left atrium (LA). The same depth and sector width is used for the stress images.

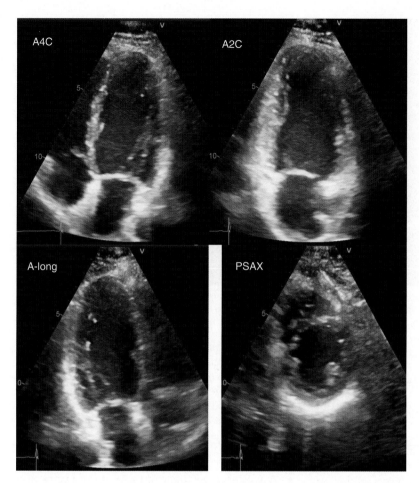

Fig. 8.6 **Baseline stress echo images.** The standard 2D views for stress echocardiography are the apical 4-chamber view *(A4C),* apical 2-chamber view *(A2C),* apical long-axis view *(A-long),* and parasternal short-axis view *(PSAX).* For both exercise and dobutamine stress, images are recorded in a cine loop quad-screen format, with rest and stress images shown side-by-side to allow comparison of the same myocardial segments. Several beats are acquired and the best image saved. The cine loop should only include systole (which is relatively constant in duration despite changes in heart rate) so that the rest and exercise images have the same timing. Depth and image position should be similar on baseline and stress image.

TABLE 8.1	Qualitative Scale for Assessment of Segmental Wall Motion on Echocardiography
Wall Motion	**Definition**
Normal	Normal endocardial inward motion and wall thickening in systole.
Hypokinesis	Reduced amplitude (<5 mm) and velocity of endocardial motion and wall thickening in systole. Delay in the onset of contraction and relaxation.
Akinesis	Absence of inward endocardial motion (<2 mm) or wall thickening in systole.
Dyskinesis	Outward motion or *bulging* of the segment in systole, usually associated with thin, scarred myocardium.
Aneurysmal	Diastolic contour abnormality and dyskinesis.

❑ If endocardial definition is suboptimal, left-sided echo contrast is used to improve evaluation of regional endocardial motion (Fig. 8.7).

❑ The ECG leads and gain are adjusted to show a clear signal with an adequate QRS height for accurate electrocardiography gating (Fig. 8.8).

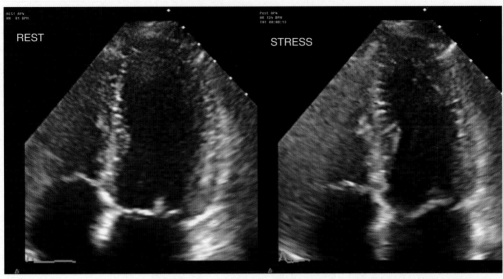

Fig. 8.7 Normal reduction in LV size with stress. As these end-systolic images at rest and peak stress in an apical 4-chamber view show, overall LV size normally decreases with stress due to a smaller diastolic LV volumes and increased endocardial motion of all segments.

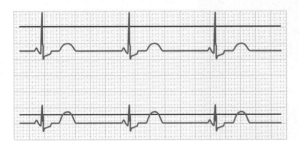

Fig. 8.8 Electrocardiographic triggering. Schematic of an appropriate electrocardiographic signal with little noise and a QRS height greater than the T wave, allowing accurate triggering for digital image acquisition and an example with the T wave equal in height to the QRS signal so that both signals will trigger image acquisition, resulting in very short cine loops that do not include the full cardiac cycle.

Step 3: Perform the Stress Protocol

❖ EXERCISE STRESS

- Any standard exercise protocol can be used with ECG and blood pressure monitoring.
- Upright treadmill exercise provides the highest workload, but images can only be obtained after exercise, so rapid image acquisition is essential.
- Supine bicycle exercise provides a lower workload, but images can be acquired during exercise using a dedicated stress echo stretcher and bicycle.

❖ KEY POINTS

- ❑ With treadmill exercise, ensure that the patient can move rapidly from the treadmill to the echo stretcher.
- ❑ In addition to echo images, the heart rate and blood pressure response to exercise, patient symptoms, arrhythmias, and ECG ST-segment changes are important clinical parameters (Fig. 8.9).

- ❑ The endpoint for a maximal exercise stress study is when the patient cannot exercise further due to shortness of breath, leg fatigue, or other symptoms.
- ❑ The exercise test also is stopped for any decline in blood pressure, significant arrhythmias, excessive increase in blood pressure, or significant ST-segment depression.

❖ DOBUTAMINE STRESS

- A typical dobutamine stress protocol begins at a does 5 μg/kg/min intravenously via a calibrated pump (if there are resting wall motion abnormalities) or 10 μg/kg/min, with an increase by 10 μg/kg/min every 3 minutes to a maximum dose of 40 μg/kg/min.
- Atropine in increments of 0.25 mg (maximum 1 mg total) may be added to achieve target heart rate, if needed.
- The primary endpoint is a heart rate 85% of the maximum predicted heart rate for age.
- Other endpoints include:
  - ○ Maximum dose allowed by the protocol
  - ○ Definite wall motion abnormality in two or more adjacent segments
  - ○ Systolic blood pressure less than 100 mm Hg or more than 200 mm Hg
  - ○ Diastolic blood pressure more than 120 mm Hg
  - ○ Significant arrhythmia
  - ○ Patient discomfort

❖ KEY POINTS

- ❑ Heart rate, blood pressure, electrocardiographic findings, and symptoms are monitored throughout the test.
- ❑ Maximum predicted heart rate is roughly 220 minus the patient's age.

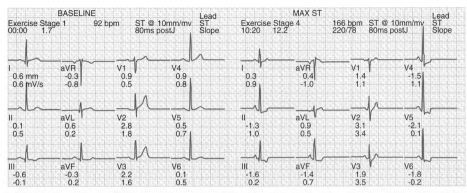

Fig. 8.9 **Exercise stress echocardiogram (ECG).** The 12-lead resting ECG leads are shown on the left and the stress ECG on the right. The numbers below each averaged ECG lead show the amount of ST depression (in mm) and the slope of the ST segment for each lead. In this 42-year-old man with multiple cardiac risk factors and chest pain symptoms, there is a 1.5- to 2-mm flat ST depression in the inferior and lateral leads consistent with myocardial ischemia.

TABLE 8.2	Patterns of Wall Motion With Dobutamine Stress Echo			
	Normal	**Ischemia**	**Stunned or Hibernating**	**Infarction**
Baseline	Normal	Normal	Hypokinetic or akinetic	Hypokinetic or akinetic
Low dose	Normal	Normal	Improved	Hypokinetic or akinetic
High dose	Hyperkinetic	Hypokinetic or akinetic	Hypokinetic or akinetic	Hypokinetic or akinetic

- ❑ About 10% of patients have a fall in blood pressure, which may necessitate ending the dobutamine infusion.
- ❑ ST-segment depression with dobutamine is not diagnostically useful. ST-segment elevation is rare but is predictive of significant coronary disease.
- ❑ Both ventricular and atrial arrhythmias may be precipitated by dobutamine and require prompt cessation of dobutamine infusion.
- ❑ When needed, the effects of dobutamine can be reversed with a rapidly acting IV beta blocker, such as esmolol or metoprolol.
- ❑ Improvement in wall motion at low-dose dobutamine of a myocardial segment that is abnormal at rest is evidence for myocardial viability.
- ❑ A biphasic response is when a myocardial segment that is abnormal at rest shows increased wall thickening at low-dose dobutamine (viability) and then worsening of wall motion at high dose (ischemia) (Table 8.2).

Step 4: Evaluate Regional and Global Left Ventricular Systolic Function at Peak Heart Rate

- Cine loop images of the ventricle are acquired at (or immediately after) peak stress using the same four image planes as the baseline images (see Fig. 8.6).
- The image depth, sector width, and electrocardiography gating on the stress images are the same as on the baseline images.
- Rest and exercise images are compared side-by-side in the cine loop format (Fig. 8.10).

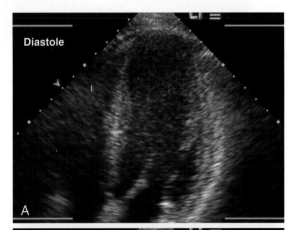
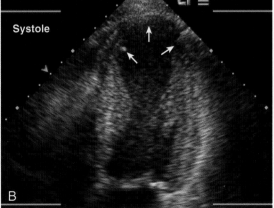

Fig. 8.10 **Inducible ischemia.** Resting myocardial wall motion was normal in this 56-year-old man with exertional chest discomfort. The immediate images after stress with the apical 4-chamber view at end-diastole (A) and end-systole (B) show akinesis of the apical lateral wall and inferior septum. These findings are consistent with inducible ischemia in the territory of the distal left anterior descending coronary artery.

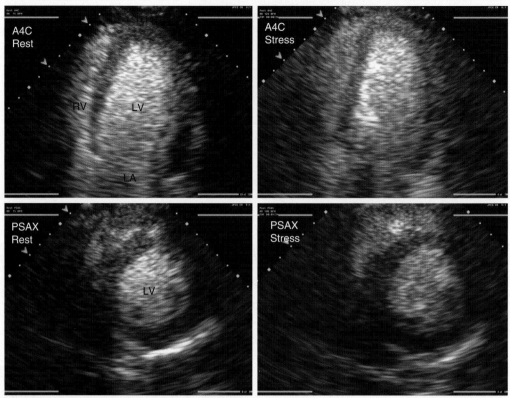

Fig. 8.11 **Multivessel coronary disease.** End-systolic images at rest *(left)* and stress *(right)* in an apical 4-chamber view *(A4C, top)* and parasternal short-axis view *(PSAX, bottom)* show little change in LV size from rest to peak stress despite reaching 90% of maximum predicted heart rate. Even though there was no regional wall motion abnormality, the failure of LV size to decrease and the absence of global hyperkinesis are strongly suggestive of multivessel coronary disease with balanced ischemia.

❖ **KEY POINTS**

❑ With exercise stress, the images are obtained as quickly as possible after exercise.

❑ With pharmacologic stress, images are acquired at each dosage stage, as well as at peak dose and heart rate.

❑ If endocardial definition is suboptimal, left-sided echo contrast is used to improve evaluation of regional endocardial motion.

❑ Several cine loops are quickly acquired in each view with subsequent selection of the best image to compare to the baseline images.

❑ Using electrocardiography gating and the same cine loop length for rest and exercise images results in the appearance of a similar timing of contraction on both images, which facilitates recognition of new wall motion abnormalities.

❑ The normal response to exercise or dobu-tamine stress is hyperkinesis of all segments with a decrease in ventricular chamber size (Fig. 8.11).

❑ Each myocardial segment is graded as hyper-kinetic, normal, hypokinetic, akinetic, or dyskinetic.

Step 5: Monitor Patient Recovery

■ The patient is monitored until all symptoms or wall motion abnormalities (if any) resolve and heart rate has returned to normal (<100 bpm).

■ If symptoms or wall motion abnormalities were seen at peak-dose dobutamine, heart rate may be slowed more rapidly with a short-acting beta blocker.

❖ **KEY POINTS**

❑ Ischemia is reversible so that stress-induced wall motion abnormalities quickly resolve as heart rate declines.

❑ Post-stress images are recorded to document that LV global and regional function has returned to baseline on completion of the study.

❑ If ischemia is induced, as evidenced by chest discomfort or wall motion abnormalities, a short-acting beta blocker (such as esmolol) is used to reduce heart rate and relieve symptoms.

Step 6: Review and Interpretation of the Stress Study

■ Baseline and stress echocardiographic images are reviewed in a side-by-side cine loop format using a systemic approach to grading wall motion for each myocardial segment.

■ The stress study interpretation depends on integration of clinical (symptoms, exercise duration), hemodynamic (blood pressure, heart rate), electrocardiographic (ST changes and arrhythmias), and ECG data.

❖ KEY POINTS

❑ The stress echo report includes the following minimal elements:
  ❑ Exercise duration or maximum dobutamine/atropine dose
  ❑ Heart rate and blood pressure at baseline and maximal stress
  ❑ ECG ST-segment changes or arrhythmias
  ❑ Symptoms
  ❑ Resting global and regional LV systolic function
  ❑ Global and regional LV systolic function at maximal stress
  ❑ Integration of these data to indicate study quality (images and maximum stress achieved), the likelihood of coronary disease, and the probable affected vessels
❑ The maximum stress achieved is a key element in interpretation; typically the study is considered nondiagnostic unless the maximum heart rate is at least 85% of the maximum predicted heart rate for that patient.
❑ An inducible wall motion abnormality is defined as hypokinesis or akinesis of a segment that was normal at rest. Failure of a normal segment to become hyperkinetic also is evidence of ischemia.
❑ ECG evidence of an inducible wall motion abnormality in one or more adjacent segments is consistent with coronary artery disease, with the probable affected coronary artery identified from the location of the wall motion abnormality (Fig. 8.12).
❑ With three-vessel coronary disease, instead of a regional wall motion abnormality, the only finding may be the absence of hyperkinesis and failure of ventricular size to decrease appropriately.
❑ Symptoms of chest discomfort accompanied by inducible wall motion abnormalities are consistent with ischemia; symptoms occurring simultaneously with normal regional function suggest noncardiac chest pain.

Acute Coronary Syndromes

Basic Principles

■ Acute coronary syndromes include patients with:
  ○ ST-segment elevation myocardial infarction (STEMI)
  ○ Non–ST-segment elevation myocardial infarction (NSTEMI)
  ○ Unstable angina (Table 8.3)

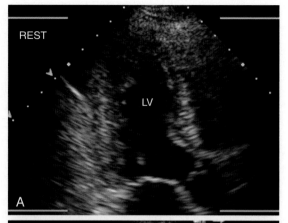
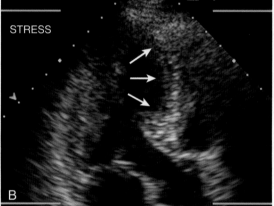

Fig. 8.12 **Abnormal exercise stress study.** Example of inducible ischemia with the apical long-axis view showing normal wall motion on this end-systolic image at rest (A), with akinesis of the mid and apical segments of the anterior septum with exercise stress (B, *arrows*).

■ Other causes of acute chest pain that require immediate intervention (Table 8.4) are:
  ○ Aortic dissection
  ○ Pericarditis
  ○ Pulmonary embolism

Step 1: Evaluate Regional Ventricular Function

■ A regional wall motion abnormality in a patient with chest pain indicates myocardial infarction or ischemia.
■ In a patient with prior coronary disease, it may be difficult to distinguish preexisting regional dysfunction from acute dysfunction.
■ Regional ventricular function may be normal between episodes of chest pain in patients with unstable angina.

❖ KEY POINTS

❑ Echocardiographic evaluation of wall motion is most helpful when ECG is nondiagnostic; prompt revascularization is appropriate in patients with STEMI.

TABLE 8.3   Coronary Artery Disease: Clinical-Echocardiographic Correlates

	Coronary Anatomy	Clinical Presentation	Echocardiographic Findings
Asymptomatic coronary disease	Coronary artery narrowing <70% Typically does not cause symptoms or myocardial ischemia	Stress echo may be requested in asymptomatic patients at high risk of coronary disease, for example, to assess risk before noncardiac surgery	A normal stress echo does not exclude atherosclerotic coronary disease but indicates a low likelihood of significant ischemia.
Chronic stable angina	Coronary stenosis ≥70% Narrowing may be asymptomatic at rest but causes symptoms with exertion	Typical angina on exertion	Normal resting LV regional and global systolic function. Stress echo shows inducible wall motion abnormalities in the distribution of the affected coronary artery.
Acute coronary syndrome	Coronary occlusion or severe stenosis with rupture of an atherosclerotic plaque and luminal thrombus	Acute chest pain Differential diagnosis includes aortic dissection, pericarditis, AS, HCM	Akinesis or hypokinesis of the myocardium supplied by the occluded vessel with normal wall thickness. With unstable angina, wall motion may be normal between pain episodes.
Old myocardial infarction	Occluded coronary with attenuated distal vessel, collateral vessels often are present	Asymptomatic if other coronary vessels are not stenosed Heart failure if significant LV dysfunction is present	Thinning increased echogenicity and akinesis in the distribution of the affected coronary artery. Ischemic MR may be present.
End-stage ischemic disease	Multiple old coronary occlusions, small distal vessels	Heart failure	Dilated LV with severely reduced ejection fraction. Areas of akinesis and areas of normal LV function are present. LV diastolic dysfunction. RV systolic function is normal, unless RV infarction is present. Ischemic MR may be present.

AS, Aortic stenosis; HCM, hypertrophic cardiomyopathy; MI, myocardial infarction; MR, mitral regurgitation.
From Otto CM: *Textbook of Clinical Echocardiography*, ed 6, Phidelphia, 2018, Elsevier.

TABLE 8.4   Medically Urgent Causes of Acute Chest Pain

Acute Coronary Syndrome
Acute ST-elevation myocardial infarction (STEMI)
Non–ST-elevation myocardial infarction (NSTEMI)
Unstable angina
Aortic dissection
Pulmonary embolus
Acute pericarditis
Esophageal rupture (Boerhaave syndrome)

□ A remote transmural myocardial infarction results in akinesis, myocardial thinning, and increased echogenicity, consistent with scar (Fig. 8.13).

□ However, with a prior NSTEMI or reperfused myocardial infarction, wall thickness may be relatively normal.

□ Normal regional myocardial function simultaneous with chest pain symptoms indicates a very low likelihood of an acute coronary syndrome.

Step 2: Estimate or Measure Ejection Fraction

■ Evaluation of overall LV systolic function is clinically useful in management of patients with acute chest pain.

■ Hospitalization and further evaluation often is needed in patients with a reduced ejection fraction, even when due to causes other than acute coronary syndrome.

❖ KEY POINTS

□ Measurement of ejection fraction using 3D volumetric imaging or the apical biplane approach is preferred when endocardial definition is adequate and there are no time constraints.

□ 3D volumetric imaging also allows analysis of regional wall motion (Figs. 8.14 and 8.15).

□ In urgent situations, a visual estimate of ejection fraction based on parasternal short-axis and apical 4-chamber, 2-chamber, and long-axis views is appropriate.

□ Left-sided echo contrast may be helpful for definition of both global and regional LV systolic function when image quality is suboptimal.

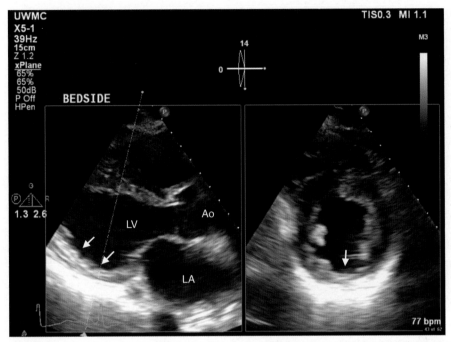

Fig. 8.13 **Myocardial infarction.** The inferior-lateral (posterior) wall is thinned, bright, and akinetic with biplane imaging in the parasternal long-axis *(left)* and short-axis *(right)* views.

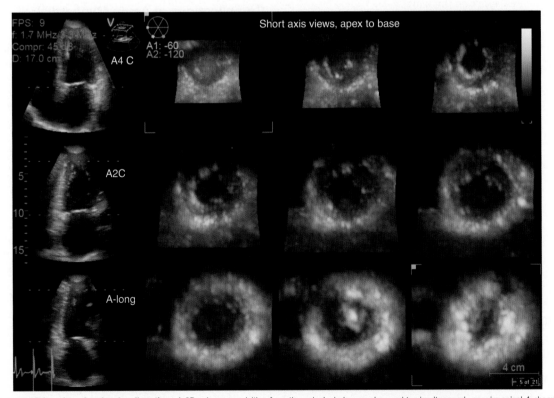

Fig. 8.14 **3D imaging of regional wall motion.** A 3D volume acquisition from the apical window can be used to simultaneously acquire apical 4-chamber *(A4C)*, apical 2-chamber *(A2C)*, and apical long-axis *(A-long)* views, as well as multiple reconstructed short-axis views of the LV for evaluation of wall motion.

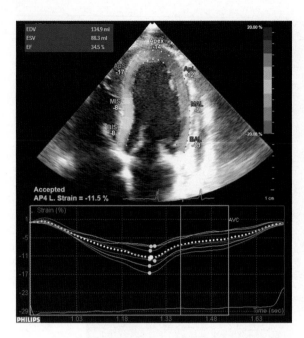

Fig. 8.15 **Longitudinal strain imaging in coronary disease.** Measurement of longitudinal strain in apical views provides another modality for evaluation of regional and global LV systolic function in patients with coronary disease. In this example, apical 4-chamber global longitudinal *(AP4 L)* strain is reduced (−11.55), and the colored coded lines shows heterogeneity in the degree and timing of regional function.

Step 3: Consider Alternate Causes of Chest Pain

- The echo may suggest other causes of chest pain when LV function is normal.
- Often additional imaging approaches are needed for further evaluation when the clinical diagnosis remains unclear.

❖ **KEY POINTS**

- ❏ Evidence of aortic dilation and aortic regurgitation in a patient with acute chest pain prompts further evaluation for aortic dissection by transesophageal echocardiography (TEE) or cardiac computed tomographic imaging.
- ❏ Although a pulmonary embolus is rarely visualized on echo, findings of pulmonary hypertension and right ventricle (RV) dilation or dysfunction suggest this diagnosis be considered.
- ❏ A pericardial effusion is consistent with the diagnosis of pericarditis but also may be seen with acute aortic dissection (with rupture into the pericardium) and with numerous systemic diseases (see Chapter 10).

Step 4: Evaluate Cardiac Hemodynamics

- Echo evaluation of cardiac hemodynamics is helpful in selected patients with acute chest pain.

❖ **KEY POINTS**

- ❏ Ischemia or infarction often is accompanied by diastolic dysfunction with evidence of elevated left atrial pressure on the Doppler LV and LA filling curves (see Chapter 7).
- ❏ Pulmonary pressures may be elevated due to elevated left-sided filling pressures.

- ❏ Cardiac output can be measured using the LV outflow tract diameter and flow velocity integral (see Chapter 6).

Complications of Acute Myocardial Infarction

- Echo provides rapid, accurate bedside diagnosis of mechanical complications of acute myocardial infarction (see the Echo Exam).
- Mechanical complications of myocardial infarction present as recurrent chest pain, new systolic murmur, heart failure, cardiogenic shock, or a systemic embolic event.
- Arrhythmias associated with acute myocardial infarction may occur in the absence of significant structural abnormalities.

Step 1: Evaluation of the Patient With Recurrent Chest Pain After Myocardial Infarction

- Recurrent chest pain after myocardial infarction may be due to recurrent ischemia, pericarditis, or noncardiac chest pain.
- ECG evaluation focuses on segmental wall motion and detection of a pericardial effusion.

❖ **KEY POINTS**

- ❏ Comparison of regional wall motion with previous studies may allow detection of recurrent ischemia in the peri-infarct region or in the distribution of a different coronary artery. However, coronary angiography often is needed for definitive diagnosis.
- ❏ The presence of a pericardial effusion is consistent with the diagnosis of pericarditis but also may be seen with acute aortic dissection (with rupture into the pericardium) or with LV rupture.

❑ LV rupture may present as transient chest pain; this diagnosis should be considered when pericardial effusion is present in a patient with a history of myocardial infarction, particularly if the episode of chest pain was accompanied by hypotension (Fig. 8.16).

Step 2: Evaluation of the Patient With a New Systolic Murmur After Myocardial Infarction

- The differential diagnosis of a new murmur that develops after myocardial infarction is:
  - Ventricular septal defect due to rupture of the septal myocardium, *or*
  - Acute mitral regurgitation (MR) due to papillary muscle rupture or dysfunction
- Imaging focuses on evaluation of segmental wall motion and detection of a pericardial effusion with Doppler evaluation for the cause of the murmur.

❖ **KEY POINTS**

❑ MR after myocardial infarction most often is due to ischemia or infarction of the papillary muscle or underlying inferior-lateral LV wall, resulting in "tethering" of the mitral leaflets with inadequate systolic coaptation (Fig. 8.17).

❑ With partial or complete papillary muscle rupture, acute severe MR occurs, with pulmonary edema and cardiogenic shock.

❑ TEE often is needed to define the mechanism and evaluate the severity of ischemic MR.

❑ Ventricular septal defects that develop after myocardial infarction are detected using color

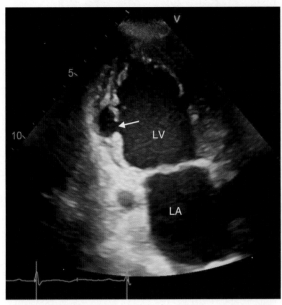

Fig. 8.16 LV rupture. In this patient with an inferior myocardial infarction, an area of discontinuity in the inferior wall *(arrow)* is seen in the apical 2-chamber view. Color Doppler showed flow into this small narrow-necked pseudo-aneurysm. The myocardial rupture is contained by pericardial adhesions, which form the wall of the pseudo-aneurysm.

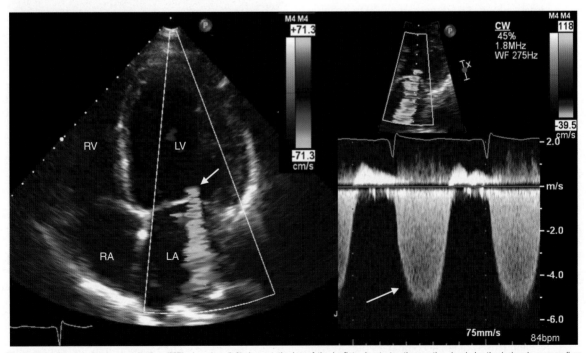

Fig. 8.17 Ischemic mitral regurgitation (MR). Imaging *(left)* shows tethering of the leaflets due to traction on the chords by the ischemic myocardium underlying the papillary muscle, resulting in a "tented" appearance of the closed valve at end-systole and central jet of MR *(arrow)* as the anterior leaflet fails to coapt completely with the relatively immobile posterior leaflet. CW Doppler *(right)* shows a dense signal of moderate regurgitation. Note that the aliasing velocity has been adjusted for vena contracta measurement.

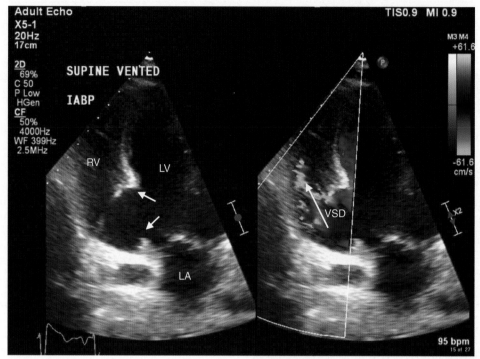

Fig. 8.18 LV pseudo-aneurysm and ventricular septal defect. This posteriorly angulated apical 4-chamber view shows a diastolic contour abnormality in the basal inferior septum with an abrupt discontinuity *(short arrows)* between normal myocardial and the dilated segment consistent with an inferior pseudo-aneurysm. However, instead of rupture into the pericardial space, the rupture is into the RV with color Doppler demonstrating a large jet of flow *(long arrow)* across the ventricular septal defect (VSD).

Doppler showing a flow disturbance on the RV side of the septum. Often the defect can be visualized on two-dimensional (2D) imaging. Continuous-wave (CW) Doppler interrogation provides information on the LV-to-RV systolic pressure difference (Fig. 8.18).

❑ With a ventricular septal defect, oxygen saturation is increased from the right atrium (RA) to the RV due to shunting of oxygenated blood from the LV to RV across the ventricular defect. If a right-sided heart catheter is in position, measurement of oxygen saturations may be helpful when the diagnosis is unclear.

Step 3: Evaluation of the Patient With Hypotension or Cardiogenic Shock After Myocardial Infarction

■ Hypotension after myocardial infarction may be due to RV infarction, LV systolic dysfunction, or myocardial rupture with pericardial tamponade.

■ Echocardiographic evaluation focuses on evaluation of global left and RV systolic function and detection of a pericardial effusion.

❖ KEY POINTS

❑ RV infarction often accompanies an inferior myocardial infarction. The typical presentation is hypotension that responds to volume loading. Echo shows a dilated hypocontractile RV, despite normal pulmonary pressures (Fig. 8.19).

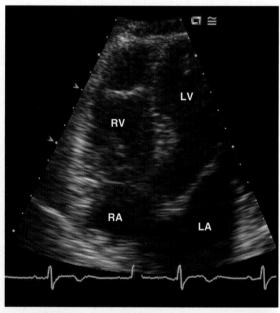

Fig. 8.19 RV infarction. RV dilation and (in real time) hypokinesis in a patient with an inferior myocardial infarction is seen in this apical 4-chamber view.

❑ With a large or recurrent myocardial infarction, LV systolic function may be significantly reduced, resulting in pulmonary edema and hypotension. Echo allows measurement (or estimation) of ejection fraction and assessment of regional ventricular function.

- Myocardial ischemia or infarction is typically accompanied by diastolic dysfunction, often with elevated LV filling pressures. Diastolic dysfunction may lead to pulmonary congestion but rarely is the primary cause of hypotension.
- LV rupture due to myocardial infarction may result in acute cardiac tamponade and death. However, in some cases the myocardial rupture is contained by a pericardial thrombus and adhesions.
- A contained LV rupture is called a *pseudo-aneurysm*, because its wall consists of pericardium (not myocardium) (Fig. 8.20).
- Typical characteristics of a pseudo-aneurysm are a narrow neck compared with its widest diameter and an abrupt transition at an acute angle between the normal myocardium and the aneurysm. Often the pseudo-aneurysm is lined with thrombus.
- Most pseudo-aneurysms require urgent surgical intervention to repair the ventricular rupture. True aneurysms typically are treated medically.

Step 4: Evaluation of Late Complications of Myocardial Infarction

- Late complications of myocardial infarction include LV aneurysm, thrombus, and systolic dysfunction.
- Echocardiographic examination includes evaluation of global and regional myocardial function, calculation of ejection fraction, assessment of diastolic dysfunction, and a diligent search for apical thrombus.

❖ KEY POINTS

- Adverse ventricular remodeling after myocardial infarction results in thinning and scar formation in areas of infarction, overall LV dilation, and a reduction in ejection fraction. Adverse remodeling is prevented, to some extent, by appropriate medical therapy.
- The myocardial thickness in diastole, wall thickening during systole, and endocardial motion are graded for each myocardial segment.
- An aneurysm is defined as a discrete area of the LV (usually the apex) with a diastolic contour abnormality and systolic dyskinesis (Fig. 8.21).
- LV ejection fraction is calculated using the biplane apical approach. Single plane or M-mode evaluation of LV function may be inaccurate due to regional ventricular dysfunction.
- Apical thrombus is best visualized in standard and oblique apical views. Identification of thrombus is enhanced by use of a higher-frequency transducer and a shallow image depth (Fig. 8.22).
- Apical trabeculation is distinguished from thrombus by the lack of mobility, linear appearance, and attachments to the LV wall.
- Left-sided ultrasound contrast may be helpful when it is difficult to distinguish apical trabeculation from thrombi (Fig. 8.23).

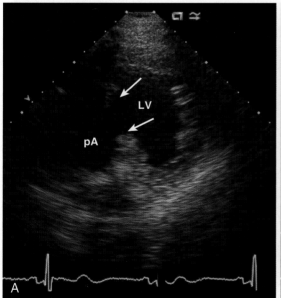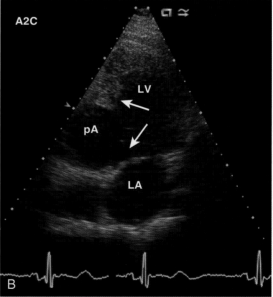

Fig. 8.20 Chronic LV pseudo-aneurysm. Characteristics include a narrow neck *(arrows)* relative to the maximum diameter of the pseudo-aneurysm, as seen in a short-axis view of the LV (A) and in the apical 2-chamber view (B). There is an abrupt transition from the normal myocardial thickness to the aneurysm, and the pseudo-aneurysm has an irregular echodensity consistent with thrombus lining the cavity. *A2C,* Apical 2-chamber; *pA,* pseudo-aneurysm.

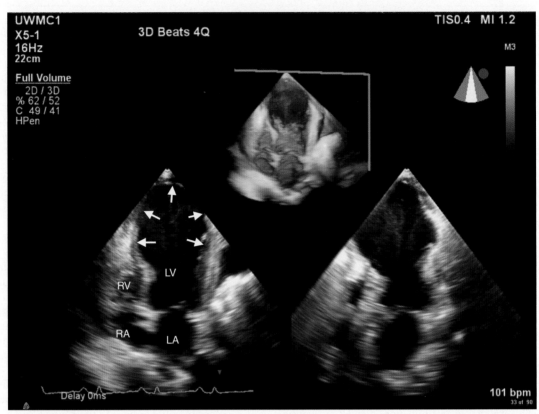

Fig. 8.21 **Apical aneurysm.** A true aneurysm is characterized by a diastolic contour abnormality with a gradual, smooth transition from normal myocardial thickness to the thin scarred myocardium of the aneurysm and with systolic dyskinesis as shown by the *arrows* in the apical 4-chamber (A4C) *(left)* with the and 2-chamber (A2C) view shown on the *right* and the full volume acquisition in the *center.*

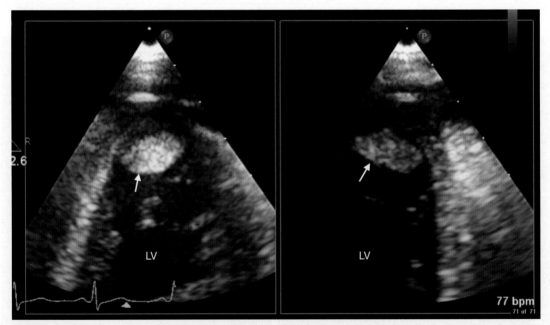

Fig. 8.22 **Apical thrombus.** This apical echodensity *(arrow)* that protrudes into the chamber in an area of dyskinesis is consistent with an apical thrombus. Biplane imaging in a zoomed view *(left)* using a high-frequency transducer and an oblique image plane through the apex *(right)* helps confirm that these echoes represent a thrombus, and not prominent trabeculation or an imaging artifact.

End-Stage Ischemic Disease

- End-stage ischemic disease, colloquially called *ischemic cardiomyopathy*, has many features in common with a dilated cardiomyopathy or ventricular

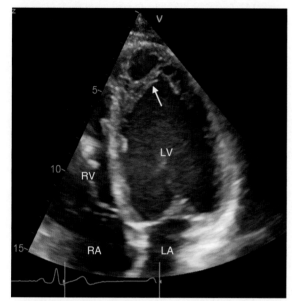

Fig. 8.23 Apical trabeculation. The apical trabeculation *(arrow)* seen in this apical 4-chamber view is distinguished from thrombus by similar echodensity to myocardium, a linear structure that connects to the myocardium at both ends and the absence of an underlying wall motion abnormality.

dysfunction due to valvular heart disease (see the Echo Exam at the end of the chapter).

- The echocardiographic features most helpful in diagnosis of end-stage ischemic disease are:
  - Definite regional wall motion abnormalities with areas of thinning and akinesis (Fig. 8.24)
  - Normal RV size and systolic function (unless RV infarction has occurred)
  - Absence of evidence for primary valvular heart disease

Step 1: Evaluate Global Left Ventricular Systolic and Diastolic Function

- Overall LV systolic function is evaluated by calculation of an apical biplane ejection fraction.
- LV diastolic function is evaluated as described in Chapter 7.

  ❖ **KEY POINTS**

  ❑ Calculation of a biplane ejection fraction is performed whenever possible. If endocardial definition is suboptimal, left-sided contrast echo provides better visualization of LV function.

  ❑ Most patients with end-stage ischemia disease have diastolic dysfunction, as well as systolic dysfunction.

  ❑ Early in the disease course, diastolic dysfunction is characterized by impaired relaxation.

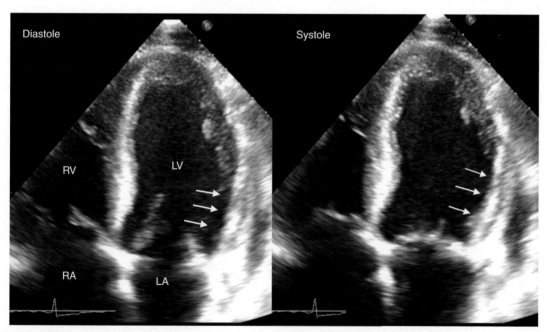

Fig. 8.24 End-stage ischemic disease. In an apical 4-chamber view, the LV chamber is dilated with severely reduced systolic function. The inferior septal and apical ½ of the lateral wall are severely hypokinetic, with an overall ejection fraction of 24%. However, the cause of LV dysfunction is coronary disease, not a dilated cardiomyopathy, because the basal ½ of the lateral wall is thin, echodense, and akinetic *(arrows)*, which is consistent with transmural infarction and scar formation. The apical 2-chamber view showed relatively normal endocardial motion and wall thickening of the basal ⅔ of the anterior wall and anterior septum, confirming regional dysfunction in a pattern consistent with coronary artery disease.

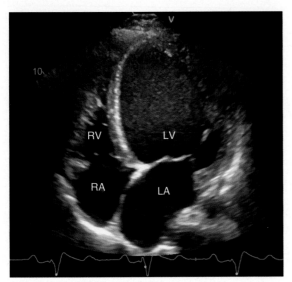

Fig. 8.25 **Normal RV with ischemic disease.** In patients with heart failure due to end-stage ischemic disease, RV size and systolic function often are normal (unless concurrent RV infarction has occurred). Compared with the dilated and hypokinetic LV, the normal RV appears relatively small and hyperdynamic.

□ However, as systolic function deteriorates, LV filling pressures may increase, LV compliance decreases, and the increased ventricular volumes result in a rightward shift along the LV diastolic pressure-volume curve.

Step 2: Evaluate Regional Left Ventricular Systolic Function

■ Regional function is evaluated by grading each myocardial segment as normal, hypokinetic, akinetic, or dyskinetic.
■ Any areas of thin, scarred myocardium are noted.

❖ **KEY POINTS**

□ A discrete area of scarring or dyskinesis is consistent with coronary disease, rather than a primary cardiomyopathy.
□ In both end-stage ischemic disease and primary cardiomyopathy, ventricular function typically is best preserved for the inferior-lateral and lateral basal segments of the LV.
□ LV global and regional strain measurements may be helpful in evaluation of end-stage ischemic disease.

Step 3: Evaluate Right Ventricular Size and Systolic Function

■ RV size and systolic function are qualitatively evaluated as discussed in Chapter 6.
■ RV systolic function typically is normal in patients with end-stage ischemic disease, so that the RV appears small and hypercontractile compared with the dilated, hypokinetic LV (Fig. 8.25).

❖ **KEY POINTS**

□ When the RV is proportionate to the LV, the degree of RV dilation is similar to the degree of LV dilation.
□ When RV systolic function appears similar to LV function, the degree of dysfunction is the same for both ventricles.
□ RV function may be impaired in patients with coronary disease and a prior RV infarction.

Step 4: Estimate Cardiac Hemodynamics

■ Pulmonary artery systolic pressure is estimated from the velocity of the tricuspid regurgitant jet and the appearance and respiratory variation of the inferior vena cava, as discussed in Chapter 6.
■ Evidence for elevated left atrial pressure includes a prolonged and high-velocity pulmonary vein a-wave reversal and a high ratio of transmitral flow to tissue Doppler velocity in early diastole (see Chapter 7).

❖ **KEY POINTS**

□ Pulmonary pressures may be elevated due to LV dysfunction, leading to chronic elevation of LA pressure and consequent pulmonary hypertension.
□ Evidence for elevated filling pressures may no longer be present after optimization of medical therapy.

Step 5: Identify and Evaluate Any Associated Valve Disease

■ LV dilation and systolic dysfunction due to chronic valve disease may be difficult to distinguish from a primary cardiomyopathy or end-stage ischemic heart disease.
■ LV systolic dysfunction of any cause often is accompanied by significant mitral valve regurgitation due to displacement of the papillary muscle, leaflet tethering, and annular dilation.

❖ **KEY POINTS**

□ Primary mitral valve disease is characterized by abnormalities of the valve leaflets or chordae—for example, myxomatous or rheumatic valve disease.
□ With secondary MR, the mitral valve apparatus is anatomically normal, but geometric relationships are altered by the dilated LV.
□ MR due to ischemic heart disease may improve with medical or interventional approaches for relief of ischemia.
□ Coronary angiography may be needed to determine the contribution of coronary disease to the clinical cardiac dysfunction.

THE ECHO EXAM: CORONARY ARTERY DISEASE

Echocardiographic Diagnosis of Coronary Disease

Modality	Clinical Utility	Echocardiographic Findings	Recording	Interpretation
Resting regional wall motion	• Acute coronary syndrome • Chronic CAD	• Akinesis or hypokinesis of infarcted or acutely ischemic regions	• 2D or 3D imaging of the LV. • Optimize endocardial definition. • Use contrast if images are suboptimal.	• Use standard wall segment nomenclature for location. • Categorize wall motion as normal, hypo- or akinetic. • Use 3D display when possible.
Exercise stress echocardiography	• Diagnosis of CAD • Evaluation for ischemia with known CAD	• Normal wall motion at rest • Hypokinesis or akinesis with stress in ischemic segments • Return of normal wall motion with rest	• Depth that includes only LV, optimize endocardial definition, use contrast if needed. • Same depth as baseline, optimize endocardial definition, use contrast if needed. • Select optimal image from series of digital cine loops.	• Include exercise duration, blood pressure and heart rate response, symptoms, and ECG changes in report. • Compare baseline and stress images in same views. • Maximal work load affects accuracy of echo results for detection of ischemia.
Dobutamine stress echocardiography	• Diagnosis and evaluation of CAD in patients unable to exercise	• Normal wall motion at rest • Hypokinesis or akinesis with stress in ischemic segments • Return of normal wall motion with rest	• Depth that includes only LV, optimize endocardial definition, use contrast if needed. • Same depth as baseline, optimize endocardial definition, use contrast if needed. • Select optimal image from series of digital cine loops.	• Include symptoms and peak heart rate as percent of maximum predicted in report. • Blood pressure response and ECG changes are not diagnostic for CAD. • Compare baseline and stress images in same views. • Maximal work load affects accuracy of echo results for detection of ischemia.
Myocardial viability	• Diagnosis of hibernating or stunned myocardium	• Biphasic response on DSE	• Standard DSE protocol with additional low dose stages	• Improvement in wall thickening at low dose followed by ischemia at high dose. • DSE is consistent with viable myocardium supplied by a stenosed vessel.
Overall LV systolic function	• All CAD patients	• Ejection fraction by 2D and 3D imaging • dP/dt	• 3D biplane apical ejection fraction • CWD mitral regurgitant jet	• The degree of reduction in EF after acute MI depends on infarct size and success of reperfusion.
LV diastolic function	• All CAD patients	• Diastolic dysfunction and elevated filling pressures depend on type and severity of CAD	• Standard approaches to evaluation of LV diastolic function and filling pressures (see Chapter 7)	• Transient diastolic dysfunction with ischemia. • End-stage CAD is associated with severe diastolic dysfunction.

CAD, Coronary artery disease; *DSE*, dobutamine stress echocardiography; *ECG*, electrocardiogram; *EF*, ejection fraction; *MI*, myocardial infarction.

Complications of Acute Myocardial Infarction

Complication	Echocardiographic Findings	Imaging Approach
Pericardial effusion	• Small circumferential pericardial effusion	• Standard views for evaluation of effusion • Larger effusion raises concern for LV rupture
RV infarction	• Dilated hypo- or akinetic RV • Infarction of adjacent inferior LV wall	• Apical and subcostal views to evaluate RV free wall motion • Measure TAPSE, DTI S-velocity, fractional area change
Ischemic MR	• Tethering of posterior leaflet with posteriorly directed MR • Papillary muscle rupture (rare) with mass attached to flail leaflet • Moderate to severe MR (may be intermittent, present only during ischemic episodes)	• Evaluate mitral valve anatomy in standard views • Evaluate and quantitate mitral regurgitant severity (see Chapter 12) • TEE and 3D imaging often needed to identify cause of MR
Ventricular septal defect	• Discrete septal defect in area of akinesis with left to right flow seen on color and CW Doppler	• Use color Doppler to detect VSD in focal region of akinesis or when imaging suggests discontinuity in septum • CW Doppler confirms velocity and direction of blood flow
Free wall rupture and tamponade	• Large pericardial effusion with tamponade • Acute fatal event unless temporarily sealed by fibrinous pericardial adhesions	• Pericardial hematoma or localized effusion after MI should be promptly reported to referring MD • Use color Doppler to search for communication from LV to pericardial space; subcostal views helpful
LV pseudoaneurysm	• Abrupt transition from normal myocardium to aneurysm • Acute angle between myocardium and aneurysm • Narrow neck • Ratio of neck diameter to aneurysm diameter <0.5 • Often lined with thrombus	• Most often located at inferior base of LV • Parasternal views and apical 2-chamber views are helpful • TEE imaging often needed for diagnosis
LV aneurysm	• Thin, bright, dyskinetic LV segment with a diastolic contour abnormality • Often with associated thrombus	• Most often located at LV apex • Best seen in apical views or with 3D imaging from apex
LV thrombus	• Echogenic mass, distinct from myocardium, often protruding into the chamber, with underlying akinesis, typically at the apex	• Use high frequency transducer, zoom mode, adjust gain and instrument settings; off-axis lateral apical views are helpful • Contrast to opacify the LV better demonstrates the thrombus • Apical thrombi may be missed on TEE
LV systolic dysfunction	• Location and size of the regional wall motion abnormalities correspond to infarct size • Overall ejection fraction also reflects adverse LV remodeling	• 3D or 2D biplane ejection fraction calculations

DTI, Doppler tissue imaging; *TAPSE*, tricuspid annular plane systolic excursion; *MR*, mitral regurgitation; *VSD*, ventricular septal defect.

Coronary Anatomy and Echo Wall Segments

Coronary Artery	Echo Wall Segments	Variations
Left anterior descending (LAD)	Anterior septum Anterior wall Apex	Diagonal branches of the LAD may supply some segments of the lateral wall. Extension of the LAD around the LV apex is variable.
Circumflex (Cx)	Anterior-lateral wall Posterior-lateral wall	The number and distribution of obtuse marginal branches supplying the lateral wall is variable.
Posterior descending artery (PDA)	Inferior wall Inferior septum	The PDA arises from the right coronary in about 80% of patients. Length of the PDA is variable, extending to the apex in some patients. An LV extension branch from the PDA may supply parts of the lateral wall.

Differentiation of Left Ventricular Systolic Dysfunction Due to End-Stage Ischemic Disease from Dilated Cardiomyopathy or Chronic Valvular Disease

Findings	End-Stage Ischemic Disease	Dilated Cardiomyopathy	Chronic Valvular Disease
Left-ventricular ejection fraction	Moderate-severely depressed	Moderate-severely depressed	Moderate-severely depressed
Segmental wall motion abnormalities	May be present	Absent	Absent
RV systolic function	Normal	Decreased	Variable
Pulmonary artery pressures	Elevated	Elevated	Elevated
Mitral regurgitation	Moderate	Moderate	Moderate-severe
Aortic regurgitation	Not significant	Not significant	Moderate-severe

SELF-ASSESSMENT QUESTIONS

Question 1

A 56-year-old woman with no medical history presents with precordial chest discomfort and dyspnea. Blood pressure is 86/50 mm Hg with a heart rate of 115 bpm. Physical examination reveals jugular venous distention and bibasilar lung crackles. There is a systolic murmur at the cardiac apex radiating toward the left axilla. TTE reveals a hypokinetic inferior wall with an ejection fraction of 40%. There is moderate, posteriorly directed mitral regurgitation (MR). The tricuspid regurgitant jet velocity is 3.4 m/s and the inferior vena cava diameter measures 2.1 cm with minimal inspiratory collapse. You suspect myocardial ischemia in which coronary distribution?

A. Anterior septal perforator
B. Left circumflex artery
C. Posterior descending artery
D. Left anterior descending artery

Question 2

Which of the following is the earliest manifestation of myocardial ischemia detectable during stress echo?

A. Anginal chest discomfort
B. ECG ischemic changes
C. Regional coronary hypoperfusion
D. Segmental wall motion abnormality

Question 3

You are evaluating a 64-year-old man who had an anterior myocardial infarction and underwent placement of a drug-eluting stent in his left anterior descending artery 1 week ago. He was discharged home on aspirin, clopidogrel, a beta blocker, and a statin medication. He presents now with dyspnea and the following image is obtained (Fig. 8.26). What do you refer the patient for next?

A. Repeat coronary angiogram
B. Pericardiocentesis
C. Pulmonary angiogram
D. Intra-aortic balloon pump

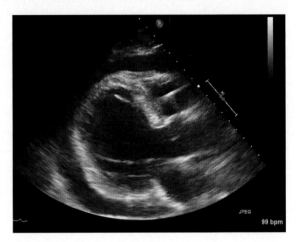

Fig. 8.26

Question 4

A 62-year-old man presents with progressive dyspnea. The following apical 2-chamber view is obtained on TTE (Fig. 8.27). The image is most consistent with:

  A. Myocardial rupture
  B. Chagas disease
  C. Cardiac sarcoidosis
  D. LV aneurysm
  E. Endomyocardial fibrosis

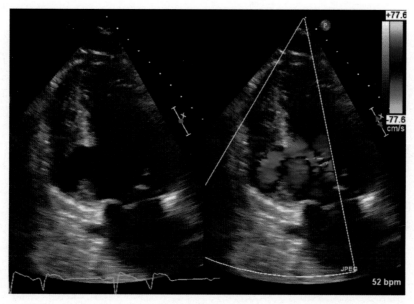

Fig. 8.27

Question 5

A 71-year-old man presented with recurrent ventricular tachycardia. He had a history of myocardial infarction 1 year prior from an occluded posterior descending artery. Parasternal long-axis views in diastole and systole (Fig. 8.28) demonstrate which abnormality?

  A. Pericardial hematoma
  B. Ventricular aneurysm
  C. Ischemic inferolateral wall
  D. Papillary muscle rupture

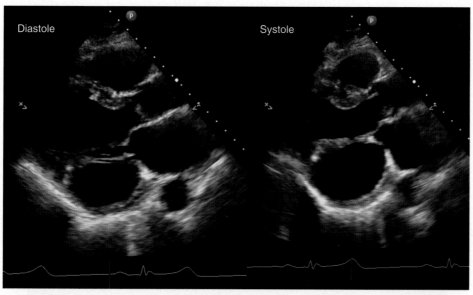

Fig. 8.28

Question 6

A 29-year-old woman underwent transthoracic echo-cardiography for palpitations. She had a normal elec-trocardiogram (ECG). A parasternal short axis with slight superior angulation at the level of the aorta and pulsed-wave (PW) Doppler sampled in the region of the asterisk (*) is shown (Fig. 8.29). This image and Doppler flow is most consistent with:

A. Anomalous left main coronary artery
B. Ventricular septal defect
C. Aortic abscess
D. Ventricular pseudoaneurysm
E. Posteriorly directed circumflex of the right coronary artery

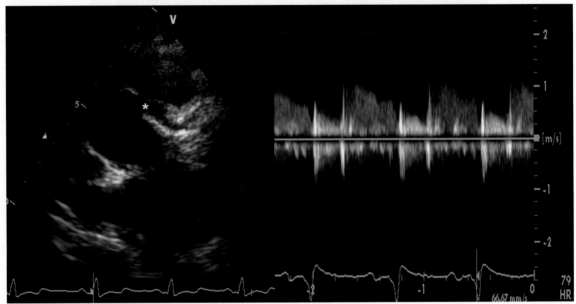

Fig. 8.29

Question 7

A 63-year-old woman had dyspnea on exertion and lower extremity edema 2 months after a myocardial infarction from an occluded distal right coronary artery. An echocardiogram was performed. Based on end-diastole and systole (Fig. 8.30) apical images, the most likely diagnosis is which of the following?

A. Apical aneurysm
B. Ruptured papillary muscle
C. Ventricular septal defect
D. RV infarction
E. Secondary mitral regurgitation

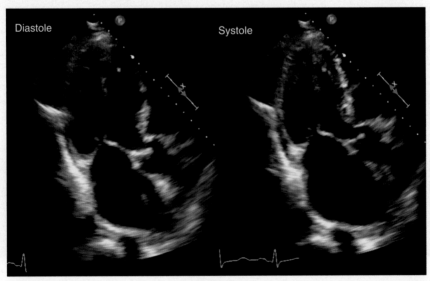

Fig. 8.30

Question 8

A 68-year-old woman presents to the emergency department with precordial chest discomfort that developed suddenly during a protracted argument with her estranged son. The patient has hypertension and is a nonsmoker. Physical examination reveals flat neck veins. Her blood pressure is 158/98 mm Hg. Her lungs are clear and no murmurs are heard. The ECG shows diffuse ST-elevation and her troponin is mildly elevated at 2.5 ng/mL (normal <0.5 ng/mL) with a normal B-type natriuretic peptide level. What would likely be seen on transthoracic imaging?

- **A.** RV free wall hypokinesis
- **B.** Basal segment hyperkinesis
- **C.** Inter-ventricular septal dyskinesis
- **D.** Apical segment hyperkinesis

Question 9

You are asked to evaluate a 68-year-old man who presented to the neurology service following a left middle cerebral artery stroke. Past medical history includes a left anterior descending coronary distribution myocardial infarct 4 weeks ago, and the patient underwent stent placement. TTE is completed (Fig. 8.31). You refer the patient for:

- **A.** Initiation of vitamin K antagonist
- **B.** Patent foramen ovale closure
- **C.** Surgical pseudoaneurysm repair
- **D.** Cardiac magnetic resonance imaging

Question 10

A 70-year-old woman with chest pain and bilateral hip-arthritis is referred for dobutamine stress echocardiography. At baseline the patient's blood pressure was 110/70 mm Hg and heart rate 65 beats per minute. The baseline electrocardiogram (ECG) showed normal sinus rhythm with non-specific ST changes. After 3 minutes at an infusion dose of 20 μg/kg/min, the patient's heart rate is 75% of the patient's maximum predicted heart and blood pressure is 120/60 mm Hg. The ECG shows rare premature ventricular contractions with 0.5 mm ST depression. Wall motion remains normal. Which of the following is the next best step?

- **A.** End the study because target heart rate has been reached.
- **B.** Terminate the study due to the inadequate increase in blood pressure
- **C.** Increase the dobutamine dose.
- **D.** Stop the study due to ECG findings.
- **E.** Ask the patient to do side leg raises.

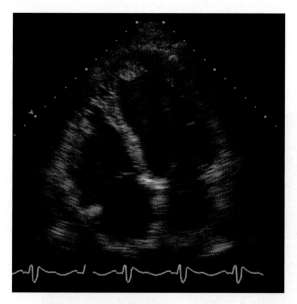

Fig. 8.31

Question 11

A 58-year-old man is preparing for hospital discharge following a myocardial infarct. He had presented with stuttering chest discomfort over 3 to 4 days and subsequently received a drug-eluting stent in the right coronary artery. Before discharge, TTE is completed. Images from the short-axis view are shown (Fig. 8.32). Based on the images provided, which of the following additional findings would you expect on the echocardiogram?

A. Pulmonary to systemic shunt ratio = 2.4
B. Septal E' velocity = 0.1 m/s
C. Tricuspid regurgitant velocity = 2.1 m/s
D. Wall motion score index = 1

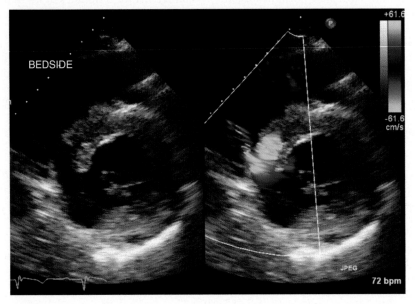

Fig. 8.32

Question 12

A 68-year-old man presents for dobutamine stress echo. Image quality was not optimal and transpulmonary microbubble contrast was used. Resting LV function is normal with an ejection fraction of 60%. The end-systolic images in the apical 4-chamber view at rest (Fig. 8.33A) and at peak dobutamine infusion (see Fig. 8.33B) are presented. The LV response to dobutamine in this case is best described as:

A. Akinetic
B. Biphasic
C. Hyperdynamic
D. Tethered

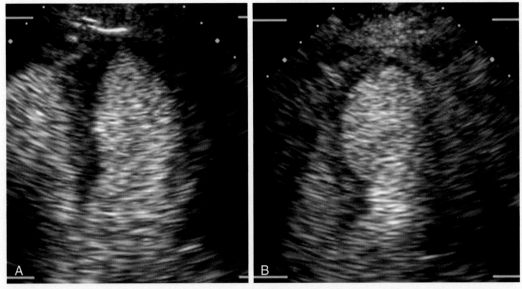

Fig. 8.33

ANSWERS

Answer 1: C

This patient's clinical presentation (with cardiogenic shock, chest discomfort, and echocardiographic findings) is consistent with an acute coronary syndrome. The patient has inferior wall motion abnormalities and significant mitral regurgitation (MR). MR coincident with ischemia suggests papillary muscle dysfunction, which would correlate with dyspnea. The posteromedial papillary muscle is typically supplied by a single coronary artery, the posterior descending artery. Ischemia and dysfunction of the posteromedial papillary muscle tethers the posterior leaflet, resulting in posteriorly directed MR. In this patient, ischemia has involved the RV as well, exacerbating hemodynamic instability. In contrast, the anterolateral papillary muscle is typically supplied by both the left anterior descending and left circumflex arteries, making it less susceptible to ischemia. The septal perforator arteries do not supply the papillary muscles.

Answer 2: C

The sequential progression of myocardial ischemia during stress echo is initiated by relative regional hypoperfusion distal to a coronary occlusion provoked by increased myocardial oxygen demand. With regional hypoperfusion, metabolic changes occur within the affected myocardium. Following this, there are alterations in LV diastolic function. With continued ischemia, there is impaired systolic function in the ischemic region. Only with prolonged ischemia are characteristic ECG changes, such as horizontal ST depression, and onset of typical angina. On a standard stress echo, regional coronary hypoperfusion cannot be visualized so the earliest change seen is segmental wall motion abnormalities. Although evaluation of diastolic function during stress echo is conceptually possible, practical application of diastolic interrogation is difficult to routinely implement.

Answer 3: B

The parasternal long-axis view shows a moderate circumferential pericardial effusion. This was a new effusion that developed after the infarction. An inflammatory pericardial effusion may complicate myocardial infarction and typically presents several days after the infarct. The patient is symptomatic (dyspnea) with rapid accumulation of fluid in a relatively short time frame. Additional spectral Doppler imaging showed respiratory variation in tricuspid and mitral inflow, as well as increased central venous pressure. He was referred for pericardiocentesis with drainage of 1100 mL of clear fluid and resolution of symptoms.

Answer 4: A

The apical 2-chamber view shows myocardial discontinuity at the base of the inferior wall. The echolucency in this region is a contained myocardial rupture (pseudoaneurysm). This is a late complication of myocardial infarction and is most common in the basal inferior wall following a right coronary artery distribution infarction. Because an LV pseudoaneurysm is an LV rupture that has been contained by pericardium, prompt surgical intervention is needed. Extension of necrotic tissue to the inferior septum may also lead to rupture of the interventricular septum and a septal defect. This is in contrast to true LV aneurysms, with myocardial thinning and dilation, but with preserved myocardial continuity. The walls of a true LV aneurysm are thinned and scarred myocardium (not pericardium as with a pseudoaneurysm), and there is a smooth transition from normal to infarcted myocardium with a wide neck of the aneurysm. Chagas disease is a cause of nonischemic cardiomyopathy, most commonly seen in Latin America; a clinical manifestation of Chagas disease is LV apical aneurysm formation. The inflammatory lesions in cardiac sarcoid typically occur in a noncoronary distribution, predominantly in the endocardium of the anteroseptum and apex of the LV, with focal hypokinesis of affected regions. Endomyocardial fibrosis is characterized by fibrosis of the left and/or right apices (with akinesis or dyskinesis), often with associated apical thrombi.

Answer 5: B

The patient has a LV aneurysm of the inferolateral wall as a complication of posterior myocardial infarction. There is a diastolic contour abnormality in the inferolateral wall which demonstrates thinning and dyskinesis when compared to the anteroseptal wall during systole. LV aneurysm can be a late complication of acute myocardial infarction and be associated with ventricular tachycardia. Pericardial hematoma (answer A) would be an acute complication from free wall rupture that would demonstrate pericardial echogenic fluid and discontinuity of the ventricular wall. An ischemic wall would demonstrate a hypokinetic wall segment with reduced amplitude and wall thickening, not dyskinesis with enlargement of the ventricular cavity. Papillary muscle rupture is a complication of acute inferior and posterior myocardial infarctions but has an acute presentation with decompensated heart failure and shock. The papillary muscle and chordae mitral valve attachments are intact in the figure.

Answer 6: A

The patient has anomalous ostia of a left main coronary artery with an anterior take-off that traverses anteriorly around the aortic valve. The ostia of the right and left main coronary arteries can be directly visualized with echocardiography, but the origin and course of this vessel do not follow normal anatomy (see Figs. 8.2 and 8.3). The pulsed-wave (PW) demonstrates flow velocity primarily in diastole consistent with coronary flow. The location is too superior for a ventricular septal defect (answer B), which would have more prominent systolic velocities. An aortic abscess (answer C) can appear adjacent to the aortic valve and aorta as an echolucent structure. However, the clinical scenario is not consistent with aortic valve endocarditis and flow is usually not detected in an abscess cavity. A ventricular pseudoaneurysm (answer D) has bidirectional flow and would be more inferior in location. A more common anomalous coronary artery variant with the circumflex traveling posterior from the right coronary artery (answer E) would be posterior to the aorta.

Answer 7: E

Fig. 8.30 shows an akinetic inferolateral wall with incomplete coaptation of the mitral valve due to leaflet tethering. Secondary mitral regurgitation (MR) from inferior myocardial infarction is frequently posteriorly directed (Fig. 8.34) and associated with left atrial enlargement. MR may be due to papillary muscle dysfunction, abnormalities in wall motion, or less commonly papillary muscle rupture. A papillary muscle rupture (answer B) would demonstrate a flail leaflet with papillary muscle tissue in the LA during systole. (See Fig. 8.23 in Otto CM: *Textbook of Clinical Echocardiography*, ed 6, Philadelphia, 2018, Elsevier.)

Apical aneurysm (answer A) or a ventricular septal defect (answer C) may be seen in anterior myocardial infarctions, but Fig. 8.30 demonstrates normal systolic anteroseptal and apical motion with inward endocardial movement and wall thickening. A RV infarction (answer D) may occur from a proximal right coronary occlusion proximal to the RV marginal branches, the RV is not well evaluated in an apical long-axis view.

Answer 8: B

This woman's presentation is consistent with stress cardiomyopathy, an acute cardiac syndrome also termed *Takotsubo cardiomyopathy* with acute chest pain or dyspnea following a significant emotional or physiologic stress. The clinical manifestation is transient akinesis or dyskinesis of the apical and midventricular segments of the LV, which extend beyond a single epicardial coronary distribution. Basal segments are hyperdynamic. An image from this patient's ventriculogram is presented (Fig. 8.35).

Angiography in patients with stress cardiomyopathy demonstrates an absence of obstructive coronary disease. Stress cardiomyopathy has a strong female predominance (>90%). Catecholamine excess in the setting of microvascular disease has been implicated. Although the wall motion abnormality findings might be consistent with multivessel disease (more than one epicardial coronary distribution), with diffuse ST-segment elevation on ECG that exceeds biomarker measurement of necrosis, findings are discordant with the relatively low serum biomarker values for myocardial necrosis. The outcome of stress cardiomyopathy is generally good, and LV functional recovery is likely with supportive care.

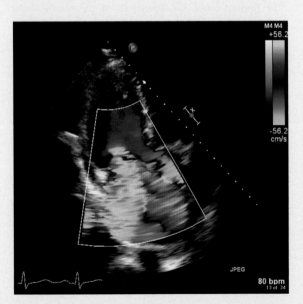

Fig. 8.34

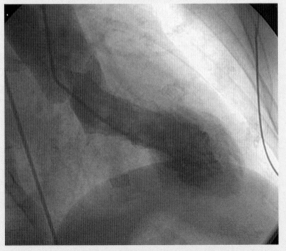

Fig. 8.35

Answer 9: A

The image shows an apical 4-chamber view of the LV with a large apical thrombus. The patient's left anterior descending artery infarction likely resulted in anteroapical akinesis. Blood stasis in the akinetic apex can lead to thrombus formation, which can subsequently embolize. Vitamin K antagonist therapy (warfarin) is indicated for 3 to 6 months with a follow-up echocardiogram to monitor for thrombus resolution. An embolic stroke may result from a paradoxical embolus via a patent foramen ovale. However, in this case, therapy for the LV thrombus is indicated, regardless of whether a patent foramen ovale (PFO) is present. A pseudoaneurysm is a mechanical complication of myocardial infarction where myocardial necrosis leads to a contained ventricular rupture. In patients where apical thrombus is suspected, transpulmonary microbubble contrast may help delineate the thrombus. In this case, the thrombus is well visualized without the need for echocontrast.

Answer 10: C

The patient has a normal response to dobutamine infusion but has not yet reached the target of 85% maximum predicted heart rate. Inotropy is increased with dobutamine doses up to 20 µg/kg/min; chronotropic changes are prominent above 20 µg/kg/min with the protocol maximum typically set at 40 µg/kg/min. Supine exercises such as leg raises (answer E) are an alternative option to reach target heart rate, but this patient has limiting hip arthritis. Dobutamine stress testing should be discontinued early with excessive elevations of blood pressure (systolic blood pressure >220 mm Hg or diastolic blood pressure >120 mm Hg). Study termination also may be required if significant hypotension occurs, but, unlike exercise testing, a small increase or fall in blood pressure does not indicate a worse prognosis or suggest the presence of severe coronary artery disease. Significant ventricular arrhythmia (non-sustained ventricular tachycardia or frequent polymorphic ventricular beats) and ST-segment elevation warrant termination of the study for safety considerations. Continued titration of dobutamine is appropriate with normal wall motion and no chest pain when only minor ST segment depression is present (answer D).

Answer 11: A

This is a subcostal short-axis view of the heart. The interventricular septum is thin, bright, and scarred, consistent with prior infarct. Color Doppler imaging shows flow toward the transducer across the infarct, consistent with ventricular septal rupture. The ratio of the stroke volume in the pulmonary artery (Qp) to the stroke volume in the LV outflow tract (Qs) would be increased, representing the additional volume of flow across the defect from the higher pressure LV

into the RV. Ischemic ventricular septal rupture is a rare complication after a myocardial infarct and typically occurs several days after the event. Most patients present with acute cardiac symptoms and hypotension but some patients are relatively asymptomatic initially. The rupture may be evident as a systolic murmur on physical examination; echo usually is diagnostic. A septal E' velocity = 0.1 m/s implies normal septal tissue velocity. With a septal infarct, myocardial velocity should be severely reduced, generally less than 0.05 m/s. With the left to right shunt, RV systolic pressure should be increased whereas a tricuspid jet velocity of only 2.1 m/s implies a normal pressure gradient. The wall motion score index is a quantitative measure of regional wall motion, based on the mean wall motion score for all myocardial segments, using a grade of 1 and 4 where 1 is normal motion, 2 is hypokinetic, 3 is akinetic, and 4 is dyskinetic; a wall motion score index of 1 implies normal LV function in all segments, and would not be consistent with a myocardial infarction.

Answer 12: A

This is an abnormal stress echocardiogram. During imaging, microbubble transpulmonary contrast was used to aid endocardial border definition. The resting image shows a normal LV contour and wall thickness consistent with normal endocardial motion. At peak stress, there is a contour abnormality of the apical two-thirds of the inferior septum and the entire apex with a lack of systolic inward motion. In contrast, the basal two-thirds of the lateral wall showed increased inward motion on the stress image compared to baseline. Subsequent coronary angiography in this patient demonstrated a 90% right coronary artery occlusion and an 80% left anterior descending artery occlusion. A biphasic response is the LV response of hibernating myocardium to low dose dobutamine where, in patients with severe LV dysfunction and akinetic regions at rest, an initial increase in contractility of the akinetic zones at very low doses of dobutamine (≈5 µg/kg/min) is followed by akinesis in these regions at higher infusion doses (≈20 to 30 µg/kg/min). A biphasic response is the effect of severely ischemic but not infarcted myocardium, which responds with increased inotropy at a very low dose of dobutamine but becomes frankly ischemic at higher dobutamine doses. A hyperdynamic LV response is increased endocardial motion and a decrease in systolic LV cavity size, which is normal and consistent with no impairment in coronary flow. In patients with a prior transmural infarct, normal myocardium adjacent to infarcted tissue may have decreased systolic motion due to "tethering" from the akinetic, infarcted region. In this case, resting LV function was normal without infarction at baseline.

9 Cardiomyopathies, Hypertensive, and Pulmonary Heart Disease

CARDIOMYOPATHIES

General Step-By-Step Approach

An overall approach to patients with a known or suspected cardiomyopathy is reviewed, followed by specific features of each type of cardiomyopathy.

Step 1: Measure Left Ventricular Chamber Size and Systolic Function

❖ LEFT VENTRICULAR CHAMBER SIZE

- Two-dimensional (2D) guided M-mode measurement of left ventricle (LV) minor axis internal dimensions at end-diastole and end-systole.
- Three-dimensional (3D) volumetric or apical biplane calculation of end-diastolic and end-systolic ventricular volumes (Figs. 9.1 and 9.2).

❖ KEY POINTS

- ❑ 3D volumetric LV volumes indexed to body size are the most accurate approach for evaluation of LV dilation because the pattern of dilation may not be reflected in basal minor axis dimensions.
- ❑ 2D LV internal dimensions are measured from the parasternal window, because the ultrasound beam is perpendicular to the blood-myocardial interface, providing high axial resolution.
- ❑ 2D imaging in long-and short-axis views will ensure that the dimension is measured in the minor axis of the ventricle (not at an oblique angle, which would overestimate size).
- ❑ On 2D images, the white–black (tissue–blood) interface is used to measure LV dimensions.
- ❑ The rapid sampling rate of M-mode (compared with the slow frame rate of 2D imaging) provides more accurate identification of the endocardial borders (Fig. 9.3).
- ❑ 2D guided M-mode measurements are most accurate when the ultrasound beam can be aligned perpendicular to the LV wall of interest.
- ❑ For sequential studies, measurements should be made with the same method at the same location.

❖ LEFT VENTRICULAR SYSTOLIC FUNCTION

- LV ejection fraction is calculated using 3D volumes or the 2D apical biplane approach.
- Global longitudinal strain is measured using speckle tracking imaging.
- LV dP/dt is calculated from the mitral regurgitation velocity curve (Fig. 9.4).
- Forward stroke volume is measured in the LV outflow tract and indexed to body size.
- Regional ventricular function is evaluated qualitatively as normal, hypokinetic, or akinetic for each myocardial segment (see Chapter 8).

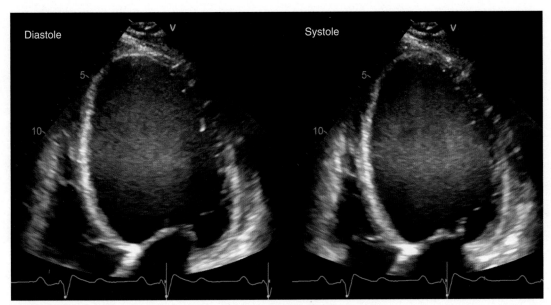

Fig. 9.1 Dilated cardiomyopathy. Apical biplane calculation of ejection fraction is based on tracing endocardial borders at end-diastole *(left)* and end-systole *(right)* in the 4-chamber view *(as shown)* and in the 2-chamber view. Foreshortened apical views are avoided by positioning the patient in a steep left lateral position with an apical cutout in the stretcher to allow the transducer to be positioned on the true apex and after moving the transducer down one or more interspaces.

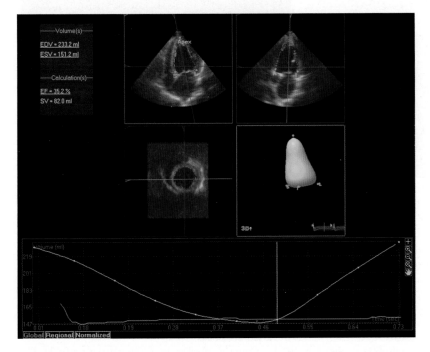

Fig. 9.2 3D measurement of LV ejection fraction in dilated cardiomyopathy. A full volume acquisition from the apical window is used to measure endocardial borders in three orthogonal views to generate the 3D volume reconstruction. The time-volume curve is shown at the bottom of the figure with the calculated volumes and ejection fraction (EF) in the upper left. Volumes are increased and EF reduced in this patient with dilated cardiomyopathy.

❖ KEY POINTS

❑ Ejection fraction measured by the apical biplane method is confirmed by a visual estimate to ensure image quality is adequate for quantitation.

❑ The traced endocardial borders are reviewed for accuracy and retraced if the estimated and measured ejection fractions differ by more than 10 ejection fraction units.

❑ Echo-contrast is used to enhance identification of endocardial borders when image quality is suboptimal.

❑ Measured ejection fraction is reported whenever possible. The estimated ejection fraction is

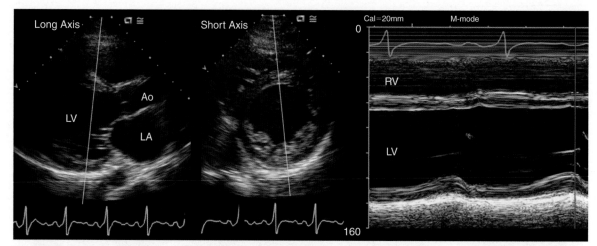

Fig. 9.3 M-mode tracing of the LV. The 2D image is used to ensure the M-line is perpendicular to the long axis of the LV in the parasternal long-axis view and in the middle of the chamber in the short-axis view. The rapid sampling rate of the M-mode recording (time on the horizontal axis) provides more accurate identification and measurement of septal and posterior wall thickness and ventricular chamber dimensions at end-diastole (onset of QRS) and end-systole (maximum posterior motion of septum). *Ao,* Aorta.

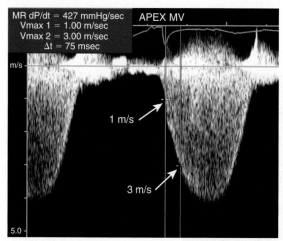

Fig. 9.4 Rate of LV pressure increase. The rate of increase in velocity of the mitral regurgitant jet is markedly reduced in early systole. The calculated *dP/dt* of 427 mm Hg/s indicated severely reduced LV contractility.

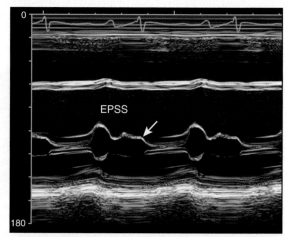

Fig. 9.5 E-point septal separation (EPSS). M-mode tracing at the level of the mitral valve shows a marked increase in the EPSS consistent with severe LV systolic dysfunction. There also is delayed mitral valve closure *(arrow)*—an AC shoulder or B-bump—which is a sign of an elevated LV filling pressure.

reported only if endocardial borders cannot be traced accurately or a 3D measurement is not possible.

❏ Ejection fraction is an imperfect measure of contractility because it is affected by loading conditions. Even so, ejection fraction is useful for clinical decision making.

❏ LV *dP/dt* and forward stroke volume are other useful parameters of LV systolic function (see Chapter 6).

❏ Indirect qualitative indicators of LV systolic dysfunction include M-mode findings of reduced aortic root motion and increased E-point septal separation (Fig. 9.5).

❏ Global longitudinal strain is more independent of loading conditions and more sensitive for detection of early LV systolic dysfunction.

❖ **EVALUATE FOR OTHER CAUSE OF LEFT VENTRICULAR DILATION AND SYSTOLIC DYSFUNCTION**

■ A cardiomyopathy is defined as a primary disease of the myocardium in the absence of coronary or valvular disease.

■ Evaluate for evidence of other causes of LV dilation and dysfunction, specifically valve disease (aortic stenosis, mitral regurgitation, or aortic regurgitation) and coronary artery disease.

❖ **KEY POINTS**

❏ LV dilation and dysfunction due to coronary disease with myocardial infarction or hibernation can be difficult to distinguish from a primary cardiomyopathy.

- Mitral regurgitation may be a cause or a consequence of LV dilation and dysfunction. When more than mild mitral regurgitation (vena contracta >3 mm) is present, careful quantitative evaluation is helpful (see Chapter 12) (Fig. 9.6).
- The degree of aortic valve leaflet opening is reduced when LV dysfunction is present, making it difficult to separate severe aortic stenosis resulting in LV dysfunction from moderate aortic stenosis with coincidental LV dysfunction (see Chapter 11) (Fig. 9.7).

Step 2: Evaluate for the Presence and Pattern of Ventricular Hypertrophy

❖ PRESENCE AND SEVERITY OF LEFT VENTRICULAR HYPERTROPHY

- 2D guided M-mode measurement of LV wall thickness
- Calculation of LV mass in selected cases

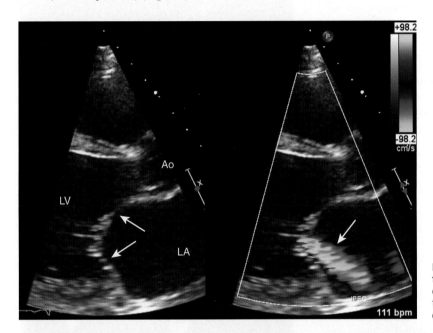

Fig. 9.6 **Secondary mitral regurgitation.** Mitral regurgitation in a patient with dilated cardiomyopathy due to tethering of the leaflets *(arrows)* with central to posteriorly directed regurgitant jet. *Ao,* Aorta.

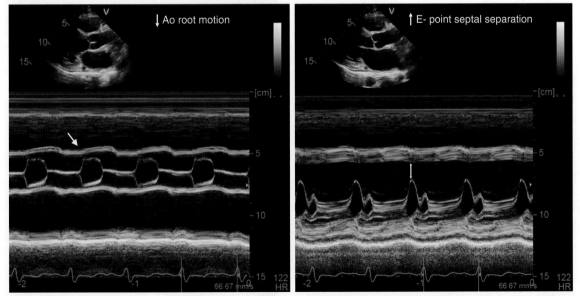

Fig. 9.7 **Aortic (Ao) root and mitral valve motion in dilated cardiomyopathy.** In this M-mode recording in a patient with a dilated cardiomyopathy, the aortic tracing *(left)* shows reduced anterior-posterior motion of the root due to a reduced cardiac output. The mitral M-mode shows increased E-point septal separation due to LV dilation and systolic dysfunction and a delayed mitral closure due to high filling pressures.

❖ **KEY POINTS**

❑ 2D guided M-mode measurement of LV wall thickness at end-systole (onset of the QRS) is adequate in most cases.

❑ Calculation of LV mass from traced 2D endocardial and epicardial borders is largely limited to research applications.

❖ **PATTERN OF LEFT VENTRICULAR HYPERTROPHY**

▪ Long-axis, short-axis, and apical views are used to evaluate the pattern of ventricular hypertrophy (Fig. 9.8).

❖ **KEY POINTS**

❑ 2D imaging allows evaluation of the pattern of hypertrophy in all myocardial segments.

❑ When hypertrophy is concentric, LV wall thickness measurements at one site adequately represent the degree of hypertrophy.

❑ When hypertrophy is asymmetric, measurements at key sites are reported, particularly the diastolic septal thickness in patients with hypertrophic cardiomyopathy.

❑ 2D guided M-mode measurements are most accurate when the ultrasound beam can be aligned perpendicular to the LV wall of interest. Otherwise, 2D measurements at end-diastole are reported.

Step 3: Assess Left Ventricular Diastolic Function (see Chapter 7)

▪ LV and LA inflow patterns (Fig. 9.9)
▪ Tissue Doppler at the mitral annulus (Fig. 9.10)
▪ Isovolumic relaxation time (Fig. 9.11)

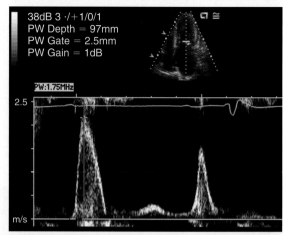

Fig. 9.9 Severe LV diastolic dysfunction. LV diastolic filling in a 62-year-old patient with a dilated cardiomyopathy showing an increased E/A ratio with a steep early diastolic deceleration slope. The E is greater than A in this patient older than age 50, in association with a steep deceleration slope, suggests severe LV diastolic dysfunction with elevated filling pressures.

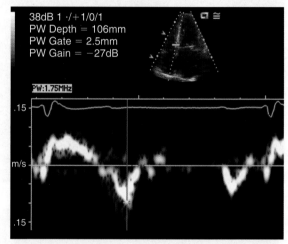

Fig. 9.10 Tissue Doppler at the mitral annulus. This tracing shows an E′ less than 0.10 m/s, with an E′ greater than A′, in the same patient as Fig. 9.9. The ratio of transmitral E velocity to tissue Doppler E′ velocity is 2.2/0.10 = 22, which is severely elevated, consistent with a high LA pressure.

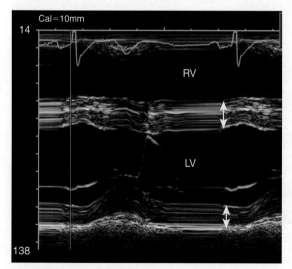

Fig. 9.8 Concentric LV hypertrophy. This M-mode tracing shows increased wall thickness of both the septum and posterior wall.

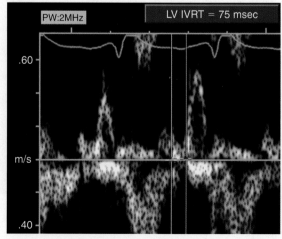

Fig. 9.11 Isovolumic relaxation time (IVRT). The IVRT, measured from the end of aortic ejection flow to the onset of mitral inflow, is normal at 75 ms.

❖ KEY POINTS

- ▫ Systolic LV dysfunction typically is accompanied by some degree of diastolic dysfunction.
- ▫ Classification of the degree of diastolic dysfunction as mild (impaired relaxation) versus severe (decreased compliance) is used in clinical decision making.
- ▫ LV filling pressures are estimated whenever systolic dysfunction is present.

Step 4: Estimate Pulmonary Artery Pressures (see Chapter 6)

- ■ Pulmonary systolic pressure is estimated from the tricuspid regurgitant (TR) jet velocity and estimated right ventricular (RA) pressure (Figs. 9.12 and 9.13).
- ■ Other signs of pulmonary hypertension include a short time to peak velocity in the pulmonary artery velocity curve, paradoxical septal motion, and a high end-diastolic pulmonic regurgitant velocity.

❖ KEY POINTS

- ▫ Pulmonary pressures often are elevated in patients with heart failure due to a cardiomyopathy.
- ▫ Pulmonary pressures may be reduced with effective medical therapy, in conjunction with a decrease in left atrium (LA) (or LV filling) pressure.
- ▫ When pulmonary pressures are elevated disproportionately to the degree of left-sided heart dysfunction, concurrent primary pulmonary disease or pulmonary thromboembolism may be present.

Step 5: Evaluate Right Ventricular Size and Systolic Function

- ■ RV size and systolic function are assessed from parasternal, apical, and subcostal views (Fig. 9.14).
- ■ Standard measures of RV size and function are used (see Chapter 6).

❖ KEY POINTS

- ▫ RV systolic dysfunction may be due to primary myocardial disease affecting both ventricles or to the effects of pulmonary hypertension.
- ▫ Qualitative assessment of RV size and function takes into account the degree of LV dilation and dysfunction. RV lengthwise systolic shortening and tricuspid annular plane systolic excursion (TAPSE) are reduced when RV dysfunction is present.

Step 6: Evaluate the Severity of Mitral and Tricuspid Regurgitation (see Chapter 12)

- ■ Mitral and tricuspid regurgitation often are present in patients with a cardiomyopathy.

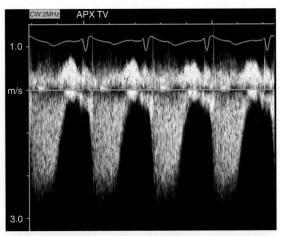

Fig. 9.12 Estimates of pulmonary systolic pressure. This tricuspid regurgitant (TR) jet velocity obtained from an apical view (APX TV) has a peak somewhere around 2.5 m/s. This signal is not ideal because the peak is not well defined. This likely is due to the position of the ultrasound beam relative to the jet and the use of color coding (instead of gray scale) for the spectral display, which often obscures the peak velocity with superimposed noise. However, the peak velocity of about 2.4 m/s indicates a RV-to-RA systolic pressure difference of 23 mm Hg.

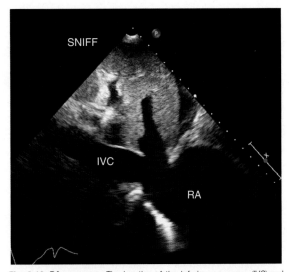

Fig. 9.13 RA pressure. The junction of the inferior vena cava *(IVC)* and RA is visualized from the subcostal window for estimating RA pressure. In this patient, the IVC diameter is about 2.5 cm and collapses less than 50% with rapid inspiration (SNIFF), which is consistent with an RA pressure of 10 to 15 mm Hg.

- ■ Regurgitant severity is evaluated using standard approaches, starting with the color Doppler vena contracta and the continuous-wave (CW) Doppler velocity curve.
- ■ The mechanism of regurgitation is evaluated using 2D imaging from multiple views; typically regurgitation is secondary to ventricular dilation and dysfunction, but some patients have concurrent structural valve disease.

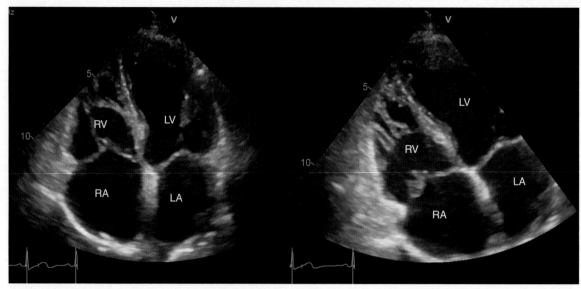

Fig. 9.14 RV size. The RV is imaged from the apical 4-chamber view *(left)* by tilting the transducer toward the RV and optimizing visualization of the RV free wall *(right)*. Typical measurements include the basal diastolic RV diameter.

Fig. 9.15 Mitral leaflet tethering. Schematic diagram showing leaflet tethering with dilated cardiomyopathy due to lateral displacement of the papillary muscles, resulting in an oblique angle to the mitral annulus. *MR,* Mitral regurgitation.

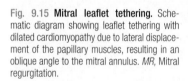

Normal

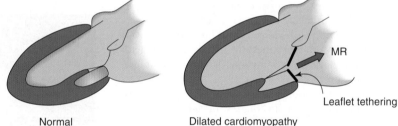

Dilated cardiomyopathy

❖ **KEY POINTS**

- ❏ Mitral and tricuspid regurgitation due to LV dilation and dysfunction are common.
- ❏ The mechanism of atrioventricular valve regurgitation is *tethering* of the mitral leaflets resulting in incomplete systolic coaptation. This also has been described as an increased angle between the papillary muscles so that the leaflets are "pulled apart" relative to the mitral annulus (Fig. 9.15).
- ❏ The degree of annular dilation is variable, with a variable contribution to the degree of mitral regurgitation.
- ❏ Mitral regurgitation severity may decrease with effective therapy for heart failure.

Step 7: Evaluate Left Atrium Size (see Chapter 2)

- ■ LA size typically is increased either due to chronic elevation of LV filling pressures or to coexisting mitral regurgitation (see Fig. 2.22).
- ■ LA size can be evaluated qualitatively, using a simple anterior-posterior dimension, or by calculation of atrial volume from apical views.

❖ **KEY POINTS**

- ❏ LA anterior-posterior dimension is measured in a long-axis view at end-systole (maximum LA dimension).
- ❏ Although atrial volumes are predictive of clinical outcome, simpler measures of atrial size suffice for clinical decision making in many cases.
- ❏ When clinically indicated, LA volume is calculated from tracing the LA border at end-systole in apical 4-chamber and 2-chamber views. LA volume then is indexed for body size.
- ❏ RA size also may be increased and is evaluated qualitatively (as mild, moderately, or severely dilated) in comparison to the other cardiac chambers.

Additional Steps

Dilated Cardiomyopathy

- ■ Evaluate for LV apical thrombus (Fig. 9.16).
- ■ Differentiate from end-stage coronary disease (Table 9.1).

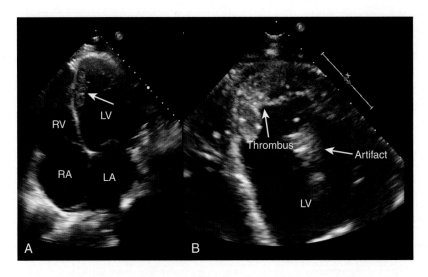

Fig. 9.16 **LV apical thrombus.** (A) In the apical 4-chamber view, the LV is dilated with marked thickening along the apical septum suggestive of thrombus. (B) Using a higher transducer frequency and shallow image depth, the laminated thrombus filling the apex is better visualized. At this depth, a ring-down artifact also is seen overlying the LV chamber.

TABLE 9.1	Cardiomyopathies: Clinical Echocardiographic Correlation		
Cardiomyopathy	**Pathophysiology**	**Clinical Presentation**	**Echocardiographic Findings**
Dilated			
Idiopathic	Primary myocardial dysfunction of unknown cause	• Heart failure signs and symptoms	• Dilation of all four chambers with RV and LV systolic dysfunction • Secondary mitral regurgitation in some patients, but valve leaflets are normal • LV thrombus can occur with severe LV dysfunction • Elevated LV filling pressures with variable elevation in PA pressures
Familial	Inherited primary myocardial dysfunction	• Heart failure signs and symptoms	• Dilation of all four chambers with RV and LV systolic dysfunction • Secondary mitral regurgitation may be present, but valve leaflets are normal • LV thrombus can occur with severe LV dysfunction • Elevated LV filling pressures with variable elevation in PA pressures
Chagas	Protozoan infection, due to *Trypanosoma cruzi,* that affects the heart, esophagus, and colon	• Acute phase is characterized by fever, myalgias, hepatospleno-megaly, and myocarditis. • Chronic Chagas heart disease has a high mortality rate (44% at 4 years) due to sudden death (55%-65%), heart failure (25%-30%), and stroke (10%-15%)	• LV dilation and systolic dysfunction, ranging from mild to severe • Wall motion may be regional but not in a pattern consistent with coronary artery disease • Apical abnormalities are common: with apical aneurysm in about 5% of asymptomatic patients and about 55% of those with heart failure
Duchenne MD	Inherited myopathic disorder that affects both skeletal and cardiac muscle	• Often have asymptomatic LV dysfunction, likely due to limited physical activity • Late in disease, heart failure and arrhythmias are seen	• Echocardiography is consistent with a dilated cardiomyopathy

Continued

TABLE 9.1	Cardiomyopathies: Clinical Echocardiographic Correlation—cont'd		
Cardiomyopathy	**Pathophysiology**	**Clinical Presentation**	**Echocardiographic Findings**
Hypertrophic			
Hypertrophic	Inherited autosomal-dominant myocardial disease	• Wide age range of clinical presentation • Often diagnosed in asymptomatic patients on screening echo • Present with symptoms of heart failure and angina or as sudden death with no previous diagnosis	• Asymmetric LV hypertrophy with normal systolic function but abnormal diastolic function • About 1/3 have resting dynamic outflow obstruction, and 1/3 have a provoked gradient with exercise
Fabry	Inherited X-linked glycolipid storage disease, now recognized in women as well as men	• Presents in boys under age 10 years with skin and neurologic findings • Presents in women later in life with unexplained LV hypertrophy • Diagnosis based on plasma alpha-galactosidase A activity • Conduction system abnormalities and arrhythmias are common	• LV hypertrophy may be asymmetric but in an atypical pattern for HCM • Endocardial hyperechoic layer is typical for Fabry heart disease • About 50% have aortic and mitral valve thickening and mild regurgitation
Restrictive			
Amyloid	Extracellular tissue deposition of serum protein subunit fibrils—cardiac involvement in 50% of primary AL amyloidosis (monoclonal light chains) cases but only 5% with secondary AA amyloidosis	• Conduction system disease • Myocardial involvement	• Increased LV and RV wall thickness with increased myocardial echogenicity, but "sparkling" appearance is not specific or sensitive for diagnosis • Progressive diastolic dysfunction • Valve thickening • Intracardiac thrombus • Strain pattern with preserved apical function
Sarcoidosis	Systemic disease with pulmonary involvement in most patients Subclinical cardiac involvement in up to 20% of patients	• Cardiac involvement most often results in conduction system abnormalities, ventricular arrhythmias or heart failure	• Nonspecific • Regional wall motion abnormalities in a noncoronary disease pattern • LV systolic and diastolic dysfunction
Other			
Isolated LV non-compaction	Rare, primary genetic cardiomyopathy	• Clinical presentation with heart failure, angina, arrhythmias, and thromboembolic events	• Deep ventricular trabeculations, particularly in the inferior and lateral walls • Color Doppler shows communication between intertrabecular recesses and LV chamber • Ejection fraction may be reduced • Ratio of noncompacted to compacted myocardium >2:1 at end-systole in short-axis view
Takotsubo (stress-induced cardiomyopathy)	Catecholamine-induced acute myocardial dysfunction	• Sudden onset of chest pain, dyspnea, ECG changes, and elevated cardiac enzymes with normal coronary arteries • Occurs in the setting of intense emotional or physical stress or with an acute medical illness • Over 80% of cases are women, typically age 50-75 years	• Apical dilation and systolic dysfunction resulting in a significant reduction in LV ejection fraction • Pattern of regional myocardial dysfunction is atypical for coronary disease • LV systolic function typically returns to normal in 1 to 4 weeks, although recurrences have been reported

TABLE 9.1 Cardiomyopathies: Clinical Echocardiographic Correlation—cont'd

Cardiomyopathy	Pathophysiology	Clinical Presentation	Echocardiographic Findings
Arrhythmogenic RV cardiomyopathy	Familial inheritance in at least 30%, most often in an autosomal-dominant pattern Autosomal-recessive inheritance also has been described	• Presents with sudden cardiac death or ventricular arrhythmias	• RV dilation and systolic dysfunction • Echo findings are nonspecific; diagnosis depends on MRI and electrophysiologic evaluation

AL, Amyloid light-chain; *ECG,* electrocardiogram; *HCM,* hypertrophic cardiomyopathy; *MD,* muscular dystrophy; *MRI,* magnetic resonance imaging; *PA,* pulmonary artery.
From Otto CM: Cardiomyopathies, hypertensive and pulmonary heart disease. In *Textbook of clinical echocardiography,* ed 6, Philadelphia, 2018, Elsevier.

- Differentiate LV dysfunction due to severe mitral regurgitation from a primary cardiomyopathy with secondary mitral regurgitation.
- Ensure an accurate ejection fraction calculation.

❖ **KEY POINTS**

- ❑ Decision making for placement of an automated implanted defibrillator is based on the calculated ejection fraction, with the breakpoint typically at an ejection fraction less than 35% after optimization of medical therapy.
- ❑ Examination for LV apical thrombus includes oblique views of the LV apex using a high-frequency transducer and shallow image depth. Contrast imaging may be helpful to exclude thrombus when standard imaging is not diagnostic.
- ❑ Transesophageal echocardiography (TEE) is not useful to evaluate for apical thrombus due to the distance of the apex from the transducer and the likelihood that the true apex may be missed from this approach.
- ❑ LV systolic dysfunction due to coronary disease and to a primary cardiomyopathy may look similar on echocardiography. Both may show wall motion that is best preserved at the inferior-lateral base.
- ❑ Features that suggest end-stage coronary disease include definite evidence for myocardial infarction (segmental thinning and akinesis) and normal RV size and systolic function. However, direct visualization of coronary anatomy by conventional catheter or computed tomographic angiography typically is needed.
- ❑ Stress echocardiography is difficult to interpret with significant resting LV systolic dysfunction with a suboptimal sensitivity and specificity for detection of ischemia.
- ❑ Speckle-tracking strain imaging provides a more quantitative evaluation of global and regional function in patients with a cardiomyopathy.

Hypertrophic Cardiomyopathy

❖ **STEP 1: LEFT VENTRICULAR HYPERTROPHY**

- Describe the anatomic pattern of hypertrophy (Fig. 9.17).
- Evaluate the end-diastolic wall thickness of the basal posterior wall.
- Measure the maximal end-diastolic septal thickness. Wall thickness measurements should be taken from both long-axis and short-axis views of the ventricle.

❖ **KEY POINTS**

- ❑ The most common pattern of hypertrophy involves the ventricular septum with a normal posterior LV wall.
- ❑ Apical hypertrophy may be missed unless echo-contrast is used to opacify the ventricle, because the endocardial border in the mid-LV may be difficult to visualize (Fig. 9.18).
- ❑ Even with atypical patterns of hypertrophy, the basal posterior wall thickness typically is normal in patients with hypertrophic cardiomyopathy.
- ❑ Maximal septal thickness is a predictor of sudden death risk. Septal thickness is measured at end-diastole, taking care to exclude RV trabeculations from the measurement.

❖ **STEP 2: DYNAMIC SUBAORTIC OUTFLOW OBSTRUCTION**

- Evaluate dynamic subaortic outflow obstruction.
- Evaluate the mechanism and severity of mitral regurgitation.

❖ **KEY POINTS**

- ❑ Subaortic obstruction is due to systolic anterior motion (SAM) of the mitral leaflet and a hypertrophied septum.
- ❑ The Doppler velocity curve peaks in late systole, instead of in mid-systole as seen with valvular obstruction (Fig. 9.19).

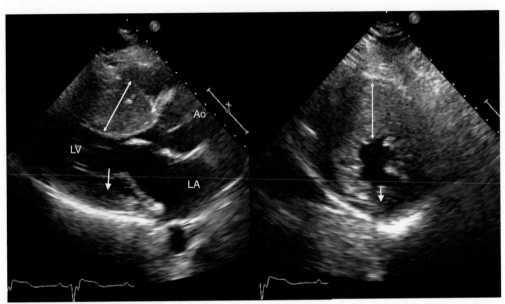

Fig. 9.17 Hypertrophic cardiomyopathy with septal hypertrophy. These parasternal long-axis views at end diastole in a long-axis *(left)* and short-axis *(right)* image plane show marked increased thickness of the interventricular septum *(double headed arrows)* with a normal thickness of the posterior wall *(short arrow)*.

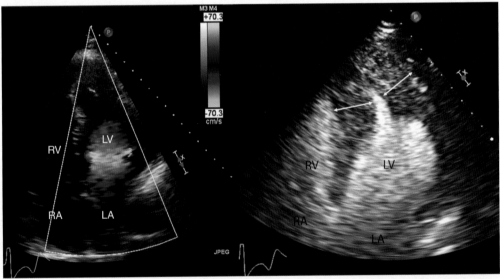

Fig. 9.18 Apical hypertrophic cardiomyopathy. The apical 4-chamber view *(left)* in patients with apical hypertrophic cardiomyopathy often shows poor visualization of the apical myocardium with wall motion sometimes mistaken for apical akinesis. Contrast enhancement of the LV chamber *(right)* shows the small LV chamber with marked hypertrophy of the apical segments of the septum and lateral wall *(arrows)*

- The level of obstruction is established with pulsed or high-pulse repetition frequency Doppler, with CW Doppler used to measure the maximum velocity.
- The severity of obstruction varies with loading conditions, increasing when afterload is decreased or when ventricular volume is reduced.
- If resting outflow obstruction is not present (peak gradient less than 30 mm Hg), exercise

testing may be used to detect latent obstruction, which is defined as an increase in subaortic maximum gradient to at least 50 mm Hg with exercise.
- Mitral regurgitation may be due to SAM of the mitral leaflet, resulting in inadequate coaptation with a typical posterior-directed regurgitant jet (Fig. 9.20).

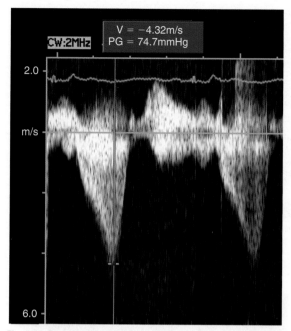

Fig. 9.19 Dynamic subaortic obstruction. CW Doppler recording from an apical approach of outflow velocity in a patient with hypertrophic cardiomyopathy. This waveform is consistent with dynamic obstruction with a late-peaking high-velocity systolic signal. The level of obstruction is not defined using CW Doppler, because the signal includes velocities from the entire length of the ultrasound beam. A step-by-step pulsed Doppler evaluation moving the sample volume from the LV toward the aortic valve allows localization of the site of obstruction.

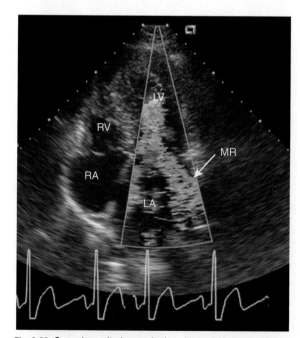

Fig. 9.20 Secondary mitral regurgitation. Mitral regurgitation *(MR)* in a patient with hypertrophic cardiomyopathy and dynamic subaortic obstruction. The mitral regurgitant posterior-lateral jet direction is demonstrated in this apical 4-chamber view.

❖ **STEP 3: DISTINGUISH FROM HYPERTENSIVE HEART DISEASE AND NORMAL AGING CHANGES**

- Hypertensive heart disease may be mistaken for hypertrophic cardiomyopathy.
- LV hypertrophy in a patient with a clinical history of hypertension most often is due to hypertensive heart disease.
- With aging, dilation and tortuosity of the ascending aorta result in an increased angle between the basal septum and aortic root, with *bulging* of the septum into the LV outflow tract.

❖ **KEY POINTS**

- ❑ Hypertension results in concentric LV hypertrophy; even the basal posterior wall is thickened.
- ❑ Dynamic outflow obstruction may occur with hypertensive heart disease, but the location of obstruction is midventricular and SAM occurs in the mitral chordal region, instead of at the leaflet level.
- ❑ Age-related bulging of the basal septum can be difficult to distinguish from hypertrophic cardiomyopathy; diagnosis depends on associated echocardiographic and clinical findings, as well as genetic and family studies.

Restrictive Cardiomyopathy

- Evaluate for LV hypertrophy and systolic function (Fig. 9.21)
- Perform a more detailed evaluation of LV diastolic function (Fig. 9.22).
- Differentiate restrictive cardiomyopathy from constrictive pericarditis (see Chapter 10).

❖ **KEY POINTS**

- ❑ Restrictive cardiomyopathy is a primary disease of the myocardium, which is often related to an infiltrative or inflammatory process.
- ❑ Restrictive cardiomyopathy is characterized by predominant diastolic, rather than systolic, dysfunction so that detailed evaluation of diastolic function is helpful.
- ❑ Restrictive cardiomyopathy and constrictive pericarditis result in similar changes in ventricular filling but can be differentiated based on several features (see Table 10.2).
- ❑ LV systolic dysfunction may also be present, especially late in the disease course.
- ❑ Pulmonary systolic pressure usually is moderately to severely elevated.
- ❑ Amyloid heart disease is characterization by an LV strain pattern with preserved function at the apex ("apical sparing") (see Fig. 9.21).
- ❑ Sarcoid heart disease may present with regional wall motion abnormalities in a noncoronary distribution.

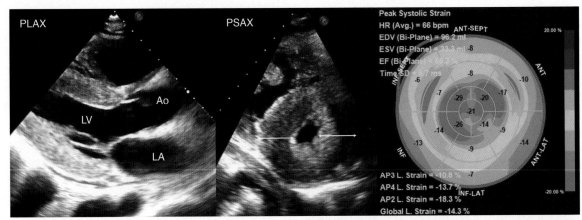

Fig. 9.21 Amyloid heart disease. Amyloid heart disease is characterized by concentric LV hypertrophy and mild valve thickening as seen in these parasternal long-axis *(left)* and short-axis *(right)* views. In the short-axis view, there is shadowing of the lateral wall, so the true thickness *(arrows)* might be underestimated. The speckle-tracking strain imaging display shows strain values from the apex *(in the center)* to the base in color and with numeric values. This pattern of preserved apical function with reduced basal function (sometimes called "apical sparing") is typical for amyloid heart disease.

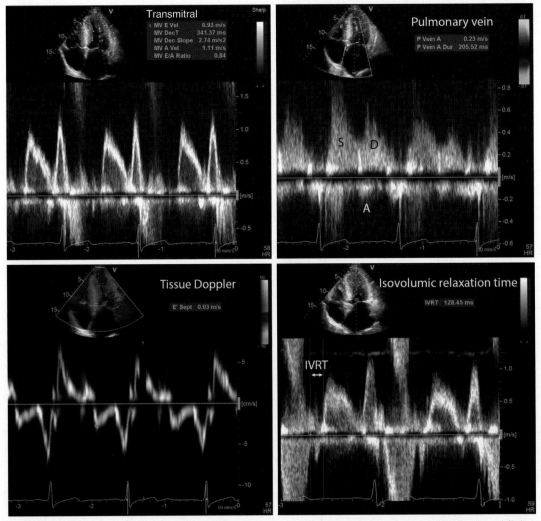

Fig. 9.22 Diastolic dysfunction. Evaluation of diastolic function in a patient with a restrictive cardiomyopathy includes transmitral flow *(upper left)*, tissue Doppler velocity at the mitral annulus *(lower left)*, pulmonary vein flow *(upper right)*, and the isovolumic relaxation time *(lower right)*. These tracings show impaired diastolic relaxation (transmitral and tissue Doppler E less than A, prolonged deceleration time, reduced diastolic pulmonary venous flow, and prolonged isovolumic relaxation time [IVRT]). Measures of LA pressure include an E/E′ greater than 30, even though the pulmonary venous a-wave is low velocity and short in duration.

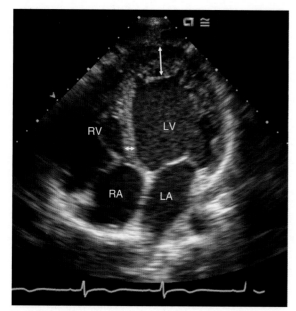

Fig. 9.23 **LV noncompaction.** Apical 4-chamber view showing LV non-compaction, particularly in the apex *(arrow)* with increased thickness of the trabeculated myocardium.

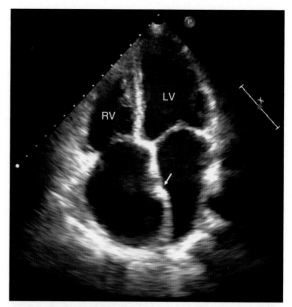

Fig. 9.24 **After heart transplantation.** In this patient with biatrial anasto-moses at heart transplantation, the enlarged left and right atria, caused by suturing of the native and donor atrium *(arrows; shows suture line)*, are seen in the apical 4-chamber view.

❏ Additional evaluation with cardiac magnetic resonance imaging (MRI) may be helpful in patients with a restrictive cardiomyopathy.

Other Cardiomyopathies

- Arrhythmogenic right ventricular dysplasia (ARVD) is a genetic cardiomyopathy with fibro-fatty replacement of the RV resulting in arrhythmias, dilation, and systolic dysfunction.
- LV noncompaction is characterized by areas of prominent trabeculation and hypokinesis, typically located in the LV apex and mid-LV segments of the lateral and inferior walls (Fig. 9.23).
- Chagas disease is due to a parasitic infection resulting in apical aneurysm formation in about 50% of patients and global hypokinesis in those with advanced disease.
- Takotsubo cardiomyopathy is an acute stress-related cause of heart failure with apical dilation and dyskinesis (apical "ballooning").

ADVANCED HEART FAILURE THERAPIES

Posttransplant Heart Disease

- Evaluation of the patient after heart transplantation follows the general approach outlined for a patient with a cardiomyopathy.
- Early after heart transplantation, the major issues are surgical (e.g., pericardial effusion) and myocardial preservation (e.g., RV and LV systolic function).

- Echocardiographic signs of transplant rejection include diastolic and systolic LV dysfunction.
- After transplant, long-term follow-up of patients includes dobutamine stress echocardiography for detection of graft coronary artery disease.

❖ KEY POINTS

- ❏ Biatrial enlargement is typical after heart transplantation, with sometimes massive atrial enlargement with biatrial anastomotic suture lines (Fig. 9.24).
- ❏ Complications of percutaneous myocardial biopsy include (1) cardiac perforation, resulting in pericardial effusion and tamponade, and (2) tricuspid valve damage resulting in regurgitation.
- ❏ New systolic dysfunction, even if mild, may indicate acute rejection and requires prompt evaluation by the transplant team.
- ❏ When dobutamine stress echocardiography is performed after heart transplantation, atropine may not increase heart rate due to cardiac denervation.

Left Ventricular Assist Devices

- End-stage heart failure may be treated acutely or chronically with an implanted continuous flow device.
- The most common type of left ventricular assist devices (LVADs) has an inflow cannula in the LV apex and an outflow cannula in the ascending aorta.

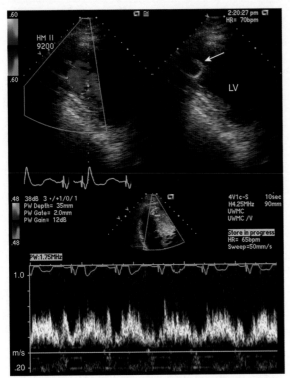

Fig. 9.25 **Left ventricular assist device (LVAD).** The LVAD inflow cannula *(arrow)* is seen in the apical view. Pulsed Doppler shows continuous low velocity flow into the LVAD cannula.

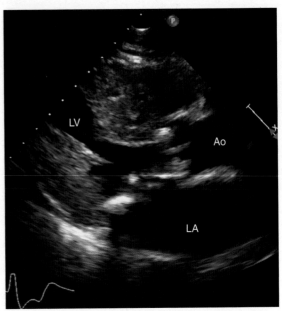

Fig. 9.26 **Hypertensive heart disease.** Parasternal long-axis view in a patient with hypertension, showing mild ventricular hypertrophy, aortic valve sclerosis, and mild mitral annular calcification. *Ao,* Aorta.

- Echocardiography allows detection of LVAD complications.
- Measurements of LV size and the degree of aortic valve opening may be used to optimize LVAD flow rates.

❖ **KEY POINTS**

- ❑ The aortic valve leaflets may remain closed, open partially or open intermittently in patients with an LVAD. M-mode echocardiography allows recording of the pattern and extent of leaflet motion for several beats (longer than a 2-beat cine image).
- ❑ Flow signals in the inflow and outflow cannula can be helpful for diagnosis of obstruction of the cannula (Fig. 9.25).
- ❑ A health care provider experienced in management of LVAD patients is present during the echocardiographic study if measurements at different LVAD flow rates are needed.
- ❑ Evaluation of RV size and systolic function is important when an LVAD is present.

HYPERTENSIVE HEART DISEASE

- Evaluation of the patient with hypertensive heart disease follows the general approach outlined for a patient with a cardiomyopathy.

- Blood pressure should be recorded at the time of every echocardiographic examination.

❖ **KEY POINTS**

- ❑ Hypertension results in LV hypertrophy with impaired diastolic relaxation.
- ❑ Prolonged poorly controlled hypertension may eventually result in more severe diastolic dysfunction and in superimposed systolic dysfunction.
- ❑ Effective treatment of hypertension results in regression of LV hypertrophy.
- ❑ LV hypertrophy may be accompanied by dynamic midcavity obstruction due to a small, thick-walled, hyperdynamic ventricle.
- ❑ Obstruction may only be present or may increase with hypovolemia or hyperdynamic states (such as anemia, fever, sepsis).
- ❑ Aortic valve sclerosis and mitral annular calcification are typically seen in patients with hypertensive heart disease (Fig. 9.26).
- ❑ Hypertension, like aging, is associated with dilation and increased tortuosity of the ascending aorta, resulting in a more acute angle between the ventricular septum and the aortic root, sometimes mistaken for focal basal septal thickening (Fig. 9.27).

PULMONARY HEART DISEASE

- Pulmonary hypertension in the absence of significant left-sided heart disease indicates primary pulmonary or pulmonary vascular disease.

- The effects of pulmonary hypertension on the right heart result in pulmonary heart disease (or cor pulmonale) (Fig. 9.28).
- New onset of increased pulmonary pressures in a patient with acute chest pain or shortness of breath suggests the possibility of acute pulmonary embolism.

Step-by-Step Approach

Step 1: Estimate Pulmonary Pressure

- Pulmonary systolic pressure is determined based on the velocity in the TR jet and the estimated RA pressure (see Chapter 6) (Fig. 9.29).
- Additional signs of pulmonary hypertension also are evaluated.

❖ KEY POINTS

- ❑ When 2D echocardiography findings show right heart dysfunction, a diligent search for the highest-velocity TR jet is especially important.
- ❑ Other findings that suggest pulmonary hypertension include a short time to peak velocity and mid-systolic deceleration of the pulmonary artery velocity curve and paradoxical septal motion (Fig. 9.30).
- ❑ The velocity of the TR jet reflects the systolic pressure difference between the RV and RA, not the volume of regurgitation. Thus, severe pulmonary hypertension may be present with only mild TR.
- ❑ Overestimation of pulmonary pressures is avoided by using a gray-scale velocity display, increasing the high-pass (or wall) filter and adjusting the gain level appropriately. The low-intensity linear signals outside the edge of the

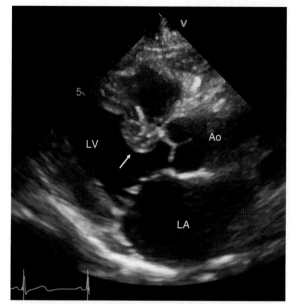

Fig. 9.27 Basal LV septal prominence. Parasternal long-axis view in an elderly patient showing prominence of the base of the septum (sometimes called a *septal knuckle; arrow*) due to an increased angle between the long axes of the aorta and LV. Mild mitral annular calcification and left atrial enlargement are present.

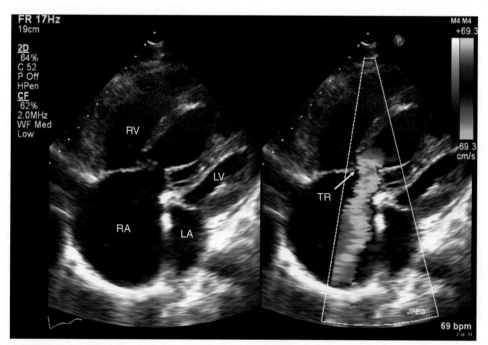

Fig. 9.28 Cor pulmonale. In this patient with severe pulmonary hypertension, there is severe RV hypertrophy and dilation with severely reduced RV systolic function. The RA is severely enlarged, with bulging of the atrial septum from right to left, suggesting that RA pressure is higher than LA pressure. Color Doppler shows severe tricuspid regurgitation due to annular dilation and RV dysfunction with a vena contracta width *(arrow)* greater than 7 mm. *TR,* Tricuspid regurgitation.

velocity envelope are not included in the velocity measurement.

❑ Pulmonary vascular resistance (PVR; in Wood units) can be estimated from the tricuspid regurgitant peak velocity (V_{TR}) and the velocity-time integral of flow in the RV outflow tract (VTI_{RVOT}) using the equation:

$$PVR = 10\,(V_{TR}/VTI_{RVOT})$$

Step 2: Evaluate Right Ventricular Size and Systolic Function

■ The RV responds to chronic pressure overload with dilation of the chamber, in addition to hypertrophy of the wall, often accompanied by systolic dysfunction.

■ RV size is measured as described in Chapter 6.

■ RV systolic function is evaluated using the TAPSE and the Doppler tissue annular systolic velocity.

■ The pattern of ventricular septal motion is evaluated in a parasternal short-axis view.

❖ **KEY POINTS**

❑ Visually, if the LV is normal in size, the RV is severely dilated if the 2D area in a 4-chamber view is larger than the LV; moderately dilated if equal to the LV; and mildly dilated if greater than normal but not equal to the LV.

❑ RV size and systolic function are evaluated based on parasternal, apical, and subcostal views.

❑ RV size and function often are best evaluated from the subcostal window, because the RV is seen in oblique image planes from the parasternal view and the RV free wall may be difficult to visualize on apical views.

❑ Elevated RV pressure results in flattening of the ventricular septum during both systole and diastole, whereas right heart volume overload results in flattening mostly during diastole.

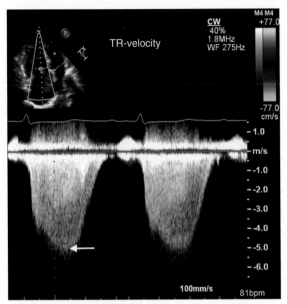

Fig. 9.29 Pulmonary hypertension. Tricuspid regurgitant *(TR)* jet in the same patient as Fig. 9.28 recorded with CW Doppler from an apical window. This recording shows a well-defined peak velocity with a dark band of velocities along the outer edge of the velocity curve, consistent with a good-quality signal. Even though color Doppler was used to guide placement of the CW Doppler ultrasound beam, a nonparallel intercept angle cannot be excluded with certainty. However, this TR velocity of 5.2 m/s indicates an RV-to-RA systolic pressure difference of 108 mm Hg, consistent with severe pulmonary hypertension.

Step 3: Evaluate the Severity of Tricuspid Regurgitation

■ Pulmonary hypertension often results in dilation of the tricuspid annulus with inadequate leaflet coaptation and tricuspid regurgitation.

■ Tricuspid regurgitation severity is evaluated based on the vena contracta width of the regurgitant jet, the density of the CW Doppler velocity curve, and the pattern of flow in the hepatic veins.

❖ **KEY POINTS**

❑ Vena contracta width is best measured in the parasternal RV inflow view; a width greater than 7 mm indicates severe regurgitation.

❑ The density of the CW Doppler signal is compared with antegrade flow: equal density indicates severe regurgitation.

❑ The normal hepatic vein pattern of systolic flow into the RA is reversed when tricuspid regurgitation is severe. However, systolic flow reversal also may be seen when the patient is not in sinus rhythm, even when regurgitation is not severe.

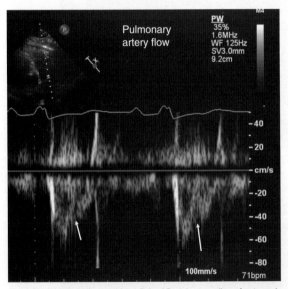

Fig. 9.30 Mid-systolic notching. Pulsed Doppler recording of antegrade flow in the pulmonary artery from the parasternal RV outflow view, in the same patient as Fig. 9.29, shows a short time to peak velocity and a mid-systolic notch *(arrows)* in the velocity curve, which are specific for severe pulmonary hypertension.

Step 4: Exclude Other Causes of Pulmonary Hypertension or Right Heart Enlargement

- Pulmonary hypertension and right heart enlargement also may be due to left-sided heart disease or congenital heart disease.
- Right heart enlargement without severe pulmonary hypertension is seen with volume overload due to valve regurgitation or a left to right shunt.

❖ **KEY POINTS**

❑ Left-sided or congenital heart disease results in secondary pulmonary hypertension, which is easily distinguished from primary pulmonary disease.

❑ Right-sided volume overload in the absence of an obvious atrial septal defect or severe right-sided valve regurgitation prompts TEE examination to exclude a sinus venous atrial septal defect or partial anomalous pulmonary venous return.

THE ECHO EXAM

Possible Diagnoses in Patient Referred for "Heart Failure"

Ischemic disease
Valvular disease
Hypertensive heart disease
Cardiomyopathy
    Dilated
    Hypertrophic
    Restrictive
    Other
Pericardial disease
    Constriction
    Tamponade
Pulmonary heart disease

Typical Cause of Increased Wall Thickness

	Hypertensive Heart Disease	Hypertrophic Cardiomyopathy	Restrictive Cardiomyopathy
LV hypertrophy	Present	Present	Present
Pattern of hypertrophy	Concentric	Asymmetrical	Concentric
Clinical history of hypertension	Present	Absent	Absent
Outflow obstruction	Mid-ventricular cavity obliteration	Dynamic subaortic obstruction	Absent
RV hypertrophy	Absent	May be present	Present
Pulmonary hypertension	Mild	Mild	Moderate
LV systolic function	Normal initially but reduced late in disease course	Normal	Normal initially but reduced late in disease course
LV diastolic function	Abnormal	Abnormal	Abnormal

+, Present.

Cardiomyopathies: Typical Features

	Dilated	Hypertrophic	Restrictive	Athlete's Heart
LV systolic function	Moderately-severely ↓	Normal	Normal	Normal
LV diastolic function	May be abnormal	Abnormal	Abnormal	Normal
LV hypertrophy	↑ LV mass due to LV dilation with normal wall thickness	Asymmetrical LV hypertrophy	Concentric LV hypertrophy	Normal wall thickness
Chamber dilation	All four chambers	LA and RA dilation if MR is present	LA and RA dilation	LV dilation
Outflow tract obstruction	Absent	Dynamic LV outflow tract obstruction in some patients	Absent	Absent
LV end-diastolic pressure	Elevated	Elevated	Elevated	Normal
Pulmonary artery pressures	Elevated	Elevated	Elevated	Normal

MR, Mitral regurgitation.

Echo Approach to the Cardiomyopathies

Modality	Echo Views and Flows	Measurements
Imaging	LV size and systolic function	LV-EDV, LV-ESV Apical biplane EF
	Degree and pattern of LV hypertrophy	LV mass
	Evidence for dynamic outflow tract obstruction	SAM of the mitral valve Aortic valve mid-systolic closure
	RV size and systolic function	
	LA size	
Doppler echo	Associated valvular regurgitation	Measure vena contracta, quantitate if more than mild
	LV diastolic function	Standard diastolic function evaluation with classification of severity and estimate of LV-EDP
	LV systolic function	dP/dt from MR jet Calculation of cardiac output
	Pulmonary pressures	TR jet and IVC for PA systolic pressure Evaluate PR jet for PA diastolic pressure Estimate pulmonary resistance
	Color, pulsed, and CW Doppler to quantitate outflow obstruction	Maximum outflow tract gradient

EF, Ejection fraction; *LV-EDV,* left ventricular end-diastolic volume; *LV-ESV,* left ventricular end-systolic volume; *MR,* mitral regurgitation; *PA,* pulmonary artery; *PR,* pulmonic regurgitation; *SAM,* systolic anterior motion; *TR,* tricuspid regurgitation.

SELF-ASSESSMENT QUESTIONS

Question 1

A 61-year-old man with history of heart block, paroxysmal atrial fibrillation, and bilateral hand tingling complained of shortness of breath. The patient had an unremarkable echocardiogram reported 5 years prior when he was being evaluated for a possible pacemaker. The patient has no other known cardiovascular history. Based on the echocardiogram (Fig. 9.31), the most likely diagnosis is which of the following?

A. Amyloidosis
B. Cor pulmonale
C. Hypertrophic cardiomyopathy
D. Hypertensive heart disease

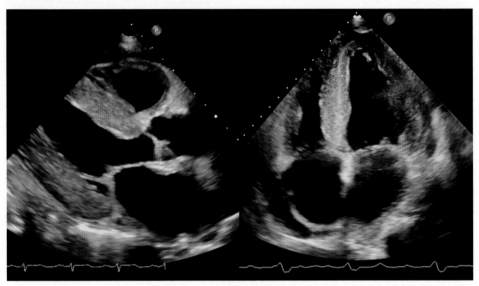

Fig. 9.31

Question 2

A 36-year-old man with hypertrophic cardiomyopathy is evaluated with echocardiography. Doppler tracings are obtained (Fig. 9.32). Which features of the Doppler signal are the most helpful in distinguishing the LV outflow velocity from mitral regurgitation?

A. Duration of flow
B. Maximum velocity
C. Accompanying diastolic flow velocity
D. Color imaging of jet direction

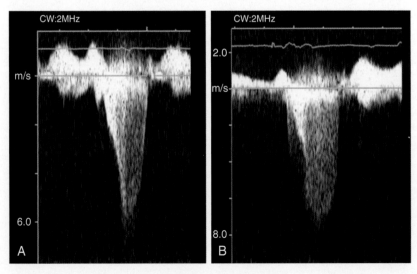

Fig. 9.32

Question 3

Which of the following is most consistent with RV systolic dysfunction?

- **A.** Tissue Doppler tricuspid annulus systolic velocity = 5 cm/s
- **B.** Tricuspid annular plane systolic excursion (TAPSE) = 3.0 cm
- **C.** RV annular diameter = 3.0 cm
- **D.** Tricuspid regurgitant (TR) jet acceleration slope = 1500 mm Hg/second

Question 4

An 83-year-old man with peripheral edema was evaluated for lower extremity edema. He has long-standing high blood pressure but no other significant medical or family history. An electrocardiogram (ECG) was unremarkable. An echocardiogram was obtained (Fig. 9.33) with a septal thickness measuring 2 cm as shown. The patient was noted to have normal systolic function and impaired relaxation. What diagnosis is most likely?

- **A.** Hypertrophic cardiomyopathy
- **B.** Discrete subaortic stenosis
- **C.** Sarcoidosis
- **D.** Normal age-related changes

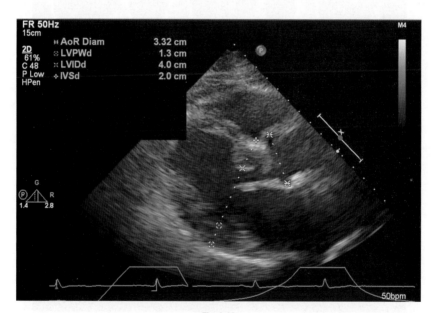

Fig. 9.33

Question 5

A 62-year-old patient status post-cardiac transplantation 12 years ago for a familial cardiomyopathy is referred for echocardiography. The following measurements are recorded:

LV dimension, end-diastole/ end-systole	5.0 cm/3.5 cm
Ejection fraction	62%
LA dimension	5.2 cm
Tricuspid regurgitant (TR) jet	2.1 m/s

His LV inflow (A), tissue Doppler (B), and LA inflow velocities (C) are shown (Fig. 9.34). These findings are most consistent with:

A. Transplant rejection
B. Coronary vasculopathy
C. Pericardial constriction
D. Normal heart

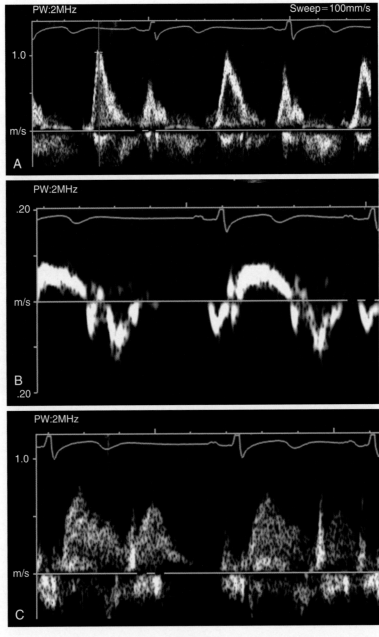

Fig. 9.34

Question 6

A 42-year-old woman presents for evaluation of exertional dyspnea. The following pulmonic valve M-mode tracing was obtained. (Fig. 9.35). Based on the finding *(arrows)* indicated, an additional echocardiographic finding that you would expect to see in this patient would be:

A. Prominent LV apical trabeculations

B. Interventricular septal flattening

C. Systolic anterior motion (SAM) of mitral valve chordae

D. Severe biatrial enlargement

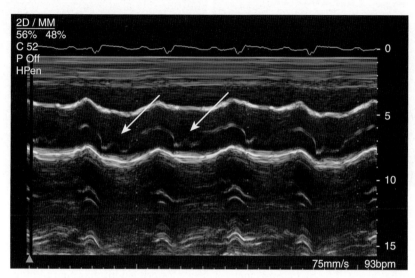

Fig. 9.35

Question 7

A 62-year-old man with a history of heart failure has this M-mode tracing recorded (Fig. 9.36). What is the mostly likely explanation for this finding?

A. Hypertrophic cardiomyopathy

B. Aortic stenosis

C. Left ventricular assist device (LVAD)

D. Normal functioning cardiac allograft

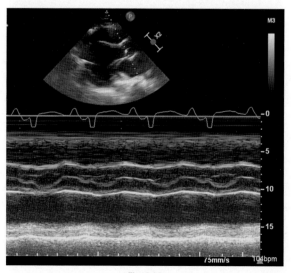

Fig. 9.36

Question 8

A patient is referred for echocardiography for a newly diagnosed systolic murmur (Fig. 9.37). These images are most consistent with:

A. Mitral valve prolapse
B. Dilated cardiomyopathy
C. Hypertrophic cardiomyopathy
D. Aortic stenosis

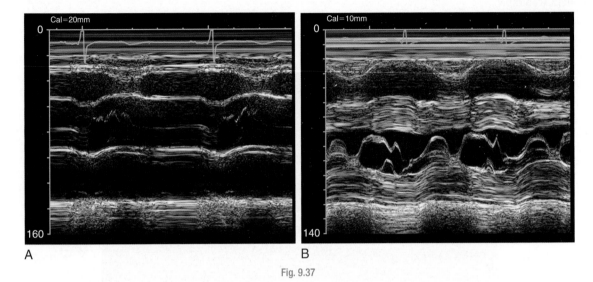

Fig. 9.37

Question 9

A 62-year-old man presents to the emergency department following cardiac arrest. The ECG shows tachycardia with frequent ectopic beats and non-specific ST-T wave changes. Troponin-I is elevated at 2.0 ng/mL. A transthoracic echocardiogram is obtained (Fig. 9.38). LV ejection fraction is measured at 65% by the apical biplane method without regional wall motion abnormalities. Urgent coronary angiography is negative for critical intracoronary lesions. The most likely diagnosis is:

A. Cardiac tamponade
B. Takotsubo cardiomyopathy
C. Aortic dissection
D. Pulmonary embolism

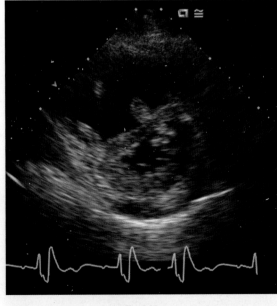

Fig. 9.38

Question 10

A 66-year-old woman with primary pulmonary hypertension confirmed by right heart catheterization is referred for echocardiography to determine if there has been interval improvement in pulmonary pressures since starting medical therapy. On her prior study, comment was made that peak tricuspid regurgitant (TR) jet was faint and unmeasurable. To evaluate RV pressure you recommend:

A. Doppler tracing pulmonary valve
B. Qp/Qs measurement
C. 2D imaging inferior vena cava (IVC)
D. Doppler tracing pulmonary branches

Question 11

A 59-year-old woman with no prior history of heart disease or recent travel presented to the hospital with shortness of breath and anxiety after a recent death in the family. The patient had diffuse T-wave inversion and mild pulmonary edema. The patient underwent echocardiogram with representative images in diastole (Fig. 9.39, *left*) and systole (see Fig. 9.39, *right*) shown. The most likely diagnosis is which of the following:

A. Spontaneous coronary artery dissection
B. Takotsubo cardiomyopathy
C. Chagas disease
D. Arrhythmic RV cardiomyopathy
E. Pulmonary embolism

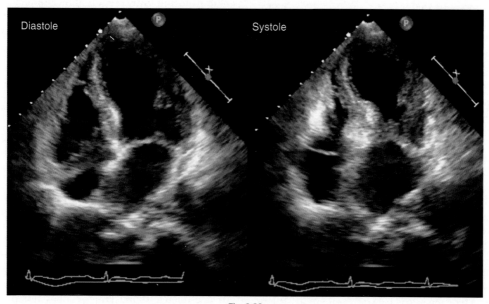

Fig. 9.39

Question 12

A 22-year-old male college football player was evaluated by his primary physician for bradycardia. The patient's blood pressure was 102/66 mm Hg. Electrocardiogram demonstrated sinus bradycardia at 42 beats per minute, LV hypertrophy voltage criteria, and 2 mm upsloping ST-elevation in precordial leads. An echocardiogram was ordered and noted 4-chamber enlargement with a dilated LV cavity at 5.7 cm and wall thickness of 1.5 cm. Systolic function was in a low-normal range at 52% and elevated early inflow mitral velocity (E) and tissue Doppler (E′). Based on these findings, the best assessment is which of the following?

A. Cardiac MRI to rule out hypertrophic cardiomyopathy
B. Reassurance of normal findings for the patient
C. Cardiac biopsy to establish diagnosis of infiltrative cardiomyopathy
D. Continuous ambulatory blood pressure monitoring to rule out hypertensive disease

ANSWERS

Answer 1: A

The patient's echocardiogram shows biventricular hypertrophy, enlarged atrium, small pericardial effusion, and valvular thickening consistent with an infiltrative cardiomyopathy. Given a clinical presentation of conduction deficit and peripheral neuropathy, this is most consistent with amyloidosis. The myocardium has a characteristic increased "sparkling" echogenicity that can be seen in amyloidosis. However, sparkling myocardium is not specific, and definitive evaluation is with a cardiac biopsy. Cor pulmonale (answer B) would be consistent with an acute or chronic pulmonary process without left-sided heart involvement. Hypertrophic cardiomyopathy (answer C) would be less likely in this patient with a normal echocardiogram 5 years prior. Valvular thickening is not part of myocardial hypertrophic disease, but mitral valve abnormalities (such as leaflet elongation with systolic anterior motion [SAM]) are frequently present. The history of heart block is also more often seen with infiltrative and inflammatory diseases. The patient has no prior history of hypertension (answer D) and thickening of the RV free wall and septum would not be attributed to systemic blood pressure.

Answer 2: B

It can be challenging to separate the velocity signal from the mitral regurgitant jet from the LV outflow signal in patients with hypertrophic cardiomyopathy when dynamic LV outflow obstruction is present. All of the listed features can be helpful, but maximum velocity, when both signals are recorded, is most reliable. The mitral regurgitant velocity must be higher than the LV outflow velocity, because the LV to LA pressure difference is always higher than the LV to aortic pressure difference. However, the signals may overlap because the jet direction may be similar, with an anteriorly directed mitral regurgitant jet due to systolic anterior motion (SAM) of the mitral valve. Examination of flow duration may aid in differentiation given that LV outflow starts after isovolumic contraction, whereas mitral regurgitation starts at mitral valve closure; however, flow duration may be misleading if onset of mitral regurgitation is delayed (late-systolic flow) following SAM of the mitral leaflets. The diastolic Doppler mitral inflow signal is typically recorded on both LV outflow and mitral valve inflow tracings, so it would not definitively differentiate between them. With obstruction, turbulent systolic flow in the LV outflow tract with aliasing of the color Doppler signal often obscures clear visualization of the mitral regurgitation jet.

Answer 3: A

Pulsed tissue Doppler interrogation of the tricuspid annulus assesses basal RV function. A peak systolic velocity (S′) greater than 10 cm/s is consistent with normal RV systolic function. As with all Doppler interrogation, nonparallel alignment with flow will lead to underestimation of peak velocities. Tricuspid annular plane systolic excursion (TAPSE) measures the distance of longitudinal systolic motion of the RV just below the tricuspid valve annulus, and is typically obtained from M-mode imaging from an apical 4-chamber view, taking care to align the transducer parallel with maximal systolic motion. Global RV function is inferred from the motion of the segment interrogated, so TAPSE would not be a valid measure of regional RV dysfunction. A TAPSE of greater than 1.8 cm is consistent with normal RV systolic function. RV annular diameter should be measured from an RV focused apical 4-chamber view. The upper reference size for RV basal diameter is 4.2 cm, so a diameter of 3.0 cm would fall in the normal range. Analogous to dP/dt from the mitral regurgitant Doppler jet for LV systolic function, RV dP/dt is not routinely measured, because it is load dependent and is less accurate with increasing tricuspid regurgitation severity (commonly coincident with worsening RV function).

Answer 4: D

The patient has normal age-related changes in an 83-year-old man. The patient has isolated proximal septal thickening commonly described as a "knuckle" or "bulge." This is a common finding in older individuals and likely related to an increasing acute angle between the basal septum and the aortic root as seen in the figure. The patient's age, isolated septal prominence, and long-standing hypertension should distinguish this condition from hypertrophic cardiomyopathy (answer A). Discrete subaortic stenosis (answer B) would demonstrate thin membranes an either aortic obstruction or aortic valvular regurgitation. A membrane is more easily visualized with TEE. An age-related septal knuckle does not prove clinically important stenosis. Sarcoidosis (answer C) has nonspecific findings but is more associated with heart block, pericardial effusions, systolic dysfunction, and possible regional wall motion abnormalities, which are not present in this patient.

Answer 5: D

The tissue Doppler sample (B) demonstrates a higher myocardial E wave velocity, implying normal myocardial motion and a normal E/E′ ratio (normal LA pressure). Cardiac donor hearts usually come from younger, previously healthy donors. Echocardiography is utilized to monitor for posttransplant complications. The Doppler LV inflow pattern (A) seen in this case is comparable to a young individual, with a relatively higher E/A ratio. In young hearts, the majority of LV inflow occurs early in diastole with a relatively small contribution of LV filling by atrial contraction. Left atrial enlargement was the result of suturing the native and donor atria rather than increased LA pressure.

Echocardiographic markers of cardiac transplant rejection are usually absent in the early stages. However, with progression, myocardial inflammation may lead to increased wall thickness (hypertrophy), evidence of diastolic dysfunction with restrictive ventricular filling and, in advanced cases, systolic dysfunction. Coronary vasculopathy would manifest with regional wall motion abnormalities in the myocardial distributions affected by the vasculopathy. With diffuse microvascular disease, systolic dysfunction may be global in nature. Pericardial constriction following cardiac transplantation is rare given that the native pericardium is not resewn following transplant.

Answer 6: B

The M-mode tracing is taken across the RV outflow tract and pulmonic valve. During systole, there is mid-systolic notching (*arrows;* termed *flying W*) of the posterior pulmonary valve cusp consistent with pulmonary hypertension. Other characteristic echo findings in severe pulmonary hypertension include RV chamber enlargement with flattening of the interventricular septum, RV hypertrophy, and systolic dysfunction. Pulmonary arterial hypertension also results in an asymmetrical Doppler envelope and decreased time to peak velocity or acceleration time to less than 60 ms. Prominent apical trabeculations are seen in patients with LV noncompaction. In patients with hypertrophy cardiomyopathy, dynamic subaortic LV outflow obstruction is associated with mid-systolic closure of the aortic (not pulmonic) valve and with systolic anterior motion (SAM) of the mitral valve. Severe biatrial enlargement is a hallmark feature of restrictive cardiomyopathy with restricted ventricular diastolic filling and high atrial pressures.

Answer 7: C

The patient has a variable incomplete opening of the aortic valve with a regular rhythm and reduced anterior-posterior aortic root motion consistent with the presence of a left ventricular assist device (LVAD) for dilated cardiomyopathy. The ventricular assist device decompresses the LV and pumps blood into the ascending aorta bypassing the aortic valve. The aortic valve may remain closed through the cardiac cycle or have variable incomplete opening depending on the blood flow diverted to the LVAD. Hypertrophic cardiomyopathy would demonstrate complete early opening of an aortic valve but with mid-systolic partial closure and coarse fluttering due to dynamic obstruction. Patients with aortic stenosis have calcified and thickened aortic valves that would have similar fixed reduced opening between cardiac cycles

(answer B). A normal functioning cardiac allograft would be expected to have normal anterior-posterior aortic root motion with systolic function and left atrial enlargement. The left atrial diameter is not significantly dilated, measuring under 4 cm.

Answer 8: C

A newly diagnosed systolic murmur is a common clinical indication for a TTE. M-mode tracings across the aortic valve (A) and mitral valve (B) for this patient are shown. M-mode tracings of the mitral valve in patients with significant obstruction in the LV outflow tract show early closure of the aortic valve *(arrow)* as was seen in this case below (Fig. 9.40A). M-mode tracings across septum and mitral valve show a severely thickened septum and systolic anterior motion (SAM) of the anterior mitral valve leaflet *(arrow)* (see Fig. 9.40B). These echocardiographic findings are consistent with hypertrophic cardiomyopathy. A systolic murmur is common in hypertrophic cardiomyopathy, due to turbulent flow in the LV outflow tract.

The murmur of mitral valve prolapse is due to mitral regurgitation. M-mode tracings of the mitral valve leaflets in mitral valve prolapse show late-systolic posterior buckling into the LA.

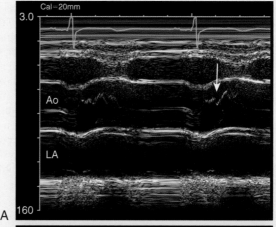

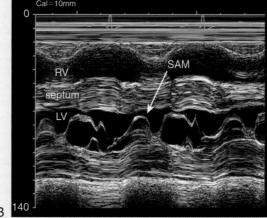

Fig. 9.40

Patients with dilated cardiomyopathy often have significant functional mitral regurgitation due to dilation of the valve annulus and resultant poor leaflet coaptation. M-mode tracings of these patients show enlargement of the LV and increased E point septal separation. In calcific aortic stenosis, there is thickening and heavy calcification of the aortic valve. In advanced cases, there is poor systolic opening of the leaflets throughout systole. The aortic valve leaflets in this M-mode tracing appear thin and mobile, not consistent with aortic stenosis.

Answer 9: D

This parasternal short-axis view shows interventricular septal flattening, consistent with RV enlargement. The echocardiogram and clinical presentation are most consistent with pulmonary embolism with acute RV strain. Although increased cardiac biomarkers suggest acute myocardial injury, LV systolic function is preserved without regional wall motion abnormalities, and the troponin is only minimally elevated. Coronary angiography is negative, excluding a transmural myocardial infarction. The clinical presentation of takotsubo cardiomyopathy is chest pain or dyspnea following a significant emotional or physiological stress, manifested as transient akinesis of the apical and mid-LV segments with regional wall motion abnormalities that extend beyond a single epicardial coronary arterial distribution. Normal LV chamber size and systolic function, as was seen in this case, is not consistent with takotsubo cardiomyopathy. There is no pericardial effusion seen on the image provided to suggest cardiac tamponade. Although the clinical presentation could be concordant with aortic dissection, the aorta is not seen on this image and there are no findings to suggest a complication of dissection, such as a pericardial effusion.

Answer 10: A

This patient's peak tricuspid regurgitant (TR) jet was faint and unmeasurable, making estimation of RV systolic pressure by echocardiography limited on repeat studies. In the absence of pulmonic stenosis, the RV end-diastolic pressure can be estimated from the pulmonic regurgitant jet (Fig. 9.41). The RV diastolic pressure is calculated as $4V^2$, where (V) is the peak end-diastolic velocity measured from the pulmonic valve Doppler regurgitant jet. Analogous to pulmonary artery systolic pressure estimates, the pulmonary artery diastolic pressure is the sum of the RV diastolic pressure and the RA pressure estimate, which is inferior vena cava (IVC) diameter at rest and following inspiration. The diameter of the IVC, as assessed by 2D imaging, provides an estimate of right atrial pressure (not RV pressure, the

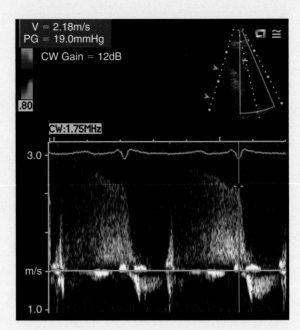

Fig. 9.41

question in this case). The pulmonic volume flow rate (Qp) measurement is the product of the RV outflow tract Doppler velocity time integral and the cross-sectional area at the RV outflow tract. The systemic volume flow rate (Qs) is the product of the LV outflow tract Doppler velocity time integral and the cross-sectional area at the LV outflow tract. Qp/Qs ratio is a calculation of the comparative volume flow between the RV and LV to quantitate the severity of an intracardiac shunt. Antegrade Doppler tracing of the pulmonary branches would provide hemodynamic data for the pressure gradient at the point of interrogation (i.e., pulmonary artery branch stenosis) and would not provide data on RV chamber pressure in systole.

Answer 11: B

The echocardiogram demonstrates hyperdynamic basal systolic function with diffuse apical dilation and dysfunction after a stressful event most consistent with takotsubo cardiomyopathy (stress-induced cardiomyopathy). Regional wall motion abnormalities of middle to apical segment in the septal and lateral walls are not consistent with a coronary artery distribution (answer A). Chagas disease (answer C) is a protozoan infection with frequent systemic findings, travel to endemic areas for *Trypanosoma curzi*, and apical aneurysms. Arrhythmic right ventricular cardiomyopathy (answer D) would be associated with right ventricular enlargement and dysfunction, which are not appreciated in the figure.

Answer 12: B

The patient has normal findings of an athlete's heart. Regular intensive athletic training produces alterations in myocardial structure with chamber dilation and wall thickening. Distinguishing between physiologic phenotypic changes with exercise and cardiomyopathy is important to prevent unnecessary testing in healthy adults, yet identifying at risk patients with potential cardiomyopathy. Athletes typically have normal systolic and diastolic function unlike hypertrophic cardiomyopathy of infiltrative disease (answers A and C). The patient has normal blood pressure at a young age, and screening for hypertension with continuous ambulatory monitoring is not warranted. Hypertensive heart disease is less likely to lead to biatrial enlargement and normal diastolic function in this young patient. Furthermore, hypertension would need to be severe to produce such morphological changes at an early age.

10 Pericardial Disease

STEP-BY-STEP APPROACH

Pericardial Effusion

- There are numerous causes for accumulation of fluid in the pericardial space (Table 10.1).
- A pericardial effusion may be asymptomatic or may be associated with pericarditis or with tamponade physiology.
- Pericarditis is a clinical diagnosis based on the triad of typical pericardial pain, a pericardial rub, and diffuse ST elevation on the electrocardiogram (ECG) (Fig. 10.1).
- Tamponade physiology is present when systemic blood pressure or cardiac output is reduced due to compression of the cardiac chambers by the pericardial fluid.

❖ KEY POINTS

- ❑ In patients with pericarditis, the effusion ranges from absent to large in size.
- ❑ The presence of a pericardial rub does not correlate with the size of the effusion.
- ❑ In a patient with a large pericardial effusion and hypotension or a low cardiac output, tamponade physiology likely is present, even if other echocardiographic signs are not seen.

Step 1: Record Blood Pressure and Heart Rate

- The first step in echocardiographic evaluation of a patient with suspected pericardial disease is to

measure and record blood pressure and heart rate (as for any echocardiographic examination).
- Pulsus paradoxus is a decline in the systolic blood pressure by more than 20 mm Hg with inspiration (Fig. 10.2).

❖ KEY POINTS

- ❑ Hypotension and tachycardia are nonspecific but are seen in patients with tamponade physiology.
- ❑ To measure pulsus paradoxus, the blood pressure cuff is deflated until the first Korotkoff sound is intermittently heard during expiration. The cuff is then slowly deflated until the Korotkoff sound is heard on every beat. The difference between these two pressures is the paradoxical pulse.
- ❑ A physician should be present for the echocardiographic study when the patient is hemodynamically compromised (i.e., hypotension or significant tachycardia).

Step 2: Evaluate for the Presence of Pericardial Fluid

- An echo-free space adjacent to the heart is consistent with a pericardial effusion (Fig. 10.3).
- The pericardial sac extends completely around both the left ventricle (LV) and right ventricle (RV), from the apex to the base, and extends around the right atrium (RA) to the bases of the superior and inferior vena cava.

TABLE 10.1   Pericardial Disease: Clinical-Echocardiographic Correlates

	Clinical Presentation	Echocardiographic Findings
Constrictive pericarditis	Dyspnea on exertion and signs of venous congestion (elevated venous pressure, ascites, and edema)	• Ventricular septal shift • Hepatic vein diastolic flow reversals in expiration • Preserved or increased medial E' velocity, often with medial E' > lateral E' velocities • Respiratory variation in mitral E velocities • Plethora of the IVC • Decreased lateral longitudinal strain, as compared to medial
Pericardial effusion	Variable depending on cause; often asymptomatic and incidentally discovered	• Pericardial effusion size ranges from trivial to very large; location is circumferential or loculated; fluid echo-brightness will vary with characteristics (transudative, exudative, or frankly bloody)
Tamponade	Variable; often nonspecific; including hypotension, tachycardia, elevated venous pressure, and pulsus paradoxus	• Chamber collapse • Plethora of the IVC • Respiratory variation in right- and left-heart filling and venous flow patterns
Acute pericarditis	Characteristic chest pain and ECG changes; pericardial friction rub on auscultation	• Effusion sometimes present, and helps secure the diagnosis • Ventricular regional wall motion abnormalities suggest associated myocarditis or an alternative diagnosis • Tamponade or constrictive physiology can occur

ECG, Electrocardiogram; *IVC,* inferior vena cava.
From Otto CM: *The practice of clinical echocardiography,* ed 6, Philadelphia, 2018, Elsevier.

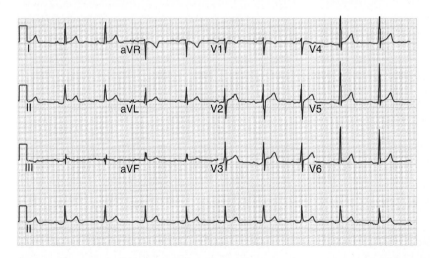

Fig. 10.1 **ECG in pericarditis.** This 12-lead electrocardiogram (ECG) shows diffuse upsloping ST elevation and PR segment depression, consistent with pericarditis in this 42-year-old man with a 2-week history of persistent dull chest pain and a pericardial rub on physical examination.

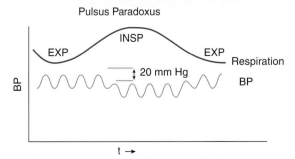

Fig. 10.2 **Pulsus paradoxus.** This schematic shows that with inspiration, systolic blood pressure falls by at least 20 mm Hg when pulsus paradoxus is present. *BP,* Blood pressure; *EXP,* expiration; *INSP,* inspiration.

■ The pericardial sac extends posterior to the left atrium (LA), between the pulmonary vein orifices (the oblique sinus of the pericardium), and there is a small cuff of pericardial space around the base of the great vessels (the transverse sinus) (Fig. 10.4).

❖ **KEY POINTS**

❑ An isolated anterior, relatively echo-free space usually is due to the normal epicardial fat pad. With an effusion, the echo-free space usually is seen both anteriorly and posteriorly (Fig. 10.5)

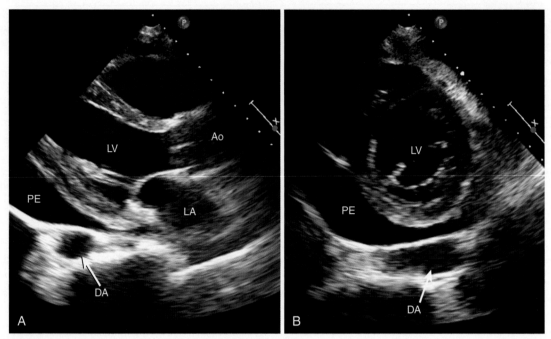

Fig. 10.3 Pericardial effusion. An echo-free space consistent with a pericardial effusion is seen posterior to the LV in both the parasternal long-axis view (**A**) and in the short-axis view at the midventricular level (**B**). *Ao,* Aorta; *DA,* descending aorta; *PE,* pericardial effusion.

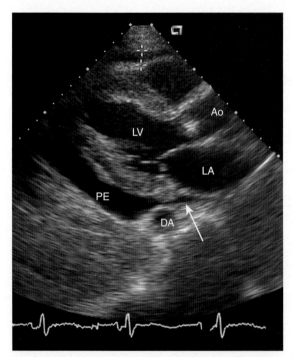

Fig. 10.4 Pericardial fluid in the oblique sinus of the pericardium. A small echo-free space is seen posterior to the LA *(arrow)* in this parasternal long-axis view. This is clearly a pericardial effusion, not pleural fluid, as it tracks anteriorly to the descending aorta. *Ao,* Aorta; *DA,* descending aorta; *PE,* pericardial effusion.

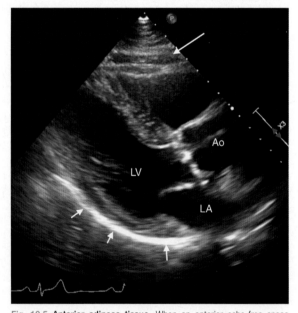

Fig. 10.5 Anterior adipose tissue. When an anterior echo-free space *(long arrow)* is seen, as in this parasternal long-axis view, without evidence for posterior effusion *(short arrows),* the most likely diagnosis is normal epicardial adipose tissue or a "fat pad." This patient also has aortic valve stenosis. *Ao,* Aorta

❑ A pleural effusion is seen anterior to the descending thoracic aorta, whereas a pleural effusion extends posteriorly to the descending aorta (Fig. 10.6)

❑ Fluid adjacent to the RA in the apical 4-chamber view may be due to pericardial or pleural fluid. The specific diagnosis is based on evidence of pericardial or pleural fluid in other views.

❑ If the pericardial fluid contains thrombus or fibrinous debris, the effusion may be echogenic instead of echolucent (Fig. 10.7).

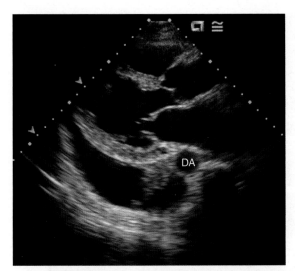

Fig. 10.6 **Pleural effusion.** A large left pleural effusion is seen in this parasternal long-axis view. The pleural effusion extends posterior to the descending thoracic aorta. *DA,* Descending aorta.

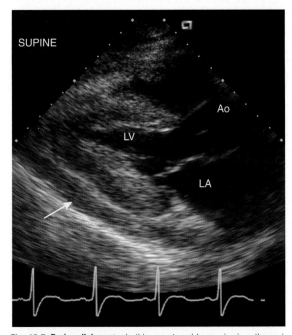

Fig. 10.7 **Pericardial mass.** In this parasternal long-axis view, the pericardial space *(arrow)* is filled with echo-dense material, consistent with hematoma, tumor, or fibrinous debris. *Ao,* Aorta.

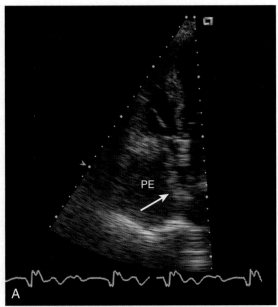

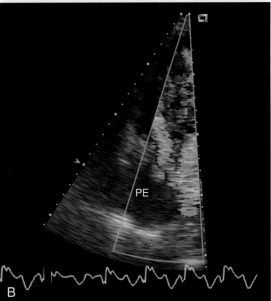

Fig. 10.8 **Loculated pericardial effusion.** In an apical 4-chamber orientation, the sector has been narrowed to focus on the right side of the heart. The RV is small, with a catheter seen in the chamber. **(A)** The area normally occupied by the RA consists primarily of loculated pericardial effusion with the RA free wall *(arrow)* compressed so that is almost touches the interatrial septum. **(B)** Color Doppler confirms the severe compression of the RA with a very narrow flow stream into the RV. *PE,* Pericardial effusion.

Step 3: Evaluate the Distribution of Pericardial Fluid

- Effusions may be circumferential or loculated so that evaluation in multiple views from parasternal, apical, and subcostal windows is essential.
- Loculation of fluid due to adhesions often is seen after cardiac surgery or trauma or with malignant effusions.

❖ **KEY POINTS**

- ❑ Loculated fluid may be missed unless multiple views are examined; sometimes transesophageal echocardiography (TEE) is needed to identify loculated fluid posterior to the LA (Fig. 10.8).
- ❑ Loculated fluid occasionally may be mistaken for a normal cardiac chamber (e.g., when loculated fluid compresses the LA or RA).

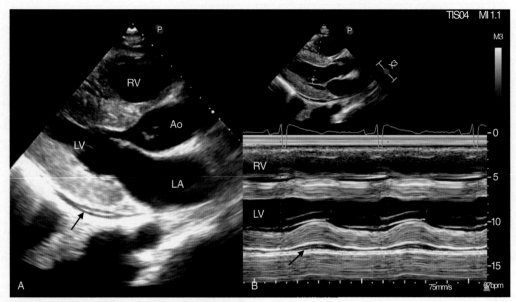

Fig. 10.9 M-mode tracing of pericardial effusion. (A) A very small pericardial effusion is seen on 2D imaging posterior to the LV *(arrow).* (B) The M-mode tracing demonstrates the small effusion more clearly with flat motion of the parietal pericardium so that there is a more prominent posterior echo-free space in systole than diastole *(arrow);* the posterior wall moves anteriorly while the pericardial line remains flat during systole.

Step 4: Estimate the Size of the Pericardial Effusion

- A small amount of pericardial fluid is normal, appearing as a trivial or absent effusion on echocardiography.
- The volume of an abnormal pericardial effusion ranges from 50 mL to more than 1 L.
- The size of the effusion is qualitatively graded as small, moderate, or large.

❖ **KEY POINTS**

- A small effusion on two-dimensional (2D) imaging can be confirmed by the M-mode finding of flat motion of the parietal pericardium with systolic separation of the epicardium (Fig. 10.9).
- There is no precise approach to estimation of pericardial fluid volume by echocardiography.
- One useful approach is to consider the effusion small if the distance between the epicardium and pericardium is less than 0.5 cm, moderate if 0.5 to 2 cm, and large if more than 2 cm (Fig. 10.10).
- With loculated effusions, size is described in a similar fashion along with the location of the fluid.
- Evaluation from the subcostal view is especially important because this approach often is used for pericardiocentesis (Fig. 10.11).

Tamponade Physiology

- Pericardial pressure depends on both the volume and rate of accumulation of pericardial fluid.
- Tamponade physiology occurs when pericardial pressure exceeds intracardiac pressure.

- With tamponade physiology, cardiac output and blood pressure are reduced due to impaired cardiac filling due to compression of the cardiac chambers.
- Pulsus paradoxus is an excessive fall (>20 mm Hg) in systolic blood pressure with inspiration, due to the fall in cardiac output with inspiration.

❖ **KEY POINTS**

- Tamponade physiology may occur with a rapidly accumulating moderate-sized effusion (e.g., with aortic dissection or trauma) but may not occur even with very large effusions if the rate of increase in size was gradual.
- Thin-walled, low-pressure cardiac chambers (e.g., the RA) are compressed at lower pericardial pressures than thicker-walled chambers (e.g., the RV).
- Cardiac compression is most evident during the phase of the cardiac cycle when the chamber pressure is low (e.g., systole for the atrial chambers, diastole for the RV).
- With inspiration, intrathoracic pressure falls, resulting in increased filling of the right heart. If total cardiac volume is fixed (as with tamponade physiology), the increased filling of the right heart limits filling of the left heart, resulting in a lower forward stroke volume and blood pressure.
- If the patient has a low cardiac output or hypotension and a large pericardial effusion is present, further echocardiographic evaluation is not needed; prompt therapy is more appropriate.

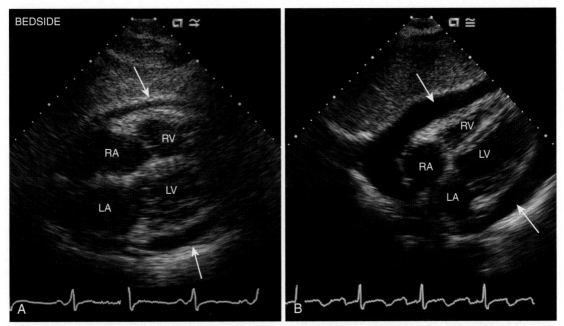

Fig. 10.10 Size of pericardial effusion. The size of a pericardial effusion is graded qualitatively, but measurement of the distance between the epicardium and pericardium is helpful. On a subcostal view, both these patients have circumferential pericardial effusion, with a moderate effusion **(A)** showing between 0.5 and 2 cm maximal pericardial separation compared to more than 2 cm with a large effusion *(arrows)* **(B)**.

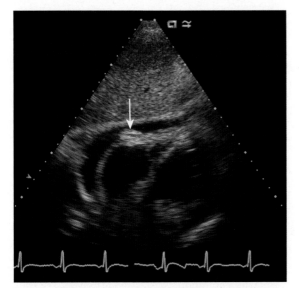

Fig. 10.11 Subcostal view of pericardial effusion. This approach often is used for drainage of pericardial fluid. In this patient, the effusion between the liver and right side of the heart is seen. The normal adipose tissue at the right atrioventricular groove *(arrow)* often is well seen when a pericardial effusion is present. If pericardiocentesis is planned, a transducer position where the effusion is closer to the site of needle entry, with less intervening hepatic tissue, is preferred. This effusion is quite small, so many clinicians would defer pericardiocentesis.

Step 1: Look for Right Atrium Systolic Collapse

- When intrapericardial pressure exceeds RA pressure, the RA free wall collapses in systole (Fig. 10.12).

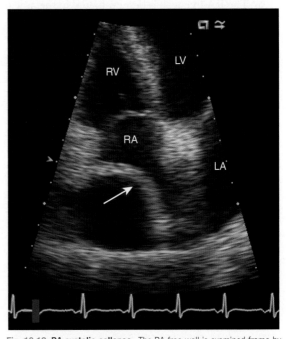

Fig. 10.12 RA systolic collapse. The RA free wall is examined frame by frame in the apical 4-chamber plane using zoom mode and a narrow sector. This end-systolic frame shows persistent systolic compression (or collapse) of the RA free wall *(arrow)* consistent with tamponade physiology.

- RA free wall inversion for more than one-third of systole is sensitive and specific for the diagnosis of tamponade physiology.

❖ **KEY POINTS**

  ▫ Brief systolic inversion of the RA free wall may be seen without tamponade physiology.

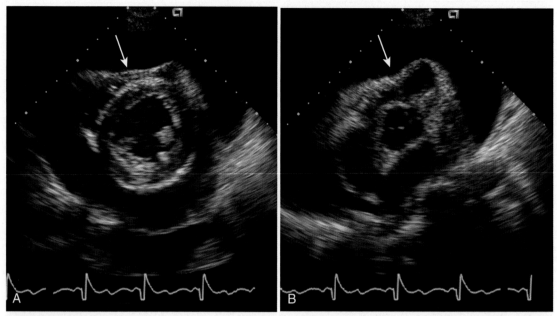

Fig. 10.13 **RV diastolic collapse.** Parasternal short-axis views in mid-diastole in a patient with a large pericardial effusion show RV diastolic collapse at the midventricular **(A)** and RV outflow tract **(B)** levels *(arrows)*. The RV chamber is very small, with a convex indentation of the RV free wall by the pericardial effusion.

❑ The RA free wall is best evaluated in the apical and subcostal 4-chamber views.

❑ Zoom mode provides optimal image resolution; a narrow 2D sector improves frame rate.

❑ Frame-by-frame analysis, to determine the number of frames with free wall inversion compared with the total frames in systole, improves the accuracy of this approach.

Step 2: Evaluate Right Ventricular Diastolic Collapse

■ When intrapericardial pressure exceeds RV diastolic pressure, the RV free wall collapses in diastole (Fig. 10.13).

■ RV diastolic collapse is less sensitive but more specific than brief RA systolic collapse for the diagnosis of pericardial tamponade.

❖ KEY POINTS

❑ Frame-by-frame analysis or use of an M-mode cursor through the RV free wall may be helpful for evaluation of the timing of RV free wall motion.

❑ RV diastolic collapse may be appreciated in parasternal long- and short-axis and in apical and subcostal 4-chamber views.

❑ If the RV free wall is thickened due to hypertrophy or an infiltrative process, diastolic collapse may not occur even with elevated pericardial pressures.

❑ RV diastolic collapse will not occur if RV diastolic pressure exceeds pericardial pressure, as can happen in severe pulmonary hypertension.

Step 3: Examine for Reciprocal Respiratory Changes in Right and Left Ventricular Volumes

■ An effusion with tamponade physiology results in a fixed total cardiac volume.

■ With a fixed total volume, the increase in right-sided filling with inspiration is matched by a reciprocal decrease in left-sided volumes.

■ Conversely, with expiration there is a relative increase in left, compared with right, heart filling.

❖ KEY POINTS

❑ The reciprocal changes in right- and left-filling with respiration are best seen on 2D imaging in a 4-chamber view.

❑ With inspiration, the ventricular septum shifts to the left, followed by a shift toward the right with expiration.

❑ An M-mode tracing of the septum from the parasternal window also may be helpful.

Step 4: Evaluate for Reciprocal Respiratory Changes in Right and Left Ventricular Filling Velocities

■ Analogous to the changes in RV and LV volumes with respiration, the volume of inflow across the atrioventricular valves varies with respiration.

■ With inspiration, there is an increase (>25%) in RV diastolic filling; with expiration, LV diastolic filling increases by >25% (Fig. 10.14).

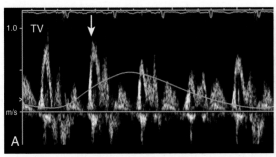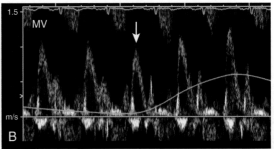

Fig. 10.14 **Inflow velocities with tamponade.** In this patient with a large pericardial effusion, ventricular inflow velocities across the tricuspid valve *(TV)* and mitral valve *(MV)* were recorded at a slow sweep speed simultaneously with a respirometer tracing. The cyan-colored respirometer tracing indicates inspiration as an upward deflection and expiration as a downward deflection. **(A)** The TV tracing shows that the inflow velocity increases with inspiration with a peak velocity of only 0.29 m/s in expiration and 0.75 m/s with inspiration *(arrow)*. **(B)** There are reciprocal changes in transmitral flow, with the peak velocity decreasing from 1.2 m/s during expiration to 0.9 m/s on the first beat after inspiration *(arrow)*.

❖ **KEY POINTS**

❏ The phase of respiration is recorded (using a respirometer) simultaneously with the ECG and Doppler velocity data.

❏ A slow sweep speed is used to include more than one respiratory cycle on the recording.

❏ The Doppler sample volume is positioned, and a 2D image is recorded for several beats to ensure that the intercept angle between the Doppler beam and the direction of inflow does not vary significantly with respiration. If there is a significant variation in the intercept angle, observed differences in velocity with respiration may be an artifact due to assuming a constant angle in the Doppler equation.

❏ With tamponade physiology, RV diastolic filling increases and LV diastolic filling decreases on the first beat after inspiration.

❏ Evaluation of filling dynamics is challenging, so that an apparent lack of respiratory variation does not exclude the possibility of tamponade physiology.

Step 5: Determine If Right Atrium Filling Pressures Are Elevated

■ Elevated RA filling pressures are a sensitive, but not specific, sign of cardiac tamponade.

■ Echocardiographic evaluation of RA filling pressure is based on the size and respiratory variation of the inferior vena cava; a dilated vena cava without respiratory variation and with dilated hepatic veins is called *plethora of the inferior vena cava* (Fig. 10.15).

❖ **KEY POINTS**

❏ Images of the inferior vena cava are obtained from the subcostal view in spontaneously breathing patients.

❏ This method is not applicable in patients on positive pressure mechanical ventilation.

❏ There are many other causes for elevated RA pressures, other than tamponade physiology, so this finding is interpreted in the context of the other imaging findings.

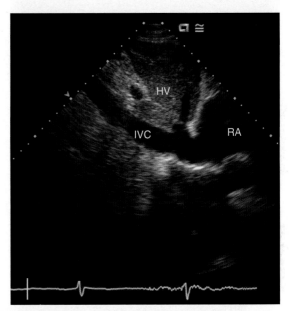

Fig. 10.15 **Inferior vena caval (IVC) dilation.** Subcostal view showing a dilated IVC and hepatic vein in a patient with pericardial tamponade. With inspiration, there was no change in IVC diameter. *HV,* Hepatic vein.

❏ Tamponade may be present without plethora of the inferior vena cava if the patient is hypovolemic.

Step 6: Perform Echo-Guided Pericardiocentesis If Clinically Indicated

■ Echocardiography may be used to guide the percutaneous pericardiocentesis procedure either to define the best approach to percutaneous drainage or to confirm the needle position in the pericardial space (Fig. 10.16).

■ Echocardiography is used after pericardiocentesis to assess the amount of residual fluid (Fig. 10.17).

❖ **KEY POINTS**

❏ Evaluation from parasternal, apical, and subcostal approaches demonstrates the depth and amount of pericardial fluid relative to the position of the transducer.

- Visualization of the tip of the needle is problematic because any segment of the needle passing through the 2D image plane may be mistaken for the tip; therefore three-dimensional (3D) imaging may be helpful.

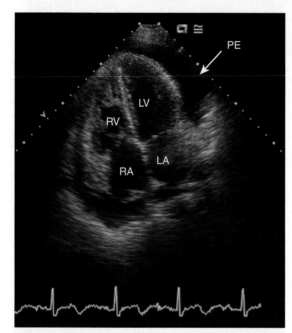

Fig. 10.16 **Large pericardial effusion.** Apical 4-chamber view showing a large circumferential pericardial effusion, with relatively more fluid posterior and lateral to the LV, as is typical on echocardiography. Fluid is seen adjacent to the RA, and a small amount of fluid is seen superior to the LA, in the oblique sinus of the pericardium that extends between the right and left pulmonary veins. *PE,* Pericardial effusion.

- The position of the needle is confirmed by injection of a small amount of agitated saline to produce a contrast effect.

Pericardial Constriction

- Pericardial constriction is the result of pericardial thickening and fibrosis with fusion of the parietal and visceral pericardium.
- The thickened and rigid pericardium constricts the cardiac chambers, resulting in a limited total cardiac volume and a reduced cardiac output.

❖ **KEY POINTS**

- Common causes of pericardial constriction include prior cardiac surgery or trauma, radiation therapy, and recurrent pericarditis.
- Like tamponade physiology, the fixed total cardiac volume with pericardial constriction results in reciprocal changes in right- and left-heart filling (Fig. 10.18).
- Typically there is no significant pericardial effusion when constrictive pericarditis is present, although there are rare cases of effusive constrictive physiology.
- Clinically the differentiation of constrictive pericarditis (which is treated by pericardiotomy) and restrictive cardiomyopathy (which is treated medically) is problematic.

Step 1: Look for Evidence of Pericardial Thickening

- Pericardial thickening may be evident on 2D echocardiography as areas of increased echogenicity in the pericardial region (Fig. 10.19).

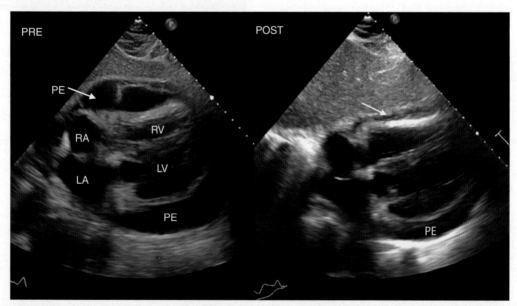

Fig. 10.17 **Echocardiographic monitoring of pericardiocentesis in the cardiac catheterization lab.** At baseline *(PRE),* a subcostal 4-chamber view shows a large pericardial effusion with some fibrinous stands. After drainage of 1 L of fluid *(POST),* repeat imaging shows a much smaller effusion along the RV free wall, although some fluid persists posterior to the LV. If needle position is uncertain, a small amount of sterile saline can be injected to produce a contrast effect, confirming the needle tip is in the pericardial space. *PE,* Pericardial effusion.

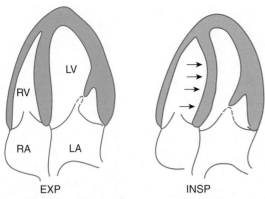

Fig. 10.18 **Pericardial constriction.** Schematic diagram showing an apical 4-chamber view at end-expiration *(EXP)* and during inspiration *(INSP)* with pericardial constriction. The increase in RV filling with inspiration results in a compensatory decrease in LV size, as the total cardiac volume is constrained by the thickened and adherent pericardium. This results in "septal shift" with inspiration.

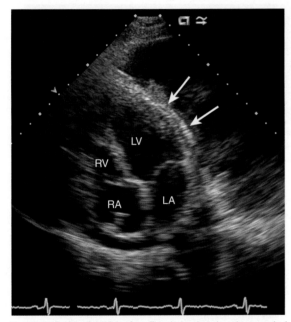

Fig. 10.19 **Pericardial thickening.** This 4-chamber view shows marked thickening of the pericardium lateral to the LV *(arrows)* in a patient later diagnosed with constrictive pericarditis. Pericardial thickening is differentiated from effusion by the echogenicity of the pericardial space.

■ On M-mode tracings, pericardial thickening is evident as multiple dense parallel lines posterior to the LV endocardium that persist even with low gain settings (Fig. 10.20).

❖ **KEY POINTS**

❑ Echocardiography is not sensitive for detection of pericardial thickening; cardiac computed tomography or cardiac magnetic resonance imaging is preferred when measurement of pericardial thickness is needed.

❑ Pericardial thickening may be asymmetric so that a complete evaluation includes evaluation from parasternal, apical, and subcostal windows.

Step 2: Evaluate for Anatomic Evidence of Constriction

■ Typical findings in patients with pericardial constriction are enlarged atria (due to chronically elevated filling pressures) and small ventricles with normal systolic function.

■ M-mode findings in constrictive pericarditis include reduced posterior motion of the LV posterior wall endocardium in diastole (<2 mm) and a brief rapid posterior motion of the ventricular septum in early diastole.

❖ **KEY POINTS**

❑ There are no specific 2D imaging findings in patients with constrictive pericarditis.

❑ The diagnosis of constrictive pericarditis should be considered in the appropriate clinical setting (cardiac symptoms in a patient at risk of constrictive disease) if the echocardiogram does not show other causes for the patient's symptoms.

❑ Constrictive pericarditis most often is diagnosed in patients with unremarkable echocardiographic images.

Step 3: Perform Doppler Studies to Diagnose Constriction

■ Reciprocal respiratory changes in RV and LV diastolic filling, in the absence of a pericardial effusion, suggest the diagnosis of constrictive pericarditis (Fig. 10.21).

■ Typically, pulmonary pressures are normal in patients with constrictive pericarditis but elevated (>60 mm Hg) in those with restrictive cardiomyopathy.

■ Tissue Doppler E′ velocity is increased with constrictive pericarditis compared to a decreased E′ velocity (<8 cm/s) with restrictive cardiomyopathy.

❖ **KEY POINTS**

❑ With pericardial constriction, the normal myocardium allows rapid early diastolic filling of the chamber with normal relaxation and compliance. Once the chamber has reached the limit of total cardiac volume imposed by the rigid pericardium, ventricular filling abruptly halts.

❑ The ventricular inflow pattern shows a prominent early (E) filling velocity, a normal deceleration slope, and a very small atrial contribution to filling (due to elevated end-diastolic LV pressures).

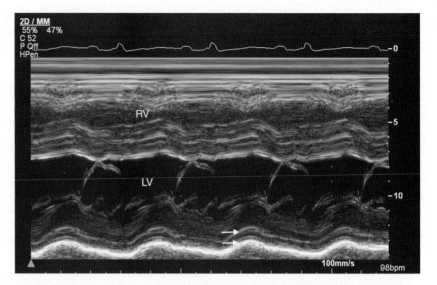

Fig. 10.20 **M-mode of pericardial thickening.** A band of multiple echo densities moving together posterior to the LV on M-mode is consistent with a thick posterior pericardium that moves with the epicardium during the cardiac cycle. Pericardial thickening in the areas between the two *arrows.* A pericardium effusion would be echo-free in this space and the posterior pericardial line would be flat. *PW,* Posterior wall.

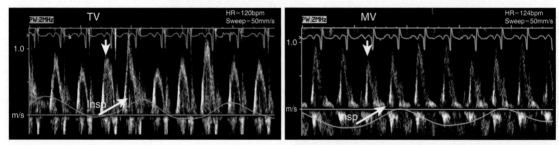

Fig. 10.21 **Inflow velocities with constriction.** A marked (>25%) increase in RV filling is seen across the tricuspid valve *(TV)* during inspiration (Insp; *arrow)* with a reciprocal respiratory decrease (>25%) in LV diastolic filling across the mitral valve *(MV).*

- ❏ The RA inflow (hepatic vein) pattern shows a prominent atrial reversal, with prominent diastolic (and blunted systolic) ventricular filling.
- ❏ Pulmonary pressures are estimated based on the velocity in the tricuspid regurgitant jet and an estimate of RA pressure.

Step 4: Measure Septal and Lateral Wall Tissue Doppler Velocities

- ■ Normally, the tissue Doppler E′ velocity is higher when recorded from the lateral side of the mitral annulus compared recordings made medially, at the septum in the 4-chamber view.
- ■ With constrictive pericarditis, this pattern is reversed with a higher septal, compared to medial, tissue Doppler E′ velocity, often called *annulus reversus* (Fig. 10.22).

❖ **KEY POINTS**

- ❏ The likely explanation for this finding is restricted diastolic expansion of the lateral LV wall by the adherent pericardium.
- ❏ This pattern also may be seen on speckle tracking strain imaging. Global longitudinal strain is normal but reduced focally along the free wall of the LV (anterior, lateral, and posterior).

Step 5: Distinguish Constrictive Pericarditis from Restrictive Cardiomyopathy

- ■ Echocardiography alone often is inadequate to distinguish constrictive pericarditis from restrictive cardiomyopathy (Table 10.2).
- ■ However, the possibility of these diagnoses often is first suggested by the echocardiographic findings.

❖ **KEY POINTS**

- ❏ RA and LA filling pressures are increased in both conditions.
- ❏ RV and LV diastolic pressures are equal, even after volume loading, when constrictive pericarditis is present.
- ❏ Pulmonary systolic pressure typically is severely elevated with a restrictive cardiomyopathy.
- ❏ Severe biatrial enlargement is typical with restrictive cardiomyopathy.
- ❏ Early diastolic filling is rapid with constrictive pericarditis and is reduced with restrictive cardiomyopathy early in the disease course.
- ❏ However, with advanced restrictive physiology, ventricular compliance is reduced so that early diastolic filling may appear similar to the pattern seen with constrictive pericarditis.

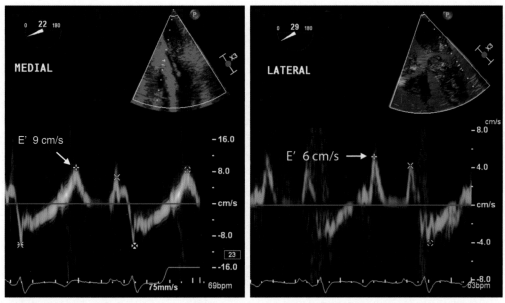

Fig. 10.22 **Annulus reversus.** On TEE images recorded just before surgery for pericardial constriction, tissue Doppler imaging at the medial annulus *(left)* shows a higher early diastolic (E′) velocity than the tissue Doppler E′ velocity at the lateral annulus *(right)*. The relative medial-lateral velocities are the opposite of normal; often called *annulus reversus.*

TABLE 10.2	Comparison of Pericardial Tamponade, Constriction, and Restrictive Cardiomyopathy		
	Pericardial Tamponade	**Constrictive Pericarditis**	**Restrictive Cardiomyopathy**
Hemodynamics			
RA pressure	↑	↑	↑
RV/LV filling pressures	↑, RV = LV	↑, RV = LV	↑, LV > RV
Pulmonary artery pressures	Normal	Mild elevation (35-40 mm Hg systolic)	Moderate-severe elevation (≥60 mm Hg systolic)
RV diastolic pressure plateau		>⅓ peak RV pressure	>⅓ peak RV pressure
Radionuclide Diastolic Filling			
		Rapid early filling, impaired late filling	Impaired early filling
2D Echo			
	Moderate-large PE IVC plethora	Pericardial thickening without effusion	LV hypertrophy Normal systolic function
	Small ventricular chambers RV diastolic and RA systolic collapse	Respiratory ventricular septal shift	No respiratory change in septal motion
Doppler Echo			
	Reciprocal respiratory changes in RV and LV filling	E > a on LV inflow Prominent y-descent in hepatic vein Pulmonary venous flow = prominent a-wave, reduced systolic phase Respiratory variation in IVRT and in E velocity	1. Early in disease e < A on LV inflow 2. Late in disease E > a 3. Constant IVRT 4. Absence of significant respiratory variation

Continued

TABLE 10.2	Comparison of Pericardial Tamponade, Constriction, and Restrictive Cardiomyopathy—cont'd		
Tissue Doppler			
	↓ E' without respiratory variation	↑ E' Lateral E' < septal E'	E' <8 cm/s with S' <8 cm/s Lateral E' > septal E'
Global Longitudinal Strain			
		Normal	Globally decreased
Other Diagnostic Tests			
	Therapeutic/diagnostic pericardiocentesis	CT or CMR for pericardial thickening	Endomyocardial biopsy

CMR, Cardiac magnetic resonance imaging; *IVC,* inferior vena cava; *IVRT,* isovolumic relaxation time; *PE,* pericardial effusion.
From Otto CM: *Textbook of clinical echocardiography,* ed 6, Philadelphia, 2018, Elsevier.

❑ The LV myocardium is normal with constrictive pericarditis. With restrictive cardiomyopathy, LV wall thickness often is increased.
❑ The ratio of septal to lateral annular tissue Doppler E' velocity can help distinguish constrictive pericarditis from restrictive cardiomyopathy.

❑ Additional helpful studies are CT and/or CMR direct imaging of pericardial thickness, cardiac catheterization for simultaneous measurement of LV and RV diastolic pressures, and endomyocardial biopsy.

THE ECHO EXAM

Pericardial Disease

Pericardial Effusion

Views
    Parasternal
    Apical
    Subcostal
Distinguish from pleural fluid
Size
    Small (<0.5 cm)
    Moderate (0.5-2.0 cm)
    Large (>2.0 cm)
Diffuse versus loculated
Evaluate for tamponade physiology if moderate or large
TEE if needed, especially in postoperative patients

Pericardial Tamponade

Clinical Findings

Low cardiac output
Elevated venous pressures
Pulsus paradoxus
Hypotension

2D-Echo

Moderate-large pericardial effusion
RA systolic collapse (duration greater than ⅓ of systole)
RV diastolic collapse
Reciprocal respiratory changes in RV and LV volumes
Inferior vena cava (IVC) plethora

Doppler

Respiratory variation in RV and LV diastolic filling
Increased RV filling on first beat after inspiration
Decreased LV filling on first beat after inspiration

Constrictive Pericarditis

Imaging

Pericardial thickening
Normal LV size and systolic function
LA enlargement
Flattened diastolic wall motion
Abrupt posterior motion of the ventricular septum in
    early diastole
Dilated inferior vena cava (IVC) and hepatic veins

Doppler

Prominent Y-descent on hepatic vein or superior vena
    cava (SVC) flow pattern
LV inflow shows prominent E velocity with a rapid early
    diastolic deceleration slope and a small or absent A
    velocity
Increase in LV-IVRT by >20% on first beat after inspiration
Respiratory variations in RV/LV diastolic filling (dif-
    ference >25%) with inspiratory ↑RV ↓LV filling with
    inspiration
Tissue Doppler ↑ E′ >8 cm/s with S′ >8 cm/s
Annulus reversus with septal E′ > lateral E′
Pulmonary venous flow shows prominent a-wave and
    blunting of systolic phase

IVRT, Isovolumetric relaxation time.

LV Pseudoaneurysm

Abrupt transition from normal myocardium to aneurysm
Acute angle between myocardium and aneurysm
Narrow neck
Ratio of neck diameter to aneurysm diameter <0.5
Often lined with thrombus

SELF-ASSESSMENT QUESTIONS

Question 1

Identify the numbered structures in Fig. 10.23:

1. _____
2. _____
3. _____
4. _____
5. _____
6. _____

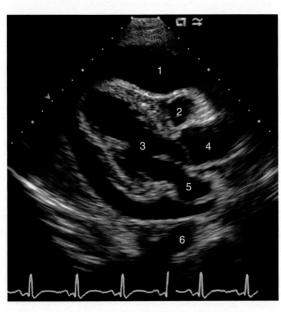

Fig. 10.23

Question 2

Identify the numbered structures in Fig. 10.24:

1. _____
2. _____
3. _____
4. _____

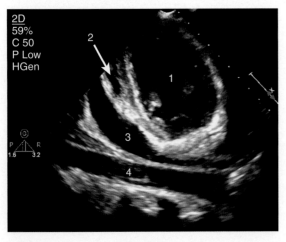

Fig. 10.24

Question 3

A 57-year-old man complained of lightheadedness and shortness of breath 2 months after coronary artery bypass grafting. The patient's blood pressure was 89/69 mm Hg and heart rate was 95 beats per minute. An echocardiogram was performed (Fig. 10.25). Which of the following is the next best step in management?

    A. Pericardiocentesis
    B. Transesophageal echo
    C. Pericardiectomy
    D. Diuretic medications
    E. Computed tomography of the chest

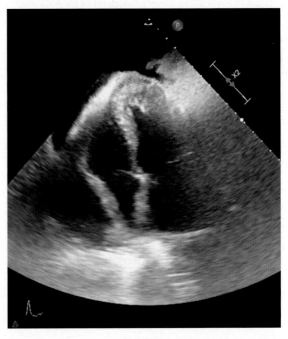

Fig. 10.25

Question 4

A 34-year-old woman underwent TEE after onset of symptoms consistent with a transient ischemic attack. The structure identified (Fig. 10.26) with the *asterisk* is which of the following based on the 2D and color Doppler images?

A. Coronary artery aneurysm
B. Aortic abscess
C. Transverse pericardial sinus
D. Left atrial appendage
E. Sinus of Valsalva aneurysm

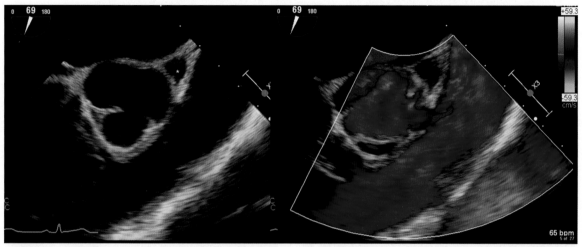

Fig. 10.26

Question 5

A 55-year-old woman presents with a 3-month history of progressive pedal edema and exertional dyspnea. She has no significant past medical history. Data from her transthoracic echocardiogram are as follows:

LV end-diastolic volume	100 mL
LV posterior diastolic wall thickness	1.2 cm
LV ejection fraction	59%
LA indexed volume	45 mL/m²
Mitral valve E-wave velocity	1.7 m/s
Tissue Doppler E′ velocity	0.05 m/s
Inferior vena cava (IVC) diameter	2.0 cm
Tricuspid regurgitant (TR) jet velocity	3.6 m/s

You conclude that the data are most consistent with:
A. Pericardial constriction
B. Dilated cardiomyopathy
C. Restrictive cardiomyopathy
D. Chronic obstructive pulmonary disease

Question 6

A 54-year-old woman with acute myeloid leukemia presents with dyspnea. Based on the image in Fig. 10.27, the next best step in patient management is:

A. Pericardiocentesis
B. Thoracentesis
C. Ligation of the persistent left superior vena cava
D. Pericardial stripping

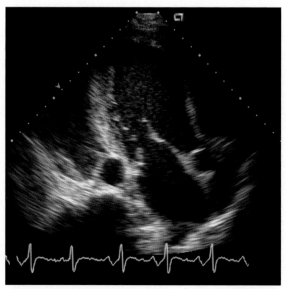

Fig. 10.27

Question 7

The Doppler flow data as shown in Fig. 10.28 were obtained in patient with dyspnea. These tracings are most consistent with:

   A. Normal respiratory variation
   B. Pericardial constriction
   C. Restrictive cardiomyopathy
   D. Chronic obstructive pulmonary disease

Question 8

A 55-year-old woman becomes hypotensive during a percutaneous coronary intervention and an urgent echocardiogram is obtained (Fig. 10.29); the most likely diagnosis is:

   A. Acute myocardial infarction
   B. Cardiac tamponade
   C. Hypovolemia
   D. Papillary muscle rupture
   E. Pericardial hematoma

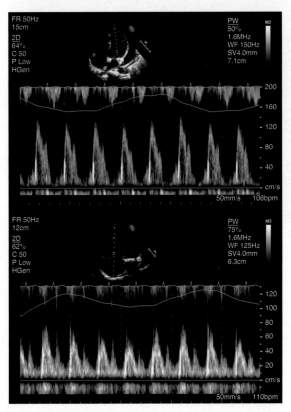

Fig. 10.28

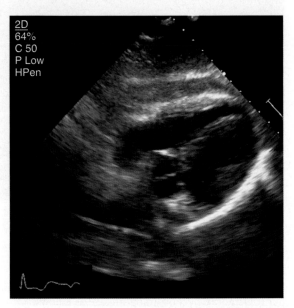

Fig. 10.29

Question 9

A 62-year-old man was referred for echocardiogram (ECG) by his hepatologist. The patient had been evaluated for decompensated cirrhosis with ascites and lower extremity edema that had been refractory to diuretic use over the last year. Based on the echocardiographic images and Doppler flow signal (Fig. 10.30), which of the following would be most likely?

A. A septal E′ of 6 cm/s
B. An inferior vena cava diameter of 1.7 cm
C. A transmitral E/A ratio of 0.9
D. A pericardial thickness of 4 mm
E. Anterior septal motion during early diastole with inspiration

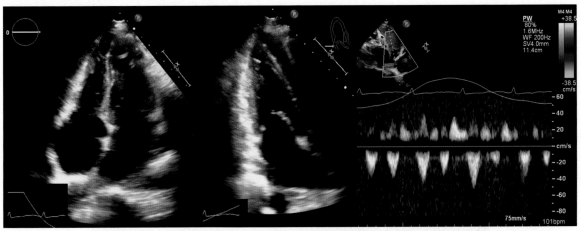

Fig. 10.30

Question 10

The following pulsed Doppler tracings were recorded (Fig. 10.31). The upper portion of the figure is the Doppler flow across the mitral valve, and the bottom portion of the figure is Doppler flow across the tricuspid valve. The most likely diagnosis for this patient is:

A. Chronic obstructive pulmonary disease
B. Normal respiratory variation
C. Pericardial tamponade
D. Positive pressure ventilation

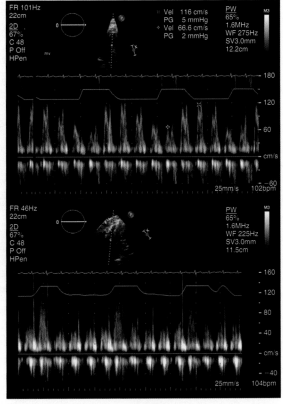

Fig. 10.31

Question 11

A 78-year-old man presents with exertional dyspnea 6 years after coronary artery bypass grafting. Coronary angiography documents occlusion of one of his four bypass grafts. A TTE (Fig. 10.32) is ordered and compared with a study he had done 5 years earlier.

Of the following options, what additional finding would most likely be present?

A. IVRT respiratory variation
B. Indexed LA volume 43 cm³
C. LV *dP/dt* 800 mm Hg/s
D. Inferior vena cava diameter 1.5 cm

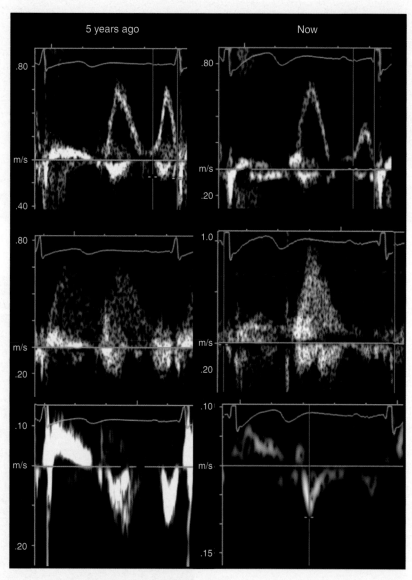

Fig. 10.32

Question 12

A 42-year-old obese, diabetic man with nonalcoholic fatty liver disease underwent echocardiogram (ECG) for evaluation of liver transplantation. The patient had no cardiovascular signs or symptoms. The finding labeled with the *asterisk* on Fig. 10.33 is most likely which of the following?

A. Pericardial effusion
B. Pericardial cyst
C. Hematoma
D. Metastatic tumor
E. Epicardial fat

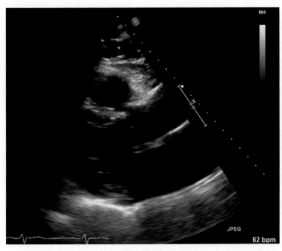

Fig. 10.33

ANSWERS

Answer 1

Fig 10.23 is a parasternal long-axis view in a patient with a large pericardial effusion *(1)*, which is also seen posterior to the LV. The RV outflow tract *(2)* is small and compressed due to tamponade physiology. LV *(3)* size is relatively normal, but the LA *(5)* appears small and underfilled compared to the normal-sized aorta *(4)*. The position of the effusion anterior to the descending thoracic aorta *(6)* confirms that the fluid is pericardial, not pleural.

Answer 2

Fig. 10.24 is an apical view of the LV *(1)* with the image plane angulated posterior to the standard 4-chamber view and then rotated to show the descending thoracic aorta *(4)* in long axis. Only a small segment of the RV *(2)* is seen but a pericardial effusion *(3)* is present.

Answer 3: A

This 4-chamber view (see Fig. 10.25) was recorded during echo-guided pericardiocentesis with injection of agitated saline, which is seen along the apical lateral wall, confirming the correct location of the needle. There is a large pericardial effusion with a 4 cm echolucent space surrounding the heart with right atrial collapse with inversion of the RA free wall in late systole. In the setting of a large pericardial effusion, right atrial collapse, and symptomatic hypotension, cardiac tamponade is confirmed and pericardiocentesis is warranted. TEE (answer B) may be needed in rare cases when there is isolated posterior loculated effusion after bypass surgery that cannot be visualized with transthoracic echocardiography. A pericardiectomy (answer C) may be considered in recurrent symptomatic pericardial effusions or pericardial constriction but not as first-line treatment for acute tamponade. Tamponade leads to impaired cardiac filling. Increasing preload with intravenous fluids may be considered as a temporizing measure, but diuretic medication (answer D) would further decrease cardiac output. Alternative imaging, such as computed tomography (answer E), may be needed for evaluation of constriction or pericardial masses leading to extrinsic cardiac compression; however, the presence of an effusion confirms the diagnosis and would make further imaging unnecessary.

Answer 4: C

Fig. 10.26 demonstrates a normal mid-esophageal short-axis view of the aortic and pulmonic valves. Color Doppler highlights systolic flow in the aorta and pulmonic artery with absence of color in an echolucent space posterior to the great vessels and

anterior to the LA. This is the transverse sinus and is a normal finding. The pericardium extends superiorly around the great vessels to form this pocket of fluid that can be seen using TEE. A coronary aneurysm (answer A) may be seen in this view but would have an ostium connecting to the aorta and would have color flow. An aortic abscess (answer B) may appear as an echolucent structure next to the aortic annulus, but clinical findings of endocarditis, system infection, and conduction block are more commonly seen. The left atrial appendage (answer D) and epicardial fat may occasionally be visualized within this space and be confused for thrombus; however, the marked figure is echolucent without any appendage present. A sinus of Valsalva aneurysm (answer E) may be seen in this view but would appear as a thin, long, mobile, convoluted sac, similar to a wind-sock that would have color flow.

Answer 5: C

This is a patient with restrictive cardiomyopathy. Patients with restrictive cardiomyopathy have relatively normal systolic function with significant diastolic dysfunction, often in the setting of increased LV wall thickness. This study shows decreased ventricular compliance and severely elevated LV filling pressure as reflected in the elevated E-wave velocity of 1.7 m/s and a severely elevated E/E' of 34. The elevated LV filling pressure is also reflected in the severely elevated indexed LA volume (normal <30 mL/m^2) and pulmonary hypertension. LV chamber size (indexed diastolic LV volume) is normal, with preserved systolic function and mild hypertrophy of the chamber walls, also characteristic of restrictive cardiomyopathy. For pericardial constriction, elevation in RV filling pressure is more pronounced than the increase in LV filling pressure, evidenced by dilation of the inferior vena cava, which is not seen in this case. Also, in constriction, myocardial tissue Doppler typically shows a tissue Doppler E' > 8 cm/s and a S' > 8 cm/s with only mildly increased pulmonary pressures. This patient does not have a dilated cardiomyopathy; LV volume would be increased, with a decreased ejection fraction. Chronic obstructive pulmonary disease is not associated with LV diastolic dysfunction, and the severity of pulmonary hypertension is greater than expected for this diagnosis.

Answer 6: B

This patient has a large left-sided pleural effusion. Fig. 10.27 is an apical long-axis view of the heart. The LV is closest to the transducer. Posterior to the heart, there is an echolucent space consistent with fluid. The circular structure is the descending thoracic aorta seen in cross section. Tracking posterior to the descending thoracic aorta is a large pleural effusion. A pleural and pericardial effusion can be differentiated by the tissue planes that bound the fluid collection. Fluid that tracks anterior to the descending aorta is pericardial. In this example, there is a trivial pericardial stripe seen just along the epicardial border, which is normal thickness. The descending aorta might be mistaken for a dilated coronary sinus, as seen in patients with a persistent left superior vena cava. However, the coronary sinus is not well seen on this image; it typically is closer to the atrioventricular groove and slightly superior to the descending aorta in this view. A persistent left superior vena cava is a normal variant and does not cause symptoms or require intervention. Pericardial stripping refers to surgical removal of a thickened pericardial when pericardial constriction is present.

Answer 7: A

Fig. 10.28 shows pulsed Doppler flow signals across the mitral *(top)* and tricuspid *(bottom)* valves in a patient with a moderate to large pericardial effusion. The *green line* shows inspiration *(up)* and expiration *(down)*. With inspiration, intrathoracic pressure becomes negative, resulting in an increase in RV inflow (tricuspid E-wave velocity). With pericardial tamponade or constriction, respiratory variation in ventricular inflow is greater than 25% between the first beat after inspiration and the first beat after expiration with LV inflow changing in the opposite direction (reciprocal changes). With exaggerated respiratory effort, as can occur with chronic obstructive pulmonary disease, respiratory variation in inflow to the thinner-walled RV is commonly seen, but without external cardiac constraint, reciprocal changes in LV filling are not seen. In restrictive cardiomyopathy, there is no external constraint on the heart and, although diastolic LV function is abnormal, reciprocal respiratory changes in ventricular filling are not seen.

Answer 8: E

This subcostal 4-chamber view (see Fig. 10.29) shows a large hematoma in the pericardial space, between the liver and RV. This acute, echodense pericardial hematoma is the most likely cause of hypotension due to decreased cardiac output, due to compression of the right heart. An acute myocardial infarction due to stent thrombosis results in a regional wall motion abnormality of the LV. Cardiac tamponade presents with an echolucent pericardial effusion and signs of tamponade physiology. Hypovolemia is diagnosed on echocardiography when the LV is small and underfilled. Papillary muscle rupture results in acute severe mitral regurgitation.

Answer 9: D

The patient's echocardiogram (ECG) shows a thickened and increased echogenicity of the pericardium

characteristic of pericardial constriction (see Fig. 10.30). The ventricular chambers have a triangular deformation in diastole from the constricting pericardium along with enlarged atrium from elevated filling pressures. The hepatic vein Doppler shows increased systolic, diastolic, and atrial reversal flows with inspiration consistent with constriction physiology. Pericardial evaluation with either CT or MRI should be obtained to evaluate the thickness and calcification of the pericardium (Fig. 10.34). Pericardial thickness and calcification exceeding 2 mm (answer D) with the echocardiographic findings and hemodynamic consequences confirmed the diagnosis and etiology of the patient's cardiac cirrhosis. The underlying myocardium is normal in constriction with a normal early diastolic septal velocity above 8 cm/s (answer A) that usually exceeds lateral septal wall motion (annulus reversus). This patient's septal E′ was 13.2 cm/s and lateral E′ was 11.5 cm/s. Pericardial constriction leads to elevated ventricular filling pressures producing elevated E/A ratios above 2 (answer C) and inferior vena cava (IVC) plethora with diameters above 2.1 cm (answer B). With pericardial constriction inspiration increases right-sided ventricular filling compared to LV filling leading to posterior septal shifting toward the LV (answer E).

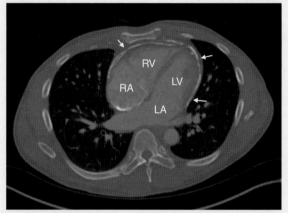

Fig. 10.34

Answer 10: C

These tracings show mitral *(top)* and tricuspid *(bottom)* inflow velocities with the *green line* indicating inspiration *(up)* and expiration *(down)*. These findings are consistent with pericardial tamponade with a significant (>25%) decrease in the mitral E-wave velocity on first beat after inspiration. The tricuspid velocities also show an exaggerated change with respiration, with decreased LV filling during inspiration and increased LV filling during expiration. The mechanism for these changes is that negative intrathoracic pressure with normal inspiration allows increased RV inflow. Because total heart volume is limited due to compression by the pericardial fluid, the increase in RV size

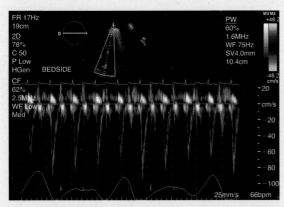

Fig. 10.35

results in a decrease in LV size and a reduction in LV filling with inspiration. The opposite changes occur during expiration, and these changes exceed the normal degree of variation in RV and LV inflow with respiration. The changes in LV filling are then reflected in forward cardiac output across the aortic valve (Fig. 10.35), resulting in the physical examination finding of pulsus paradoxus with a 20 mm Hg or greater decline in systolic blood pressure with inspiration.

With exaggerated respiratory effort, as can occur with chronic obstructive pulmonary disease, respiratory variation in inflow to the thinner-walled RV is commonly seen, but without external cardiac constraint, reciprocal changes in LV filling are not seen. In myocardial restriction, there is no external constraint on the heart and, although diastolic LV function is abnormal, reciprocal respiratory changes in ventricular filling are not seen. With positive pressure ventilation, the normal pattern of negative intrathoracic pressure is disrupted. Thus, in patients on positive pressure ventilation, changes in inferior vena cava size are not reliable for estimated right atrial pressure. Similarly, the expected respiratory changes in LV and RV filling patterns may not be present even when tamponade is present.

Answer 11: A

This patient has Doppler evidence of pericardial constriction, likely a consequence of his prior bypass grafting surgery. In addition to the findings shown, respiratory variation in LV/RV inflow and the IVRT would be present. In pericardial constriction, myocardial function is normal, with normal LV relaxation and ventricular compliance, but diastolic filling of the ventricle is constrained externally by the rigid pericardium. The early component of diastolic filling,

E-wave, is normal, but the late atrial contribution, A-wave velocity, is minimal because of elevated LV end-diastolic pressure. Therefore the E/A ratio *(top)* is increased in this patient compared with his baseline study. On the pulmonary venous tracing *(middle),* higher LV filling pressure leads to blunting of the systolic component of LA filling compared with baseline. However, because myocardial function is normal, the E/E′ ratio remains in the normal range, with a baseline E/E′ of $0.65/1.1 = 6$ and a follow-up E/E′ of $0.65/0.08 = 8$, both of which are in the normal range and within measurement variability of each other. In constriction, the thickened pericardium encases the entire heart, and biventricular size is normal or only mildly increased; an indexed LA volume of 43 cm^3 is severely increased and would be more typical of restrictive cardiomyopathy. The LV *dP/dt* is normal (>1000 mm Hg/s) with pericardial constriction, because LV systolic function is normal. Also, in constriction, return of blood is restricted, with severely increased central venous pressure, and the inferior vena cava would be dilated and plethoric, not normal caliber.

Answer 12: E

Fig. 10.33 shows a normal parasternal view with a prominent epicardial fat pad along the RV free wall. Epicardial fat is associated with higher-risk cardiometabolic profiles (such as obesity, diabetes, and fatty liver disease). The characteristic anterior location with an increased fine pattern echogenicity should be distinguished from a pericardial effusion (answer A), because there is a lack of posterior effusion and echolucency. Epicardial fat is frequently present anteriorly to the RV free wall near the aorta in this view and will move in unison with RV contraction. A pericardial cyst (answer B) is a rare echolucent cystic structure more commonly in the atrioventricular groove and RV. Hemorrhage into the pericardial space forming a hematoma (answer C) may appear to have irregular echogenic material but would be less delineated and more often be associated with fibrinous stranding and an acute symptomatic clinical scenario. Although not shown, epicardial fat will move with the cardiac cycle unlike abnormal fluid collections. Metastatic tumor (answer D) is a less common finding and has nonspecific nodular appearance, pericardial effusions, and an appropriate clinical setting. Alternative imaging (such as CT or MRI) can provide additional characteristics to distinguish fat from masses or bleeding when the clinical scenario and echocardiographic findings are more equivocal.

AORTIC STENOSIS

Step-by-Step Approach

Step 1: Determine the Etiology of Stenosis

- Parasternal two-dimensional (2D) images of the valve in long- and short-axis views (Fig. 11.1)
- Number of leaflets, mobility, thickness, and calcification
- Level of obstruction: Valvular, subvalvular, or supravalvular
- Three-dimensional (3D) transthoracic echocardiography (TTE) or transesophageal echocardiography (TEE) imaging is helpful for better definition of valve anatomy, particularly diagnosis of a unicuspid or bicuspid valve (Fig. 11.2)

❖ KEY POINTS

- ❑ Calcific changes of a trileaflet valve usually start in the central part of the leaflets, resulting in a three-pointed star-shaped orifice.
- ❑ Rheumatic aortic valve disease affects the commissures and leaflet edges, with a triangular-shaped orifice, and is accompanied by rheumatic mitral valve changes.
- ❑ A bicuspid valve may appear trileaflet in diastole due to a raphe in one leaflet; the number of leaflets must be visualized when the valve is open in systole, taking care to identify each commissure, and the points where the leaflets attach to the aortic wall.
- ❑ 3D imaging is recommended when available.

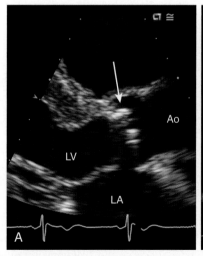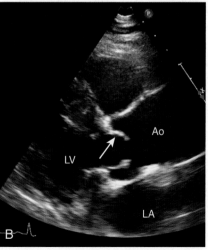

Fig. 11.1 **Etiology of aortic valve stenosis.** (A) With calcific valve disease, there is increased echogenicity of the leaflets, due to calcification and thickening, with reduced systolic opening of the leaflets. (B) In a patient with a congenitally bicuspid, noncalcified valve, the long-axis view shows thin leaflets with reduced systolic opening due to *doming* of the leaflets in systole *(arrow)*, as seen by the curve at the tips of the leaflets. *Ao,* Aorta.

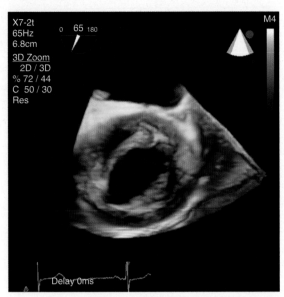

Fig. 11.2 3D TEE imaging of a bicuspid aortic valve. A 3D view of the aortic valve from the aortic side of the valve clearly shows two leaflets, with no raphe, and two commissures in systole.

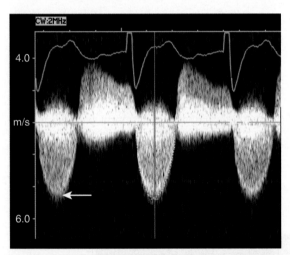

Fig. 11.3 Aortic jet velocity recorded with CW Doppler. An optimal signal-to-noise ratio is obtained using a small dedicated transducer; the small footprint of this transducer also allows optimal positioning and angulation to align the ultrasound beam parallel to the direction of the stenotic jet. In this example, the scale has been adjusted to show both aortic stenosis (AS) and regurgitation. The aortic jet should show a denser signal around the edge and a smooth velocity curve. The difficulty in identifying the maximum velocity is seen in this example, with fuzzy linear signals at peak velocity that are due to the transit time effect. Maximum velocity is measured at the edge of the denser signal, as shown by the *arrow*.

- ❑ Subvalvular or supravalvular stenosis is distinguished from valvular stenosis based on the site of the increase in velocity and on the anatomy of the outflow tract.

Step 2: Evaluate Stenosis Severity

Aortic Jet Velocity (Fig. 11.3)

- ■ Continuous-wave (CW) Doppler gray-scale spectral recording of aortic jet velocity (Tables 11.1 and 11.2)

TABLE 11.1   Other High-Velocity Systolic Jets That May Be Mistaken for Aortic Stenosis

Subaortic obstruction (fixed or dynamic)
Mitral regurgitation
Tricuspid regurgitation
Ventricular septal defect
Pulmonic or branch pulmonary artery stenosis
Peripheral vascular stenosis (e.g., subclavian artery)

From Otto CM: *Textbook of clinical echocardiography*, ed 6, Philadelphia, 2018, Elsevier.

❖ KEY POINTS

- ❑ Use multiple acoustic windows (apical, suprasternal, right parasternal) with careful patient positioning and transducer angulation to avoid underestimation of velocity.
- ❑ A dedicated small CW Doppler transducer provides the optimal signal-to-noise ratio and allows more precise angulation of the transducer.
- ❑ Decrease gain, increase wall filters, and adjust the baseline and scale to optimize identification of the maximum velocity.
- ❑ Use the gray-scale spectral displays, because with some color displays the signal-to-noise ratio is poor and the edge of the spectral envelope may be blurred, leading to overestimation of velocity.
- ❑ A smooth velocity curve with a dense outer edge and clear maximum velocity should be recorded; fine lines at the peak of the curve are due to the transit time effect and are not included in measurements.
- ❑ Color Doppler is usually not helpful for jet direction, because the jet is short with poststenotic turbulence and because the elevational plane is not visualized.

Mean Gradient

- ■ Transaortic maximum pressure gradient (ΔP) is calculated from velocity (v) using the Bernoulli equation (Fig. 11.4) as:

$$\Delta P = 4v_{max}^2 \qquad (11.1)$$

❖ KEY POINTS

- ❑ When proximal velocity (V_{prox}) is greater than 1.0 m/s, it should be included in the Bernoulli equation, so that:

$$\Delta P = 4\left(v_{max}^2 - v_{prox}^2\right) \qquad (11.2)$$

- ❑ Mean gradient is calculated by tracing the velocity curve and averaging instantaneous gradients over the systolic ejection period (Fig. 11.5).
- ❑ Any underestimation of aortic velocity results in an even greater underestimation in gradients.

TABLE 11.2 Categories of Stenosis Severity		
Aortic Stenosis Severity	**Valve Anatomy and Hemodynamics**	**LV Geometry and Function**
At risk of AS	Bicuspid valve or aortic sclerosis, V_{max} <2 m/s	Normal
Progressive AS	Mild AS: V_{max} 2.0-2.9 m/s or mean ΔP <20 mm Hg Moderate AS: V_{max} 3.0-3.9 m/s or mean ΔP 20-39 mm Hg	Mild LVH and diastolic dysfunction may be present.
Severe AS	Severe leaflet calcification with reduced systolic motion or congenital AS $V_{max} \geq 4$ m/s, or Mean $\Delta P \geq 40$ mm Hg Typically AVA ≤ 1.0 cm^2	LVH, diastolic dysfunction, systolic function usually normal. Patient may be asymptomatic or symptomatic.
Low-output low-gradient severe AS with low EF	Severely calcified aortic valve V_{max} <4 m/s (rest) AVA ≤ 1.0 cm^2	LV EF <50% DSE – $V_{max} \geq 4$ m/s with AVA ≤ 1.0 cm^2
Low-output low-gradient severe AS with normal EF	Severely calcified aortic valve. V_{max} <4 m/s (rest) AVA ≤ 1.0 cm^2 Indexed AVA ≤ 0.6 cm^2/m^2 SV index <35 mL/m^2 Measured with normal BP	Small LV chamber with increased relative wall thickness. Normal EF Restrictive diastolic filling
Mitral Stenosis Severity	**Hemodynamics**	**Associated Findings**
At risk of MS	Rheumatic leaflet changes without stenosis	
Progressive MS	Rheumatic valve disease Pressure half time <150 ms MVA >1.5 cm^2	PA systolic pressure <30 mm Hg Mild LA enlargement
Severe MS	MVA ≤ 1.5 cm^2	PA systolic pressure >30 mm Hg Moderate LA enlargement
Very severe MS	MVA ≤ 1.0 cm^2	PA systolic pressure >30 mm Hg Moderate-severe LA enlargement

AS, Aortic stenosis; *AVA,* aortic valve area; *DSE,* low-dose dobutamine stress echocardiography; *EF,* ejection fraction; *LVH,* left ventricular hypertrophy; *MS,* mitral stenosis; *MVA,* mitral valve area; *PA,* pulmonary artery.

Continuity Equation Valve Area (Fig. 11.6)

- Aortic valve area (AVA) is calculated as:

$$AVA = (CSA_{LVOT} \times VTI_{LVOT}) / VTI_{Ao} \qquad (11.3)$$

- The simplified continuity equation, which uses maximum velocities instead of velocity-time integrals (VTIs), also can be used:

$$AVA = CSA_{LVOT} \times (V_{LVOT}) / V_{Ao} \qquad (11.4)$$

❖ KEY POINTS

- ❑ Left ventricular outflow tract (LVOT) diameter is measured in the parasternal long-axis view in mid-systole using zoom mode and adjusting gain setting to optimize the blood-tissue interface (Fig. 11.7).
- ❑ Diameter (D) is measured at the basal insertion of the aortic leaflets from inner edge to inner edge of the aortic annulus. Calculate the circular cross-sectional area:

$$CSA = \pi (D/2)^2 \qquad (11.5)$$

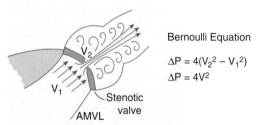

Bernoulli Equation

$$\Delta P = 4(V_2^2 - V_1^2)$$
$$\Delta P = 4V^2$$

Fig. 11.4 **Fluid dynamics of aortic stenosis (AS).** There is laminar low velocity flow on the ventricular side of the valve, a small area of acceleration into the narrow orifice, and the high-velocity jet of flow through the narrowed valve. The distal flow disturbance is shown by the *curved arrows.* The instantaneous pressure gradient (ΔP) across the valve is related to the proximal velocity (V_1) and jet velocity (V_2) as shown. Because the proximal velocity is much less than the jet velocity, and usually is less than 1 m/s, the simplified Bernoulli equitation uses only jet velocity in the equation. *AMVL,* Anterior mitral valve leaflet.

- ❑ LVOT diameter is useful for valve area calculation but should not be used for sizing of transcatheter valves because of the complex anatomy of the outflow tract and valve. CT imaging of the aortic annulus is preferred for this indication.

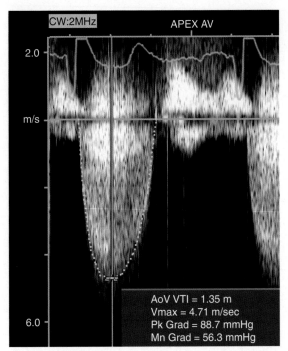

AoV VTI = 1.35 m
Vmax = 4.71 m/sec
Pk Grad = 88.7 mmHg
Mn Grad = 56.3 mmHg

Fig. 11.5 Mean transaortic pressure gradient. For accurate measurement of aortic velocity and mean gradient, the baseline is moved and the scale is adjusted so that the stenotic signal fills the vertical range of the display. The horizontal axis or "sweep speed" is adjusted to 100 mm/s to allow accurate measurement. The Doppler curve is traced along the outer edge of the dark signal to obtain the velocity-time integral (VTI). The instantaneous pressure gradients over the systolic ejection period are averaged by the analysis package to provide the mean systolic gradient. Note that the mean gradient is *not* calculated by using the mean velocity in the Bernoulli equation.

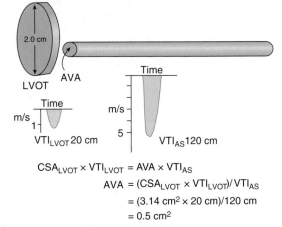

CONTINUITY EQUATION

$$CSA_{LVOT} \times VTI_{LVOT} = AVA \times VTI_{AS}$$
$$AVA = (CSA_{LVOT} \times VTI_{LVOT})/VTI_{AS}$$
$$= (3.14 \text{ cm}^2 \times 20 \text{ cm})/120 \text{ cm}$$
$$= 0.5 \text{ cm}^2$$

Fig. 11.6 Continuity equation. The basic principle is that the volume of flow proximal to and in the narrowed valve must be equal. Flow for one cardiac cycle in the left ventricular outflow tract *(LVOT)* is shown as a cylinder with a diameter equal to LVOT diameter. Length is equal to the velocity-time integral *(VTI)* of LVOT flow (because the integral of velocity over time is distance, like traveling in a car). The flow through the orifice is shown as a cylinder with the cross-section equal to aortic valve area *(AVA)* and length equal to the VTI of the aortic stenosis (AS) jet. Because the volume of both cylinders is the same, the equation is solved for AVA as shown.

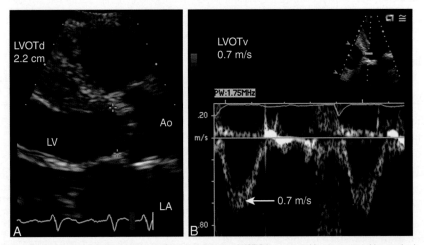

Fig. 11.7 Transaortic volume flow rate. (A) Left ventricular outflow tract diameter (LVOTd) is measured in a parasternal long-axis view in mid-systole from the inner edge of the septum to the inner edge of the anterior mitral leaflet, immediately adjacent to the aortic valve leaflets *(markers)*. A magnified image allows more accurate measurement, and typically several beats are measured to ensure a reproducible value. A typical outflow tract diameter is 2.2 to 2.6 cm in adult men and 2.0 to 2.4 cm in adult women. (B) Although LVOTd is measured from the parasternal window, to provide axial resolution of the tissue-blood interfaces, with ultrasound imaging, LVOT velocity is recorded from the apical window to allow parallel alignment between the ultrasound beam and flow direction. Pulsed Doppler is used to measure the velocity signal on the ventricular side of the aortic valve, in an anteriorly angulated 4-chamber view (as shown here) or in a long-axis view. The sample volume length or gate is adjusted to 2 to 3 mm and the sample volume is positioned as close to the valve as possible (often the closing click is seen), avoiding the small area of flow acceleration immediately adjacent to the stenotic orifice. The sample volume position should correspond to the site where LVOT diameter was measured. The velocity range and baseline are adjusted so the signal fits but fills the scale, using a fast (100 to 150 mm/s) horizontal axis scale. A smooth curve with a dense band of velocities ("envelope of flow") with a well-defined peak velocity should be seen. The midpoint of the spectral broadening at peak velocity is measured. *Ao,* Aorta.

- LVOT velocity is recorded with pulsed Doppler from the apical window with the sample volume positioned just apically from the flow acceleration into the valve. An aortic closing click on the spectral tracing indicates correct sample volume positioning.
- Move the baseline, adjust the velocity scale, and use an expanded time scale for accurate measurements.
- Trace the modal systolic velocity (VTI_{LVOT}) and measure peak velocity (V_{LVOT}).
- If LVOT diameter cannot be accurately measured, calculate the aortic valve index, which is the ratio of LVOT to aortic jet velocity:

$$\text{Aortic valve index} = V_{LVOT}/V_{AO} \qquad (11.6)$$

Planimetry of Aortic Valve Area

- Planimetry of the valve area can be helpful in selected cases with excellent images, but caution is needed due to reverberations and shadowing from leaflet calcification.
- With calcific aortic stenosis (AS), the systolic orifice is not planar, so measurement from 2D or 3D images is not recommended.
- The orifice of a unicuspid, bicuspid, or rheumatic valve may be identified using 3D TEE imaging, allowing direct measurement of valve opening (Fig. 11.8).

❖ **KEY POINTS**

- A full-volume 3D image is acquired, focused on aortic valve anatomy.
- The valve area measurement is made by adjusting the three image planes to show the valve orifice in systole.
- With congenital valve disease, the leaflets "dome" is systole with the valve orifice at the tip

of the leaflets; valve area will be overestimated if the tomographic plane is not optimally adjusted.
- Gains are adjusted to show the white–black interface to trace the valve area.
- Accuracy may be limited with extensive calcification due to shadowing and reverberation artifacts.

Step 3: Evaluate Aortic Regurgitation and Ascending Aorta

- If regurgitation is significant (vena contracta ≥3 mm), evaluate as detailed in Chapter 12.
- Dilation of the ascending aorta may accompany AS, particularly with a bicuspid valve.

❖ **KEY POINTS**

- Most patients with AS have some degree (usually mild) of regurgitation.
- With combined moderate stenosis and regurgitation, quantitation of both lesions is needed.
- The end-diastolic diameter of the aorta is measured at the sinuses, sinotubular junction, and mid-ascending aorta when aortic valve disease is present (see Chapter 16).

Step 4: Evaluate the Consequences of Chronic LV Pressure Overload

- Measure LV size and wall thickness and calculate ejection fraction as detailed in Chapter 6.
- Evaluate LV diastolic function as detailed in Chapter 7.
- Evaluate coexisting mitral regurgitation (if vena contracta ≥3 mm) as detailed in Chapter 12.
- Estimate pulmonary pressures as detailed in Chapter 6.

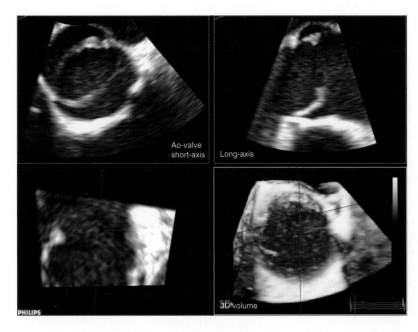

Fig. 11.8 3D measurement of aortic valve area (AVA). 3D TEE can be used to measure valve area in a patient with a bicuspid valve, using the 3D modality to ensure the measurements are made at the tips of the doming leaflets. The correctly aligned short-axis view of the open bicuspid aortic valve in systole *(green box, upper left)* obtained by adjusting the image plane using the long-axis plane *(red box, upper right)* to ensure the image plane is at the tip of the leaflets and the orthogonal plane *(blue box, lower left)* to adjust the tilt of the plane. The full volume is shown in the *lower right panel.*

TABLE 11.3	Possible Causes of Discrepancies in Measures of Aortic Stenosis Severity

Severe AS by Velocity or Gradient but Not by Valve Area (AS Velocity >4 m/s and AVA >1.0 cm^2)

LVOT diameter overestimated
LVOT velocity recorded too close to valve
High transaortic flow rate due to:
- Moderate to severe aortic regurgitation
- High output state
- Large body size

Severe AS by Valve Area But Not by Velocity or Gradient (AS Velocity ≤4 m/s and AVA ≤1.0 cm^2)

LVOT diameter underestimated
LVOT velocity recorded too far from valve
Small body size
Low transaortic flow volume due to:
- Low ejection fraction
- Small ventricular chamber
- Moderate to severe mitral regurgitation
- Moderate to severe mitral stenosis

AS, Aortic stenosis; *AVA,* aortic valve area; *LVOT,* left ventricular outflow tract.
From Otto CM: *Textbook of clinical echocardiography,* ed 6, Philadelphia, 2018, Elsevier.

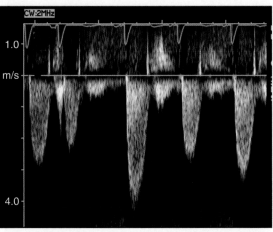

Fig. 11.9 **Effect of variable heart rate on aortic velocity.** When the cardiac rhythm is irregular, the velocity (and pressure gradient) across a stenotic valve varies with the length of the R-R interval because of an increased stroke volume (SV) with a longer diastolic filling period. This example shows the variation in aortic jet velocity (at a slow sweep speed to include multiple beats) in a patient in atrial fibrillation. Ideally, heart rate should be controlled before evaluation of stenosis severity is performed. Several beats are then averaged for each measurement. Signal quality in this example is suboptimal so additional efforts to improve patient and/or transducer positioning are needed.

❖ KEY POINTS

- ❑ AS typically results in concentric LV hypertrophy.
- ❑ Systolic function and ejection fraction remain normal in most patients but, occasionally, systolic dysfunction is identified in an asymptomatic patient.
- ❑ Diastolic dysfunction, usually impaired relaxation, is common.
- ❑ Pulmonary pressures may be elevated with longstanding severe AS.

Step 5: Additional Evaluation for Low-Output Low-Gradient Aortic Stenosis

- ■ Additional evaluation may be needed when clinical evaluation suggests AS may be more severe than indicated by standard measures of stenosis severity (Table 11.3).
- ■ With a calcified aortic valve and a valve area ≤1.0 cm^2 but a velocity <4 m/s in conjunction with an LV ejection fraction less than 50%, dobutamine stress echo should be considered.
- ■ With a calcified aortic valve and a valve area ≤1.0 cm^2 but a velocity <4 m/s and a normal ejection fraction, an integrative approach to evaluation is needed.

❖ KEY POINTS

- ❑ The degree of valve calcification (mild, moderate, severe) is a simple, important parameter that is predictive of clinical outcome.
- ❑ The aortic valve index (the dimensionless ratio of outflow tract to aortic jet velocity) provides a simple index of stenosis severity (normal, 1.0; mild, 0.5; severe, 0.25).

- ❑ Blood pressure should be recorded at the time of the velocity data acquisition; stenosis severity may be underestimated in hypertensive patients, so measurement should be repeated after effective treatment of hypertension.
- ❑ With atrial fibrillation, several beats should be averaged for each measurement (Fig. 11.9).
- ❑ With low output AS and a low LV ejection fraction, a velocity ≥4 m/s with an AVA ≤1.0 cm^2 on dobutamine stress echocardiography is consistent with severe AS (Fig. 11.10).

▍ MITRAL STENOSIS

Step-by-Step Approach

Step 1: Evaluate Mitral Valve Morphology

- ■ Use long- and short-axis views of the mitral valve to demonstrate the typical findings of rheumatic valve disease (Fig. 11.11):
  - ○ Commissural fusion resulting in diastolic doming
  - ○ Chordal shortening and fusion
- ■ Evaluate mitral valve leaflet mobility, thickening, calcification, and subvalvular disease.
- ■ Use 3D imaging for better evaluation of the symmetry of commissural fusion (Fig. 11.12).

❖ KEY POINTS

- ❑ Rheumatic valve disease is the most common cause of mitral stenosis.
- ❑ Rarely, severe mitral annular calcification encroaches on the mitral orifice, but calcific stenosis is rarely severe.

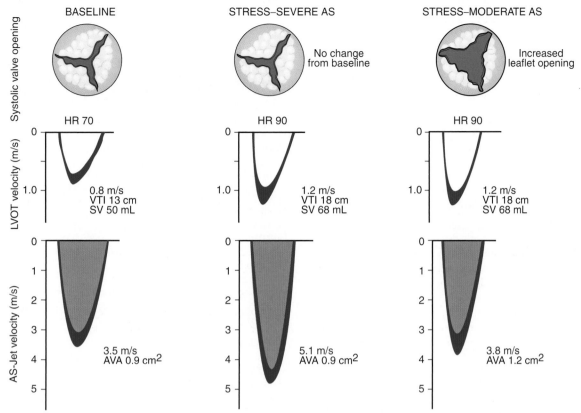

Fig. 11.10 **Low-output low-gradient aortic stenosis (AS).** Changes in aortic valve opening and Doppler flows with dobutamine stress echocardiography for low-output low-gradient AS. The baseline data show a hypothetical patient with an ejection fraction (EF) of 35% and limited aortic valve systolic opening, an aortic jet velocity (AS-jet) of 3.5 m/s, and aortic valve area (AVA) of 0.9 cm^2. If true, severe AS is present (*middle panel*), as EF increases from 35% to 45%, transaortic flow rate increases but aortic opening is fixed, resulting in a marked increase in aortic velocity (and pressure gradient) with no change in valve area. In a patient with the same baseline data but "pseudo-severe AS," the increase in EF and transaortic stroke volume (SV) "push" the aortic leaflets to open more so there is a smaller increase in aortic velocity in association with an increase in AVA. Current diagnostic testing relies on Doppler data with dobutamine stress testing, because direct imaging of valve anatomy is not adequate for visualization of the exact systolic orifice. *VTI,* Velocity-time integral. *(From Otto CM, Owens DS: Stress testing for structural heart disease. In Gillam LD, Otto CM:* Advanced approaches in echocardiography: practical echocardiography series, *Philadelphia, 2013, Elsevier.)*

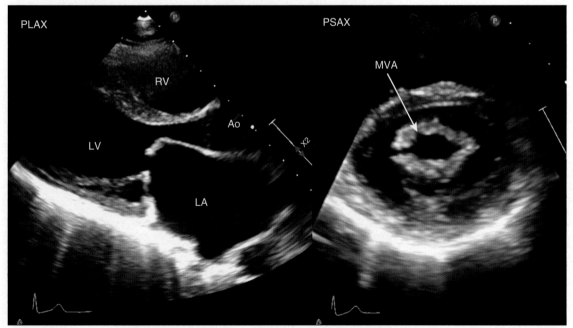

Fig. 11.11 **Rheumatic mitral stenosis.** In the parasternal long-axis view (*PLAX*), the typical changes of rheumatic mitral stenosis are seen with thickening of the leaflet tips, diastolic doming of the anterior mitral leaflet due to commissural fusion, and chordal shortening and fusion. In the parasternal short-axis view (*PSAX*), the rheumatic mitral valve area (*MVA*) can be measured, ensuring the image plane is at the leaflet tips by scanning from apex toward base to identify the smallest area of the funnel-shaped stenotic orifice. The inner edge of the white-dark interface is traced to obtain valve area. The distance between the LV wall and the edge of the orifice reflects the degree of commissural fusion both medially and laterally. The accuracy of 2D MVA planimetry depends on the experience and skill of the sonographer in obtaining the correct image plane *Ao,* Aorta.

❑ In addition to a numerical score, a narrative description of valve anatomy is helpful for deciding on the optimal intervention.

❑ The extent of commissural calcification and asymmetry of leaflet calcification should be noted.

❑ The subvalvular apparatus may be best seen on apical views (and poorly visualized on TEE).

Step 2: Evaluate the Severity of Mitral Stenosis

3D and 2D Planimetry of Valve Area

■ Valve area is measured directly by tracing the orifice in a short-axis view at the leaflet tips (Table 11.4).

■ Mitral valve area (MVA) may be measured accurately with 2D imaging by experienced sonographers, but ensuring measurement at the mitral leaflet tips is more reliable with 3D imaging.

❖ **KEY POINTS**

❑ With 2D imaging, starting in a parasternal short-axis orientation, the image plane is slowly moved from the apex toward the base to identify the orifice of the funnel-shaped stenotic valve.

❑ The zoom mode is used to focus on the valve orifice, with the gain reduced to clearly show the tissue–blood interface.

TABLE 11.4	Pitfalls in Evaluation of Mitral Stenosis Severity
Pressure Gradient	
Intercept angle between mitral stenosis jet and ultrasound beam Beat-to-beat variability in atrial fibrillation Dependence on transvalvular volume flow rate (e.g., exercise, coexisting mitral regurgitation)	
2D or 3D Valve Area	
Image orientation Tomographic plane 2D gain settings Intraobserver and interobserver variability in planimetry of orifice Poor acoustic access Deformed valve anatomy post-commissurotomy	
T½ Valve Area	
Definition of V_{max} and early-diastolic slope Nonlinear early-diastolic velocity slope Sinus rhythm with A-wave superimposed on early-diastolic slope Influence of coexisting aortic regurgitation Changing LV and LA compliances immediately after commissurotomy	
Continuity Equation Mitral Valve Area	
Accurate measurement of transmitral stroke volume (SV)	

From Otto CM: *Textbook of clinical echocardiography*, ed 6, Philadelphia, 2018, Elsevier.

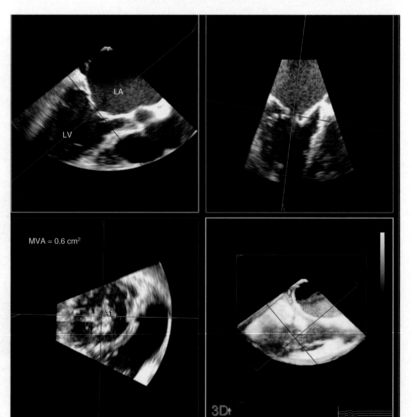

Fig. 11.12 3D measurement of mitral valve area (MVA). Using 3D TEE volumetric data, images are shown in three planes identified by *green, blue,* and *red.* The plane for each color box is shown as a line in the other two views. The blue box at *lower left* is the short-axis view of the mitral orifice. This view was obtained by aligned the red image plane *(upper right box, line in upper and lower left images)* in the center of the orifice and the blue image plane *(lines in upper left and upper right images)* at the leaflet tips. These planes are adjusted iteratively on the mid-diastolic imaging until the minimal orifice at the leaflet tips was visualized. The short-axis image of the orifice then is traced from the inner edge of the white-black interface. Measurement of MVA by 3D planimetry is less dependent than 2D imaging on operator skill and experience.

- With 3D imaging, a 3D volume is acquired from the parasternal window, taking care that the volume includes the orifice and avoiding stitch artifact.
- The 3D volume is used to obtain a short-axis view at the leaflet tips using three orthogonal image planes.
- The inner border of the black–white interface is traced to obtain valve area.
- The orifice typically is a smooth, elliptical shape in patients with no prior procedures.
- After percutaneous or surgical valvotomy, the orifice is more irregular due to splitting of the fused commissures.

Mean Gradient (Fig. 11.13)

- The Doppler velocity curve across the narrowed mitral orifice is recorded from the apical window.
- Mean gradient is determined using the Bernoulli equation to average the instantaneous pressures gradients over the diastolic filling period.

❖ KEY POINTS

- The mitral stenosis jet is directed toward the apex, so only minor adjustment of transducer position and angulation is needed to obtain a parallel angle between the Doppler beam and mitral jet; color flow Doppler can help with alignment.
- Transducer position and gain are adjusted to demonstrate a clear outer boundary of the velocity curve with a well-defined peak and a linear deceleration slope.
- The baseline is moved toward the edge of the display, the scale adjusted so that the Doppler

curve fits but fills the space, and gain and wall filters adjusted to decrease signal noise.
- Pulsed or high-pulse repetition frequency (HPRF) Doppler may provide a more clearly defined velocity curve than CW Doppler.
- Movement of the heart with respiration may result in variation in the Doppler curve due to a variation in the intercept angle; if so, have the patient suspend respiration briefly during data recording.

Pressure Half-Time Valve Area (Fig. 11.14)

- The pressure half-time is calculated from the Doppler curve at the time interval between peak velocity and the peak velocity divided by 1.4.
- The empiric constant 220 is divided by the pressure half-time ($T\frac{1}{2}$ in milliseconds) to estimate MVA in cm^2:

$$MVA = T\frac{1}{2}/220 \qquad (11.7)$$

Step 1: Identify the peak early diastolic velocity.

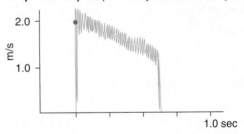

Step 2: Draw a line along the diastolic deceleration slope.

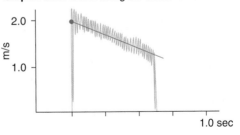

Step 3: The pressure half time ($T\frac{1}{2}$) is the time interval in milliseconds between the peak velocity and the point on the deceleration line equal to the peak velocity divided by 1.4 (the square root of 2).

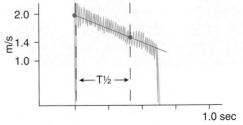

Fig. 11.14 Mitral pressure half-time measurement. In this example, the pressure half-time is 320 ms. The mitral valve area (MVA) is 220/320 = 0.7 cm^2, consistent with severe stenosis.

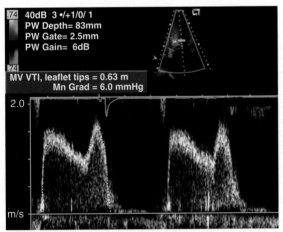

Fig. 11.13 Mean transmitral pressure gradient in mitral stenosis. The transmitral velocity is recorded with pulsed Doppler (including HPRF) or CW Doppler if needed to prevent signal aliasing, from an apical window with the baseline shifted and the velocity scale adjusted so that the Doppler velocity fits the vertical axis of the tracing. The time scale is set at 100 to 150 mm/s with the electrocardiogram included for timing. After a smooth Doppler curve with a narrow band along the outer edge and a clearly defined peak is obtained, the outer edge of the signal is traced. The analysis package averages the instantaneous gradients over the diastolic filling period. This patient is in sinus rhythm, which does not affect the accuracy of Doppler evaluation of stenosis severity.

❖ **KEY POINTS**

❑ The peak velocity occurs at the onset of diastole with flow deceleration in mid-diastole.

❑ A clearly defined peak velocity is needed for an accurate pressure half-time measurement (Fig. 11.15).

❑ The diastolic slope should be linear with a clearly defined edge; if a nonlinear slope is obtained, the mid-diastolic segment of the curve should be used for the pressure half-time calculation (Fig. 11.16).

❑ The pressure half-time may be inaccurate if left atrium (LA) or LV compliance is abnormal.

❑ If an atrial contraction is present, only the early diastolic portion of the curve is included in the pressure half-time calculation.

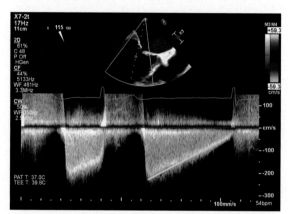

Fig. 11.15 Pressure half-time example. On this TEE study, CW Doppler was used to record the diastolic flow profile across the stenotic mitral valve. Pulsed Doppler was not used due to signal aliasing of the velocity signal. The pressure half-time is measured by identifying the peak early diastolic velocity and then placing a line along the mid-diastolic deceleration slope, as shown by the yellow line. The pressure half-time is the time interval between the peak gradient and ½ the peak gradient. The empiric constant 220 is divided by the pressure half-time by to obtain the valve area. In this example, the pressure half-time was 350 msec and valve area 0.6 cm². The longer diastolic interval is more accurate for measurement of pressure half-time because the diastolic slope is better demonstrated than on the shorter diastolic flow signal.

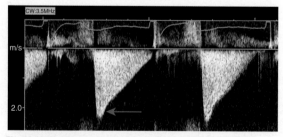

Fig. 11.16 Nonlinear diastolic velocity curve. TEE imaging in a 64-year-old woman with rheumatic mitral valve disease shows CW Doppler antegrade flow (away from the transducer) across the stenotic mitral valve. The initial diastolic slope *(arrow)* is steeper than the mid-diastolic slope. When there is an initial steep decline in velocity (often called a "ski-slope" pattern) with a flatter mid-diastolic slope, the pressure half-time is measured along the mid-diastolic portion of the curve, as shown on the second beat, extrapolating back to the onset of flow.

Continuity Equation Valve Area

■ If further evaluation of mitral stenosis severity is needed, a continuity equation valve area can be calculated.

■ Transmitral stroke volume (SV) is divided by the velocity-time integral of the mitral stenosis (VTI_{MS}) jet to obtain MVA:

$$MVA = SV_{mitral}/VTI_{MS} \qquad (11.8)$$

❖ **KEY POINTS**

❑ Transmitral SV is determined in the LVOT or across the pulmonic valve.

❑ This approach is only accurate when there is no mitral regurgitation.

Step 3: Evaluate Mitral Regurgitation (Fig. 11.17)

■ If regurgitation is significant (vena contracta ≥3 mm), evaluate as detailed in Chapter 12.

❖ **KEY POINTS**

❑ Most patients with rheumatic mitral stenosis have some degree of mitral regurgitation.

❑ With combined moderate stenosis and regurgitation, quantitation of both lesions is needed.

❑ The degree of mitral regurgitation may need to be evaluated by TEE, because moderate or greater regurgitation is a contraindication to percutaneous valvotomy.

Step 4: Examine Aortic and Tricuspid Valves for Rheumatic Involvement

■ When rheumatic mitral stenosis is present, careful evaluation of aortic and tricuspid valves is needed to detect rheumatic involvement.

❖ **KEY POINTS**

❑ Rheumatic disease typically affects the mitral valve first, causing stenosis and/or regurgitation.

❑ The aortic valve is affected in about 35% of patients and the tricuspid valve in about 6% of patients with rheumatic mitral valve disease.

❑ The appearance of rheumatic disease affecting the aortic and tricuspid valves is similar to the mitral valve, with commissural fusion being the most consistent feature.

Step 5: Evaluate the Consequences of Mitral Valve Obstruction

■ Measure LA size (Fig. 11.18).

■ Evaluate for LA thrombus on TEE if a valve procedure is considered (Fig. 11.19).

■ Estimate pulmonary pressures as detailed in Chapter 6.

■ Evaluate right ventricle (RV) size and systolic function.

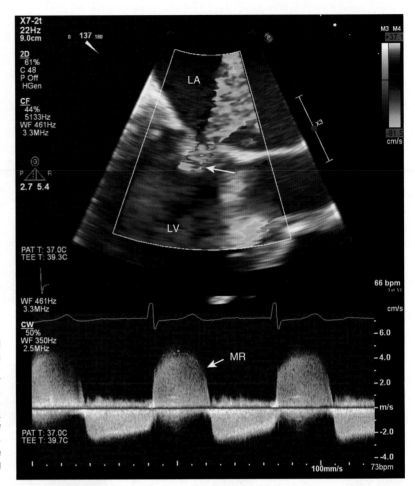

Fig. 11.17 **Coexisting rheumatic mitral regurgitation.** TEE imaging in a patient with rheumatic mitral stenosis shows concurrent mitral regurgitation on this systolic color Doppler image *(top)* and CW Doppler recording *(bottom)*. MR severity is graded as mild-moderate based on the vena contracta width (4 mm; *arrow*) and relative low density of the CW Doppler regurgitant signal. Quantitation of regurgitation by the proximal isovelocity surface area method confirmed this qualitative grading with a regurgitant volume of only 8 mL.

❖ **KEY POINTS**

❑ LA enlargement is usually present in patients with mitral stenosis and is related to the severity and chronicity of mitral valve obstruction.

❑ Patients with rheumatic mitral valve disease have a high risk of atrial thrombus, even if in sinus rhythm.

❑ Pulmonary pressures are elevated passively due to the increased LA pressure. In addition, reactive pulmonary hypertension is seen with changes in the pulmonary vasculature that may persist after relief of mitral stenosis

❑ RV enlargement and systolic dysfunction in patients with mitral stenosis may be due to pulmonary hypertension (pressure overload) or to rheumatic tricuspid regurgitation (volume overload).

TRICUSPID STENOSIS

■ Tricuspid stenosis is uncommon and usually is due to rheumatic tricuspid valve involvement in patients with mitral stenosis.

■ Evaluation of rheumatic tricuspid stenosis is similar to evaluation of mitral stenosis.

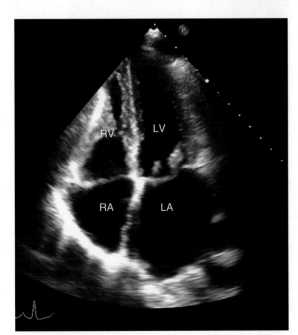

Fig. 11.18 **LA enlargement.** The marked degree of LA enlargement in this patient with rheumatic mitral stenosis is seen in an apical 4-chamber view. The LA area appears larger than the LV area in this frame.

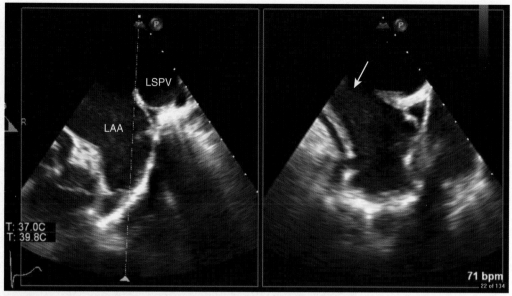

Fig. 11.19 LA appendage spontaneous contrast. In this patient with mitral stenosis, the LA is severely enlarged on TEE imaging. Although a thrombus is not seen in these biplane views of the LV appendage, there is marked spontaneous contrast with low-velocity swirling blood flow *(arrow)* consistent with a high risk of thromboembolism. *LAA,* Left atrial appendage; *LSPV,* left superior pulmonary vein.

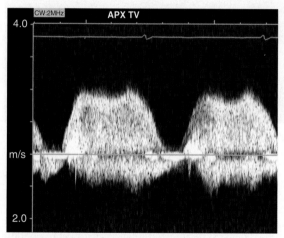

Fig. 11.20 Tricuspid stenosis. Antegrade flow across a stenotic tricuspid valve recorded with CW Doppler from an apical view. The velocity is markedly increased, with a mean gradient of 12 mm Hg, and the diastolic slope is very flat with a pressure half-time of 400 ms and a valve area of 0.6 cm^2.

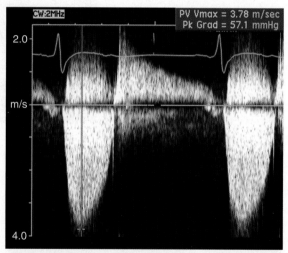

Fig. 11.21 Pulmonic stenosis. CW Doppler recording of pulmonary valve flow showing an antegrade velocity of 3.2 m/s, consistent with a maximum gradient of 41 mm Hg, or moderate pulmonic stenosis. Pulmonary regurgitation is seen above the baseline and appears to be moderate based on the relative density of retrograde versus antegrade flow. Pulmonary pressures are low, based on the low end-diastolic velocity of the regurgitant signal.

❖ **KEY POINTS**

❑ Rheumatic tricuspid stenosis appears similar to mitral stenosis, with commissural fusion and diastolic bowing of the leaflets.

❑ Carcinoid disease can cause tricuspid stenosis with thickened, shortened leaflets.

❑ The antegrade tricuspid velocity curve, recorded from an RV inflow view or an apical approach, allows measurement of mean gradient and pressure half-time.

❑ Diastolic pressure gradients may be lower for the tricuspid, compared with mitral stenosis (Fig. 11.20).

❑ Planimetry of the stenotic tricuspid orifice rarely is possible with 2D imaging; 3D imaging may be helpful in some cases.

PULMONIC STENOSIS (FIG. 11.21)

■ The velocity across the pulmonic valve is recorded using pulsed or CW Doppler from a parasternal approach.

■ Maximum gradient is calculated using the Bernoulli equation.

- Coexisting pulmonic regurgitation is evaluated by color and CW Doppler.

❖ KEY POINTS

- ❏ Pulmonic stenosis usually is due to congenital heart disease and may be an isolated defect or a component of more complex congenital disease, such as tetralogy of Fallot.
- ❏ Visualization of the pulmonic valve is challenging on both transthoracic and TEE imaging in adults; often Doppler data are used to infer valve pathology.
- ❏ Grading of stenosis severity is based on the maximum transvalvular pressure gradient (mild

<25 mm Hg; moderate 25 to 50 mm Hg; severe >50 mm Hg).
- ❏ Pulmonic stenosis often is accompanied by significant pulmonic regurgitation, particularly if there has been a prior surgical or percutaneous procedure.
- ❏ Branch pulmonary artery stenosis may also be present and is difficult to evaluate by echocardiography, although evaluation of the proximal right and left pulmonary may be possible from a high parasternal short-axis view.

THE ECHO EXAM

Aortic Stenosis: Key Measures

Parameter	Key Measures	Clinical Decision Thresholds
Valve anatomy	Calcific Bicuspid (two leaflets in systole) Rheumatic	
Stenosis severity	Jet velocity (V_{max}) Mean pressure gradient (ΔP_{mean}) LVOT/AS velocity ratio Aortic valve area (AVA)	$\geq$4 m/s (severe) $\geq$5 m/s (very severe) $\geq$40 mm Hg $\leq$0.25 <1.0 cm^2 <0.6 cm^2/m
Stroke volume (SV)	SV index	<35 ml/m^2
Rate of progression	Annual changes in V_{max} on serial studies	$\geq$0.3 m/s/yr
Coexisting aortic regurgitation	Qualitative evaluation of severity	
LV response	LV hypertrophy LV dimensions or volumes LV ejection fraction	 <50%
Other findings	Pulmonary pressures Mitral regurgitation	

LVOT, Left ventricular outflow tract.

Technical Details for Quantitation of Aortic Stenosis Severity

Components	Modality	View	Recording	Measurements
LVOT diameter $LVOT_D$	2D	Parasternal long-axis	Adjust depth, optimize endocardial definition, zoom mode.	Inner edge to inner edge of LVOT, parallel and adjacent to aortic valve, mid-systole
LVOT flow V_{LVOT} VTI_{LVOT}	Pulsed Doppler	Apical 4-chamber (anteriorly angulated)	Sample volume 2-3 mm, envelope of flow with defined peak, start with sample volume at valve and move apically	Trace modal velocity of spectral velocity curve.
AS jet V_{max} $VTI_{AS\text{-}jet}$	CW Doppler	Apical, SSN, other	Examination from multiple windows, careful positioning, and transducer angulation to obtain highest-velocity signal	Measure maximum velocities at edge of intense velocity signal.
Pressure gradient			$\Delta P_{max} = 4(V_{max})^2$	
Continuity equation			$AVA\ (cm^2) = [\pi\ (LVOT_D/2)^2 \times VTI_{LVOT}]/VTI_{AS\text{-}Jet}$	
Simplified continuity equation			$AVA\ (cm^2) = [\pi\ (LVOT_D/2)^2 \times V_{LVOT}]/V_{AS\text{-}Jet}$	
Velocity ratio			Velocity ratio $= V_{LVOT}/V_{AS\text{-}Jet}$	
Stroke volume (SV) index			$SV_i = [\pi\ (LVOT_D/2)^2 \times VTI_{LVOT}]/BSA$	

AS, Aortic stenosis; *AVA,* aortic valve area; *BSA,* body surface area; *LVOT,* left ventricular outflow tract; *SSN,* suprasternal notch; *V,* velocity, *VTI,* velocity time integral.

Mitral Stenosis: Key Measures

Parameter	Key Measures	Clinical Decision Thresholds
Valve anatomy	Valve thickness and mobility Calcification Commissural fusion Subvalvular involvement	
Stenosis severity	2D or 3D valve area Mean pressure gradient Pressure half-time valve area	MVA ≤1.5 cm² (severe) MVA ≤1.0 cm² (very severe) Variable depending on flow rate ≥150 msec (severe) ≥220 msec (very severe)
LA	Size (dimension or volume) TEE for thrombus before transcatheter balloon commis- surotomy	
Coexisting mitral regurgitation	Qualitative and quantitative evaluation of severity	
Pulmonary vasculature	Pulmonary systolic pressure RV size and function	>30 mm Hg
Other findings	Aortic valve involvement LV size and systolic function	

MVA, Mitral valve area.

Technical Details for Quantitation of Mitral Stenosis Severity

Parameter	Modality	View	Recording	Measurements
2D planimetry of valve area MVA$_{2D}$	2D	Parasternal short-axis	Scan from apex to base in order to identify minimal valve area	Planimetry of inner edge of dark-light interface
2D planimetry of valve area MVA$_{3D}$	3D full volume acquisition	TTE or TEE	Acquire full volume of mitral valve with analysis in x, y, z planes after acquisition	Adjust image planes to obtain planar view of mitral orifice at leaflet tips; trace white-black interface
Mean gradient Mean ΔP	Pulsed (HPRF) or CW Doppler	Apical 4-chamber or long-axis	Align Doppler beam parallel to MS jet Adjust angle to obtain smooth envelope, clear peak, and linear deceleration slope	Trace maximum velocity of spectral velocity curve
Pressure half-time T½	Pulsed (HPRF) or CW Doppler	Apical 4-chamber or long-axis	Same as mean gradient; adjust scale so velocity curve fills the screen HPRF Doppler often has less noise than CW Doppler signal	Place line from maximum velocity along mid-diastolic linear slope. MVA = 220/T½

HPRF, High-pulse repetition frequency; *MVA,* mitral valve area.

SELF-ASSESSMENT QUESTIONS

Question 1

Match the phenotypic manifestation (1 to 4) with the clinical condidtion (A to D):

1. Noncoronary cusp calcium
2. Leaflet edge thickening
3. Early systolic cusp closure
4. Commissural raphe
   - **A.** Hypertrophic cardiomyopathy
   - **B.** Aortic sclerosis
   - **C.** Rheumatic valve disease
   - **D.** Congenitally bicuspid valve

Question 2

A 52-year-old man with reduced exercise tolerance and a systolic murmur is referred for transesophageal imaging. The image in Fig. 11.22 is most consistent with:

- **A.** Subaortic membrane
- **B.** Hypertrophic cardiomyopathy
- **C.** Calcific aortic valve disease
- **D.** Bicuspid aortic valve
- **E.** Supravalvular stenosis

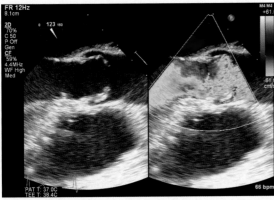

Fig. 11.22

Question 3

In an 82-year-old woman with a loud systolic murmur on exam, you suspect that peak aortic jet velocity is underestimated on the apical Doppler recording. Which of the following views would be most likely to help identify the peak aortic jet velocity?

- **A.** Left parasternal view
- **B.** Subcostal 4-chamber view
- **C.** Suprasternal notch view
- **D.** Parasternal long-axis view

Question 4

This TEE image (Fig. 11.23) was obtained in an 82-year-old man with shortness of breath. The next best step for quantitation of aortic stenosis severity in this patient is:

- **A.** 3D TEE imaging
- **B.** Dobutamine stress echocardiography
- **C.** Transgastric CW Doppler aortic velocity
- **D.** TTE Doppler echocardiography
- **E.** LV speckle tracking stain imaging

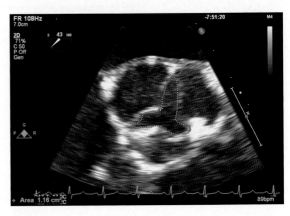

Fig. 11.23

Question 5

An asymptomatic patient with rheumatic mitral stenosis is seen for a routine follow-up. The diastolic flow curve shows an increased velocity and flat diastolic slope with the following measurements:

Maximum velocity	2.0 m/s

The time intervals between maximum velocity and various points on the diastolic flow curve are measured as follows:

1.8 m/s	190 ms
1.4 m/s	225 ms
1.0 m/s	240 ms
0.6 m/s	280 ms

Calculate the mitral valve area (MVA) _____

Question 6

The following parasternal long-axis view M-mode image is consistent with (Fig. 11.24):
- **A.** Mitral stenosis
- **B.** Aortic stenosis
- **C.** Tricuspid stenosis
- **D.** Pulmonic stenosis

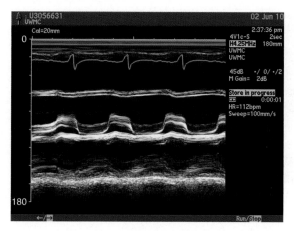

Fig. 11.24

Question 7

A 34-year-old woman presents for clinical evaluation, and the following image is obtained (Fig. 11.25). Based on this image, which additional echocardiographic finding is likely?
- **A.** Holodiastolic flow reversal abdominal aorta
- **B.** Dilated left ventricle
- **C.** Pulmonary vein systolic flow reversal
- **D.** Dilated inferior vena cava

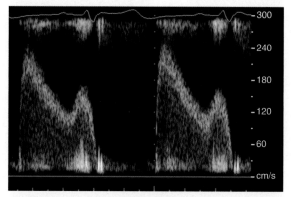

Fig. 11.25

Question 8

A 44-year-old woman is referred for echocardiography for new-onset atrial fibrillation. She lives in a rural area and has not seen care providers regularly due to lack of insurance. The following image is obtained (Fig. 11.26). The most likely cause of the abnormalities seen here is the following:
- **A.** Rheumatic valve disease
- **B.** Bacterial endocarditis
- **C.** Senile calcific valve disease
- **D.** End-stage renal disease

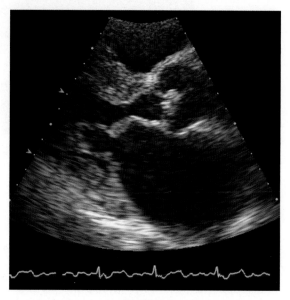

Fig. 11.26

Question 9

An 82-year-old man with prior ischemic heart disease presents for evaluation. Echocardiography demonstrates a heavily calcified aortic valve, an EF of 24%, and regional wall motion abnormalities in the anterior wall, inferior wall, and apex. The LV outflow tract (LVOT) diameter measures 2.4 cm. The following data were obtained from a dobutamine stress echocardiogram at an infusion rate of 20 μg/kg/m:

	Baseline	Dobutamine
Ejection fraction (%)	24	38
LVOT velocity (m/s)	0.7	1.2
Aortic maximum velocity (m/s)	3.6	4.4
Mean aortic gradient (mm Hg)	32	38

Calculate the aortic valve area (cm^2) at baseline and during dobutamine stress:
Aortic valve area _____ _____

Question 10

A 60-year-old woman with tricuspid valve stenosis is admitted to the hospital with dyspnea and pedal edema. The trans-tricuspid Doppler tracing is shown (Fig. 11.27). In this case, the severity of stenosis is best assessed by measuring:

A. Average of peak gradient three cardiac cycles
B. Mean gradient of longest Doppler signal
C. Average of mean gradient three cardiac cycles
D. Peak gradient of highest Doppler signal

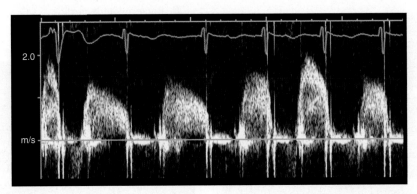

Fig. 11.27

Question 11

An 82-year-old woman is referred for progressive exertional dyspnea. She has a known history of moderate aortic stenosis. A myocardial perfusion study did not show evidence of myocardial ischemia. Prior TTE done 2 years ago demonstrated an ejection fraction of 68% without regional wall motion abnormalities; the aortic valve was calcified with peak aortic jet velocity of 3.6 m/s. She recently underwent transthoracic echo at a different medical center and the following aortic jet velocity was obtained (Fig. 11.28). The most appropriate next step in patient management is:

A. Transesophageal echocardiography
B. Repeat transthoracic echocardiography
C. Dobutamine stress echocardiography
D. Coronary angiography

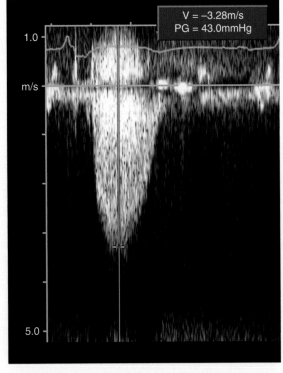

Fig. 11.28

Question 12

An 84-year-old man with a history of hypertension presented with worsening shortness of breath and systolic murmur, and underwent echocardiography. He had a blood pressure of 128/92 mm Hg, a heart rate of 70 beats per minute, and a body surface area of 2.1 m². Ejection fraction was 60%, and there was moderate mitral regurgitation. Measurement of the LV outflow tract (LVOT) diameter was 2.3 cm with a velocity time integral of 17 cm. Based on the additional information in Fig. 11.29, the stage of aortic stenosis (AS) is:

  A. Severe symptomatic low gradient AS with paradoxical low flow (Stage D3)

  B. Severe symptomatic low flow/low gradient AS with reduced LV ejection fraction (Stage D2)

  C. Severe symptomatic high gradient AS (Stage D1)

  D. Severe asymptomatic AS (Stage C)

  E. Moderate AS (Stage B)

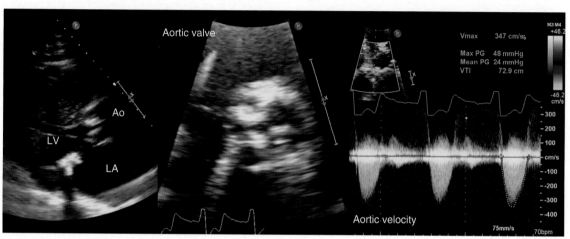

Fig. 11.29

ANSWERS

Answer 1

1. **B**—Aortic sclerosis, or "senile calcification," is a slowly progressive process that affects the aortic valve. In more prominent cases, calcification can lead to aortic stenosis (AS) with hemodynamic obstruction of aortic outflow. Most commonly, sclerotic changes of the aortic valve occur at the base of the cusps, initially in the noncoronary cusp with progressive involvement of the other cusps over time.

2. **C**—Rheumatic valve disease is the result of leaflet scarring and chronic inflammation from an autoimmune reaction triggered by recurrent infections with group A Streptococci. This is manifest by inflammation along leaflet coaptation. Progression can lead to commissural fusion and leaflet retraction, producing a stenotic, triangular valve orifice.

3. **A**—Ejection of blood through the left ventricular outflow tract (LVOT) may be impeded in the setting of hypertrophic cardiomyopathy with significant subaortic obstruction. With anterior motion of the anterior mitral valve leaflet and LV outflow obstruction in middle to late systole, there is a relative decrease in the pressure gradient above the obstruction, below the aortic valve, leading to early systolic closure of the aortic valve. This is typically best seen with M-mode imaging of the aortic valve from the parasternal long-axis view.

4. **D**—A congenitally bicuspid aortic valve may appear as two symmetrical cusps, or asymmetric cusps with a raphe or ridge replacing what would have been a commissure. On short-axis views of the aortic valve in diastole, these valves may appear tricuspid, but are revealed as bicuspid in systole, with visualization of the raphe.

Answer 2: D

This is a long-axis view of the left ventricular outflow tract (LVOT). In the 2D image on the left, the aortic valve leaflets show systolic doming, typical for bicuspid aortic valve disease. Color Doppler flow imaging in the right panel shows a laminar flow profile in the LVOT with flow acceleration at the level of the valve orifice leading to a mosaic pattern of distal flow disturbance. Hypertrophic cardiomyopathy typically appears as asymmetric septal thickening; there is often accompanying systolic anterior motion of the mitral subvalvular apparatus resulting in subaortic obstruction with color Doppler showing the increase in velocity proximal to the aortic valve. A subaortic membrane typically appears as a thin echogenic line in the LVOT with associated obstruction on color Doppler imaging. The ascending aorta is normal caliber without evidence of supravalvular stenosis.

Answer 3: C

To identify the peak aortic jet velocity, the transducer must be optimally aligned parallel to blood flow. As described in the Doppler equation, nonparallel alignment of the ultrasound beam with flow will underestimate peak velocity. Because of slight variation in peak aortic flow trajectory from person-to-person, several views are needed to ensure that the maximum aortic jet velocity is recorded. Typically, peak aortic jet flow is obtained from the suprasternal notch or right parasternal window, or from the apical 4-chamber view. For both the subcostal 4-chamber view and parasternal long-axis view, flow across the aortic valve is perpendicular to the transducer, and peak velocity will be underestimated.

Answer 4: D

This short-axis TEE view of a calcified trileaflet aortic valve with shows planimetry of apparent aortic leaflet opening in systole with a measured area of 1.2 cm^2. 2D planimetry is rarely reliable for quantitation of aortic stenosis (AS) due to several factors including shadowing and reverberations from valve calcification, inadequate visualization of the valve orifice, differences between anatomic and effective orifice area, and the inability to measure a 3D structure in a single 2D plane. 3D TEE imaging may be helpful in patients with a congenital bicuspid valve, because the systolic orifice can be identified more accurately from a 3D volumetric data acquisition. However, this approach is still suboptimal in patients with calcific disease as in this case. Dobutamine stress echocardiography is helpful in patients with LV dysfunction to distinguish moderate from severe aortic stenosis (AS) but would not be appropriate without a prior complete resting hemodynamic study in this patient. In some patients, the Doppler CW beam can be aligned with the aortic jet from a transgastric approach, but this method is prone to underestimation of stenosis severity due to a nonparallel intercept angle. LV speckle tracking strain imaging is abnormal in adults with AS but does replace hemodynamic evaluation for clinical decision making. The clinical standard for evaluation of AS severity is transthoracic Doppler echocardiography (answer D) with measurement of maximum aortic velocity, mean transaortic gradient and calculation of continuity equation valve area. Additional measurements, such as stroke volume (SV) index, are needed in selected patients.

Answer 5: 1.0 cm^2

The pressure half time is the time required for the pressure gradient across an obstruction to decrease to half of its maximal value. Velocity is squared in the Bernoulli equation to calculate pressure gradient, so to calculate the velocity on the curve where the gradient is half the maximum gradient, maximum velocity is divided by 1.4 (because 1.4 is the square root of 2). In this case, 2.0 m/s divided by 1.4 equals 1.4 m/s, so the T½ is 225 ms. Then mitral valve area (MVA) is calculated by the equation $220/T½$, in this case $220/225 = 0.98$ cm^2. Valve area calculations are only accurate to one decimal point, so this calculation should be rounded up and reported at 1.0 cm^2, which is consistent with severe mitral stenosis.

Answer 6: A

This is an M-mode tracing through the mitral valve leaflets. In this view, the pulmonic and tricuspid valves are not visualized. At this level, the aortic valve is not seen. The aortic valve would be seen if the M-mode ultrasound beam were moved closer to the base of the heart. Mitral valve motion is shown against time on the horizontal axis. Just following systole, the mitral valve is closed in the midportion of the image. There is only a small opening of the anterior and posterior mitral valve leaflet tips in diastole.

Answer 7: D

This is a transmitral Doppler tracing taken from an apical window with flow directed toward the transducer during diastole. The Doppler pattern is consistent with atrioventricular valve inflow and the prolonged diastolic deceleration slope consistent with mitral stenosis. Obstruction of LV inflow leads to pulmonary hypertension and volume overload, resulting in an elevated right atrial pressure and dilation of the inferior vena cava. Holodiastolic flow reversal (upstream reversal of flow) in the abdominal aorta would be seen with severe aortic regurgitation. Similarly, pulmonary vein systolic reversal would be seen in the setting of significant mitral regurgitation. In patients with mitral valve stenosis, LV size typically is small with an under-filled left ventricle. LV dilation would be expected only if the patient had mixed stenosis and regurgitation, which is not evident on this Doppler recording.

Answer 8: A

This parasternal long-axis image shows thickening of both the aortic and mitral valves. There is diastolic doming of the anterior mitral valve leaflet, and the LA is severely enlarged. The aortic valve is thickened with leaflet tip retraction at the coaptation. Atrial fibrillation can be a presenting symptom with rheumatic valve disease. In the United States, many patients initially present at age 50 to 60 years, with about 80% of cases occurring in women. In immigrants from countries with a higher prevalence of rheumatic fever, valve disease presents at a younger age. Endocarditis results in valvular vegetations, leaflet destruction, and abscess formation (not commissural fusion). Calcific aortic valve disease affects the body of the leaflet, not the leaflet edges or commissures, and in this case the

mitral valve is also involved. End-stage renal disease is associated with both mitral annular calcification and calcific aortic valve disease.

Answer 9:

$$CSA_{LVOT} = \pi(LVOT_D/2)^2 = 3.14(2.4/2)^2$$
$$= 4.5 cm^2$$

Baseline AVA
$$= CSA^{LVOT} \times V^{LVOT}/V^{AS}$$
$$= (4.5 cm^2 \times 0.7 m/s)/3.6 m/s$$
$$= 0.9 cm^2$$

Dobutamine AVA
$$= CSA_{LVOT} \times V_{LVOT}/V_{AS}$$
$$= (4.5 cm^2 \times 1.2 m/s)/4.4 m/s$$
$$= 1.2 cm^2$$

Resting data are consistent with low-output, low-gradient aortic stenosis (AS) with dobutamine stress showing a normal contractile response with an increase in stroke volume (SV; left ventricular outflow tract [LVOT] velocity increases from 0.7 m/s to 1.2 m/s) and ejection fraction from 24% to 38%. Aortic velocity increases as expected at the higher flow rate but aortic valve area (AVA) also increases from 0.9 cm^2 to 1.2 cm^2. These findings are consistent moderate AS. In this situation, there is an inadequate forward SV at rest to fully open the thickened, calcified leaflets, resulting in an apparently small aortic valve orifice area at rest. However, following dobutamine infusion, there is greater leaflet opening and a larger valve area at the higher flow rate. A lack of contractile reserve would lead to no change in ejection fraction or SV with dobutamine, not the situation in this case. If severe AS were present, valve area would remain less than 1.0 cm^2, with an increase in aortic velocity to 4 m/s or higher with dobutamine.

Answer 10: C

Tricuspid valve stenosis is nearly uniformly caused by rheumatic valve disease. The patient is in atrial fibrillation with variability in the R to R interval. With a shorter cardiac cycle, less time is spent in diastole, and diastolic LV filling is completed in a shorter interval. For these shorter cardiac cycles, the peak early inflow velocity is higher than in Doppler signals with longer cardiac cycle duration. Because mean gradient averages the instantaneous gradients over the flow duration, the mean gradient with be higher on shorter cycle lengths and lower on long cycle lengths. In clinical practice, when significant variation in heart rate is present, any measurements of peak and mean gradients are averaged over several cardiac cycles. For mitral or tricuspid stenosis, mean gradients are more representative of stenosis severity than peak gradients.

Answer 11: B

The original echo report describes normal systolic function and aortic stenosis (AS), with a calcified, immobile valve. The current aortic Doppler data are incongruent because they are lower than the peak velocity obtained on the prior study. Given progression in the patient's symptoms, a repeat transthoracic study is indicated. TEE is helpful for visualization of valve anatomy and allows planimetry of valve area, but Doppler data obtained by TEE are suboptimal as it is difficult to align the transducer with the jet due to transducer position constraints in the esophagus. Dobutamine stress echocardiography may aid in differentiating low-gradient severe AS, but systolic function was preserved on the prior study, making interval development of significant LV dysfunction less likely. The yield of coronary angiography is low at this time to determine etiology of symptoms given the negative myocardial stress perfusion study, but would be appropriate prior to aortic valve replacement if planned in the future. For the repeat study, Doppler interrogation of the aortic valve should be taken from multiple views such as apical, suprasternal, high right parasternal and subcostal views, with careful patient positioning ensuring careful transducer angulation to align the beam parallel with flow. On the Doppler recording from the question above, taken from the apical window, a peak velocity of 3.3 m/s suggested only moderate range stenosis but is incongruent with the prior TTE results and with patient symptoms. In this case, a higher velocity (>4.3 m/s) was obtained from a right parasternal window consistent with severe AS.

Answer 12: A

This patient has a heavily calcified aortic valve and left ventricular hypertrophy; thus, his symptoms of shortness of breath may be due to aortic stenosis (AS). In this setting, quantitation of stenosis severity is important for clinical decision making. With a maximum aortic velocity of 3.4 m/s and a mean gradient of 24 mm Hg he does not have severe high gradient AS (Stage D1) which is defined as a maximum aortic velocity is of 4.0 m/s or higher. However, calculation of valve area is needed because some patients have severe stenosis with only a moderate gradient due to a low transaortic flow rate, defined as a stroke volume (SV) index <35 mL/m². The next step in evaluation of this patient is calculation of SV index:

$$\text{Transaortic stroke volume (SV)}$$
$$= \pi (\text{LVOT}_D/2)^2 \times \text{VTI}_{\text{LVOT}}$$
$$= 4.15 \text{ cm}^2 \times 14 \text{ cm}$$
$$= 58 \text{ cm}^3 = 58 \text{ mL}$$

$$\text{Stroke Volume Index (SVI)} = \text{SV/BSA}$$
$$= 58 \text{ mL}/2.1 \text{ m}^2 = 28 \text{ mL/m}^2$$

Then aortic valve area (AVA) is calculated.

$$\text{AVA} = \text{SV/VTI}_{\text{AS}} = 58 \text{ cm}^3/73 \text{ cm} = 0.79 \text{ cm}^2$$

Thus, although the mean gradient and peak aortic velocity are in a moderate range (Stage B), valve area is severely reduced consistent with low-flow, low-gradient severe aortic stenosis (AS). This patient's ejection fraction is normal, so he has severe low-gradient AS with normal LV ejection fraction (Stage D3) rather than Stage D2, which is defined by an ejection fraction <50%. Given a severely calcified valve with these hemodynamics, it is very likely his symptoms are due to severe AS. In practice, this diagnosis can be challenging, and careful attention to avoid measurement error is needed when low-flow AS is a possibility. Additional quantitation of valve calcification with computed tomographic imaging may be helpful in select cases.

12 Valvular Regurgitation

BASIC PRINCIPLES

Etiology and Severity of Valve Regurgitation

- The cause of valve regurgitation often can be inferred from the anatomy and motion of the valve and supporting structures.
- Measurement of regurgitant severity is based on the fluid dynamics of flow across the regurgitant orifice (Table 12.1).

❖ KEY POINTS

- ❑ Inadequate leaflet coaptation results in valve leakage, with severity best defined by the size of the regurgitant orifice area (ROA).
- ❑ Upstream from the orifice, flow accelerates in the proximal convergence zone.
- ❑ In the orifice, flow is a laminar with a high velocity, reflecting the pressure difference between the two chambers on either side of the valve.
- ❑ Downstream from the orifice, flow is disturbed with the direction, size, and shape of the regurgitant jet dependent on several factors (Table 12.2).

Vena Contracta (Fig. 12.1)

- Narrowest width of the regurgitant jet, measured using color Doppler flow imaging.

- Also may be measured with three-dimensional (3D) color imaging.

❖ KEY POINTS

- ❑ Optimal color flow images show flow acceleration proximal to the regurgitant valve and distal jet expansion in the receiving chamber, with the vena contracta being the narrow neck between them.
- ❑ Vena contracta measurements are most accurate with:
  - ❑ The flow signal in the near field of the image (e.g., transthoracic parasternal long-axis views)
  - ❑ A narrow sector width to optimize frame rate
  - ❑ Zoom mode to increase image size
- ❑ Small differences in vena contracta width correspond to substantial changes in regurgitant severity grade so that if a precise and accurate measurement is not possible, other approaches should be used (Table 12.3).
- ❑ 3D imaging of vena contracta area is a promising new approach but remains limited by low temporal resolution.

Proximal Isovelocity Surface Area

- Blood flow accelerates proximal to a regurgitant orifice.

TABLE 12.1   Relationship Between Fluid Dynamics of Valvular Regurgitation and Diagnostic Approach

Fluid Dynamic Characteristic	Diagnostic Approach
Conservation of mass through the regurgitant orifice	Continuity equation for regurgitant orifice area (ROA)
High-velocity jet in regurgitant orifice	Pressure-velocity relationship of CW Doppler curve
Proximal flow convergence	Proximal isovelocity surface area (PISA)
Downstream flow disturbance	Jet area in chamber receiving regurgitant flow
Increased volume flow across valve	Stroke volume (SV) across regurgitant minus competent valve

From Otto, CM: *Textbook of clinical echocardiography,* ed 6, Philadelphia, 2018, Elsevier.

TABLE 12.2   Factors That Affect Regurgitant Jet Size and Shape

Physiologic
Regurgitant volume
Driving pressure
Size and shape of regurgitant orifice
Receiving chamber constraint
Wall impingement
Timing relative to the cardiac cycle
Influence of coexisting jets or flow streams

Technical
Ultrasound system gain
Nyquist limit (pulse repetition frequency)
Transducer frequency
Frame rate
Image plane
Depth
Signal strength

From Otto, CM: *Textbook of clinical echocardiography,* ed 6, Philadelphia, 2018, Elsevier.

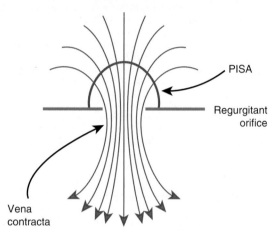

Fig. 12.1 **Fluid dynamics of valve regurgitation.** Streamlines of blood flow are shown in red. Flow proximal to the regurgitant orifice increases in velocity as the flow stream narrows into the regurgitant orifice. A proximal isovelocity surface area *(PISA)* is represented by the blue line that connects points with the same velocity on each stream line. Multiple PISA are present proximal to the orifice; the PISA seen with color flow depends on the aliasing velocity of the color scale. The flow stream continues to narrow beyond the orifice with the narrowest point or vena contracta reflecting regurgitant severity.

■ The aliasing velocity on color Doppler flow imaging provides visualization of a contour where all the blood cells have the same velocity (isovelocity) (Fig. 12.2).

■ The shape of this proximal isovelocity contour typically is a hemisphere so that the proximal isovelcity surface area (PISA) is:

$$\text{PISA }(\text{cm}^2) = 2\pi r^2 \qquad (12.1)$$

■ Volume flow rate is area times velocity (in this case, the PISA and aliasing velocity):

$$\text{Instantaneous flow rate }(\text{cm}^3/\text{s}) = \text{PISA }(\text{cm}^2) \times V_{\text{aliasing}}\ (\text{cm}/\text{s}) \qquad (12.2)$$

❖ **KEY POINTS**

❑ The PISA is best visualized from a window where the ultrasound beam is parallel to the flow direction, typically the apical long-axis or 4-chamber view for mitral regurgitation.

❑ The aliasing velocity is decreased to 30 to 40 cm/s in the direction of flow by shifting the Doppler baseline, which enhances PISA visualization.

❑ Both a narrow color sector and zoom mode are used for accurate measurement.

❑ PISA measures instantaneous flow rate (cm³/s). PISA must be integrated over the flow period to obtain flow volume (cm³ or mL).

❑ PISA may be inaccurate when the proximal flow field is not hemispherical, so this approach is more useful for central jets compared with eccentric jets.

❑ It is more difficult to visualize the PISA when regurgitation is mild, and it is more difficult to visualize a PISA for aortic, compared with mitral, regurgitation.

❑ Identification of the valve plane by two-dimensional (2D) or 3D imaging is critical, because the PISA measurement is from the aliasing velocity to the valve orifice.

TABLE 12.3   Doppler Evaluation of Valvular Regurgitation

Method	Doppler Parameters	Limitations	Correlation with Other Imaging Modalities
Color flow imaging	• Jet origin • Jet direction • Jet size	• Variation with technical and physiologic factors	• LV or aortic angiography • CMR flow visualization
CW Doppler	• Signal intensity • Shape of velocity curve	• Qualitative	• Invasive hemodynamics • CMR velocity data
Vena contracta width	• Width of jet origin	• Small values, careful measurement needed	• CMR flow visualization
Proximal isovelocity surface area (PISA)	• Calculation of RVol and ROA	• Less accurate with eccentric jets • Peak values only	• CMR flow visualization
Volume flow at two sites	• Calculation of RVol and ROA	• Tedious	• Invasive RVol and RF • CMR measurement of volume flow rates. • CMR LV and RV SVs
Distal flow reversals	• Pulmonary vein (MR), aorta (AR) or hepatic vein (TR)	• Qualitative, affected by filing pressures, AF	• None

AF, Atrial fibrillation; *AR,* aortic regurgitation; *CMR,* cardiac magnetic resonance; *MR,* mitral regurgitation; *RF,* regurgitant fraction; *ROA,* regurgitant orifice area; *RVol,* regurgitant volume; *SV,* stroke volume; *TR,* tricuspid regurgitation.
From Otto, CM: *Textbook of clinical echocardiography,* ed 6, Philadelphia, 2018, Elsevier.

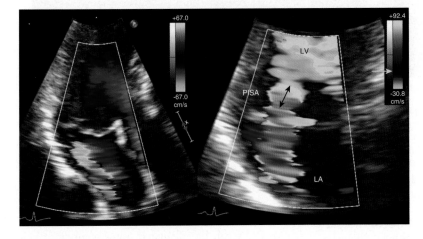

Fig. 12.2 **Proximal isovelocity surface area (PISA).** In an apical 4-chamber view at a standard depth *(left),* mitral valve prolapse is seen with a color jet of mitral regurgitation in the LA. This view is helpful for determining the presence and etiology of regurgitation. With the depth reduced and the image zoomed on the mitral valve *(right),* the Doppler aliasing velocity is reduced to 30 to 40 cm/s in the direction of flow (away from the transducer on TTE imaging) by moving the baseline *(yellow arrow)* with the image plane adjusted to visualize the proximal isovelocity surgical area *(double arrow)* and vena contracta.

Regurgitant Volume (Fig. 12.3)

■ Regurgitant volume is the amount of blood that flows backward across the valve, measured in cm³ or mL.

■ Regurgitant volume can be calculated by subtracting the stroke volume (SV) across a competent valve (forward SV) from the antegrade volume flow rate across the regurgitant valve (total SV):

$$\text{Regurgitant volume} = \text{Total SV} - \text{Forward SV} \quad (12.3)$$

■ Total SV also can be calculated by 2D or 3D echocardiographic measurement of LV SV.

❖ **KEY POINTS**

❑ Transvalvular volume flow rate calculations are based on diameter measurements (using a circular cross-sectional area [CSA]) and the velocity-time integral (VTI) of flow at that site:

$$\text{SV} = \text{CSA} \times \text{VTI} = \pi \left(D/2 \right)^2 \times \text{VTI} \quad (12.4)$$

❑ Small errors in diameter measurement lead to large errors in calculated SV.

❑ The largest source of error is ensuring that diameter is measured at the same level as the VTI recording; this is particularly problematic for transmitral volume flow.

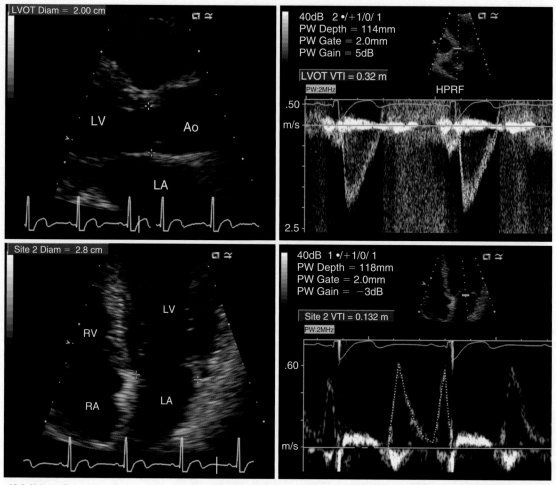

Fig. 12.3 Volume flow at two sites. In this patient with aortic regurgitation, regurgitant volume is calculated as the difference between total stroke volume (SV) across the aortic valve and forward SV across the mitral valve. The diameter *(D, left)* and velocity-time integral (VTI) *(right)* for transaortic *(top)* and transmitral *(bottom)* flow are shown. Transaortic (total) stroke volume (TSV) is LVOT cross-sectional area (CSA = πr^2 = 3.14[2 cm/2]² = 3.14 cm²) times the VTI (TSV = 3.14 cm² × 32 cm = 100 mL). Transmitral (forward) stroke volume (FSV) is π(2.8 cm /2)² × 13.2 cm = 81 mL. Then regurgitant volume (RVol) is TSV – FSV or 100 mL – 81 mL = 19 mL. Regurgitant fraction is 19 mL / 100 mL × 100% = 19%. These findings suggest mild regurgitation. *Ao,* Aorta; *LVOT,* left ventricular outflow tract; *VTI,* velocity-time integral.

- ❏ When both aortic and mitral valves are regurgitant, pulmonic valve flow rate can be used for forward SV.
- ❏ 2D LV volumes provide total SV when image planes and endocardial definition are adequate, but volumes may be underestimated if apical views are foreshortened.

Regurgitant Orifice Area

- ■ Conceptually, the regurgitant orifice area (ROA) is the size of the defect in the closed valve that allows valve regurgitation.
- ■ The actual anatomy of the regurgitant orifice may be complex, sometimes with multiple sites of backflow across the valve.
- ■ The continuity equation applies to both antegrade and retrograde flow across a valve.
- ■ Thus, ROA can be calculated from regurgitant volume (RVol) and the VTI of the regurgitant jet (RJ) as:

$$\text{ROA }(\text{cm}^3) = \text{RVol} / \text{VTI}_{RJ} \qquad (12.5)$$

❖ KEY POINTS

- ❏ ROA can be calculated using regurgitant volume calculated by any method.
- ❏ The continuous-wave (CW) recording of the regurgitant jet is used to trace the VTI (Fig. 12.4) to go with the regurgitant volume calculation from Fig. 12.3.
- ❏ Instantaneous ROA also can be estimated using the PISA approach by dividing the PISA instantaneous volume flow rate by the maximum regurgitant jet velocity:

$$\text{ROA }(\text{cm}^3) = \text{PISA }(\text{cm}^3/\text{s}) / V_{RJ} (\text{cm/s}) \qquad (12.6)$$

- ❏ The PISA-estimated ROA reflects the instantaneous ROA only; thus, it is most useful for regurgitation that occurs equally throughout the flow period.

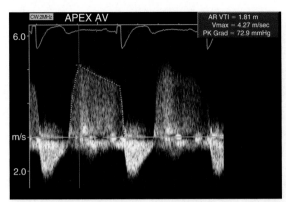

Fig. 12.4 Regurgitant orifice area (ROA) calculation. The velocity-time integral *(VTI)* of aortic regurgitant flow in the same patient shown in Fig. 12.3 is used to calculate ROA as the RVol/VTI = 18 cm³ /181 cm = 0.1 cm², consistent with mild regurgitation.

- ▫ In clinical practice, ROA should be calculated by more than one method, if possible, to ensure validity.

Distal Flow Reversals

- ■ The direction of blood flow distal to a regurgitant valve is reversed from normal when regurgitation is severe.
  - ○ With severe mitral regurgitation, there is systolic flow reversal in the pulmonary veins, but this finding is not specific unless the rhythm is normal sinus.
  - ○ With severe aortic regurgitation, there is holodiastolic flow reversal in the aorta (Fig. 12.5).
  - ○ With severe tricuspid regurgitation, there is systolic flow reversal in the hepatic veins (Fig. 12.6), but this finding is not specific unless the rhythm is normal sinus.
- ■ This qualitative indicator is integrated with other findings in classifying overall regurgitant severity.

❖ **KEY POINTS**

- ▫ These findings are more specific when flow reversal is more distal (e.g., abdominal compared with thoracic aorta for aortic regurgitation) and more severe (e.g., reversed versus blunted pulmonary vein systolic flow in mitral regurgitation).
- ▫ Normal atrial filling during ventricular systole (atrial diastole) depends on normal atrial contraction timing and force. Thus, flow reversal is sometimes seen even when regurgitation is not severe.
- ▫ Causes of false-positive systolic flow reversal include atrial fibrillation or ventricular pacing, resulting in systolic reversal in hepatic and pulmonary veins even when regurgitation is not severe.
- ▫ Diastolic flow reversal in the descending aorta also is seen with a patent ductus arteriosus.

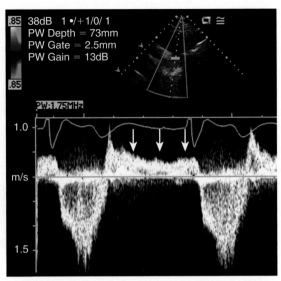

Fig. 12.5 Holodiastolic flow reversal in the descending thoracic aorta. In this patient with moderate to severe aortic regurgitation (AR), a suprasternal notch window was used to record pulsed Doppler flow in the descending thoracic aorta. Holodiastolic flow reversal *(arrows)* also may be seen with other causes of diastolic flow exiting the proximal aorta, including a patent ductus arteriosus or a large arteriovenous fistula in an upper extremity.

- ▫ Flow reversal is best detected with low wall filter settings, gain reduced to avoid channel crosstalk, and with the scale adjusted to the velocity range of interest.
- ▫ Normal patterns of flow sometimes are mistaken for flow reversal.
  - ▫ In the descending aorta, early diastolic flow reversal is normal.
  - ▫ In the hepatic veins, the atrial reversal can be prominent and may appear to extend into early systole.

Continuous-Wave Doppler Signal (Fig. 12.7)

- ■ The shape of the CW Doppler signal reflects the instantaneous pressure differences between the two chambers.
- ■ The density of the CW Doppler signal, relative to antegrade flow, reflects the volume of regurgitant flow.

❖ **KEY POINTS**

- ▫ The diastolic deceleration slope (or pressure halftime) of the aortic regurgitant signal is steeper (shorter) with more severe aortic regurgitation.
- ▫ A late systolic decline in velocity with mitral regurgitation reflects a rise in LA pressure, suggestive of a v-wave.
- ▫ Care is needed to ensure the Doppler recording is made with the ultrasound beam parallel to the direction of the regurgitant jet at the vena contracta.
- ▫ Optimal CW recordings of the regurgitant jets show a smooth velocity curve with a dense signal along the outer edge of the spectral signal.

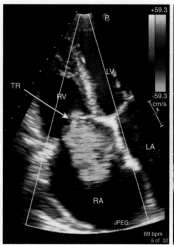
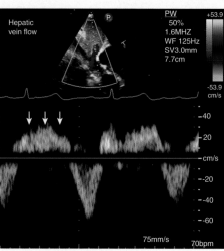

Fig. 12.6 Hepatic vein systolic flow reversal. Color Doppler imaging in a 4-chamber view *(left)* shows a large jet of tricuspid regurgitation (TR) with a wide vena contracta width (about 8 mm). The hepatic vein flow signal, recorded from the subcostal window in the central hepatic vein *(right)*, shows flow toward the transducer in systole *(arrows)*, also called *systolic flow reversal*, consistent with severe tricuspid regurgitation.

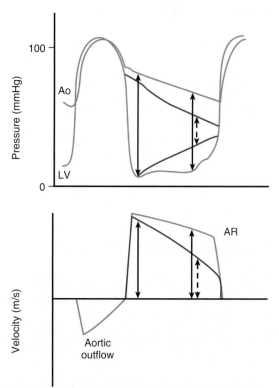

Fig. 12.7 Regurgitation hemodynamics. The shape of the CW Doppler velocity curve reflects the instantaneous pressure differences between the aorta and LV in diastole, with the relationship between LV and aortic pressures *(top)* and Doppler velocities *(bottom)* shown for chronic *(green)* and acute *(blue)* aortic regurgitation *(AR)*. *Ao,* Aorta. (From Otto, CM: *Textbook of clinical echocardiography, ed 6,* Philadelphia, 2018, Elsevier.)

❑ Recordings are enhanced using gray-scale spectral analysis with the velocity scale adjusted to the range of interest, the wall filters increased to improve the signal-to-noise ratio, and gains lowered to avoid overestimation of velocities.

▍ AORTIC REGURGITATION

Step-by-Step Approach

Step 1: Determine the Etiology of Regurgitation

- Aortic regurgitation is due either to disease of the valve leaflets or abnormalities of the aortic root (Fig. 12.8).
- Primary causes of aortic leaflet dysfunction include bicuspid valve, rheumatic disease, endocarditis, calcific disease, and some systemic diseases.
- Aortic root enlargement resulting in aortic regurgitation may be due to Marfan syndrome, familial aortic aneurysm, hypertension, or aortic dissection.

❖ KEY POINTS

- ❑ Long- and short-axis images of the aortic valve allow identification of a bicuspid aortic valve (two leaflets in systole), rheumatic disease (commissural fusion), vegetations, and calcific changes (Fig. 12.9).
- ❑ Leaflet perforation or fenestration cannot be visualized but is inferred from the location of the regurgitant jet orifice identified by color Doppler.
- ❑ When aortic regurgitation is more than mild, Doppler flow in the aorta should be measured at several sites as detailed in Chapter 16. The transducer is moved cephalad to visualize the ascending aorta.
- ❑ Marfan syndrome is characterized by loss of the normal acute angle at the sinotubular junction.
- ❑ Systemic inflammatory diseases associated with aortic regurgitation cause dilation of the aorta and thickening of the posterior aortic root extending onto the base of the anterior mitral leaflet.

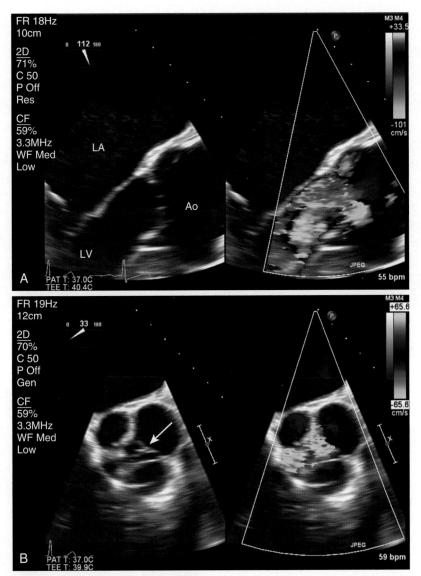

Fig. 12.8 Aortic regurgitation. (A) TEE imaging shows an eccentric aortic regurgitant jet with a vena contracta of 5 mm. (B) Short-axis views shows non-coaptation *(arrow)* of a trileaflet valve due to dilation of the aortic sinuses resulting in aortic regurgitation. *Ao,* Aorta.

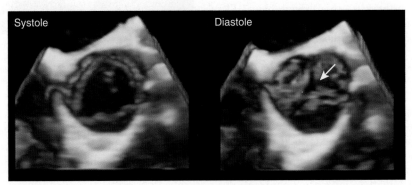

Fig. 12.9 3D aortic valve imaging. In the same patient as Fig. 12.8, 3D imaging shows a trileaflet valve in systole *(left)* with non-coaptation of the leaflets *(arrow)* in diastole *(right).*

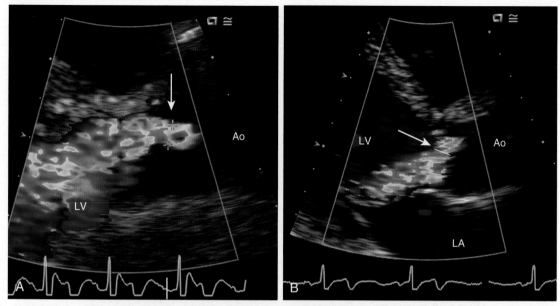

Fig. 12.10 **Aortic regurgitation vena contracta.** Examples of measuring vena contracta width with a centrally *(left)* and eccentrically *(right)* directed jet of aortic regurgitation. Vena contracta width in aortic regurgitation is best recorded in the parasternal long-axis view using zoom mode to focus on the aortic valve. The narrowest width of the regurgitant jet is measured, ideally with the proximal flow acceleration and distal jet expansion regions seen. Vena contracta width is measured perpendicular to the jet direction; with an eccentrically directed jet, this measurement is not perpendicular to the LV outflow tract. *Ao,* Aorta.

Step 2: Determine the Severity of Regurgitation

- Regurgitant severity is evaluated using a stepwise approach with integration of several types of data.
- In addition to Doppler measures of regurgitant severity, the cause of regurgitation, and LV size and systolic function are important parameters in clinical decision making.

Step 2A: Measurement of Vena Contracta Width Is the Initial Step in Evaluation of Aortic Regurgitation (Fig. 12.10)

❖ **KEY POINTS**

- ❑ With aortic regurgitation vena contracta usually is best measured in the parasternal long-axis view on transthoracic echocardiography (TTE) or the long-axis view at about 120° rotation on transesophageal echocardiography (TEE).
- ❑ Vena contracta is measured as the smallest width of the jet, taking care with eccentric jets to avoid an oblique diameter measurement.
- ❑ A vena contracta width less than 0.3 cm indicates mild regurgitation; a vena contracta width greater than 0.6 cm indicates severe regurgitation.
- ❑ Further evaluation is needed when vena contracta is 0.3 to 0.6 cm, when images of the vena contracta are suboptimal, or when further quantitation is needed for clinical decision making.

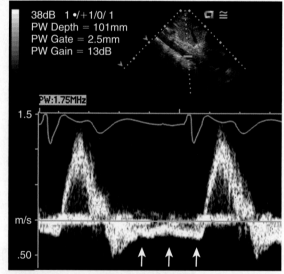

Fig. 12.11 **Proximal abdominal aorta holodiastolic flow reversal.** With severe aortic regurgitation (AR), flow in the proximal abdominal aorta, recorded from the subcostal window, shows antegrade flow in systole with retrograde flow throughout diastole *(arrows)*, reflecting severe backflow across the aortic valve.

Step 2B: Evaluation of Diastolic Flow Reversal in the Descending Aorta Is a Simple, Reliable Approach to Evaluation of Aortic Regurgitant Severity

❖ **KEY POINTS**

- ❑ Holodiastolic flow reversal in the proximal abdominal aorta is highly specific for severe aortic regurgitation (Fig. 12.11).

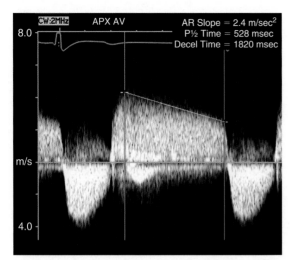

Fig. 12.12 CW Doppler evaluation of aortic regurgitation. The CW Doppler signal provides information on (1) the velocity of antegrade flow (v) reflecting both the volume of flow and coexisting valve stenosis, (2) the relative density of the regurgitant signal compared with the density of antegrade flow, and (3) the time course of the velocity signal. In this example, the diastolic slope is 2.4 m/s², with a pressure half-time of 528 ms, and the signal is only slightly less dense than antegrade flow; both these features are consistent with moderate regurgitation. The systolic velocity indicates concurrent aortic stenosis.

- Holodiastolic flow reversal in the descending thoracic aorta is seen in some patients with moderate aortic regurgitation as well as those with severe aortic regurgitation.
- Early diastolic flow reversal in the descending aorta is normal and should not be mistaken for aortic regurgitation.
- If holodiastolic aortic flow reversal is seen, but there is no color Doppler evidence of severe aortic regurgitation, evaluate for a patent ductus arteriosus, which also causes aortic diastolic flow reversal due to flow from the aorta into the pulmonary artery.

Step 2C: CW Doppler Evaluation of Aortic Regurgitation Is a Standard Part of the Evaluation

❖ **KEY POINTS**

- Aortic regurgitation usually is best recorded from an apical approach using CW Doppler, because this window allows parallel alignment between the ultrasound beam and regurgitant jet.
- In cases with an eccentric posteriorly directed aortic regurgitant jet, the best intercept angle may be obtained from the parasternal window.
- On TEE, a transgastric apical view may allow recording of the aortic regurgitant jet, but it may not be possible to obtain a parallel intercept angle using TEE.
- The density of the velocity signal compared with the density of the antegrade signal provides a qualitative measure of regurgitant severity (Fig. 12.12).

- In general, a steep diastolic deceleration slope (pressure half-time <200 ms) is consistent with severe regurgitation, whereas a flat slope (>500 ms) indicates mild regurgitation. However, some patients with compensated severe regurgitation have a long pressure half-time.
- Pressure half-time is measured using the same approach as measurement of pressure half-time in mitral stenosis (see Chapter 11).

Step 2D: When Further Quantitation Is Needed, Regurgitant Volume and Orifice Area Can Be Calculated

❖ **KEY POINTS**

- The most common approach is to calculate total stroke volume across the aortic valve and then subtract forward stroke volume (calculated across the mitral or pulmonic valve) to determine regurgitant volume.
- Reguitant orifice area is calculated by dividing regurgitant volume by the VTI of the CW aortic regurgitation velocity curve.
- The PISA is often difficult to visualize with aortic regurgitation.

Methods to calculate regurgitant volume based on antegrade and retrograde flow in the descending aorta have been described but are not routinely used.

Step 3: Evaluate Antegrade Aortic Flow and Stenosis

- Many patients with aortic regurgitation also have some degree of aortic stenosis.
- However, antegrade aortic velocity is increased in patients with severe regurgitation because of the increased antegrade volume flow rate across the aortic valve in systole.
- Thus, in addition to velocity and mean pressure gradient, aortic valve area should be calculated using the continuity equation as described in Chapter 11.

Step 4: Evaluate the Consequences of Chronic LV Pressure and Volume Overload

- The LV dilates in response to the chronic load imposed by aortic regurgitation with the extent of LV dilation reflecting the severity of regurgitation (Fig. 12.13).
- Some patients develop irreversible LV dysfunction in the absence of symptoms so that the most important parameters to measure on echocardiography in patients with chronic severe aortic regurgitation are LV size and ejection fraction.

❖ **KEY POINTS**

- LV end-diastolic and end-systolic dimensions, volumes, and ejection fraction are key measurements, with direct side-by-side comparison to previous examinations.

- Guidelines recommend M-mode ventricular dimension measurements because of better endocardial definition due to the high sampling rate of M-mode recordings.
- When the M-line cannot be aligned perpendicular to the long and short axes of the LV, 2D measurements can be used, taking care to optimally define the endocardium and to correctly measure the LV minor axis at end-diastole and end-systole.
- Indexing LV dimensions and volumes to body surface area is especially important in women and smaller patients.
- With severe aortic regurgitation LV volumes are increased in direct proportion to the regurgitant volume; the stroke volume calculated using the biplane apical approach is the total stroke volume (forward plus regurgitant).

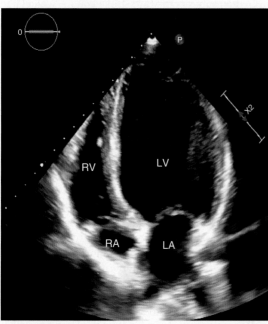

Fig. 12.13 **LV shape changes with aortic regurgitation.** In this patient with severe aortic regurgitation, the apical 4-chamber view shows a dilated LV with increased sphericity (rounded shape of the LV apex).

- The LV becomes more spherical in aortic regurgitation patients, so it is especially important to ensure that LV dimensions are measured at the same position on sequential examinations in each patient.

MITRAL REGURGITATION

Step-By-Step Approach

Step 1: Determine the Etiology of Regurgitation

- Mitral regurgitation may be primary (due to abnormalities of the valve leaflets and chordae) or secondary (due to LV dilation or dysfunction with normal leaflets).
- Primary causes of mitral leaflet and chordal dysfunction include myxomatous mitral valve disease (mitral valve prolapse), rheumatic disease, mitral annular calcification, and endocarditis (Fig. 12.14).
- LV dilation results in secondary mitral regurgitation due to annular dilation and malalignment of the papillary muscles, resulting in tethering or "tenting" of the valve leaflets in systole (Fig. 12.15).
- Ischemic mitral regurgitation may be due to papillary muscle dysfunction, regional dysfunction of the inferior-lateral wall, or diffuse LV dysfunction and dilation.
- Mitral regurgitation may be intermittent if reversible ischemia results in inadequate leaflet closure.

❖ **KEY POINTS**

- Mitral valve anatomy is evaluated in multiple 2D and 3D TTE views, including long-axis, short-axis, and 4-chamber image planes (Fig. 12.16). If better definition of valve anatomy is needed for clinical decision making, 3D TEE imaging is recommended (Fig. 12.17).
- Imaging of the mitral valve allows identification of myomatous valve disease, rheumatic disease (commissural fusion), vegetations, and calcific changes.

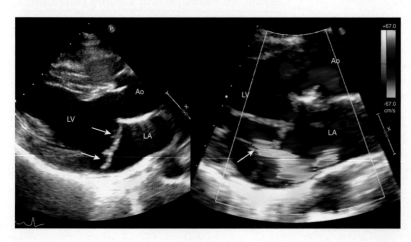

Fig. 12.14 **Primary mitral regurgitation.** In a parasternal long-axis view *(left)*, myxomatous mitral valve disease is present with prolapse of both leaflets *(arrows)* beyond the mitral annular plane in systole. Color Doppler *(right)* shows posteriorly directed mitral regurgitation with a wide vena contracta on this end-systolic frame. *Ao,* Aorta.

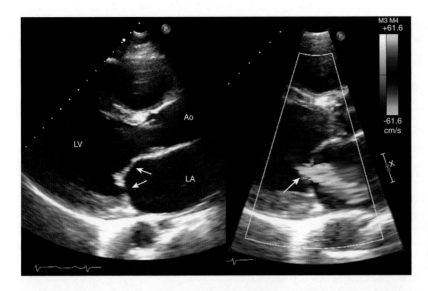

Fig. 12.15 Secondary mitral regurgitation. In a parasternal long-axis view *(left)* in a patient with a dilated cardiomyopathy, only mild leaflet thickening in present but the leaflets are "tented" or tethered *(arrows)* resulting in secondary mitral regurgitation *(arrow)* seen with color Doppler *(right). Ao,* Aorta.

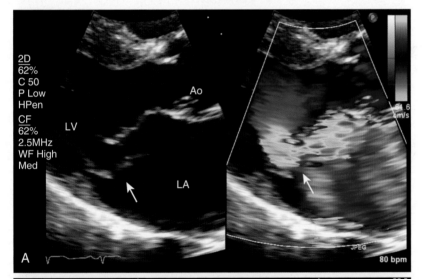

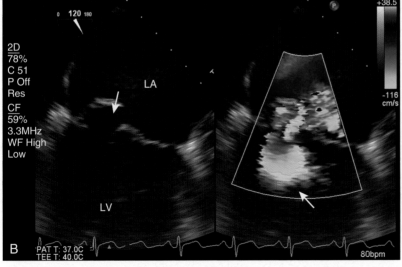

Fig. 12.16 Comparison of TTE and TEE evaluation of mitral regurgitation. (A) On TTE imaging, posterior mitral leaflet prolapse and a possible flail segment *(arrow)* are seen with color Doppler showing anteriorly directed mitral regurgitation *(arrow)* with a wide vena contracta. (B) TEE in a long-axis view shows severe prolapse of the posterior mitral leaflet *(arrow)* with severe mitral regurgitation with a wide vena contracta and large proximal isovelocity surface area (PISA) with the aliasing velocity set to 38.5 cm/s in the direction of flow. *Ao,* Aorta.

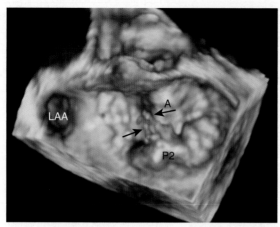

Fig. 12.17 3D TEE imaging of a flail posterior mitral leaflet. In the same patient as in Fig. 12.16, 3D imaging shows ruptured chords *(arrows)* prolapsing into the LA in systole at the lateral aspect of the central posterior leaflet scallop *(P2)*. The mitral valve is viewed from the perspective of the LA with the anterior (A) mitral leaflet shown superiorly and the LA appendage at the left of the screen. *LAA,* Left atrial appendage.

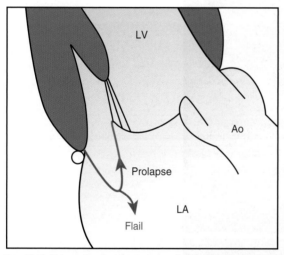

Fig. 12.18 Schematic of prolapse versus flail leaflet. The term *pro-lapse* of the mitral leaflet indicates that the chordal connections of the leaflet to the papillary muscle are intact so that, regardless of the severity of prolapse, the tip of the leaflet still points toward the LV apex. With chordal rupture, the mitral leaflet segment becomes "flail" and the tip of the flail segment points toward the roof of the LA. *Ao,* Aorta. (From Otto, CM: *Textbook of clinical echocardiography, ed 6,* Philadelphia, 2018, Elsevier.)

- With myxomatous mitral valve disease, the degree of thickening, redundancy, and prolapse of each leaflet is described.
- The tip of a flail leaflet segment points toward the roof of the LA in systole; a severely prolapsing segment is curved so that the tip points toward the LV apex (Fig. 12.18).
- Restricted leaflet motion is characteristic of secondary mitral regurgitation. The area defined by the tented leaflets and the annular plane at end-systole provides an index of the severity of restricted motion.

- 3D TEE is especially useful for evaluation of prolapse and chordal rupture in patients with myxomatous mitral valve disease.

Step 2: Determine the Severity of Regurgitation

- Regurgitant severity is evaluated using a stepwise approach with integration of several types of data.
- In addition to Doppler measures of regurgitant severity, the cause of regurgitation, LV size and systolic function, LA size, and pulmonary pressures are important parameters in clinical decision making.

Step 2A: Measurement of Vena Contracta Width Is the Initial Step in Evaluation of Mitral Regurgitation (Fig. 12.19)

❖ **KEY POINTS**

- With mitral regurgitation, vena contracta usually is best measured in the parasternal long-axis view on TTE or the long-axis view at about 120° rotation on TEE.
- Vena contracta is measured as the smallest width of the jet, taking care with eccentric jets to avoid an oblique diameter measurement. Both the proximal acceleration region and the distal jet expansion should be seen to ensure the narrowest segment of the jet is measured.
  - A vena contracta width less than 0.3 cm indicates mild regurgitation; a vena contracta width of 0.7 cm or greater indicates severe regurgitation.
  - Further evaluation is needed when the vena contracta is between 0.3 and 0.7 cm, when images of the vena contracta are suboptimal, or when further quantitation is needed for clinical decision making.

Step 2B: Evaluation of Jet Direction Determines the Next Step in Evaluation of Mitral Regurgitant Severity

- Central jets typically are seen with secondary mitral regurgitation due to LV dilation.
- Ischemic mitral regurgitation often results in an eccentric posteriorly directed jet.
- Mitral valve prolapse often results in an eccentric regurgitant jet with the jet directed away from the affected leaflet (Fig. 12.20).

❖ **KEY POINTS**

- With holosystolic regurgitation and a central jet, the PISA approach to quantitation of severity is appropriate; use of the PISA approach with late systolic regurgitation or an eccentric jet is problematic.
- With an eccentric jet or late systolic regurgitation, pulsed Doppler measurement of regurgitant volume and orifice area is appropriate.

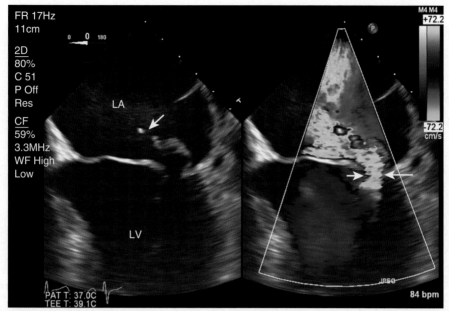

Fig. 12.19 Mitral regurgitation vena contracta width. The vena contracta *(between arrows)* is the narrow neck between the proximal acceleration on the ventricular side of the valve and jet expansion in the LA. Measurements can be made on TTE or TEE imaging.

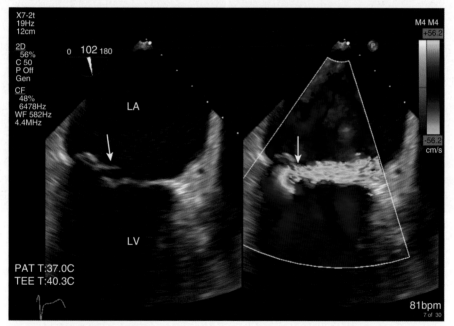

Fig. 12.20 Eccentric mitral regurgitant jet on TEE. This elderly man was admitted with acute dyspnea, thought to be due to pneumonia. However, TEE imaging shows a partial flail mitral leaflet *(left, arrow)* with an eccentric anteriorly directed mitral regurgitant jet on color Doppler imaging *(right)* with a wide vena contracta *(arrow)*. With myxomatous mitral valve disease, the direction of the jet typically is opposite the affected leaflet.

- ❑ The duration of regurgitation in systole can be visualized on frame-by-frame review of the cardiac cycle or can be inferred from the CW Doppler mitral regurgitation jet signal.

Step 2C: When Clinically Indicated, RVol and ROA Are Calculated

❖ **KEY POINTS**

- ❑ With late systolic mitral regurgitation or eccentric jets, total stroke volume is calculated across the mitral valve (SV_{Mitral}), and then forward SV (calculated across the LV outflow tract [SV_{LVOT}] or pulmonic valve) is subtracted to obtain regurgitant volume (Fig. 12.21):

$$RVol_{MR} = SV_{Mitral} - SV_{LVOT} \qquad (12.7)$$

- ❑ The 2D biplane total LV stroke volume (SV_{2D}) can be used instead of transmitral flow to calculate regurgitant volume:

$$RVol_{MR} = SV_{2D} - SV_{LVOT} \qquad (12.8)$$

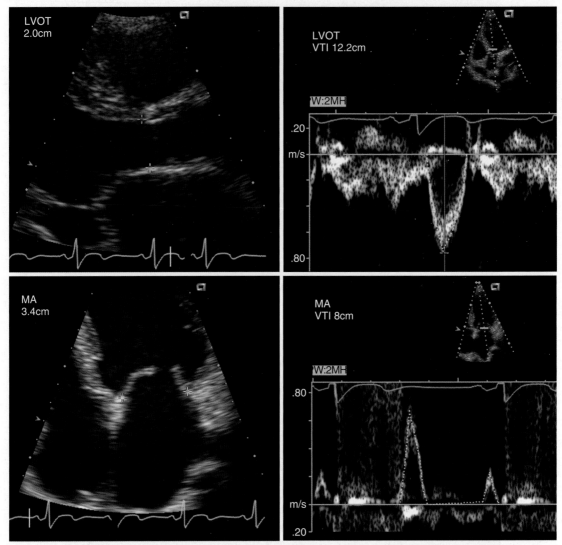

Fig. 12.21 Calculation of regurgitant volume in a patient with mitral regurgitation. Regurgitant volume is calculated from the difference between mitral *(bottom)* and aortic *(top)* volume flow rates based on measurement of annular diameters *(D, left)* and velocity-time integrals *(VTI, right)*. Total (transmitral) stroke volume (TSV) is the mitral annular cross-sectional area (CSA = πr^2 = 3.14[3.4 cm /2]² = 9.1 cm²) multiplied by the VTI (TSV = 9.1 cm² × 8 cm = 73 mL). Transaortic (forward) stroke volume VTI (TSV = 9.1 cm² × 8 cm = 73 mL). Then regurgitant volume (RVol) is TSV − FSV or 73 mL − 38 mL = 35 mL. Regurgitant fraction is 35 mL/78 mL × 100% = 48%. These findings suggest moderate regurgitation. *LVOT,* Left ventricular outflow tract; *MA,* mitral annulus.

- Regurgitant orifce area (ROA) is calculated by dividing regurgitant volume (RVol) by the velocity time integral (VTI_{MR}) of the CW Doppler mitral regurgitant velocity curve during systole:

$$\text{ROA} = \text{RVol} / \text{VTI}_{MR} \qquad (12.9)$$

- The PISA approach provides instantaneous flow rate, which is divided by the peak mitral regurgitant velocity (V_{MR}) to estimate ROA:

$$\text{ROA} = (\text{PISA} \times V_{aliasing}) / V_{MR} \qquad (12.10)$$

- The regurgitant volume can be estimated using the PISA method by multiplying the ROA by the VTI of the mitral regurgitant jet:

$$\text{RVol} = \text{ROA} \times \text{VTI}_{MR} \qquad (12.11)$$

- The PISA images are optimized using an aliasing velocity of 30 to 40 cm/s. The radius (r) of the PISA is measured from the edge of the color corresponding to the aliasing velocity to the level of the closed leaflets in systole (Fig. 12.22).
- Recording images for PISA measurement with and without color facilitates correct identification of the valve orifice plane.
- With the aliasing velocity set at about 40 cm/s and assuming a maximum regurgitant velocity of 5 m/s, quick estimate of ROA can be obtained from the PISA radius (in cm) as $r^2/2$.

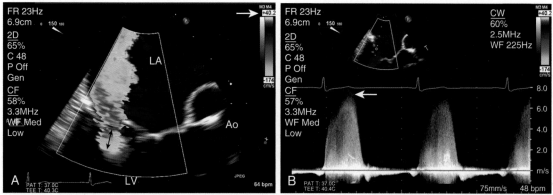

Fig. 12.22 Proximal isovelocity surface area (PISA) calculation of regurgitant volume and orifice area. (A) The PISA is seen in the long-axis TEE view in this patient; the best view will vary between patients, so careful adjustment of the image plane is needed for optimal visualization. Zoom mode is used to maximize the image size of the PISA, with a velocity scale without variance and with the baseline moved so that the aliasing velocity *(white arrow)* in the direction of flow is about 40 cm/s. In this example, the PISA diameter is 0.7 cm *(black arrow, left panel)*. The instantaneous flow rate is calculated as the surface area of the PISA ($2\pi r^2 = 2 \times 3.14 \times [0.7\ cm]^2 = 3.1\ cm^2$) times the aliasing velocity of 40 cm/s *(arrow, left panel)*, which equals 123 cm^3/s. (B) The maximum mitral regurgitant velocity recorded at the same time is 6.8 m/s (680 cm/s) *(arrow, right frame)*, then regurgitant orifice area (ROA) is (123 cm^3/s)/680 cm/s = 0.18 cm^2. Note that the high mitral regurgitation velocity indicates a severely elevated systolic blood pressure in this patient with a normal aortic valve. *Ao,* Aorta.

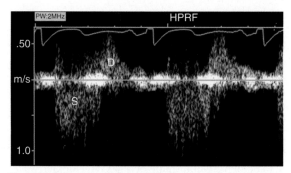

Fig. 12.23 Pulmonary vein flow systolic flow reversal. Doppler pulmonary vein flow is recorded on TTE from the apical 4-chamber view in the right superior pulmonary vein. Signal strength often is suboptimal, as in this example; even so, the flow into the LV in diastole *(D)* can be distinguished from the systolic *(S)* flow reversal due to severe mitral regurgitation.

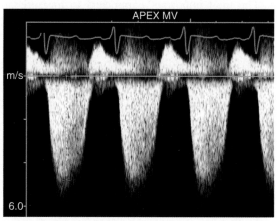

Fig. 12.24 CW Doppler recording of the mitral regurgitant velocity. This signal is evaluated for (1) the velocity and deceleration curve of the antegrade flow in diastole, (2) the relative density of the retrograde flow compared with antegrade flow, and (3) the shape and timing of the regurgitant velocity curve. In this example, the antegrade flow is normal velocity (<1 m/s) with a steep deceleration curve indicating the absence of mitral stenosis. The regurgitant signal is almost as dense as antegrade flow and is holosystolic, consistent with severe regurgitation. In addition, the falloff in velocity in late systole suggests that LA pressure is elevated in late systole, consistent with a v-wave and acute regurgitation.

Step 2D: Additional Simple Measures of Regurgitant Severity Include Pulmonary Vein Systolic Flow Reversal and the Density of the CW Doppler Signal

- Reversal or blunting of the normal pattern of pulmonary venous inflow into the LA in systole is seen in most patients with severe mitral regurgitation (Fig. 12.23).
- Pulmonary vein systolic flow reversal is specific for severe regurgitation only when sinus rhythm is present.
- The density of the CW Doppler mitral regurgitant curve, compared with the density of antegrade flow, indicates relative mitral regurgitant severity (Fig. 12.24).

❖ KEY POINTS

- ❏ The specific location of systolic flow reversal depends on jet direction, so TEE imaging may be needed to evaluate all four pulmonary veins; absence of systolic flow reversal on TTE does not exclude severe regurgitation.

- ❏ Systolic flow reversal may be present even when regurgitation is not severe in patients with atrial arrhythmias or other factors that affect normal atrial filling patterns.
- ❏ The CW Doppler mitral regurgitant jet usually is best recorded from an apical approach on TTE or a 4-chamber view on TEE, because these windows allow parallel alignment between the ultrasound beam and regurgitant jet.
- ❏ In cases with an eccentric posteriorly directed regurgitant jet, the best intercept angle may be obtained from the parasternal window or occasionally from a suprasternal approach.

Step 3: Evaluate Antegrade Mitral Flow and Stenosis

- Patients with rheumatic mitral regurgitation often have some degree of mitral stenosis.
- All patients with severe mitral regurgitation have an elevated antegrade mitral velocity because of the increased antegrade volume flow rate across the mitral valve in diastole.
- Mitral stenosis is distinguished from a high-volume flow rate by the mitral pressure half-time.

Step 4: Evaluate the Consequences of Chronic LV Volume Overload

- The LV dilates in response to the chronic load imposed by mitral regurgitation. However, the extent of LV dilation is much less than seen with aortic regurgitation because aortic regurgitation results in pressure and volume overload, whereas mitral regurgitation predominantly imposes a volume overload.
- The most important parameters to measure on echocardiography in patients with chronic severe mitral regurgitation are LV size and ejection fraction, because some patients develop irreversible LV dysfunction in the absence of symptoms.

❖ KEY POINTS

- ❑ LV end-diastole and end-systolic dimensions and volumes should be measured and compared side by side with previous examinations.
- ❑ Even a slight increase in systolic size is clinically significant, because the threshold for intervention is close to the upper normal limit for LV size (>40 mm).
- ❑ Guidelines recommend M-mode ventricular dimension measurements because of better endocardial definition due to the high sampling rate of M-mode recordings.
- ❑ When the M-line cannot be aligned perpendicular to the long and short axes of the LV, 2D measurements can be used, taking care to optimally define the endocardium and to correctly measure the LV minor axis at end-diastole and end-systole.
- ❑ LV end-diastolic and end-systolic volumes and ejection fraction are measured using 3D imaging or the 2D apical biplane method.
- ❑ With severe mitral regurgitation, LV volumes are increased in direct proportion to the regurgitant volume; stroke volume calculated using the biplane apical approach is the total stroke volume (forward plus regurgitant volume).
- ❑ Ejection fraction measurement is accurate in patients with mitral regurgitation. However, even a small decline in ejection fraction has important clinical implications for optimal timing of valve surgery, so precise measurement is essential.
- ❑ Measurement of LV dP/dt (rate of rise in pressure) from the mitral regurgitation jet is useful (see Chapter 6).

Step 5: Evaluate Other Consequences of Mitral Regurgitation

- LA enlargement is assessed as described in Chapter 2.
- Pulmonary systolic pressures are estimated as described in Chapter 6.
- RV size and systolic function are evaluated as described in Chapter 6.

PULMONIC REGURGITATION

Step-By-Step Approach

Step 1: Determine the Etiology of Regurgitation

- A small amount of pulmonic regurgitation is seen in most individuals (Fig. 12.25).
- Pathologic regurgitation most often is due to congenital heart disease, such as a repaired tetralogy of Fallot.

❖ KEY POINTS

- ❑ Imaging the pulmonic valve is difficult in adult patients.
- ❑ Thickened, deformed leaflets may be seen with congenital pulmonic valve disease (Fig. 12.26).

Step 2: Evaluate the Severity of Pulmonic Regurgitation

- Vena contracta width is helpful for evaluation of pulmonic regurgitation.
- The density and shape of the CW Doppler waveform are diagnostic (Fig. 12.27).

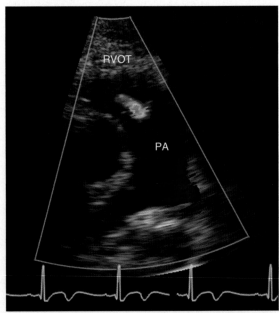

Fig. 12.25 **Color Doppler image of pulmonic regurgitation.** Pulmonic regurgitation is evaluated in the parasternal short-axis view on this diastolic image. The vena contracta is narrow, reflecting mild regurgitation. *PA,* Pulmonary artery; *RVOT,* right ventricular outflow tract.

- Further quantitation of pulmonic regurgitation is challenging but rarely needed for clinical decision making.

❖ **KEY POINTS**

- Pulmonic regurgitation is low velocity (if pulmonary diastolic pressure is normal), so the color Doppler display may show uniform laminar flow in diastole in the RV outflow tract (see Fig. 12.27A).

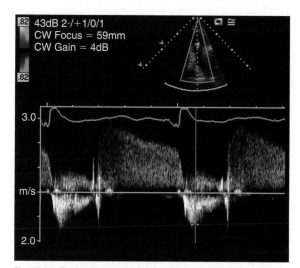

Fig. 12.26 CW Doppler recording of pulmonic regurgitation. The signal is much less dense than antegrade flow, consistent with mild regurgitation. A prominent pulmonic closing click is followed by an area of signal dropout, probably due to initial competence of the valve in early diastole, followed by the typical low-velocity diastolic curve of pulmonic regurgitation. The velocity-time course reflects the pulmonary artery-to-right ventricular pressure difference in diastole. Low-velocity flow is consistent with a small pressure gradient and thus normal pulmonary diastolic pressures.

- The CW Doppler curve is especially helpful for detection of severe pulmonic regurgitation showing a dense signal with a steep deceleration slope that reaches the baseline at end-diastole (see Fig. 12.27B).

Step 3: Evaluate the Consequences of RV Volume Overload

- Severe pulmonic regurgitation results in RV dilation and eventual systolic dysfunction.
- Timing of intervention for pulmonic regurgitation is based on the RV response, as well as regurgitant severity.

❖ **KEY POINTS**

- Evaluation of RV size and systolic function by echocardiography is largely based on qualitative evaluation of 2D images, using a scale of normal, mild, moderate, and severely abnormal.
- Sequential studies are helpful in distinguishing residual RV dilation or dysfunction after repair of tetralogy of Fallot from progressive postoperative changes.
- Cardiac magnetic resonance imaging allows quantitation of RV volumes and ejection fraction.

▌ TRICUSPID REGURGITATION

Step-By-Step Approach

Step 1: Evaluate the Etiology of Tricuspid Regurgitation

- Tricuspid regurgitation may be due to primary valve disease or may be secondary to annular dilation.

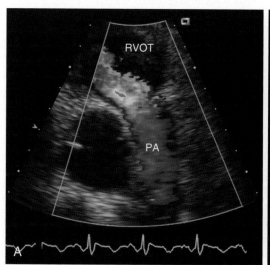

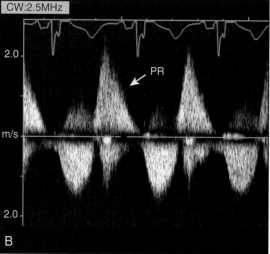

Fig. 12.27 Severe pulmonic valve regurgitation. (A) Color Doppler evaluation of the pulmonic valve in a parasternal short-axis view shows laminar flow filling the right ventricular outflow tract *(RVOT)* in diastole, consistent with severe pulmonic regurgitation. Because flow velocities are low, there is little variance, so that regurgitation may be missed on cine images but is evident on a frame-by-frame review. (B) The CW Doppler recording shows that the density of retrograde flow across the valve (above the baseline) is equal to the density of antegrade flow in systole. In addition, the end-diastolic velocity of the pulmonic regurgitation approaches zero, indicating equalization of diastolic pressures in the pulmonary artery and RV. *PA,* Pulmonary artery; *PR,* pulmonic regurgitation.

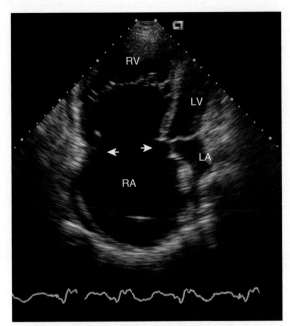

Fig. 12.28 **Ebstein anomaly of the tricuspid valve.** In the apical 4-chamber view the tricuspid valve leaflets are apically displaced so that the portion of the RV between the leaflets and the tricuspid annulus *(arrows)* has a RA pressure. Severe tricuspid regurgitation results in severe RA and RV enlargement. This patient has an intact atrial septum.

■ Primary causes of tricuspid regurgitation include endocarditis, Ebstein anomaly, rheumatic disease, carcinoid, and myxomatous disease (Fig. 12.28).

■ Secondary tricuspid regurgitation is seen with pulmonary hypertension of any cause, including mitral valve disease, pulmonary parenchymal disease, or primary pulmonary hypertension.

❖ **KEY POINTS**

❑ With Ebstein anomaly there is apical displacement (insertion of tricuspid leaflet greater than 10 mm apical from mitral valve leaflets) of one or more valve leaflets.

❑ Carcinoid results in short, thick, and immobile valve leaflets.

❑ Rheumatic tricuspid disease occurs in 20% to 30% of patients with rheumatic mitral disease.

❑ The diagnosis of secondary tricuspid regurgitation is based on the presence of pulmonary hypertension and the absence of structural abnormalities of the leaflets.

Step 2: Evaluate the Severity of Tricuspid Regurgitation

■ Vena contracta width is the key step in evaluation of tricuspid regurgitant severity.

■ Density of the CW Doppler velocity curve, relative to antegrade flow, is also helpful.

■ Systolic flow reversal in the hepatic veins indicates severe tricuspid regurgitation in patients in normal sinus rhythm.

❖ **KEY POINTS**

❑ A vena contracta greater than 0.7 cm is specific for severe tricuspid regurgitation (Fig. 12.29).

❑ Vena contracta width is best measured in the parasternal short-axis or RV inflow view.

❑ A dense CW Doppler signal is seen with severe tricuspid regurgitation, but velocity reflects the RV-to-RA systolic pressure gradient, not regurgitant severity (Fig. 12.30).

❑ Evaluation of hepatic vein flow patterns is problematic unless sinus rhythm is present.

Step 3: Evaluate the Consequences of RV Volume Overload

■ Severe chronic tricuspid regurgitation is associated with RV enlargement.

■ RV systolic function may be normal or may be reduced with chronic tricuspid regurgitation.

■ RV size and systolic function are evaluated qualitatively as described in Chapter 6.

■ RA size is increased with chronic tricuspid regurgitation.

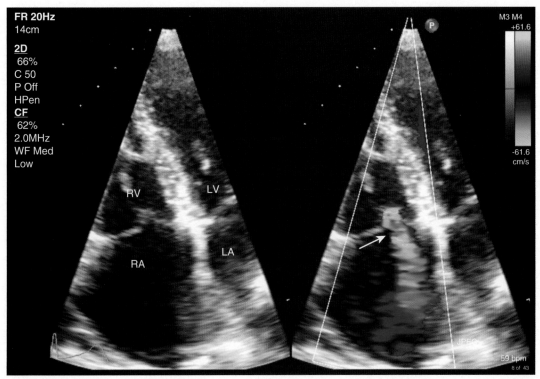

Fig. 12.29 **Vena contracta of the tricuspid regurgitant jet.** In the apical 4-chamber view, the image plane is adjusted to optimize views of the RV and tricuspid valve. Color Doppler shows tricuspid regurgitation with imaging focused on the proximal jet geometry. In this example, vena contract width is 5 mm, consistent with moderate regurgitation. Evaluation of the vena contracta is more accurate than visualization of the size of the flow disturbance in the RA for quantitation of tricuspid regurgitation.

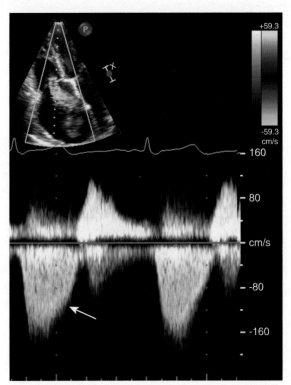

Fig. 12.30 **CW Doppler of severe tricuspid regurgitation.** In the same patient as Fig. 12.6, the CW Doppler shows a dense systolic signal with a low peak velocity. The low velocity reflects the low-pressure difference between the normal pressure in the RV and the elevated pressure in the RA. The high signal strength (or density on the spectral tracing) reflects the severity of regurgitation. Flow velocity is related to the pressure gradient as stated in the Bernoulli equation; high-volume flow rates increase velocity only slightly. Severe tricuspid regurgitation most often occurs in the absence of a severely elevated right ventricular (or pulmonary artery) pressure.

THE ECHO EXAM: VALVE REGURGITATION

Aortic Regurgitation: Echo Approach

Parameter	Key Measures	Clinical Decision Thresholds
Cause	Valve abnormality	
	Dilated aorta	
Severity of regurgitation	Vena contracta width	>0.6 cm
	Descending aorta holosystolic flow reversal	
	CW Doppler deceleration slope	PHT <200 ms
	Calculation of RVol, RF, and ROA	RVol ≥60 mL RF ≥50% ROA ≥0.3 cm^2
Coexisting aortic stenosis	Aortic jet velocity	
LV response	LV dimensions or volumes	LV-ESD >50 mm
	LV ejection fraction dP/dt	LV-EF <50%
Other findings	Dilation of sinuses or ascending aorta	>45, 50 or 55, depending on etiology and concurrent surgery (see Chapter 16)
	Aortic coarctation (with bicuspid valve)	

EF, Ejection fraction; *ESD,* end-systolic dimension; *PHT,* pressure half time; *RF,* regurgitant fraction; *ROA,* regurgitant orifice area; *RVol,* regurgitant volume.

Quantitation of Aortic Regurgitation Severity

Parameter	Modality	View	Recording	Measurements and Calculations
Vena contracta width	Color flow imaging	Parasternal long-axis	Angulate, decrease depth, narrow sector, zoom	Narrowest segment of regurgitant jet between proximal flow convergence and distal jet expansion
Descending aortic diastolic flow reversal	Pulsed Doppler	Subcostal and SSN	Sample volume 2-3 mm, decrease wall filters, adjust scale	Evidence for holodiastolic flow reversal
CW Doppler signal (intensity, slope, VTI)	CW Doppler	Apical	Careful positioning and transducer angulation to obtain clear signal	Compare signal intensity of retrograde to antegrade flow, measure slope along edge of dense signal
Volume flow at two sites (RVol, RF, ROA)	2D and pulsed Doppler	Parasternal (2D) and apical	LVOT diameter and VTI Mitral annulus diameter and VTI	$TSV = SV_{LVOT} = (CSA_{LVOT} \times VTI_{LVOT})$ $FSV = SV_{MA} = (CSA_{MA} \times VTI_{MA})$ $RVol = TSV - FSV$ $ROA = RVol/VTI_{AR}$

CSA, Cross-sectional area; *FSV,* forward stroke volume; *LVOT,* Left ventricular outflow tract; *MA,* mitral annulus; *RF,* regurgitant fraction; *ROA,* regurgitant orifice area; *RVol,* regurgitant volume; *SSN,* suprasternal notch; *SV,* stroke volume; *VTI,* velocity-time integral.

Mitral Regurgitation: Echo Approach

Parameter	Key Measures	Clinical Decision Thresholds
Cause	Primary valve disease	
	Secondary (functional)	
Severity of regurgitation	Vena contracta width	≥0.7 cm
	Jet direction (central, eccentric)	
	CW Doppler signal	
	Calculation of RVol, RF, and ROA	ROA >0.4 cm^2 RVol ≥60 mL RF ≥50%
	Pulmonary vein flow reversal	
LV response	LV dimensions or volumes	LV-ESD ≥40 mm
	LV ejection fraction	LV-EF ≤60%
	dP/dt	
Pulmonary vasculature	Pulmonary systolic pressure RV size and systolic function	
Other findings	LA size	

EF, Ejection fraction; *ESD*, end-systolic dimension; *RF*, regurgitant fraction; *ROA*, regurgitant orifice area; *RVol*, regurgitant volume.

Quantitation of Mitral Regurgitation Severity

Parameter	Modality	View(s)	Recording	Measurements and Calculations
Vena contracta width	Color flow imaging	Parasternal long-axis	Angulate, decrease depth, narrow sector, zoom	Narrowest segment proximal flow convergence and distal jet expansion
Color flow imaging	Color flow imaging	Parasternal and apical	Narrow sector, decrease depth	Central vs. eccentric, anterior vs. posterior
CW Doppler signal	CW Doppler	Apical	Careful positioning and transducer angulation to obtain clear signal	Compare signal intensity of retrograde to antegrade flow
Proximal isovelocity surface area (PISA)	Color flow imaging	Apical 4-chamber or apical long-axis	Decrease depth, narrow sector, zoom, adjust aliasing velocity Adjust aliasing velocity so PISA is hemispherical	$PISA = 2\pi r^2$ $R_{FR} = PISA \times V_{aliasing}$ $ROA_{max} = R_{FR}/V_{MR}$ $RVol = ROA \times VTI_{MR}$
Volume flow at two sites	2D and pulsed Doppler	Parasternal (2D) and apical	LVOT diameter and VTI Mitral annulus diameter and VTI	$TSV = SV_{MA} = (CSA_{MA} \times VTI_{MA})$ $FSV = SV_{LVOT} = (CSA_{LVOT} \times VTI_{LVOT})$ $RVol = TSV - FSV$ $ROA = RVol/VTI_{MR}$
2D LV total and Doppler LVOT forward SV	2D and pulsed Doppler	Parasternal (2D) and apical	LVOT diameter and VTI Apical biplane LV volumes	$TSV = EDV - ESV$ (on 2D LV volumes) $FSV = SV_{LVOT} = (CSA_{LVOT} \times VTI_{LVOT})$ $RVol = TSV - FSV$ $ROA = RVol/VTI_{MR}$
Pulmonary vein systolic flow reversal	Pulsed Doppler	Apical 4-chamber on TTE or TEE	Pulmonary vein flow in all four veins	Qualitative systolic flow reversal

CSA, Cross-sectional area; *EDV*, end-diastolic volume; *ESV*, end-systolic volume; *FSV*, forward stroke volume; *LVOT*, left ventricular outflow tract; *MA*, mitral annulus; *MR*, mitral regurgitation; *R_{FR}*, regurgitant flow rate; *ROA*, regurgitant orifice area; *RVol*, regurgitant volume; *SV*, stroke volume; *TSV*, total stroke volume; *VTI*, velocity-time integral.

Tricuspid Regurgitation: Echo Approach

Parameter	Key Measures	Clinical Decision Thresholds
Cause	Primary valve disease	
	Secondary (functional)	
Severity of regurgitation	Vena contracta width	≥0.7 cm
	PISA radius	>0.9 cm (aliasing velocity 30-40 cm/s)
	CW Doppler signal	Dense, triangular shape
	Calculation of RVol, RF, and ROA	ROA>0.4 cm^3 RVol>45 mL
	Hepatic vein systolic flow reversal (NSR)	
RV	RV size	Dilated with preserved function

PISA, Proximal isovelocity surface area; *RF,* regurgitant fraction; *ROA,* regurgitant orifice area; *RVol,* regurgitant volume.

Pulmonic Regurgitation: Echo Approach

Parameter	Key Measures	Clinical Decision Thresholds
Valve anatomy	Valve abnormality	
Severity of regurgitation	Jet width/annulus	≥70%
	Early termination of PR flow	PHT <100 ms
	Diastolic flow reversal in PR branches	
	Calculation of RF	RF >40%
Coexisting pulmonic stenosis	Pulmonic systolic velocity	
RV response	RV size	
	RV systolic function	

PHT, Pressure half-time; *RF,* regurgitant fraction.

SELF-ASSESSMENT QUESTIONS

Question 1

Doppler recordings of valve flow were recorded in the same patient. For the Doppler signals shown in Fig. 12.31, match each Doppler signal with the correct diagnosis:

A. Aortic regurgitation
B. Mitral regurgitation
C. Pulmonic regurgitation
D. Tricuspid regurgitation
E. Ventricular septal defect

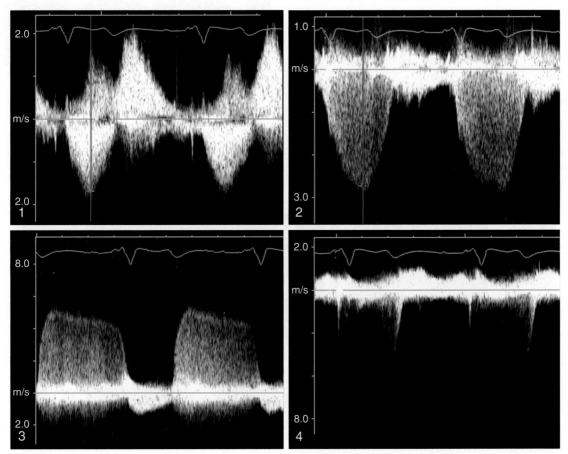

Fig. 12.31

Question 2

This Doppler signal (Fig. 12.32) was recorded on a TTE.

The most likely diagnosis is:
A. Bicuspid aortic valve
B. Mechanical prosthetic valve
C. Hypertrophic cardiomyopathy
D. Mitral valve prolapse

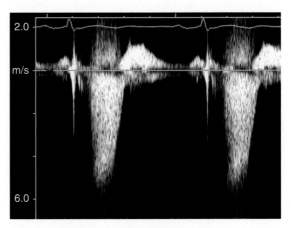

Fig. 12.32

Question 3

CW Doppler was recorded from a parasternal window (Fig. 12.33). These findings are most consistent with severe regurgitation of which valve?

A. Aortic
B. Tricuspid
C. Mitral
D. Pulmonic

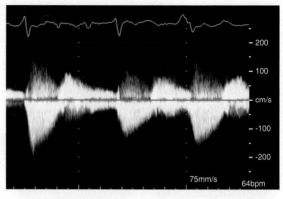

Fig. 12.33

Question 4

TEE was requested in an asymptomatic 56-year-old man with mitral regurgitation for evaluation of valve anatomy and quantitation of mitral regurgitant severity. The color and CW Doppler signals are shown in Fig. 12.34.

Calculate the following:

Regurgitant orifice area (ROA) _____

Regurgitant volume (RVol) _____

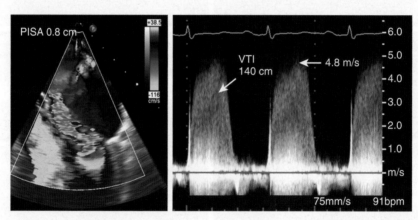

Fig. 12.34

Question 5

Which marked location on this TEE long-axis view of aortic regurgitation (Fig. 12.35) is most appropriate for measurement of the vena contracta?

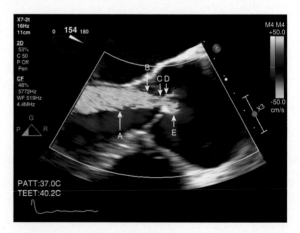

Fig. 12.35

Question 6

Based on the images in Fig. 12.36, indicate the most likely etiology of regurgitation for each image:

   A. Congenital defect
   B. Ischemic
   C. Myxomatous disease
   D. Malignancy
   E. Annular dilation
   F. Endocarditis

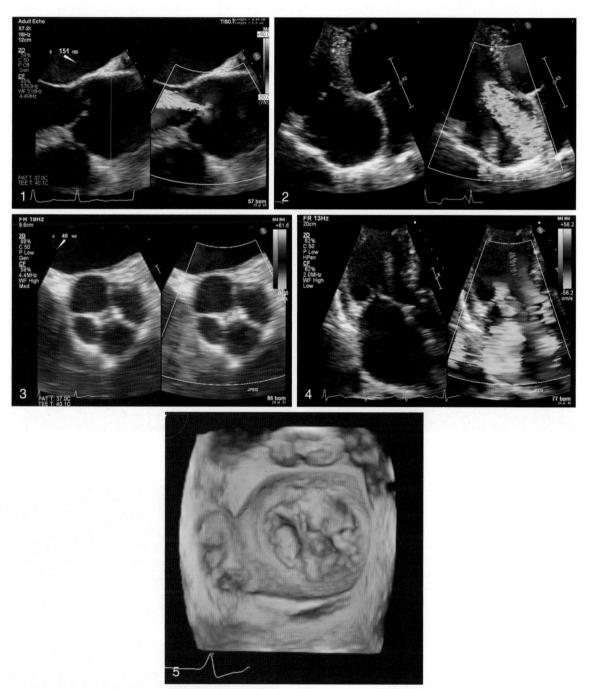

Fig. 12.36

Question 7

A 40-year-old asymptomatic man with a known bicuspid aortic valve undergoes routine TTE, and the following data are obtained:

LV dimensions, systole/diastole	4.9/7.1 cm
LV ejection fraction	48%
Tricuspid regurgitation jet velocity	3.3 m/s
Aortic sinus diameter	4.2 cm
Aortic pressure half time ($T\frac{1}{2}$)	410 ms

The most compelling finding to recommend cardiac surgery, based on these data, is:

- **A.** Vena contracta
- **B.** LV function
- **C.** Pulmonary pressure
- **D.** Ascending aorta size
- **E.** Pressure half-time ($T\frac{1}{2}$)

Question 8

Identify the red color Doppler signal (seen in Fig. 12.37).

- **A.** Aortic regurgitation
- **B.** Pulmonic regurgitation
- **C.** Ruptured sinus of Valsalva aneurysm
- **D.** Ventricular septal defect
- **E.** Coronary artery

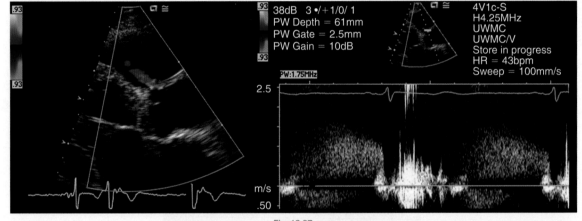

Fig. 12.37

Question 9

In an acutely ill patient admitted to the intensive care unit, a murmur is heard on physical examination, and a TTE is performed (Fig. 12.38).

The most likely diagnosis is:

- **A.** Severe mitral regurgitation
- **B.** Severe tricuspid regurgitation
- **C.** Severe aortic regurgitation
- **D.** Severe pulmonic regurgitation

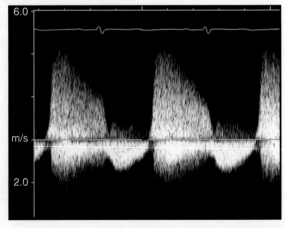

Fig. 12.38

Question 10

Echocardiographic data are recorded in a patient with a diastolic murmur (Fig. 12.39).

Mitral valve inflow VTI	15.0 cm
LV outflow tract VTI	29.0 cm
LV outflow tract diameter	2.4 cm
Mitral annular diameter	3.0 cm

Given these data, calculate the following for this patient:

Aortic regurgitant volume (RVol) _____
Aortic regurgitant fraction (RF) _____
Aortic regurgitant orifice area (ROA) _____

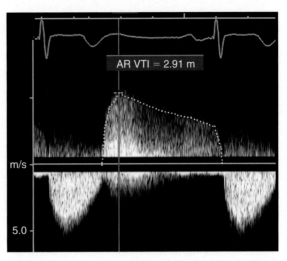

Fig. 12.39

Question 11

For each of the three Doppler flows (as shown in Fig. 12.40) indicate the most likely diagnosis using the following choices:

A. Aortic regurgitation
B. Mitral regurgitation
C. Pulmonic regurgitation
D. Tricuspid regurgitation

Question 12

This M-mode tracing (as shown in Fig. 12.41) is most consistent with:

A. Aortic regurgitation
B. Hypertrophic cardiomyopathy
C. Dilated cardiomyopathy
D. Mitral valve prolapse
E. Mitral stenosis

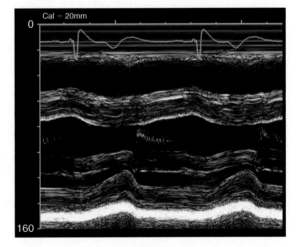

Fig. 12.41

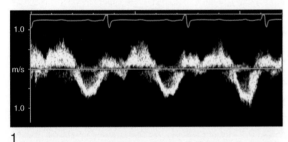

1

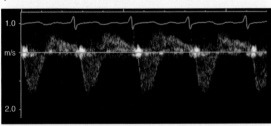

2

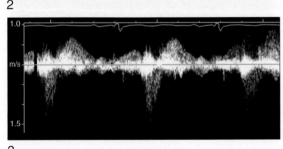

3

Fig. 12.40

ANSWERS

Answer 1

The correct answers are:

1. C
2. D
3. A
4. B

The type of valve regurgitation for each of these four Doppler signals, recorded in the same patient, can be distinguished based on the timing of the flow signal, the accompanying antegrade flow signal, and the shape and velocity of the velocity signals. The pulmonic valve (A) shows an ejection type velocity in systole, with a diastolic pulmonic regurgitation signal. This patient has severe pulmonic regurgitation with equal density of the antegrade and retrograde flow signals, a steep diastolic deceleration slope that reaches the zero baseline before the end of diastole, and an increased antegrade velocity due to the increased transpulmonic volume flow rate. Tricuspid regurgitation (B) shows a slow rate or rise in velocity, with a late peak in systole consistent with the normal RV systolic pressure increase. The peak velocity of 2.8 m/s is consistent with mildly increased RV systolic pressure. The antegrade diastolic flow signal across the tricuspid valve is not well demonstrated. The aortic regurgitant signal (C) shows a normal antegrade velocity across the aortic valve, with the velocity (over 4 m/s) and diastolic slope of the aortic regurgitant signal consistent with the aortic to LV pressure difference in diastole. Only mild aortic regurgitation is present as evidenced by the relatively low density of diastolic compared to systolic flow and the flat diastolic deceleration slope. Only trace mitral regurgitation is present with a faint signal seen at the beginning and end of systole (D). The duration of mitral regurgitation is shorter than the duration of tricuspid regurgitation because RV ejection typically is slightly longer than LV ejection.

Answer 2: D

This is a CW Doppler signal of the mitral valve taken from the apical view. The LV inflow pattern shows the early diastolic E-wave filling and the late diastolic atrial A-wave, corresponding to atrial contraction. During systole, flow is directed away from the transducer. There is absence of flow in early systole, with abrupt onset of flow in mid- to late systole. This is characteristic of mitral valve prolapse where the valve is competent earlier in systole, until buckling and prolapse of the mitral valve into the LA leads to poor leaflet coaptation and mitral regurgitation. The color M-mode tracing (as shown in Fig. 12.42) shows mitral regurgitation coinciding with prolapse of the posterior mitral valve leaflet.

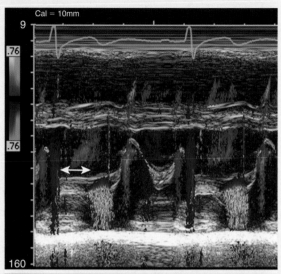

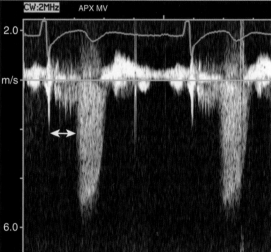

Fig. 12.42

Aortic stenosis due to a bicuspid aortic valve would show an ejection curve throughout systole and probably would show aortic regurgitation in diastole. A dynamic LV outflow gradient due to hypertrophic cardiomyopathy does peak in late systole, but flow starts with LV ejection with an upward curving or "dagger-shaped" waveform, indicative of progressive systolic obstruction rather than the abrupt late-systolic flow onset characteristic of mitral valve prolapse. A mechanical aortic or mitral prosthetic valve Doppler signal would show a bright mechanical click corresponding to opening and closing of the valve occluders. Shadowing of the LA by a prosthetic mitral valve will hinder evaluation of prosthetic regurgitation, but if prosthetic regurgitation is present, occasionally a faint holosystolic regurgitation Doppler signal can be seen during systole.

Answer 3: B

The figure demonstrates a CW Doppler from the parasternal window of a RV inflow view in a patient with severe secondary tricuspid regurgitation. The CW Doppler shows a regurgitant systolic flow that is triangular with the same density as the diastolic inflow signal consistent with severe regurgitation. The systolic flow profile might appear similar to aortic outflow; however, the low diastolic flow velocities are not consistent with aortic regurgitation (answer A). Similarly, since the view is from a parasternal approach, the flow profile would not represent a distal flow reversal in the thoracic or abdominal aorta, as those views are obtained in the suprasternal or subcostal windows, respectively. The systolic velocity with mitral regurgitation reflects the LV to LA systolic pressure difference so would be much higher, even if the patient is hypotensive or the Doppler intercept angle is not parallel (answer C). This Doppler curve is not likely to be due to severe pulmonic regurgitation (answer D), because the diastolic velocity curve does not have a steep deceleration slope and flow persists to the end of diastole. The diastolic flow signal is due to tricuspid inflow and not a regurgitation signal. This CW Doppler signal was recorded from the patient shown in Fig. 12.43, which demonstrates annular dilation, lack of tricuspid systolic coaptation, and a very wide vena contracta. A defibrillator lead can be seen traversing the tricuspid valve in this patient with a severe dilated cardiomyopathy. The rhythm strip demonstrates an irregular rhythm consistent with atrial fibrillation.

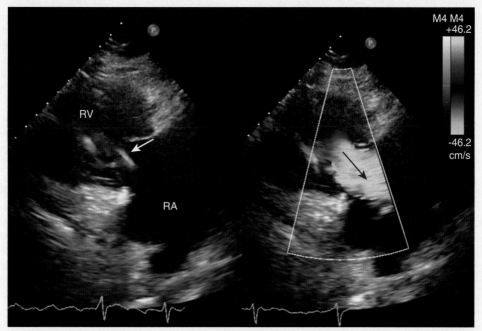

Fig. 12.43

Answer 4

Regurgitant orifice area (ROA)	0.33 cm²
Regurgitant volume (RVol)	46 mL

The first step in this calculation is to measure the proximal isovelocity surface area (PISA). This is the surface area of the 3D hemisphere on the LV side of the valve where the velocity is the same everywhere on the surface (e.g., isovelocity), defined by the color aliasing velocity. The radius of the hemisphere from the aliasing velocity to the valve plane is 0.80 cm. The surface area of a hemisphere is $2\pi r^2$. Thus:

$$PISA = 2\pi r^2 = 2\,(3.14)\,(0.80)^2 = 4.03\ cm^2 \quad (12.11)$$

The regurgitant orifice area (ROA) is calculated based on the continuity principle that the volume of blood flow through the PISA and through the regurgitant orifice are equal and that volume flow rate equals the cross-sectional area of flow times the velocity at that site. Thus, for a single point in the cardiac cycle:

$$PISA \times V_{aliasing} = ROA \times V_{MR} \quad (12.12)$$

In these images, the aliasing velocity in the direction of flow shown at the top of the color bar is 38.5 cm/s or 0.39 m/s. The maximum velocity of the mitral regurgitant jet is 4.8 m/s recorded with CW Doppler. The ROA (at that point in the cardiac cycle), then, is calculated as:

$$ROA = PISA \times (V_{aliasing}/V_{MR})$$
$$= 4.03\ cm^2 \times (0.39/4.8) = 0.33 \quad (12.13)$$

Regurgitant volume is the volume of blood that goes backward through the valve with each cardiac cycle. Regurgitant volume is calculated as the product of the velocity time integral (VTI) of the regurgitant jet and the regurgitant orifice area (ROA):

$$RVol = ROA \times VTI_{MR} = 0.33 \text{ cm}^2 \times 140 \text{ cm} \quad (12.14)$$
$$= 46 \text{ cm}^3 \text{ or } 46 \text{ mL}$$

These calculations are consistent with moderate mitral regurgitation.

Answer 5: C

Vena contracta measurements are best made from views that are perpendicular to the jet to optimize spatial resolution. The vena contracta is the narrowest diameter of the flow stream, identified as the narrow neck between the proximal flow convergence region (E) and distal flow expansion (A). Vena contracta is a useful and reproducible measure of regurgitant severity that is less dependent on technical factors, flow rates, and driving pressures compared to other color Doppler flow parameters. The vena contracta area is slightly smaller than the anatomic regurgitant orifice area (ROA) (location D) as the flow stream narrows distal to the orifice. The proximal regurgitation jet width or area (location B) as a ratio to the LV outflow diameter or area is a semi-quantitative measure that can be used to determine regurgitation severity but is larger than the vena contracta, and the jet width or area at this location can be underestimated in eccentric jets or overestimated by central jets. The distal jet expansion (location A) should be avoided when determining severity, as the length and area of the distal jet are highly dependent on instrument settings and physiologic variability that may not be indicative of severity of the regurgitation volume. The proximal flow convergence (location E) needs to be visualized to determine the vena contracta. Occasionally, the PISA method may be used to quantitate the severity of aortic regurgitation; however, it is often not feasible to obtain a hemispheric proximal isovelocity surface area (PISA) for accurate diameter measurement.

Answer 6

1: **E.** The figure demonstrates an ascending aortic aneurysm of 5.5 cm with sinotubular junction effacement. There is a lack of central aortic valve leaflet coaptation with a moderate regurgitation jet. The regurgitation is not from pathology of the leaflets but is due to annular dilation with inadequate coaptation of the stretched leaflets. Aortic root enlargement may result from connected tissue diseases (Marfan syndrome), hypertension, familial aortic aneurysms, aortitis, or cystic medical necrosis. The aortic valve may not need replacement in

some situations if aortic root surgery successfully restores valve coaptation.

2: **D.** The figure demonstrates a thickened, shortened, and immobile tricuspid valve leaflet that is consistent with carcinoid heart disease. There is severe tricuspid regurgitation present due restriction of the valve leaflets during systole. Carcinoid heart disease occurs with metastatic carcinoid tumor to the liver that secretes excess neurohormones, such as serotonin, leading to right-sided valvulopathy.

3: **A.** The figure demonstrates a congenitally abnormal aortic valve that is quadricuspid with four leaflets. Congenitally abnormal valves (unicuspid, bicuspid, and quadricuspid) lead to inadequate valvular function and shapes. While unicuspid and bicuspid valves frequently can lead to both regurgitation and stenosis, quadricuspid valves usually are associated with central regurgitation lesions.

4: **B.** The figure demonstrates a tented mitral valve with significant regurgitant jet. The inferolateral wall is akinetic without thickening in systole due to ischemic heart disease. The mitral coaptation is apically displaced with restricted closure from tethering of the valve.

5: **C.** The figure shows a surgeon's view of a 3D mitral valve with prolapse of the posterior leaflet and ruptured chords. Myxomatous disease leads to excessive motion and sagging of the leaflets into the left atrium. The aortic valve is widely open at the top of the figure during systole. The posterior P1 and P2 segments demonstrate severe prolapse into the left atrium. In addition, three small ruptured chords are seen protruding into the LA from the free edge of the central (P2) leaflet scallop. 3D echocardiography can provide localization of involved segments to assist in surgical planning and determining feasibility of surgical valvular repair.

Answer 7: B

Patients with symptomatic, severe valvular regurgitation should be referred for surgical intervention. In asymptomatic patients, evidence of the progressive effect of the regurgitant volume load with either LV dilation or a decline in systolic function is the primary criteria to prompt earlier surgical intervention. Because a small subset of patients do not develop cardiopulmonary symptoms despite LV dilation or a decline in function, periodic imaging in asymptomatic patients is indicated once regurgitation is diagnosed. Current guidelines recommend valve surgery in asymptomatic patients with severe aortic regurgitation and an end-systolic dimension of 50 mm or more, or an ejection fraction less than 50%. Surgery is recommended in this case based on the decreased ejection fraction.

A tricuspid regurgitation jet velocity of 3.3 m/s suggests that the RV systolic pressure is at least 44 mm Hg over RA pressure, supporting at least moderate pulmonary hypertension. However, pulmonary hypertension is not a primary indication for aortic valve replacement. The pressure half-time $(T^{1/2})$ is the time interval between the peak transvalvular pressure gradient and half the initial gradient. For the aortic regurgitant jet, a pressure half-time of less than 200 ms indicates rapid equalization of pressures between the aorta and LV, consistent with acute significant regurgitation. However, with chronic disease, the pressure half-time may be normal despite severe regurgitation. The vena contracta of 0.8 cm confirms that this patient has severe aortic regurgitation, which by itself is not an indication for valve surgery in the absence of symptoms. A subset of bicuspid aortic valve patients have associated dilation of the aorta, and current guidelines recommend root replacement when aortic diameter exceeds 5.5 cm. If the patient is already undergoing valve replacement for stenosis or regurgitation, replacement of the aorta should be considered at a diameter of 4.5 cm.

Answer 8: B

This color Doppler image shows an eccentric jet of pulmonic valve regurgitation as confirmed by the pulsed Doppler tracing showing the characteristic low velocity diastolic flow signal. The systolic flow signal represents normal antegrade aortic flow at a nonparallel intercept angle. Aortic regurgitation would also be diastolic but would be higher in velocity, reflecting the aortic to LV diastolic pressure difference, and the color jet would go across the valve into the LV. A ruptured sinus of Valsalva aneurysm would show high-velocity systolic (aortic to RV outflow tract pressure difference) and diastolic flow (because aortic diastolic pressure is higher than RV diastolic pressure). A ventricular septal defect would be located on the ventricular size of the aortic valve and would show high-velocity systolic flow with the shape of the flow curve similar to mitral regurgitation. Coronary artery flow occurs predominantly in diastole and is low velocity; however, an antegrade signal in systole typically also is present.

Answer 9: C

This is a CW Doppler signal showing flow away from the transducer in systole with a shape that is consistent with antegrade flow in a great vessel (aorta or pulmonary artery) or a regurgitant flow across an atrioventricular (mitral or tricuspid valve). However, the maximum velocity is less than 2 m/s, which excludes mitral regurgitation, and the shorter duration of the systolic signal suggests that tricuspid regurgitation is unlikely. The antegrade ejection velocity might be transaortic flow or transpulmonic flow. However, the diastolic signal has an initial diastolic velocity of 4 m/s, indicating a 64 mm Hg gradient between the great vessel and ventricle. Although this might be pulmonic regurgitation if severe pulmonary hypertension

were present, the timing is more consistent with aortic regurgitation. These data were recorded in a patient with acute severe aortic regurgitation. The end-diastolic velocity of the regurgitation jet, about 2 m/s, indicates the end-diastolic gradient between the aorta and LV is only 16 mm Hg, consistent with a low aortic and high LV diastolic pressure in this acutely ill patient. In addition, the diastolic regurgitant signal is as dense as antegrade systolic flow consistent with severe aortic regurgitation. The steep diastolic deceleration slope indicates rapid equalization of pressure between the aorta and LV during diastole, consistent with acute, rather than chronic, regurgitation.

Answer 10

Regurgitant volume (RVol)	25 mL
Regurgitant fraction (RF)	19%
Regurgitant orifice area (ROA)	0.09 cm^2

In this patient with aortic regurgitation, the stroke volume (SV) across the aortic valve is the sum of anterograde flow and regurgitant flow or total SV. Assuming a competent mitral valve, the anterograde flow across the mitral valve (SV_{MV}) equals forward SV. To calculate the volume flow rate (SV) at each valve, the area and velocity time integral at each site are needed. SVs are calculated by multiplying CSA (assumed to be circular using the measured diameter) and velocity time integral at that site. Thus:

$$SV_{MV} = CSA_{MV} \times VTI_{MV\ INFLOW} \\ = 3.14(3.0/2)^2 \times 15\ cm = 106\ cm^3 \quad (12.15)$$

$$SV_{LVOT} = CSA_{LVOT} \times VTI_{LVOT} \\ = \pi(D/2)^2 \times VTI_{LVOT} \\ = 3.14(2.4/2)^2 \times 29\ cm = 131\ cm^3 \quad (12.16)$$

Regurgitant volume (RV_{AR}) is the difference between SV_{LVOT} and SV_{MV}:

$$RVol_{AR} = SV_{LVOT} - SV_{MV} \\ = 131\ cm^3 - 106\ cm^3 \\ = 25\ cm^3\ or\ 25\ mL \quad (12.17)$$

The regurgitant fraction is the proportion of regurgitant volume compared with the total transaortic flow:

$$RF = RV_{AR}/SV_{LVOT} = 25\ mL/131\ mL = 19\% \quad (12.18)$$

The ROA is then calculated by dividing regurgitant SV by the VTI_{AR}.

An ROA less than 0.1 cm^2, a regurgitant volume of 25 mL, and a regurgitant fraction of 19% are all consistent with mild aortic regurgitation. These data are congruent with the visual impression from the CW Doppler signal with a faint diastolic regurgitant signal compared with antegrade flow.

Answer 11

1: D. This is a pulsed Doppler sample taken from the hepatic vein in a patient with severe tricuspid regurgitation. The image is acquired from the subcostal view with flow from the hepatic vein to the inferior vena cava directed antegrade, away from the transducer. The venous flow pattern is evident with a brief flow curve toward the transducer after atrial contraction and atrial filling during diastole. Peak flow velocities in the hepatic vein are low, and the scale is set with a maximum velocity of 0.6 m/s. With severe tricuspid regurgitation, there is systolic flow reversal in the hepatic vein, shown as flow in systole directed toward the transducer following the QRS complex instead of the normal pattern of RA filling in systole, as well as diastole. Pulmonary vein flow also shows a venous flow pattern, but diastolic filling would be directed toward the transducer from the transthoracic approach.

2: A. This is a pulsed Doppler recording taken from the descending thoracic aorta in a patient with severe aortic regurgitation. The antegrade flow in systole at 1.3 m/s with an ejection type curve that identifies this as a great artery. This is unlikely to be the pulmonary artery, because the velocity peaks in early systole and is shorter in duration and higher in velocity than typical pulmonary artery flow. The holodiastolic (extends continuously from the beginning to end of diastole) flow reversal seen as flow directed toward the transducer during diastole is consistent with moderate to severe aortic regurgitation.

3: B. This is a pulsed Doppler sample of the pulmonary vein flow in a patient with severe mitral regurgitation due to mitral valve prolapse. Diastolic LV filling with flow directed toward the transducer is seen, identifying this as pulmonary venous inflow. In systole, early systolic flow toward the transducer is seen, consistent with normal LV filling. However, in late systole, flow is reversed (directed away from the transducer), suggesting late systolic mitral regurgitation.

Answer 12: A

This is an M-mode tracing from the parasternal long-axis view. The mitral valve is seen in the midportion of the LV. During diastole, the mitral valve is open and the anterior mitral valve leaflet shows a rapid fluttering motion. This motion is the result of the aortic regurgitant jet impinging on the thin flexible anterior mitral leaflet. Regurgitation is likely only mild because the E-point septal separation is normal and there is no LV dilation. Other findings on the M-mode tracing are concentric LV hypertrophy (thick walls with a small chamber) and marked posterior pericardial thickening. With hypertrophic cardiomyopathy, asymmetric thickening of the septum compared with the posterior wall is seen, and if there is obstruction, systolic anterior motion of the mitral leaflets is present. LV chamber size is normal, not consistent with a dilated cardiomyopathy; in addition, the separation between the mitral E point and the septum is increased with LV dilation and systolic dysfunction. With mitral valve prolapse, the mitral leaflets are thickened, and there is late systolic buckling of the mitral valve leaflet posteriorly on the M-mode tracing. If mitral stenosis were present, leaflet thickening with a reduced diastolic opening and a flat diastolic leaflet slope would be seen.

13 Prosthetic Valves

BASIC PRINCIPLES

- Evaluation of prosthetic valves by echocardiography is based on the same principles as evaluation of native valve disease.
- Fluid dynamics (and Doppler flows) depend on the specific valve type and size (Fig. 13.1).
- Dysfunction of mechanical valves usually is due to valve thrombosis resulting in systemic embolism, incomplete closure (regurgitation), or inadequate opening (stenosis) (Table 13.1).
- Dysfunction of bioprosthetic valves usually is due to leaflet degeneration (regurgitation) or calcification (stenosis).
- All prosthetic valves are at risk of endocarditis, which often primarily affects the annular ring rather than the valve leaflets.

❖ KEY POINTS

- ❏ There are several types of surgically implanted bioprosthetic valves, which can be classified as stented, stentless, or combined valve-root prostheses (including homograft valves).
- ❏ Most surgically implanted bioprosthetic valves have three struts (or "stents") supporting the leaflets at the commissures.
- ❏ Stentless surgical bioprosthetic valve may be indistinguishable from a normal native valve.
- ❏ Transcatheter aortic valve implantation is usually performed via the femoral artery retrograde across the valve.
- ❏ Transcatheter bioprosthetic valves currently include balloon expandable and self-expanding types, both with a trileaflet bioprosthetic valve mounted inside a metal mesh cage or "stent" (Fig. 13.2; see Fig. 13.1).

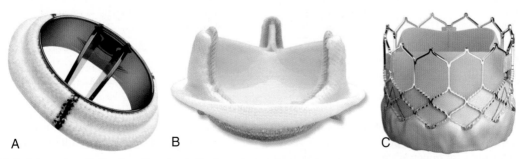

A   B   C

Fig. 13.1 **Basic types of prosthetic valves.** Examples of a bileaflet mechanical valve (A), surgical bioprosthetic valve (B), and transcatheter bioprosthetic aortic valve (C). ([A] From http://www.medtronic.com/us-en/healthcare-professionals/products/cardiovascular/heart-valves-surgical/open-pivot-mechanical-heart-valve.html. ©Medtronic 2018. [B] From https://www.edwards.com/eu/products/heartvalves/Pages/PERIMOUNTAortic.aspx. [C] From https://www.edwards.com/gb/devices/Heart-Valves/Transcatheter-Sapien-3.)

TABLE 13.1	Prosthetic Valves: Clinical Echocardiographic Correlates				
	Mechanical AVR	Surgical Bioprosthetic AVR	Transcatheter Bioprosthetic AVR	Mechanical MVR	Bioprosthetic MVR
Fluid dynamics	Complex fluid dynamics depending on valve type	Central orifice, laminar flow, blunt flow profile	Central orifice, laminar flow, blunt flow profile	Complex fluid dynamics depending on valve type	Central orifice, laminar flow, blunt flow profile
Echo imaging	Shadowing and reverberations limit valve imaging	Echogenic sewing ring and three struts. Trileaflet porcine or pericardial tissue similar to that of a native aortic valve	Increased echogenicity of aortic sinuses and annulus due to supporting stent. Biologic valve leaflets appear similar to a native aortic valve	Shadowing and reverberations limit valve imaging on TTE. Valve occluder motion well seen on TEE	Stented valve, flow directed toward septum. Trileaflet porcine or pericardial tissue similar to that of a native aortic valve
Normal Doppler findings	Antegrade velocity <3 m/s with triangular-shaped flow curve. Mild eccentric AR due to occluder closure	Antegrade velocity <3 m/s with triangular-shaped flow curve. No to trace central AR	Antegrade velocity <3 m/s with triangular-shaped flow curve. Mild valvular or paravalvular AR	Antegrade velocity <1.9 m/s with short T½. Mild eccentric MR due to occluder closure	Antegrade velocity <1.9 m/s with short T½. No to trace central MR
Advantages/disadvantages	Excellent long-term durability. Requires chronic anticoagulation	Variable durability, longer in older patients. Does not require anticoagulation	Unknown long-term durability. Currently recommended in high-risk patients. Does not require anticoagulation	Excellent long-term durability. Requires chronic anticoagulation	Variable durability, longer in older patients. Does not require anticoagulation (unless needed for AF)
Complications	Valve thrombosis. Pannus. Paravalvular AR. Endocarditis	Leaflet degeneration. Stenosis. Regurgitation. Pannus. Paravalvular AR. Endocarditis	Leaflet degeneration. Stenosis. Regurgitation. Pannus. Paravalvular AR. Endocarditis	Valve thrombosis. Pannus. Paravalvular MR. Endocarditis	Leaflet degeneration. Stenosis. Regurgitation. Pannus. Paravalvular A. Endocarditis
Echo follow-up (in addition to annual clinical evaluation)	Baseline postoperative. Changing signs or symptoms	Baseline postoperative. Changing signs or symptoms. Annual starting 5 years after implantation	Baseline postoperative. Changing signs or symptoms. Annual exams recommended at this time	Baseline postoperative. Changing signs or symptoms	Baseline postoperative. Changing signs or symptoms. Annual starting 5 years after implantation

AF, Atrial fibrillation; *AR,* aortic regurgitation; *MR,* mitral regurgitation.
From Otto CM: *Textbook of clinical echocardiography,* ed 6, Philadelphia, 2018, Elsevier.

- The most common mechanical valve now implanted is a bileaflet design with two semicircular disks that open to form a central slit-like orifice and two larger lateral openings.
- Other types of mechanical valves include single disk valves that "tilt" to open, either on a central strut or with hinges in the annular ring. Ball-cage valves may still be seen in some patients.
- On echocardiography, mechanical valves result in ultrasound reverberations and shadowing that limit direct visualization of valve function.

Step-by-Step Approach

Step 1: Review Clinical and Operative Data

- Information on the operative procedure is reviewed before the echocardiographic examination.
- The valve type and size, obtained from the medical record or the patient's valve ID card, are included on the echocardiographic report.
- Blood pressure and heart rate at the time of the echocardiogram are recorded.

❖ **KEY POINTS**

- ❏ Information in the operative report helps guide the echocardiographic image acquisition and improves the final interpretation.
- ❏ With aortic valve surgery, key features are valve replacement versus resuspension, concurrent replacement of the aortic root either above the sinotubular junction or including the sinuses of Valsalva, and surgical coronary reimplantation (with replacement of the aortic sinuses).
- ❏ With mitral valve surgery, key features are valve repair or replacement, preservation of the mitral leaflets and chords with valve replacement, amputation of the left atrial (LA) appendage, and whether a concurrent atrial ablation (e.g., maze) procedure was done.
- ❏ The valve type and size determine the expected hemodynamics and are important for distinguishing normal prosthetic Doppler data from prosthetic valve stenosis or regurgitation.
- ❏ On early postoperative studies, unexpected findings are discussed directly with the surgeon to correlate with observations during the surgical procedure.

Step 2: Obtain Images of the Prosthetic Valve

- Prosthetic aortic valves are imaged in parasternal long- and short-axis views.
- Prosthetic mitral valves are imaged in parasternal long- and short-axis views and in apical 4-chamber and long-axis views (Fig. 13.3).

- Transesophageal echocardiography (TEE) imaging is needed to evaluate the left atrium (LA) side of mechanical mitral prosthetic valves, due to shadowing from the transthoracic approach, when valve dysfunction is suspected (Fig. 13.4).
- TEE also often provides better images of the posterior aspect of aortic valve prostheses.

❖ **KEY POINTS**

- ❏ Transthoracic imaging of mechanical valves is limited by reverberations and shadowing. Even so, the leaflets and annular region may be adequately evaluated by this approach for most baseline or follow-up studies in clinically stable patients.
- ❏ Three-dimensional (3D) TEE imaging of prosthetic valves provide better spatial resolution, albeit with lower temporal resolution (see Fig 13.4).
- ❏ Bioprosthetic valves have a trileaflet structure similar to a native aortic valve. Mitral bioprosthetic valves are stented to provide support for the leaflets, with the leaflets well seen in both parasternal and apical views.
- ❏ With aortic bioprosthetic valves, support is provided either by stents, by attachment directly to the aortic wall (stentless valves), or by implanting an intact valve and root (sometimes called a "mini-root" approach). The aortic bioprosthetic prosthesis is well seen in long- and short-axis views.
- ❏ When prosthetic valve dysfunction is suspected on clinical grounds or based on transthoracic echocardiography (TTE) findings, both TTE and TEE are recommended.

Step 3: Record Prosthetic Valve Doppler Data

- Antegrade velocities across the prosthetic valve are recorded with pulsed and continuous-wave (CW) Doppler.
- Prosthetic valve regurgitation is evaluated using CW and color Doppler.

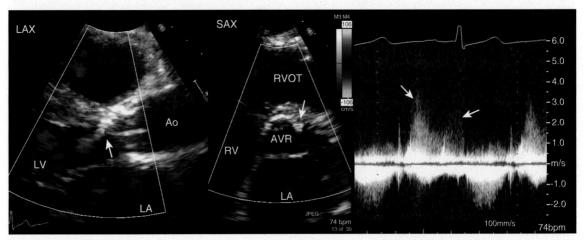

Fig. 13.2 Transcatheter aortic valve. In the parasternal long-axis *(left)* and short-axis *(center)* views, the trileaflet bioprosthetic valve is similar in appearance to a native aortic valve. Increased paravalvular echogenicity is consistent with the mesh-cage around the valve. Paravalvular regurgitation is present with an eccentric jet *(arrow)* seen *(right)*. CW Doppler shows a faint diastolic signal *(arrows)*. *Ao,* Aorta; *AVR,* aortic valve replacement; *RVOT,* right ventricular outflow tract.

❖ **KEY POINTS**

▫ Both bioprosthetic and mechanical valves are inherently stenotic compared with normal native valves.

▫ The normal antegrade velocity and pressure gradient depends on the specific valve type, valve size, heart rate, and cardiac output.

▫ Ideally, Doppler data are compared with the patient's own baseline postoperative examination, done when the patient had fully recovered from surgery and was clinically stable.

▫ If a baseline examination is not available, recorded data are compared with published data for that valve type and size.

▫ A small amount of regurgitation is normal with most prosthetic valves.

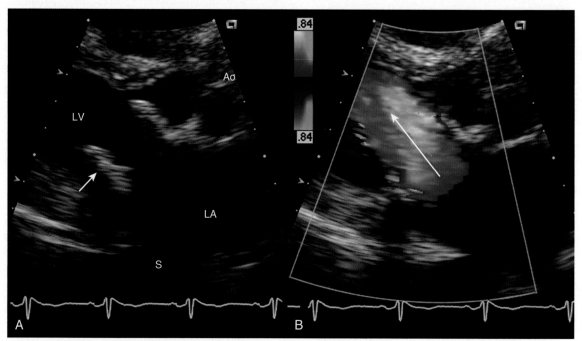

Fig. 13.3 **Stented bioprosthetic mitral valve.** (A) Parasternal long-axis view of a stented bioprosthetic mitral valve prosthesis with the typical appearance of the struts *(arrow)* protruding into the LV. Acoustic shadowing *(S)* from the valve struts results in an anechoic region in the far field. (B) Color Doppler shows the inflow stream directed toward the ventricular septum. *Ao,* Aorta.

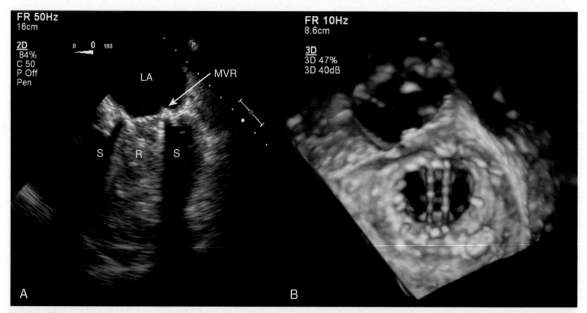

Fig. 13.4 **TEE of mechanical mitral prosthetic valve.** (A) Transesophageal 4-chamber view of a bileaflet mechanical mitral valve replacement *(MVR),* showing that with the transducer on the LA side of the valve, acoustic shadows *(S)* and reverberations *(R)* obscure the LV but not the LA side of the valve. (B) Real-time zoom 3D imaging of the valve shows the open leaflets in diastole but at a frame rate of only 10 Hz, compared to 50 Hz for 2D imaging. *([B] From Otto, CM: Textbook of clinical echocardiography, ed 5, Philadelphia, 2013, Elsevier.)*

Step 3A: Evaluate for Prosthetic Valve Stenosis (Table 13.2)

- Maximum and mean gradients are calculated with the Bernoulli equation from transvalvular velocities (Fig. 13.5).

- Continuity equation valve area can be calculated for aortic valve prostheses (Fig. 13.6).
- The mitral pressure half-time is measured for prosthetic valves in the mitral position (Fig. 13.7).

TABLE 13.2 Prosthetic Stenosis and Regurgitation: Findings Suggestive of Significant Valve Dysfunction with Stented Bioprosthetic and Mechanical Valves

	Severe Stenosis	Severe Regurgitation
AVR	V_{max} >4 m/s Mean ΔP >35 mm Hg Velocity ratio <0.25 Rounded, late peaking velocity curve shape EOA <0.8 cm^2	LV dilation AR jet width ≥65% of LVOT diameter CW Doppler signal dense with T½ <200 ms Holodiastolic flow reversal in DA RV >60 mL RF >50%
MVR	V_{max} >2.5 m/s Mean ΔP >10 mm Hg T½ >200 ms VTI$_{mitral}$/VTI$_{LVOT}$ >2.5 EOA <1.0 cm^2	LV dilation Large central MR jet or variable size wall-impinging jet Large PISA with vena contracta ≥0.6 cm CW Doppler signal dense with triangular shape Pulmonary vein systolic flow reversal Pulmonary hypertension (esp. if new) RV ≥60 mL, RF ≥50%, EROA ≥0.50 cm^2
PVR	V_{max} >3 m/s (or >2 m/s with a homograft) with a progressive increase in velocity on serial studies	RV dilation Jet width >50% of pulmonic annulus CW Doppler signal dense, steep deceleration, flow ends in mid- to late diastole Diastolic flow reversal in pulmonary artery RF >50%
TVR	V_{max} >1.7 m/s Mean ΔP ≥6 mm Hg T½ ≥230 ms	TR jet area >10 cm^2 Vena contracta width >0.7 cm CW Doppler signal dense with triangular shape Holosystolic flow reversal in hepatic veins Severe RA dilation

AR, Aortic regurgitation; *AVR,* aortic valve replacement; *DA,* descending aorta; *EOA,* effective orifice area; *EROA,* effective regurgitant orifice area; *LVOT,* left ventricular outflow tract; *Mean ΔP,* mean transvalvular pressure gradient; *MR,* mitral regurgitation; *MVR,* mitral valve replacement; *PISA,* proximal isovelocity surface area; *PVR,* pulmonary vascular resistance; *RF,* regurgitant fraction; *RV,* regurgitant volume; *TR,* tricuspid regurgitation; *TVR,* tricuspid valve replacement; V_{max}, maximum antegrade transvalvular velocity; *VTI,* velocity-time integral.

From Otto CM: *Textbook of clinical echocardiography,* ed 6, Philadelphia, 2018, Elsevier.

Summarized and modified from: Zoghbi WA, Chambers JB, Dumesnil JG, et al: Recommendations for evaluation of prosthetic valves with echocardiography and doppler ultrasound, *J Am Soc Echocardiogr* 22(9):975-1014, 2009.

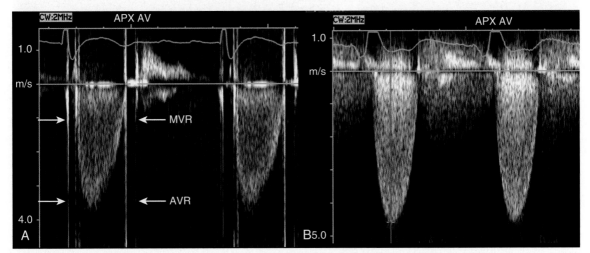

Fig. 13.5 **CW Doppler aortic valve flows.** (A) CW Doppler of antegrade flow across a normally functioning bileaflet mechanical aortic valve soon after aortic and mitral valve replacement shows an early peaking systolic antegrade velocity of 3.4 m/s. Opening and closing clicks from both valves are seen. (B) CW Doppler of a stenotic bioprosthetic valve shows a maximum velocity of 4.5 m/s. In addition, the maximum velocity occurs in mid-systole with a rounded velocity curve, consistent with an elevated mean gradient and significant valve obstruction. *AVR,* Aortic valve replacement; *MVR,* mitral valve replacement.

- LV outflow tract diameter is measured from the two-dimensional (2D) images for calculation of valve area. The valve size may differ from the subaortic anatomy and so cannot be substituted for this diameter measurement.

- When measurement of outflow tract diameter is difficult, the ratio of the velocity proximal to the valve and in the orifice is used as a measure of stenosis severity.

- With bileaflet mechanical valves, the small central orifice often results in high velocities due to local acceleration, which should not be mistaken for prosthetic valve stenosis (see Fig. 13.5A)

- The mitral pressure half-time is used to calculate valve area, as for native mitral stenosis.

$$SV_{LVOT} = SV_{AVR}$$
$$CSA_{LVOT} \times VTI_{LVOT} = EOA \times VTI_{AVR}$$
$$EOA = (CSA_{LVOT} \times VTI_{LVOT})/VTI_{AVR}$$

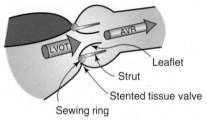

Fig. 13.6 Schematic drawing of the continuity equation with a stented bioprosthetic aortic valve replacement (AVR). Stroke volume *(SV)* proximal to the valve in the left ventricular outflow tract *(LVOT)* equals SV through the aortic valve replacement. SV at each site is equal to the cross-sectional area *(CSA)* of flow times the velocity-time integral *(VTI)* of flow at that site. LVOT flow is measured with pulsed Doppler from an apical approach. CSA$_{LVOT}$ is calculated as a circle from a mid-systolic LVOT diameter measurement, and the VTI of flow through the valve prosthesis is measured with CW Doppler, usually from the apical approach. This equation then is solved for the aortic prosthetic effective orifice area *(EOA)*.

Often the pressure half-time itself is reported.

- "Patient-prosthesis mismatch" describes a normally functioning prosthetic valve that has a valve area inadequate for the patient's body size (Fig. 13.8).

Step 3B: Evaluate for Prosthetic Valve Regurgitation

- Prosthetic valve regurgitation is evaluated using CW and color Doppler (Fig. 13.9).

- Evaluation of prosthetic mitral regurgitation requires TEE; transthoracic imaging is nondiagnostic due to shadowing and reverberation by the valve prostheses.

- A small amount of prosthetic regurgitation is normal; moderate to severe prosthetic regurgitation or any degree of paraprosthetic regurgitation is pathologic.

- Prosthetic regurgitation often is first detected with CW Doppler due to the high signal-to-noise ratio, excellent bioprosthetic penetration, and wide beam geometry of CW Doppler.

- Normal prosthetic regurgitation has a weak CW Doppler signal and typically is brief in duration.

- A dense regurgitant CW Doppler signal is an indication for further evaluation (Fig. 13.10).

- Normal prosthetic regurgitation on color Doppler is spatially localized adjacent to the valve, has a small vena contracta and jet area, is through the prosthesis (not paravalvular), and is brief in duration.

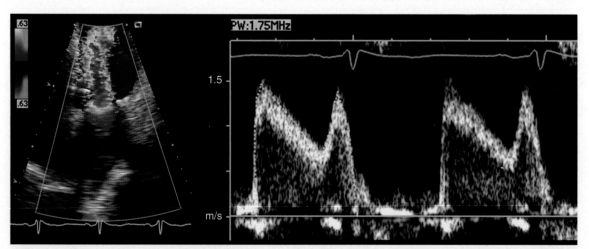

Fig. 13.7 Transmitral pulsed Doppler flow. In the apical 4-chamber view *(left)*, mitral inflow across a stented bioprosthetic valve is directed toward the ventricular septum, with a reversed direction of the normal LV diastolic flow vortex. Pulsed or CW Doppler *(right)* shows a normal inflow pattern with an E and A velocity (in sinus rhythm). The diastolic mean gradient and the pressure half-time are only slightly higher than expected for a normal native mitral valve.

- The exact pattern of normal prosthetic regurgitation depends on the valve type—for example, central with bioprosthetic valves, two eccentric jets with bileaflet mechanical valves.
- Pathologic prosthetic valve regurgitation on color Doppler often is paravalvular, has a larger vena contracta and jet area, and lasts longer during the cardiac cycle.
- Significant prosthetic regurgitation, especially of the mitral valve, may not be detectable on transthoracic imaging.

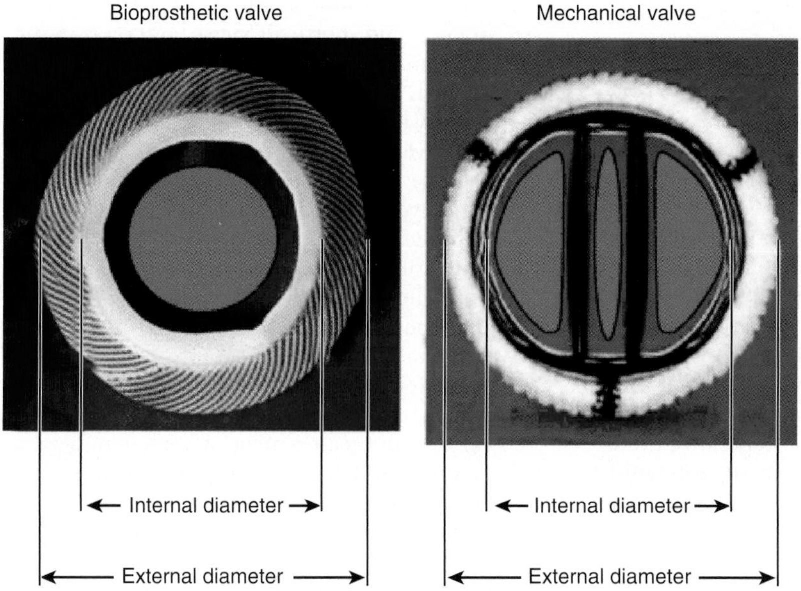

Bioprosthetic valve   **Mechanical valve**

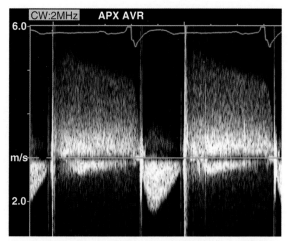

← Internal diameter →   ← Internal diameter →

← External diameter →   ← External diameter →

Fig. 13.8 **Prosthetic valve effective orifice area.** View of a bioprosthesis and a bileaflet mechanical valve with the leaflets in a fully open position. The area highlighted in pink is the effective orifice area. Patient–prosthesis mismatch is present when the effective orifice area is smaller than needed to maintain a normal cardiac output at rest and with exercise without an excessive increase in transvalvular pressure gradient. *(From Pibarot P, Dumesnil JG: Prosthesis-patient mismatch: definition, clinical impact, and prevention,* Heart *92:1022-1029, 2006.)*

Fig. 13.9 **Prosthetic aortic valve regurgitation.** CW Doppler recorded from an apical approach shows prominent valve clicks and aortic regurgitation. The diastolic aortic regurgitant signal is much less dense than the antegrade systolic signal, consistent with mild regurgitation.

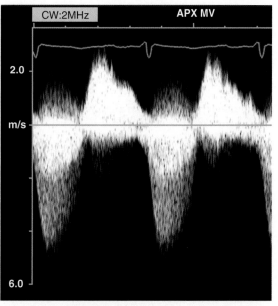

Fig. 13.10 **Transthoracic apical CW Doppler after mitral valve repair.** The antegrade flow velocity is increased to over 2 m/s, and a systolic signal is present. The systolic signal is consistent with mitral regurgitation (not LV outflow) based on the timing of flow. The density of the signal suggests that more than trivial regurgitation is present. TEE is needed for further evaluation to avoid shadowing by the annular ring.

Step 4: Evaluate Geometry and Function

- After valve surgery, LV dilation and hypertrophy typically regress, but many patients have persistent abnormalities.
- Systolic ventricular dysfunction often improves after valve surgery, but diastolic dysfunction may be evident for many years.
- LV geometry and systolic and diastolic function are evaluated in patients with prior heart valve surgery as detailed in Chapters 6 and 7.

❖ KEY POINTS

- ❑ After aortic valve replacement for aortic stenosis, left ventricular (LV) hypertrophy regresses and systolic function improves, but diastolic dysfunction may be chronic.
- ❑ After valve replacement for aortic or mitral regurgitation, LV dilation and systolic dysfunction improve in most patients, but a subset has irreversible LV dilation and systolic dysfunction.
- ❑ In patients with isolated mitral stenosis, LV size and systolic function usually are normal both before and after valve surgery.
- ❑ Comparison of the early postoperative study with the preoperative exam helps distinguish residual ventricular abnormalities from new ventricular dysfunction.

Step 5: Measure Pulmonary Pressures and Evaluate Right Heart Function

- There is an immediate decrease in pulmonary pressures after valve surgery that is directly related to the fall in LA pressure (e.g., the passive component of pulmonary hypertension).
- The late decrease in pulmonary pressures is variable and depends on the extent of irreversible changes in the pulmonary vasculature.
- Pulmonary pressures and right heart function are evaluated in patients with prior heart valve surgery as detailed in Chapters 6 and 7.

❖ KEY POINTS

- ❑ Measurement of pulmonary pressures on the early postoperative study serves as the baseline for subsequent studies.
- ❑ After mitral valve surgery, recurrent pulmonary hypertension might be due to prosthetic regurgitation, which otherwise might be missed on TTE.
- ❑ Right ventricular (RV) systolic function usually improves when pulmonary pressures decline after valve surgery.

▌ AORTIC VALVES

Bioprosthetic Aortic Valves

- Bioprosthetic aortic valves have three thin leaflets, similar to a native aortic valve.

- With surgical stented bioprosthetic valves, the three stents are seen in both long- and short-axis views.
- The flow profile and hemodynamics are similar to a native valve with only a small degree of central regurgitation.

❖ KEY POINTS

- ❑ Aortic bioprosthetic valves are well visualized in long- and short-axis views both on transthoracic imaging from a parasternal window and on TEE from a high esophageal window.
- ❑ Both TTE and TEE may be needed for complete evaluation when endocarditis is suspected, because each approach visualizes the part of the valve that is obscured by the ring shadow from the other approach.
- ❑ Antegrade flow across the valve is recorded from the apical window using CW Doppler. Alignment with flow is usually not optimal on a TEE study.
- ❑ Valve regurgitation is evaluated by color Doppler in the short- and long-axis views of the valve, with measurement of vena contracta, as described in Chapter 12 for native valves, when possible (Fig. 13.11).
- ❑ Valve regurgitation also is evaluated with CW Doppler from the apical view, with the velocity scale, gain, and filters adjusted to demonstrate the regurgitant flow signal (Fig. 13.12).

Transcatheter Aortic Valve Implantation

- TTE imaging is used to detect early complications after valve implantation.
- The echocardiographic appearance of an aortic bioprosthesis implanted by the transcatheter approach is similar to a stentless surgical bioprosthetic valve.
- Transcatheter aortic valves also may be implanted inside a dysfunctional surgical bioprosthetic valve; a "valve-in-valve" procedure.

❖ KEY POINTS

- ❑ The transaortic velocity and pressure gradient across a normal functioning transcatheter aortic valve is only slightly higher than normal due to excellent hemodynamics of this valve type; typically velocity is about 2 m/s or less.
- ❑ Paravalvular regurgitation is common after transcatheter aortic valve implantation and is a predictor of adverse outcomes (see Fig. 13.2).
- ❑ Paravalvular regurgitation after transcatheter valve implantation is described in terms of location and the extent of leak around the circumference of the valve in short-axis views.
- ❑ CW Doppler is helpful for detection of paravalvular regurgitation.

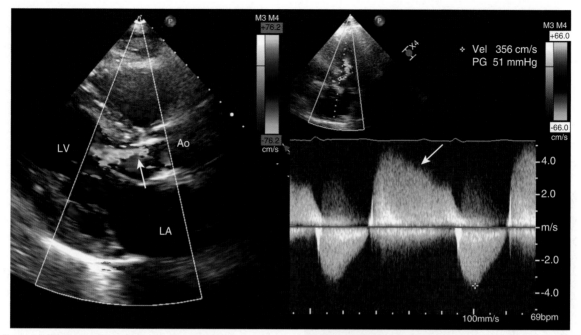

Fig. 13.11 **TTE severe bioprosthetic aortic regurgitation.** In the parasternal long-axis view *(left)*, color Doppler shows a jet of aortic regurgitation *(arrow)* that appears to originate within the sewing ring of the bioprosthetic aortic valve. Although the jet does not appear wide, the CW Doppler signal *(right)* shows a diastolic regurgitant signal *(arrow)* equal in density to antegrade flow with a steep deceleration slope, suggesting severe regurgitation. *Ao,* Aorta.

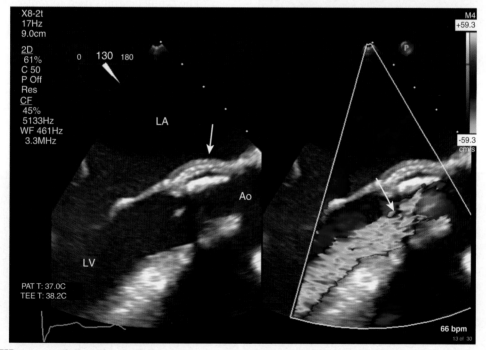

Fig. 13.12 **TEE severe prosthetic aortic regurgitation.** In the same patient as Fig. 13.11, the TEE long-axis view shows a very wide jet of aortic regurgitation originating within the prosthetic valve sewing ring, consistent with leaflet perforation due to endocarditis. Blood cultures obtained after the TTE study were positive. After appropriate antibiotic treatment, the patient underwent a second aortic valve replacement surgery. *Ao,* Aorta.

Composite Valve and Aortic Graft

- In patients with enlarged aortic sinuses and aortic valve disease, a composite valve and aortic graft is used, and the coronary arteries are re-implanted into the aortic graft (e.g., a Bentall procedure) (Fig. 13.13).

- Either a bioprosthetic or mechanical aortic valve may be used in the composite valved conduit.
- The aortic graft most often is prosthetic material, but an intact homograft valve and root may be used in some patients.

❖ **KEY POINTS**

❏ The structure and dimensions of the aorta at each level (annulus, sinuses, sinotubular junction, and mid-ascending aorta) are measured in patients who have undergone aortic valve surgery.

❏ The coronary reimplantation sites are best seen on TEE imaging.

❏ Postoperative echocardiographic findings may include paraaortic edema, hematoma, or surgical material. Review of the images with the surgical team is helpful in distinguishing expected postoperative findings from infection or bleeding (Fig. 13.14).

Valve Resuspension and Reimplantation

■ In patients undergoing graft replacement of the ascending aorta, when aortic valve and sinus anatomy are normal, the aortic valve may be "resuspended" by suturing the commissures to the proximal end of the aortic graft.

■ In patients with dilated sinuses but a normally functioning aortic valve, the native aortic valve may be sutured inside a tube graft replacement of the aortic root (called valve reimplantation or the David procedure).

❖ **KEY POINTS**

❏ Review of the operative report may be needed to determine if the aortic valve was resuspended versus reimplanted at the time of surgery.

❏ The aortic sinus anatomy and size should be evaluated carefully in patients with aortic valve resuspension because the sinuses are native tissue after this procedure.

❏ The synthetic grafts used to replace the aortic sinuses (with reimplantation of the valve) now are designed with a shape similar to the normal native sinuses.

Mechanical Aortic Valves

■ Both stenosis and regurgitation of a mechanical valve in the aortic position can be evaluated on transthoracic imaging.

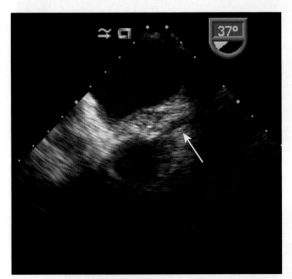

Fig. 13.13 Coronary reimplantation. In a patient with replacement of the ascending aorta and sinuses with resuspension of the native aortic valve within the conduit, TEE imaging in a short-axis view of the aorta just superior to the aortic valve showing the reimplanted left main coronary *(arrow)*.

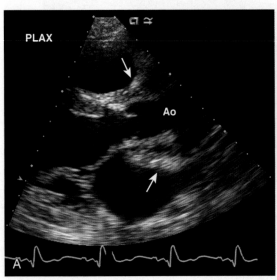
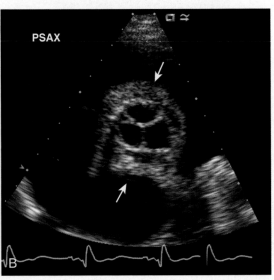

Fig. 13.14 Aortic valve resuspension. Replacement of the ascending aorta and resuspension of the aortic valve complicated by periaortic postoperative hematoma and bioprosthetic edema *(arrows)*, seen in (A) parasternal long-axis and (B) short-axis views. *Ao,* Aorta; *PLAX,* parasternal long-axis; *PSAX,* parasternal short-axis.

- TEE is needed when the indication for echocardiography is bacteremia, fever, or embolic events.
- A mechanical valve may be used in a composite aortic root and valve replacement, with coronary reimplantation (the Bentall or modified Bentall procedure).

❖ KEY POINTS

- ❏ An aortic mechanical prosthesis is best imaged in long- and short-axis views from the parasternal transthoracic or high esophageal windows by TEE.
- ❏ Infection typically involves the paravalvular region, so imaging includes evaluation of the aortic wall thickness, identification of the coronary ostium, and visualization of the paravalvular region (Fig. 13.15).
- ❏ Antegrade velocity is recorded using CW Doppler from the apical window. Prominent valve opening and closing clicks often are seen.
- ❏ A high antegrade velocity (and small calculated valve area) for a bileaflet valve in the aortic position may be due either to normal valve function (with a high velocity in the central slit-like orifice), patient prosthesis mismatch, or valve stenosis. These conditions are differentiated based on clinical information, other echocardiographic findings, and, in some cases, other diagnostic evaluations (such as computed tomographic imaging or fluoroscopy of valve motion).
- ❏ Prosthetic aortic valve regurgitation is evaluated with color Doppler in short- and long-axis views of the valve (TTE or TEE) with identification of jet origin (valvular or paravalvular) and vena contracta width.
- ❏ Normal regurgitation of a bileaflet mechanical valve typically consists of two or more eccentric small jets that originate at the closure points of the valve occluders with the sewing ring.
- ❏ CW Doppler is used to evaluate prosthetic aortic regurgitation based on the density and time course of the diastolic regurgitant signal.
- ❏ Diastolic flow reversal in the descending aorta, as with native valve regurgitation, is also useful for evaluation of prosthetic aortic regurgitation.

MITRAL VALVES

Mitral Valve Repair

- The most common mitral valve repair involves resection of a segment of the posterior leaflet, with a suture line in the midsegment of the posterior leaflet and placement of an annuloplasty ring (Fig. 13.16).
- Other procedures used for mitral valve repair include transfer of a segment of the anterior leaflet to the posterior leaflet, use of artificial chords, suturing of the anterior and posterior leaflets together in their midsegments (Alfieri repair), and a variety of other techniques.
- Percutaneous approaches to mitral valve repair include deployment of a device in the coronary sinus to mimic an annuloplasty ring and a clip or suture to mimic an Alfieri-type repair.

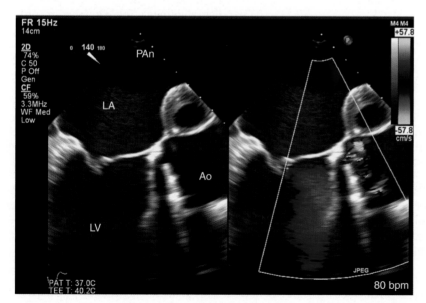

Fig. 13.15 Aortic pseudoaneurysm adjacent to mechanical aortic valve prosthesis. In a TEE long-axis view, a mechanical aortic valve prosthesis is present. There is a spherical echo-free space just superior to the valve plane, partly filled with crescent shaped echodensity. This finding is consistent with a partially thrombosed aortic pseudoaneurysm. *Ao,* Aorta.

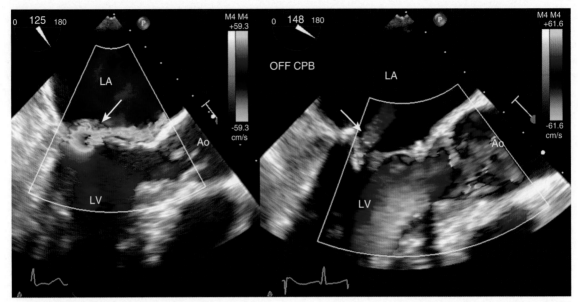

Fig. 13.16 **Mitral valve repair.** View of the mitral valve from the LA side at baseline *(left)* and after valve repair *(right)*. At baseline, severe mitral regurgitation is present with a posterior leaflet prolapse and an eccentric anteriorly directed jet *(arrow)*. After repair, an annuloplasty ring is present, and there is only a small central jet of regurgitation *(arrow)*. *Ao,* Aorta.

❖ **KEY POINTS**

❑ Knowledge of details of the repair procedure is helpful for interpreting the echocardiographic findings.

❑ The mitral annuloplasty ring causes shadows and reverberations that may obscure mitral regurgitation from the transthoracic approach; TEE is indicated when regurgitation is suspected.

❑ Mitral valve repair may be associated with a mild degree of functional stenosis, which is evaluated based on mean pressure gradient and pressure half-time valve area, as for a native valve.

❑ With a successful repair, there is no more than trace to mild (1+) residual mitral regurgitation.

❑ Recurrent mitral regurgitation after valve repair is evaluated as for a native valve.

❑ An infrequent complication of mitral valve repair is subaortic obstruction due to systolic anterior motion of the mitral leaflets. This complication is related to the size and rigidity of the annuloplasty ring.

Bioprosthetic Mitral Valves

■ Bioprosthetic mitral valves are oriented with the stents typically directed slightly toward the ventricular septum.

■ Imaging and Doppler evaluation of a bioprosthetic mitral valve are similar to evaluation of a native valve.

■ Shadowing and reverberations from the sewing ring and stents decrease the accuracy of TTE for evaluation of valve dysfunction; TEE is more

accurate when a prosthetic mitral valve is present (Fig. 13.17).

❖ **KEY POINTS**

❑ With a prosthetic mitral valve, LV inflow is directed toward the ventricular septum, the opposite of the normal diastolic vortex in the LV.

❑ Recording of antegrade flows and calculation of pressure gradient and valve area are no different than for a native mitral valve.

❑ Although the apical window usually provides a parallel alignment for Doppler recordings, in some cases the mitral inflow can be recorded from a parasternal window, depending on the orientation of the valve inflow stream.

❑ Prosthetic regurgitation is evaluated with CW and color Doppler, as for a native valve, but TEE is considered when valve dysfunction is suspected, because significant regurgitation may not be detected on TTE due to acoustic shadowing of the LA.

❑ A small amount of central regurgitation is normal for a bioprosthetic valve.

Transcatheter Bioprosthetic Valve Implantation

■ Transcatheter bioprosthetic mitral valves are in development that can be deployed in patients without a prior mitral valve ring or valve.

■ A valve-in-valve transcatheter mitral valve may be implanted in patients with degeneration of a surgical prosthetic valve.

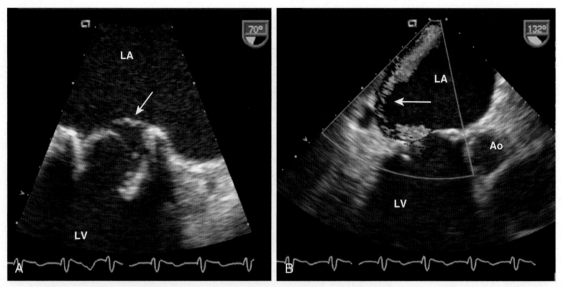

Fig. 13.17 **Flail bioprosthetic mitral valve leaflet.** A stented bioprosthetic mitral valve with (A) a flail leaflet *(arrow)* and (B) an eccentric jet of severe mitral regurgitation *(arrow)*, seen on transesophageal but not transthoracic imaging. *Ao,* Aorta.

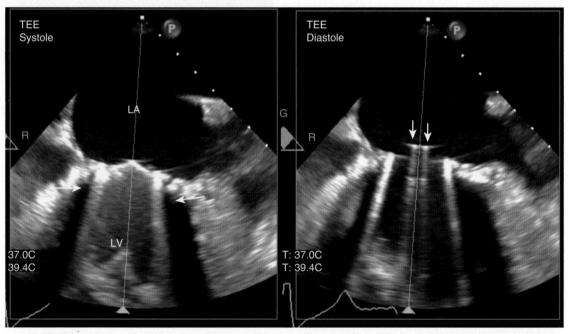

Fig. 13.18 **Bileaflet mechanical mitral valve.** Transesophageal images of a bileaflet mechanical mitral valve in systole and diastole, showing the closed occluders in systole with the two parallel *(arrows)* open occluders in diastole. The prosthetic valve casts dense shadows *(arrows)* distally obscuring the LV with reverberations distal to the closed occluders in systole.

❖ **KEY POINTS**

❑ The appearance of a transcatheter mitral valve is similar to a transcatheter aortic valve.

❑ With a transcatheter mitral valve-in-valve, additional procedures may be needed to ensure the valve does not impede LV outflow in systole.

Mechanical Mitral Valves

■ The valve occluders are best seen from the apical transthoracic or high esophageal window, using zoom mode to focus on the mitral valve (Fig. 13.18).

■ Antegrade flow across the valve is recorded from the apical window, using pulsed or CW Doppler, depending on the maximum transvalvular velocity.

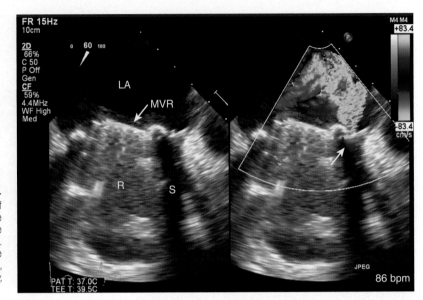

Fig. 13.19 **Paravalvular mitral regurgitation.** In a TEE 2-chamber view, a jet of mitral regurgitation is seen originating at the lateral aspect of the mechanical mitral valve replacement *(MVR)*, outside the sewing ring. Reverberations *(R)* and shadows *(S)* from the prosthetic valve obscure the LV. (From Otto, CM: *Textbook of clinical echocardiography,* ed 6, Philadelphia, 2018, Elsevier.)

- Evaluation for regurgitation requires TEE because the LA is shadowed by the prosthesis itself, both from the parasternal and apical windows.

❖ **KEY POINTS**

- ❑ Adjustments in the rotation of the image plane from the standard views may be needed to show both leaflets, from both the transthoracic and transesophageal approach.
- ❑ CW Doppler is especially important for detection of mechanical mitral valve regurgitation, because the broad CW beam may detect a regurgitant signal that is obscured by shadowing on color Doppler flow imaging.
- ❑ Other clues that suggest mitral prosthetic regurgitation on TTE include a high antegrade velocity across the mitral valve and recurrent (or persistent) pulmonary hypertension.
- ❑ TEE provides superior imaging of the posterior aspects of the prosthetic mitral valve and is more accurate than TTE for diagnosis of prosthetic regurgitation.
- ❑ Clear definition of the leaflets and annular ring allows visualization of the normal regurgitant jets that originate at the closure plane of the occluders with the sewing ring.
- ❑ Paravalvular regurgitation originates outside the sewing ring, often has an identifiable proximal isovelocity surface area on the ventricular side of the valve, and typically has a very eccentric jet direction in the LA (Fig. 13.19).
- ❑ TEE imaging is used to guide catheter-based interventions for closure of paravalvular regurgitation (Fig. 13.20).
- ❑ Pulmonary venous flow patterns in patients with mechanical mitral valves are affected by

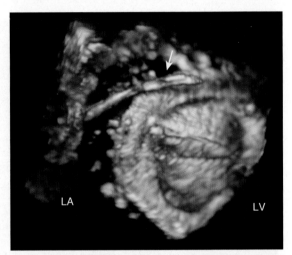

Fig. 13.20 **TEE-guided intervention for paravalvular mitral regurgitation.** 3D imaging during the procedure is used to position the guide wire across the paravalvular leak before placement of a transcatheter closure device in the same patient as in Fig. 13.19. (From Otto, CM: *Textbook of clinical echocardiography,* ed 6, Philadelphia, 2018, Elsevier.)

atrial rhythm, atrial mechanical function, and mitral valve hemodynamics, as well as by the presence of mitral regurgitation.

- ❑ Paravalvular regurgitation may be clinically important regardless of hemodynamic severity because it may be a sign of infection or may be a cause of hemolytic anemia.

TRICUSPID VALVE PROSTHESES AND RINGS

- Tricuspid valve replacement is most often performed with a bioprosthetic valve due an increased risk of valve thrombosis in the right heart (Fig. 13.21).

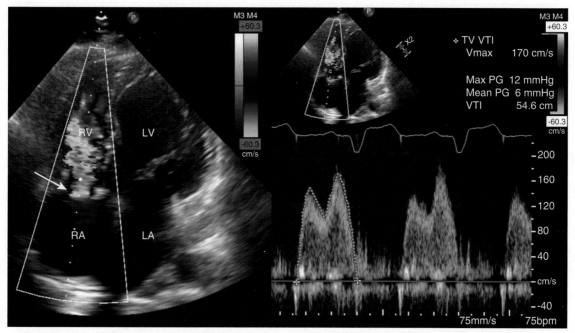

Fig. 13.21 Apical view of a bioprosthetic tricuspid valve. Color Doppler shows a normal wide-flow stream across the bioprosthetic tricuspid valve *(arrow)*. Pulsed Doppler *(right)* shows a normal inflow pattern with an E and A velocity and low diastolic gradient.

- In patients undergoing mitral valve surgery, a tricuspid valve repair and annuloplasty ring often is placed if severe tricuspid regurgitation is present or if there is annular dilation with moderate regurgitation.
- Evaluation of a prosthetic tricuspid valve is similar to evaluation of a mitral valve replacement.

❖ **KEY POINTS**

- ❑ Tricuspid valve prostheses often can be fully evaluated on TTE, because the valve is close to the chest wall and because the RA can be evaluated from the parasternal window, without shadowing by the valve prosthesis.
- ❑ TEE imaging is helpful when transthoracic images are non-diagnostic.
- ❑ Antegrade flows are recorded using pulsed or CW Doppler from the apical window for calculation of pressure gradients and pressure half-time valve area.
- ❑ Prosthetic tricuspid regurgitation is evaluated by standard approaches using CW and color Doppler.

▌ PROSTHETIC PULMONIC VALVES

- Most pulmonic valve replacements are seen in patients with congenital heart disease.
- Pulmonic valve substitutes include homografts, bioprosthetic valves (either in a conduit or isolated), and (increasingly) transcatheter valve implantation.

- Transcatheter pulmonic valves are typically placed in patients with a prior surgically implanted conduit. The transcatheter valve is analogous to a trileaflet bioprosthetic bioprosthesis mounted in an expandable stent.
- Mechanical valves are occasionally used in the pulmonic position.

❖ **KEY POINTS**

- ❑ Visualization of prosthetic pulmonic valves from either transthoracic or TEE approaches often is limited in adults. Alternate diagnostic procedures, such as cardiac magnetic resonance imaging or cardiac catheterization and angiography, often are needed.
- ❑ Antegrade velocity is recorded with pulsed or CW Doppler in the parasternal short-axis or RV outflow view.
- ❑ Pulsed and color Doppler are used to document the level of obstruction. Many of these patients also have subvalvular or supravalvular pulmonic stenosis. Stenosis also can occur at the distal anastomosis site of the conduit or in the branch pulmonary arteries.
- ❑ Severe prosthetic regurgitation is seen as to-and-fro flow on color Doppler; because the pressure difference is low, there may be little evidence of a flow disturbance.
- ❑ On CW Doppler, severe prosthetic pulmonic regurgitation is seen as a diastolic signal with a density equal to antegrade flow and a steep slope, often reaching the baseline before the end of diastole.

THE ECHO EXAM PROSTHETIC VALVES

TTE Evaluation of Prosthetic Valves

Components	Modality	View	Recording	Measurements
Antegrade flow velocity	Pulsed or CW Doppler	Apical	• Antegrade transmitral or transaortic velocity	• Peak velocity (compare to normal values for valve type and size)
Measures of valve stenosis	Pulsed and CW Doppler	Apical	• Careful positioning to obtain highest-velocity signal across prosthetic valve • LV outflow velocity proximal to aortic valve • Annular diameter	• Maximum velocity and mean gradient • Aortic valve prostheses • Continuity equation valve area (central flow) • Ratio of LVOT to aortic velocity • Acceleration time • Shape of CW Doppler curve • Mitral valve • Continuity equation valve area • Pressure half-time
Valve regurgitation	Color imaging and CW Doppler	Parasternal, apical, SSN	• Jet origin, direction, and size on color Doppler • CW Doppler of each valve • Pulmonary vein flow • Descending aorta flow	• Vena contracta width • Paravalvular regurgitation extent around valve • Intensity of CW Doppler signal • Pulmonary vein systolic flow reversal (MR) • Descending aorta flow reversal (AR)
Pulmonary pressures	CW Doppler	RV inflow and apical	• TR jet velocity • IVC size and variation	• Calculate PAP as $4v^2$ of TR jet plus estimated RA pressure.
LV	2D or 3D imaging	Apical	• Apical biplane images of LV or 3D volumetric data set	• 3D or biplane LV volumes and ejection fraction

AR, Aortic regurgitation; *IVC,* inferior vena cava; *LVOT,* left ventricular outflow tract; *MR,* mitral regurgitation; *PAP,* pulmonary artery pressure; *SSN,* suprasternal notch; *TR,* tricuspid regurgitation.

TEE Evaluation of Prosthetic Valves

Components	Modality	View	Recording	Limitations
Valve imaging	2D and 3D echo	High esophageal	• Mitral valve in high esophageal four-chamber view • Aortic valve in high esophageal long- and short-axis views	• Aortic valve prosthesis shadows anterior segments of the aortic valve • With both aortic and mitral prostheses, the aortic shadow obscures the mitral prosthesis
Antegrade flow velocity	Pulsed or CW Doppler	High esophageal or transgastric apical	• Antegrade transmitral or transaortic velocity	• Alignment of Doppler beam with transaortic valve flow is problematic; compare with TTE data
Measures of valve stenosis	Pulsed and CW Doppler	High esophageal or transgastric apical	• Careful positioning to obtain highest-velocity signal	• Maximum velocity • Mean gradient • Aortic valves: Ratio of LVOT to aortic velocity (alignment often suboptimal) • Mitral valve: Pressure half-time
Valve regurgitation	Color imaging and CW Doppler	High esophageal with rotational scan	• Document origin of jet and proximal flow acceleration, and jet size and direction	• Measure vena contracta, record pulmonary venous flow pattern, search carefully for eccentric jets
Pulmonary pressures	CW Doppler	RV inflow and apical	• TR jet velocity • IVC size and variation	• Calculate PAP as $4v^2$ of TR jet plus estimated RA pressure • Difficult to align Doppler beam parallel to TR jet; correlate with TTE data

IVC, Inferior vena cava; *LVOT*, left ventricular outflow tract; *PAP*, pulmonary artery pressure; *TR*, tricuspid regurgitation.

SELF-ASSESSMENT QUESTIONS

Question 1

An 87-year-old asymptomatic woman has relocated to your area and presents to establish care. She has a history of aortic stenosis and had undergone recent aortic valve replacement. You obtain a baseline echocardiogram (Fig. 13.22).

Based on the images provided, you conclude which of the following?

A. Endocarditis with paravalvular abscess
B. Prosthetic valve mismatch
C. Aorto-ventricular fistula
D. Normally functioning aortic valve replacement

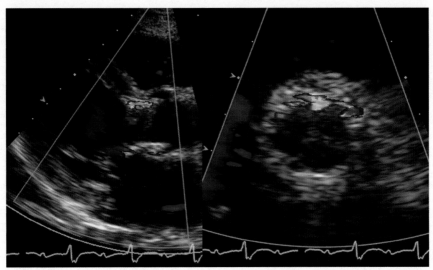

Fig. 13.22

Question 2

This echocardiographic image (Fig. 13.23) was obtained at the postoperative baseline study after bioprosthetic mitral valve replacement.

What is the most likely diagnosis for the structure indicated by the arrow?

A. Vegetation
B. Valve strut
C. Mitral valve
D. Ruptured papillary muscle
E. LV thrombus

Question 3

A 66-year-old man who had undergone mechanical mitral valve replacement for endocarditis now presents with progressive exertional dyspnea. Based on your clinical examination, you are suspicious for prosthetic valve regurgitation. What additional information from transthoracic imaging will most likely confirm your suspicion?

A. Proximal isovelocity surface area calculation
B. Pulmonary venous pulsed wave Doppler tracing
C. Transmitral CW Doppler tracing
D. Apical 4-chamber view color Doppler imaging

Question 4

A 56-year-old woman who underwent mitral valve surgery 5 years ago presents with dyspnea and a systolic

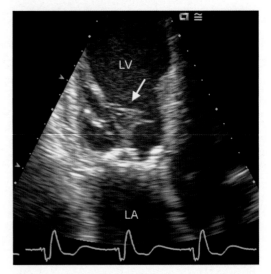

Fig. 13.23

murmur. Because of the concern for prosthetic mitral regurgitation, a TEE study is performed. This systolic TEE image (Fig. 13.24) is most consistent with:

A. A normal mechanical mitral prosthesis
B. Severe bioprosthetic mitral regurgitation
C. Residual mild regurgitation after mitral valve repair
D. Prosthetic valve endocarditis

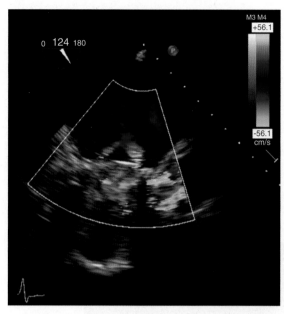

Fig. 13.24

Question 5

A patient with a mechanical aortic valve prosthesis presents with exertional dyspnea. A transthoracic echocardiogram is performed, demonstrating a peak aortic jet velocity of 3.6 m/s with an LV outflow tract velocity of 1.4 m/s. He has recently had his chronic oral anticoagulation held due to severe esophageal variceal bleeding. Prior TTE images showed a peak aortic jet velocity of 2.7 m/s with an LV outflow tract velocity of 1.0 m/s. These data are most consistent with:
- **A.** Prosthesis mismatch
- **B.** Valve thrombosis
- **C.** Bacterial endocarditis
- **D.** Hyperdynamic cardiac function

Question 6

A 71-year-old woman presented for a second opinion regarding possible prosthetic valve stenosis. She had undergone bioprosthetic aortic valve replacement 2 years ago. On exam, she is an older anxious woman with a blood pressure of 120/80 mm Hg, pulse of 72 beats/min, body surface area of 1.9 cm^2, and an aortic ejection murmur but no evidence of heart failure. Echocardiography shows a normal-appearing prosthetic valve with the following Doppler data (Fig. 13.25).

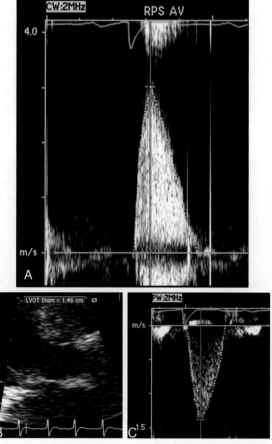

Fig. 13.25

The most likely diagnosis in this patient is:

A. No prosthetic valve dysfunction

B. Prosthetic valve stenosis

C. Prosthetic valve regurgitation

D. Patient-prosthesis mismatch

Question 7

A patient with a stentless bioprosthetic aortic valve and fevers is admitted to the inpatient service. He is referred for a TEE, and the following image (Fig. 13.26) is recorded from the midesophageal long-axis view.

Based on the imaging provided, you recommend:

A. Administer local intravenous lytic therapy

B. Broaden intravenous antibiotic therapy

C. Referral to cardiac surgery

D. Serial monitoring, repeat TEE in 1 year

Question 8

A patient with a history of prior mitral valve surgery presents with recurrent progressive dyspnea. This systolic TEE image (Fig. 13.27) is most consistent with:

A. A normal mechanical mitral prosthesis.

B. Degenerative bioprosthetic mitral regurgitation

C. Residual mild regurgitation after mitral valve repair

D. Prosthetic valve endocarditis

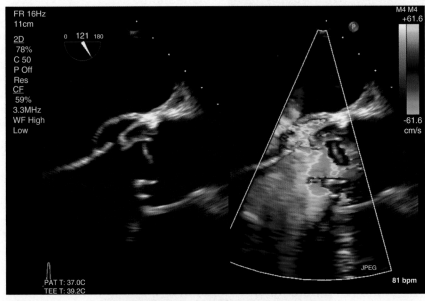

Fig. 13.26

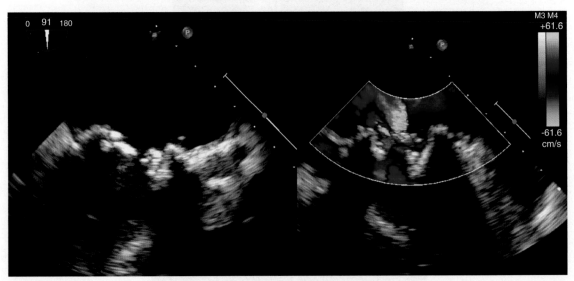

Fig. 13.27

Question 9

A 52-year-old woman with rheumatic heart disease and mitral valve replacement underwent elective cholecystectomy for biliary colic. The patient had a postoperative baseline echocardiogram 2 years prior noting normal prosthetic valve function. In preparation for surgery, the patient's warfarin was held. The patient became short of breath on the first postoperative day with a slight fever. Based on the echocardiographic images (Fig. 13.28), which of the following complications is most likely?

A. Prosthetic valve thrombosis
B. Prosthetic valve endocarditis
C. Prosthetic valve calcification
D. Patient-prosthesis mismatch

Question 10

This 88-year-old woman presented with worsening heart failure and hemoptysis. She had undergone bioprosthetic mitral valve replacement 12 years ago for severe mitral stenosis with an early postoperative baseline echocardiogram that showed normal LV and RV size and function, normal prosthetic valve function, and a pulmonary systolic pressure of 40 mm Hg. On exam now she has a blood pressure of 100/70 mm Hg, heart rate of 74 bpm with an irregular pulse, a jugular venous pressure of 20 cm H_2O, distant heart sounds, and bilateral pulmonary rales. The following Doppler tracings were recorded on the current study (Fig. 13.29).

The most likely cause of her current symptoms is:

A. Pulmonary embolus
B. LV systolic dysfunction
C. Severe mitral regurgitation
D. Rheumatic aortic valve disease
E. Mitral stenosis

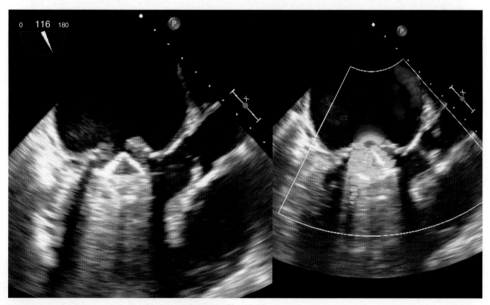

Fig. 13.28

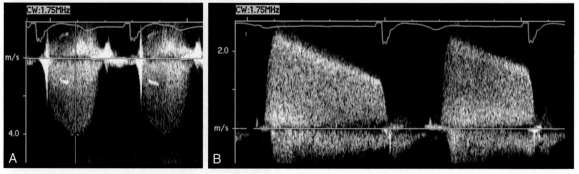

Fig. 13.29

Question 11

A 68-year-old man with a history of endocarditis requiring a mechanical mitral valve 20 years ago presented with complaints of sweating, fatigue, and jaundice. A previous baseline echocardiogram reported normal prosthetic valve function with a peak early mitral inflow velocity of 1.4 m/s and mean gradient of 4 mm Hg while the heart rate was at 80 beats per minute. The patient underwent repeat transthoracic echocardiography for evaluation of prosthetic function (Fig. 13.30). There were no other valvular abnormalities reported. Which of the following is the next best step?

A. Cardiac computed tomography to evaluate occluder motion

B. No further evaluation as gradients are due to normal flow patterns

C. Transesophageal echocardiogram to evaluate for regurgitation

D. Cardiac catheterization to measure mitral stenosis gradients

Question 12

In the patient with this echocardiographic image (Fig. 13.31), which of the following clinical findings is most likely present?

A. Elevated reticulocyte count

B. Diastolic murmur

C. Wide pulse pressure

D. S4 gallop

E. Thrombocytopenia

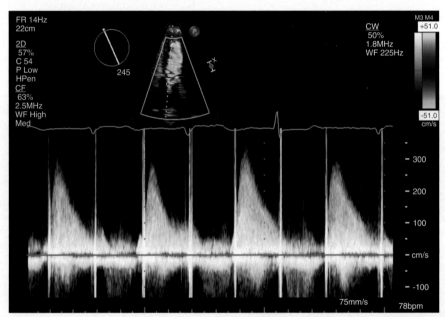

Fig. 13.30

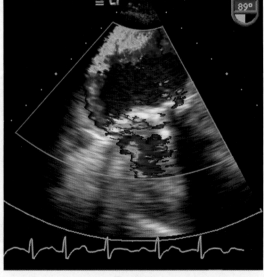

Fig. 13.31

ANSWERS

Answer 1: D

This patient has undergone transcatheter bioprosthetic aortic valve replacement (TAVR) with the valve stent visible in the long-axis view as linear bright echoes near the annulus and in the short-axis view as bright echoes in a circular shape around the annulus. Color Doppler images show paravalvular regurgitation along the anterior portion of the valve annulus. TAVR valves are positioned within the patient's native stenotic valve with the calcific leaflets pushed up against the aortic wall. In patients with heavy native valve calcification, incomplete apposition of the TAVR against the native valve may lead to a small amount of paravalvular regurgitation. Often, these jets improve or resolve with endothelialization of the prosthesis.

Spectral Doppler images in this patient demonstrated mildly increased anterograde velocities through the TAVR. This is common in TAVR valves because the maximal valve orifice size is within the native valve annulus. A peak velocity of 2.5 m/s is within expected valve hemodynamics and is not consistent with prosthetic valve mismatch. The patient is asymptomatic without clinical evidence of endocarditis, making a paravalvular abscess or aorto-ventricular fistula less likely.

Answer 2: C

This image shows the native mitral valve chords and part of the mitral leaflet, which were retained at the time of mitral valve replacement. Maintenance of mitral annular-papillary muscle continuity helps prevent loss of LV systolic contractile function with surgical mitral valve replacement. Typically the prosthetic valve is inserted centrally and the posterior leaflets and chords are left connected to the papillary muscle behind the prosthetic valve sewing ring. The anterior leaflet may be partially retained or may be resected, leaving freely mobile chordal remnants. A mitral vegetation would be more likely on the left atrial side of the valve; infection of the sewing ring with annular abscess formation instead of a typical vegetation is common with a prosthetic valve. Valve struts are more uniform in appearance and do not protrude this far into the LV cavity. A ruptured papillary muscle results in a disrupted muscle head moving freely in the LV, attached to the mitral valve; normal attachments of the chords to the papillary muscle can be seen on this image. An LV thrombus usually occurs in an area of regional dysfunction, often the apex, and is adherent to the LV myocardium.

Answer 3: C

Mechanical mitral valve occluders acoustically shadow structures distal to the valve. This often results in hindering visualization of mitral regurgitation, particularly in the apical 4-chamber view where the left atrium is in the far field relative to the mitral valve prosthesis. CW Doppler tracings are less affected by acoustic shadowing, and if a signal is detected, a diagnosis of mitral regurgitation is confirmed. Quantification of mitral regurgitation severity is relatively limited with CW tracings, but if a dense signal is identified, significant mitral regurgitation should be suspected (Fig. 13.32). In this Doppler recording, bright lines indicating valve occluder motion are seen at the beginning and end of systole with a dense systolic regurgitant signal directed away from the transducer.

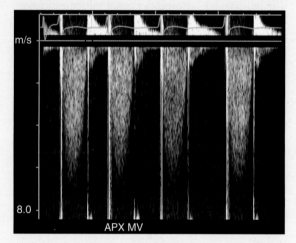

Fig. 13.32

Others signs of prosthetic mtiral regurgitation include a high early diastolic velocity and an elevated tricuspid regurgitant jet velocity, suggesting pulmonary hypertension, particularly in patients who had demonstrated normal range pulmonary pressures previously.

With significant acoustic shadowing of the left atrium, pulmonary venous tracings would be difficult to reliably record. However, if visualized, systolic flow reversal would be consistent with significant mitral regurgitation. Acoustic shadowing at the valve occluders hinders visualization of the vena contracta and a discrete proximal isovelocity surface area hemisphere is rarely visualized.

Answer 4: A

This systolic image in a TEE long-axis view shows two small crisscrossing jets of mitral regurgitation. This is a normal finding with a bileaflet mechanical valve due to displacement of a small amount of blood as the valve occluders close in systole. The bileaflet valve appears echodense with shadowing and reverberations obscuring the LV. A bioprosthetic valve in the mitral position has stents that extend into the LV chamber and thin tissue leaflets that can be seen on TEE imaging. A mitral valve repair typically results in a short, relatively immobile posterior mitral leaflet with normal anterior leaflet anatomy and motion. An annular ring is typical. With prosthetic valve endocarditis, findings might include a valvular vegetation, paravalvular abscess, or paravalvular regurgitation.

Answer 5: D

This patient presents with exertional dyspnea and has a recent history of severe bleeding; he is likely anemic. The significant interval increase in peak aortic jet velocity raises suspicion for prosthetic stenosis or obstruction. However, with anemia, cardiac function is hyperdynamic with proportional increases in both left ventricular outflow tract (LVOT) and transaortic jet velocities. The relative ratio of the LVOT to the peak aortic jet velocity ("dimensionless index") is preserved. In this case, although the aortic velocity is increased, the LVOT velocity is increased as well, thus the ratio, or dimensionless is unchanged consistent with hyperdynamic cardiac function rather than obstruction.

Answer 6: D

The Doppler data show an aortic velocity of 3.0 m/s with an LVOT diameter of only 1.5 cm and an LV outflow tract velocity of 1.4 m/s. The circular LV outflow tract cross-sectional area (CSA) is 1.8 cm². Aortic valve area calculated with the continuity equation is:

$$AVA = CSA_{LVOT} \times V_{LVOT}/V_{AS}$$
$$= 1.8 \text{ cm}^2 \times (1.4 \text{ m/s}/3.0\text{m/s}) = 0.8 \text{ cm}^2 \quad (13.1)$$

When indexed for body size:

$$\text{Indexed AVA} = 0.8 \text{ cm}^2/1.9 \text{ m}^2 = 0.43 \text{ cm}^2/\text{m}^2 \quad (13.2)$$

These data are consistent with severe patient prosthesis mismatch, with an aortic valve indexed area less than 0.65 cm²/m². Ideally, patient prosthesis mismatch is avoided by calculating the expected valve area divided by body size before valve implantation; if the expected valve area is too small, an alternate valve choice or an aortic root–enlarging procedure can be considered. Once patient prosthesis mismatch is present, decision making is more difficult because correction would require another surgical procedure. Both short- and long-term outcomes are worse when patient prosthesis mismatch is present. This patient's transvalvular mean gradient is only 14 mm Hg, and the LV outflow to aortic velocity ratio is 1.4/3.0 = 0.47, which does not support a significant hemodynamic effect from the small prosthesis. Thus, although she meets the definition for patient prosthesis mismatch, there is no significant outflow obstruction at this time.

Answer 7: C

In the images provided, the patient has a pseudoaneurysm of the aortic-mitral intervalvular fibrosis, with flow entering the pseudoaneurysm on the LV side of the aortic valve. The prosthesis is seen just anterior to the pseudoaneurysm without typical acoustic shadowing, because this is a stentless valve prosthesis. Although no obvious vegetation is seen, other views are needed to fully evaluate prosthetic valve anatomy. While broadening intravenous antibiotic therapy should be considered, the patient is demonstrating signs of active infection with fevers and paravalvular infection, so that cardiac surgery should be consulted for prosthetic valve endocarditis complicated by pseudoaneurysm. Valve thrombosis is not the key finding, so lytic therapy is not indicated.

Answer 8: B

This systolic TEE imaging in a long-axis view shows a bioprosthetic valve with thickened and calcified leaflets. Color Doppler shows a broad jet of regurgitation through the valve prosthesis, consistent with at least moderate prosthetic valve regurgitation. A mechanical valve would be echodense with shadowing and reverberations obscuring the LV. A mitral valve repair is characterized by native leaflets with an annular ring. Although endocarditis is possible, there is no definite vegetation or paravalvular abscess shown on this image.

Answer 9: A

The patient has prosthetic valve thrombosis of a mechanical mitral valve due to inadequate anti-coagulation. Fig. 13.28 shows incomplete opening of the mechanical occluder with turbulent stenotic blood flow. There is hazy opacity surrounding the area of the occluder. The patient is at high risk of prosthetic valve thrombosis with a mechanical mitral valve and requires bridging anticoagulation with heparin-based therapies for surgical procedures. The patient does not have a clear mobile vegetation or dehiscence of the prosthetic valve for endocarditis (answer B). The brightness of the valve leaflets is present from the strong reflection of a mechanical bileaflet occluder, not from calcification and leaflet failure that may occur in a bioprosthetic valve (answer C). Patient-prosthesis mismatch (answer D) occurs in normal functioning prosthetic valves that are too small for the metabolic demands of the patient.

Answer 10: E

These Doppler recordings show a high-velocity tricuspid regurgitant jet, consistent with pulmonary hypertension, and a transmitral flow signal consistent with an elevated transmitral gradient and small valve area. The tricuspid regurgitant signal is identified based on systolic flow with a long flow period relative to the QRS and with the typical rapid, followed by slow, rate of rise in velocity with a late peaking curve. The transmitral flow curve is in diastole with a typical passive flow pattern of an early diastolic peak and linear fall-off in velocity throughout diastole. Atrial fibrillation is present with no discernable a-velocity. The slow diastolic decline in velocity is consistent with mitral stenosis.

Pulmonary embolus might be associated with pulmonary hypertension, but transmitral flow would be normal. LV systolic dysfunction would result in a reduced *dP/dt* on the mitral regurgitant velocity signal, which is not shown here. Severe mitral regurgitation would result in an increased antegrade transmitral velocity, but the diastolic slope would be steep. Rheumatic aortic valve disease is present in about one-third of patients with rheumatic valve disease, and the mitral stenosis signal appears similar in shape to aortic regurgitation. However, diastolic velocities are lower across the mitral compared to aortic valve, with a diastolic blood pressure of 70 mm Hg. The initial diastolic velocity for aortic regurgitation would be about 4 m/s.

Answer 11: C

The patient has an increased peak antegrade flow of up to 3 m/s, which is a significant change from the previous reported echocardiogram. A high antegrade velocity may be due to high-flow states, stenosis, or detection of flow through the central orifice of a mechanical bileaflet valve. The deceleration slope and resulting pressure-half time of the antegrade flow for the patient is quite rapid, thus being more consistent with a high mitral flow than a prosthetic valve stenosis (answer A & D). The patient's symptoms, high flow through the mitral valve, and history of endocarditis should be further evaluated with a transesophageal echocardiogram to evaluate for potential mitral regurgitation. Paravalvular regurgitation may be shadowed from the mechanical mitral valve on transthoracic study and is better evaluated with transesophageal echocardiography. A small amount of paravalvular regurgitation can occur after surgery due to disruption of sutures from a calcified annulus; however, new paravalvular regurgitation leading to hemolysis, anemia, or heart failure needs further evaluation for potential endocarditis. Although normal bileaflet mechanical valves may have a high normal antegrade velocity through the central orifice (answer B), the patient's symptoms and change from previous baseline warrant further evaluation.

Answer 12: A

This is a TEE 2-chamber view of a patient with a mechanical mitral valve prosthesis showing an eccentric paravalvular mitral regurgitant jet. Paravalvular mitral regurgitation can cause hemolysis resulting in an elevated reticulocyte count. Most often, hemolysis is well tolerated, and the patient is able to maintain a relatively normal red blood cell count, although sometimes vitamin and iron supplements are needed. Surgical or percutaneous intervention rarely is needed to close the paravalvular leak unless there also is a large volume of regurgitant flow. This patient likely has a systolic (not diastolic) murmur. A wide pulse pressure is typical for aortic, not mitral, regurgitation. An S4 gallop will not be present as the electrocardiogram (ECG) shows atrial fibrillation. The platelet count should be normal, although blood clotting likely is abnormal due to warfarin anticoagulation for a mechanical valve and atrial fibrillation.

14 Endocarditis

BASIC PRINCIPLES

- Echocardiographic evaluation for endocarditis uses an integrated approach with transthoracic echocardiography (TTE) and transesophageal echocardiography (TEE), depending on the clinical setting and the initial echocardiographic findings.
- The modified Duke criteria for infective endocarditis are the current clinical standard.
- The primary goals of the echocardiographic examination in a patient with suspected or known endocarditis are to:
  - Detect and describe valvular vegetations
  - Quantitate degree of valve dysfunction
  - Identify paravalvular abscess or other complications
  - Evaluate hemodynamics effects of valve dysfunction on ventricular size and function and on pulmonary pressures
  - Provide prognostic data on clinical course and need for surgical intervention

❖ KEY POINTS

- Definite endocarditis is present when blood cultures are positive and diagnostic findings are present on echocardiography; these are the modified Duke major criteria for the diagnosis of endocarditis.
- Diagnostic echocardiographic findings for endocarditis are one of the following:
  - Typical vegetation on a valve or prosthetic material
  - Paravalvular abscess
  - New prosthetic valve dehiscence
  - New valvular regurgitation

- In the absence of major criteria (blood cultures and echocardiographic findings), the minor criteria for diagnosis of endocarditis are:
  - Predisposing heart condition or intravenous drug use
  - Fever
  - Vascular phenomenon (arterial emboli, mycotic aneurysm, conjunctival hemorrhage, etc.)
  - Immunologic phenomenon (glomerulonephritis, rheumatoid factor, etc.)
  - Other microbiologic evidence
- A diagnosis of definite endocarditis is based on the presence of two major, or one major plus three minor, or all five minor criteria. A diagnosis of possible endocarditis is based on one major plus one minor, or three minor criteria.

STEP-BY-STEP APPROACH

Step 1: Review the Clinical Data

- Key clinical data in the patient undergoing echocardiography for suspected endocarditis are:
  - Blood culture results
  - History of underlying cardiac disease or intravenous drug use
  - Other evidence of endocarditis (fever, embolic events, PR interval prolongation)
  - Any contraindication to TEE
- The clinical data help focus the echocardiographic examination so that particular attention is directed toward:
  - Detection of right-sided vegetations in patients with a history of intravenous drug use

○ Comparison of the current study with previous examinations in patients with underlying valve pathology

○ Additional imaging, often with TEE, of prosthetic valves and pacer leads

❖ **KEY POINTS**

❑ The sensitivity of echocardiography for detection of valve vegetations depends as much on the diligence of the exam as on image quality; therefore a pretest estimate of the likelihood of disease is helpful to the sonographer.

❑ Review of previous imaging studies before performing the exam allows quick recognition of new abnormalities.

❑ Clinical data are critical for interpretation of echocardiographic data. The echo appearance of a cardiac tumor, thrombus, and infected vegetation are similar—the final diagnosis is based on integration of echocardiographic and clinical data.

❑ Clinical data determine the urgency and most appropriate initial diagnostic modality, as well as the need for any subsequent studies.

Step 2: Choose Transthoracic and/or Transesophageal Echocardiography (Table 14.1)

■ Most centers perform TTE before TEE in patients with suspected endocarditis, but this decision depends on the clinical situation.

TABLE 14.1   Diagnostic Imaging in Infective Endocarditis

	TTE	TEE	Other	AHA/ACC 2014 ♥	ESC 2015 ♦
Diagnosis in Patients With Suspected Infective Endocarditis (IE)					
All patients with clinically suspected IE	♥♦			I (B)	I (B)
Non-diagnostic TTE		♥♦		I (B)	I (B)
Prosthetic heart valve or intracardiac device		♦			I (B)
Repeat within 5-7 days if initial study negative and clinical suspicion remains high	♦	♦			I (C)
Staphylococcus aureus bacteremia without known source	♥♦			IIa (B)	IIa (B)
Persistent fever in patient with a prosthetic valve		♥		IIa (B)	
Positive TTE (except right sided with good quality TTE)		♦			IIa (C)
Suspected paravalvular infection with suboptimal echo images			CT	IIa (B)	*
Suspected prosthetic valve endocarditis			¹⁸F-FDG PET/CT		*
Staphylococcus aureus bacteremia with known source (to detect possible cardiac involvement)	♥			IIb (B)	
Follow-up on Medical Therapy					
Change in signs or symptoms or concern for complications (new murmur, embolism, persisting fever, heart failure, abscess, AV block)	♥♦	♥♦		I (B)	I (B)
Routine follow-up for uncomplicated IE	♦	♦			IIa (B)
Perioperative Echocardiography					
Intraoperative TEE in patients undergoing valve surgery for IE		♥♦		I (B)	I (B)
Following Completion of Therapy					
Baseline study after treatment for IE is completed	♦				I (C)

FDG, Fluorodeoxyglucose; *PTE,* positron emission tomography.

♥= ACC/AHA recommendation.

♦= ESC recommendation.

*Added to ESC 2015 criteria for diagnosis of endocarditis as shown in Table 14.1. No specific class or level of evidence.

From Otto CM: *Textbook of clinical echocardiography,* ed 6, Philadelphia, 2018, Elsevier. Summarized from Nishimura RA, Otto CM, Bonow RO, Carabello BA, Erwin JP 3rd, Guyton RA, et al: 2014 AHA/ACC guideline for the management of patients with valvular heart disease, *J Am Coll Cardiol* 63(22):e57-e185, 2014; and Habib G, Lancellotti P, Antunes MJ, Bongiorni MG, Casalta JP, et al: 2015 ESC guidelines for the management of infective endocarditis, *Eur Heart J* 36(44):3075-3128, 2015.

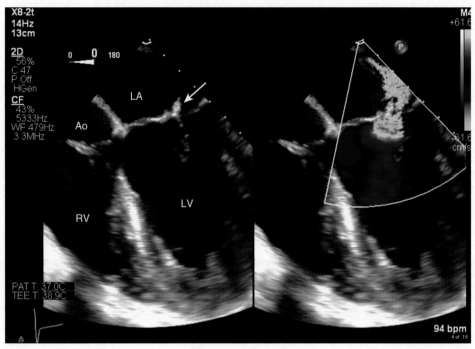

Fig. 14.1 Detection of valvular vegetations. TEE 2D *(left)* and color Doppler *(right)* views of the mitral valve in a patient with bacteremia shows a large mobile mass on the mitral valve that prolapses into the LA is systolic consistent with a vegetation. This typical vegetation is attached to the upstream side of the valve (atrial side of mitral valve), is irregular in shape, and has a chaotic pattern of motion that is separate from the normal motion of the valve tissue. Color Doppler shows associated moderate to severe regurgitation. This appearance is similar to a partial flail mitral leaflet; the final diagnosis integrates clinical and bacteriological data with the echo findings. *Ao,* Aorta.

- TTE imaging is followed by TEE if transthoracic images are nondiagnostic, if a prosthetic valve is present, or if the patient has a high risk of endocarditis.
- TEE is an appropriate initial diagnostic approach in patients with a prosthetic valve or other intracardiac devices (such as pacer leads).
- In a patient with suspected or known endocarditis, TEE is recommended if clinical data suggest paravalvular abscess.

❖ **KEY POINTS**

- ❏ TEE is more sensitive for detection of valve vegetations compared with transthoracic imaging (a sensitivity of ≈90% vs. ≈70%) (Fig. 14.1).
- ❏ TEE is more sensitive for detection of paravalvular abscess compared with transthoracic imaging (sensitivity greater than 90% vs. about 50%).
- ❏ TEE is the preferred approach in patients with prosthetic valves or other intracardiac devices (such as pacer leads) for detection of vegetations and evaluation of valve dysfunction (Fig. 14.2).
- ❏ Transthoracic imaging provides more reliable measurements of left ventricle (LV) size and

ejection fraction, because images of the LV are often oblique or foreshortened on TEE views.
- ❏ Transthoracic imaging provides more accurate Doppler evaluation of stenotic valves and estimation of pulmonary pressures, because TEE often results in a nonparallel intercept angle between the Doppler beam and high-velocity jet.
- ❏ When TEE is contraindicated but endocarditis is suspected on clinical grounds, a repeat transthoracic study in 5 to 10 days has additive value, with the prevalence of diagnostic findings increasing from 20% on the initial study to 40% on the repeat examination.

Step 3: Examine Valve Anatomy to Detect Valvular Vegetations

- Valvular vegetations on echocardiography are seen as an abnormal, irregular mass attached to the valve apparatus (Fig. 14.3).
- Valvular vegetations typically are attached to the upstream side of the valve leaflet (e.g., atrial side of the mitral or tricuspid valve, LV side of aortic valve) (Fig. 14.4).
- Motion of a vegetation typically is chaotic, with a spatial range in excess of normal valve excursion and a temporal pattern of rapid oscillations (Fig. 14.5).

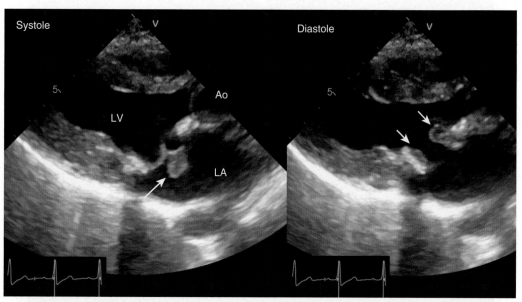

Fig. 14.2 **Prosthetic valve vegetation.** In this patient with endocarditis of a bioprosthetic mitral valve, a large mobile mass attached to the prosthetic valve leaflet prolapses into the left atrial in systole *(arrow, left)* and appears as echodensities within the valve struts in diastole *(arrows, right). Ao,* Aorta.

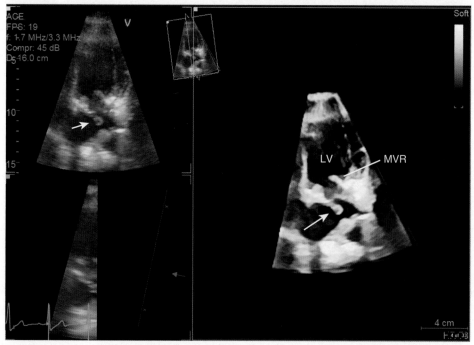

Fig. 14.3 **3D imaging of prosthetic valve vegetation.** 3D transthoracic imaging from an apical view, in the same patient as Fig. 14.2, better shows the vegetation attached to the prosthetic valve leaflets prolapsing into the left atrial in systole *(arrow). MVR,* Mitral valve replacement.

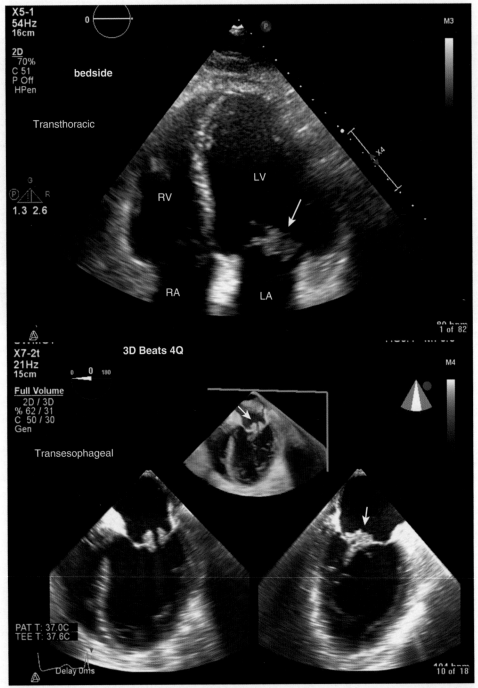

Fig. 14.4 **Mitral valve vegetation.** TTE *(top)* and TEE *(bottom)* images of the mitral valve show an echodensity on the atrial side of the leaflets, consistent with a vegetation. The TEE images more clearly show involvement of both leaflets on the biplane and 3D images. There is no evidence of paravalvular abscess.

❖ KEY POINTS

- ❏ In addition to standard views of each valve, the image plane is slowly moved from side to side (or in a rotational sweep on TEE), because vegetations often are seen only in oblique views.

- ❏ Zoom mode, a narrow sector, high transducer frequency, and harmonic imaging are used to enhance details of valve anatomy (Fig. 14.6).

- ❏ An M-mode recording through suspected vegetation seen on two-dimensional (2D) imaging helps distinguish vegetation from an artifact or valve tissue, based on the pattern and speed of motion of the structure.

- Vegetations may be missed on TTE; transesophageal imaging has a higher sensitivity for detection of vegetation due to improved image quality.
- The relationship of the vegetation to valve anatomy may be better appreciated with three-dimensional (3D) imaging, but there are no data to suggest that 3D imaging improves diagnostic accuracy for endocarditis.

- Other valve masses may be mistaken for an infected vegetation, including (Fig. 14.7):
  - Papillary fibroelastoma
  - Partial flail mitral leaflet or chord
  - Nonbacterial thrombotic endocarditis
  - Valve thrombus (especially with prosthetic valves)
  - Normal valve variants (such as Lambl excrescences)
  - Ultrasound artifacts
- Valvular vegetations tend to decrease in size and increase in echogenicity with effective therapy. However, some vegetations may still be present years after active infection.

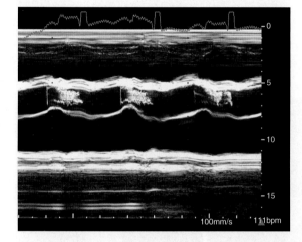

Fig. 14.5 **M-mode of aortic valve vegetation.** An indistinct echodensity adjacent to the aortic valve leaflets was seen in a patient referred for possible endocarditis. The M-mode shows fine oscillations of the mass in diastole, suggesting a vegetation rather than nonspecific leaflet thickening. *Ao,* Aorta.

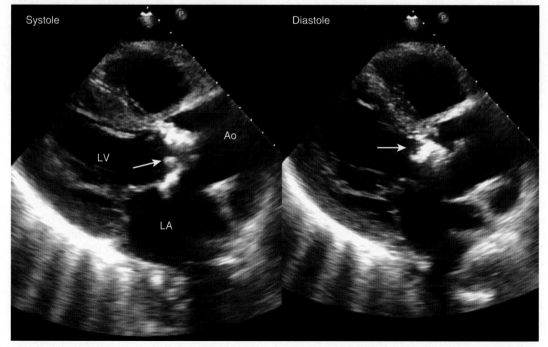

Fig. 14.6 **Aortic valve vegetation.** In a patient with a calcified bicuspid aortic valve and aortic sinus dilation, the parasternal long-axis view in systole *(left)* shows reduced systolic opening of the calcified aortic valve leaflets with a small echo density *(arrow)* on the LV side of the valve. In diastole *(right)*, a larger echo-dense mass prolapses into the LV outflow tract, which is suggestive of a vegetation or partial flail leaflet. Notice the shadowing of the LA by the calcified aortic valve. *Ao,* Aorta.

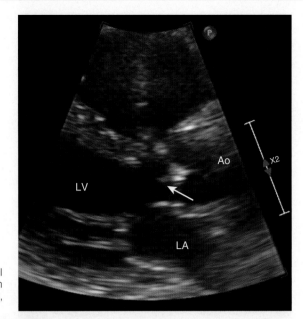

Fig. 14.7 Lambl excrescence on the aortic valve in diastole. A Lambl excrescence *(arrow)* can be difficult to distinguish from a vegetation but often is smaller, more linear and echodense, is not associated with valve dysfunction, and does not change in size or appearance on sequential studies. *Ao,* Aorta.

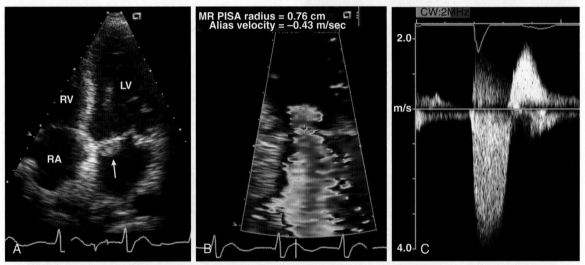

Fig. 14.8 Mitral valve vegetation and regurgitation A large mass is seen on the LA side of the mitral valve consistent with a vegetation (A). Although the mass is distant from the coaptation point, color Doppler shows significant mitral regurgitation (MR), which is quantitated with standard approaches, including the proximal isovelocity surface area (PISA) method (B) and the CW Doppler signal (C).

Step 4: Evaluate Valve Dysfunction Due to Endocarditis

- Vegetations are associated with distortion of valve anatomy and destruction of valve tissue, typically resulting in valve regurgitation (Fig. 14.8).
- The presence and severity of valve dysfunction are evaluated no differently than in a patient with valve disease of any cause (see Chapters 12 and 13).
- Valve regurgitation in a patient with endocarditis often is acute (hours to days), rather than chronic (months to years), in duration.

❖ KEY POINTS

- ❏ Vegetations may impede complete valve closure, resulting in regurgitation at the coaptation plane with either native or prosthetic valves.
- ❏ Valve destruction results in regurgitation due to leaflet perforation or deformity of the leaflet edge.
- ❏ Regurgitation of prosthetic valves often is paravalvular due to infection in the annulus with valve dehiscence (Fig. 14.9).
- ❏ About 10% of patients with endocarditis do not have significant valve regurgitation due to the location of the vegetation at the leaflet base, which does not impair valve function.
- ❏ Rarely, a large vegetation causes stenosis due to obstruction of the native or prosthetic valve orifice by the vegetation mass.
- ❏ Prosthetic valve stenosis can result from a small infected vegetation or thrombus impinging on normal disk excursion.

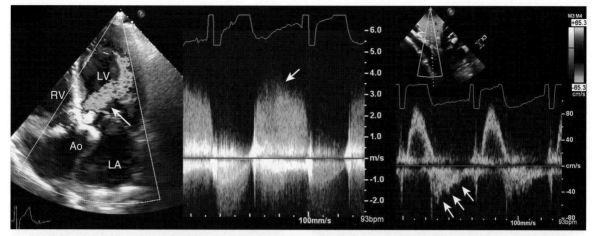

Fig. 14.9 **Aortic regurgitation due to endocarditis.** In this patient with endocarditis of a congenital bicuspid aortic valve (same patient as Fig. 14.6), color Doppler flow imaging in the apical 4-chamber view *(left)* shows a wide jet of aortic regurgitation *(arrow)*. CW Doppler *(center)* shows a diastolic regurgitant signal *(arrow)* equal in density to antegrade flow consistent with severe aortic regurgitation. Severe regurgitation is confirmed on pulsed Doppler of the proximal abdominal aorta *(right)* with holodiastolic systolic flow reversal *(arrows)*.

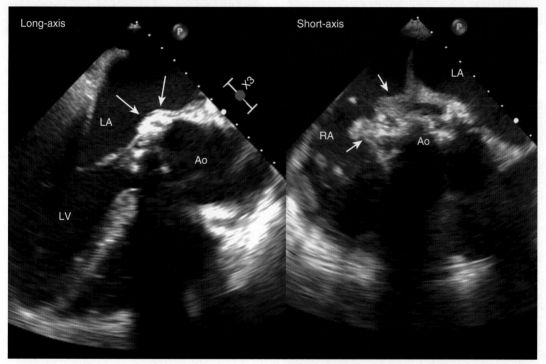

Fig. 14.10 **Paravalvular abscess.** TEE imaging in the same patient as Fig. 14.9 shows thickening and irregularity of the posterior aspect of the aortic sinuses *(arrows)* consistent with paravalvular abscess. Color Doppler suggested a small aortic to LA fistula through this region. The shadows from the calcified aortic valve now obscure the RV from this approach. *Ao,* Aorta.

Step 5: Evaluate for the Possibility of a Paravalvular Abscess or Fistula

- A paravalvular abscess is present in 20% to 60% of native aortic valve endocarditis cases and in about 15% of mitral valve infections (Fig. 14.10).
- Paravalvular infection occurs in more than 60% of prosthetic valve endocarditis cases.
- On echocardiography, a paravalvular abscess may be echolucent or echodense.
- A paravalvular aortic abscess often communicates with the aortic lumen, appearing as an aneurysm of the sinus of Valsalva (Fig. 14.11).

- Rupture of paravalvular infection into adjacent chambers results in an infected fistula (Fig. 14.12).

❖ KEY POINTS

- ❑ TEE is indicated when a paravalvular abscess is suspected, because the sensitivity of transthoracic imaging is low.
- ❑ Aortic paravalvular infection often is recognized based on distortion of the normal contours of the sinuses of Valsalva.

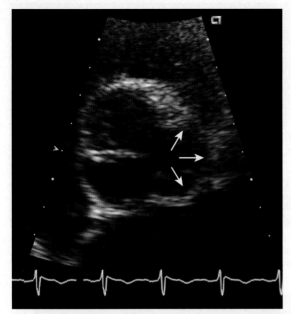

Fig. 14.11 Sinus of Valsalva aneurysm. Infection of the aortic sinuses can present as an asymmetric dilation, as seen with the left coronary sinus in this image. Comparison with previous images and TEE imaging both are helpful in distinguishing an infected sinus from benign congenital dilation.

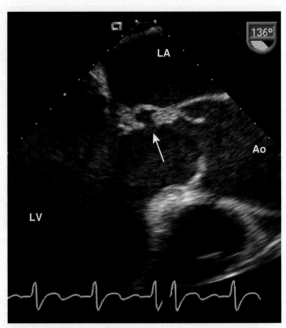

Fig. 14.13 Mitral leaflet perforation. In this patient with aortic valve endocarditis, infection has extended into the base of the adjacent anterior mitral leaflet *(arrow)* with thickening and a small perforation. *Ao,* Aorta.

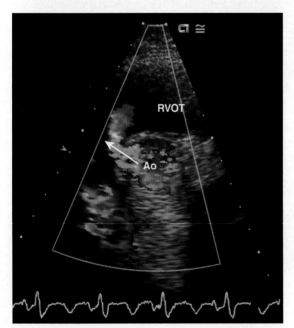

Fig. 14.12 Fistula formation. Infection of an aortic valve prosthesis resulting in a fistula from the aorta to the RV outflow tract seen on TTE in a parasternal short-axis view. The appearance is similar to a ventricular septal defect, but Doppler interrogation showed both diastolic and systolic flow more consistent with flow from the aorta into the RV. *Ao,* Aorta; *RVOT,* right ventricular outflow tract.

□ Paravalvular aortic infection may extend into the base of the anterior mitral leaflet, resulting in mitral leaflet perforation (Fig. 14.13).

□ An aortic paravalvular abscess may rupture into the LV (resulting in severe aortic regurgitation) or into the left atrium, right atrium (RA), or RV outflow tract (resulting in a fistula).

□ With prosthetic aortic valves, infection may result in an aneurysm of the aortic-mitral intervalvular

fibrosa (a space between the aortic and mitral valve that communicates with the LV) (Fig. 14.14).

□ A mitral paravalvular abscess may extend into the pericardium, resulting in purulent pericarditis.

Step 6: Measure the Hemodynamic Consequences of Valve Dysfunction

■ Valve dysfunction due to endocarditis may result in ventricular dilation and dysfunction or in pulmonary hypertension.

■ Because regurgitation often is acute, evidence of chronic volume overload may be absent even when regurgitation is severe.

❖ **KEY POINTS**

□ Evaluation of the patient with endocarditis includes measurement of LV dimensions, volumes, and ejection fraction as detailed in Chapter 6.

□ Pulmonary systolic pressure is estimated as described in Chapter 6.

□ Early (mid-diastolic) closure of the mitral valve may be seen on M-mode when acute severe aortic regurgitation is present due to the rapid rise in diastolic LV pressure.

□ The time course of the continuous-wave (CW) Doppler recording of valve regurgitation may show evidence of hemodynamic decompensation:

□ A rapid decline in velocity in late systole with mitral (or tricuspid) regurgitation suggests a left (or right) atrial v wave.

□ A steep diastolic deceleration slope with aortic regurgitation suggests acute regurgitation with an elevated LV end-diastolic pressure (Fig. 14.15).

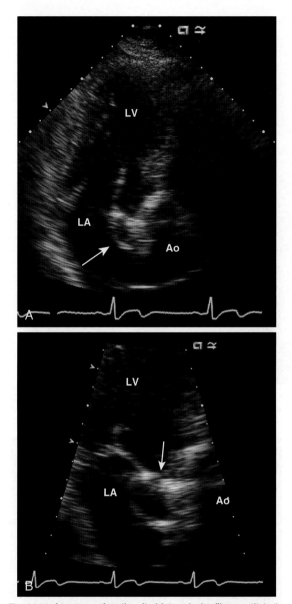

Fig. 14.14 **Aneurysm of aortic mitral intervalvular fibrosa.** (A) In the apical long-axis view, a curved pulsatile echo-free space *(arrow)* is seen between the posterior aortic root and LA. (B) Using zoom mode, the narrow neck where this aneurysm of the aortic mitral intervalvular fibrosa communicates with the LV is seen *(arrow). Ao,* Aorta.

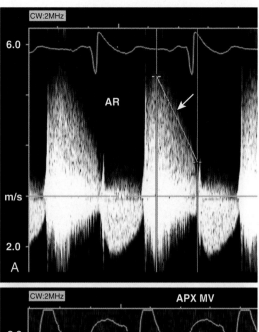

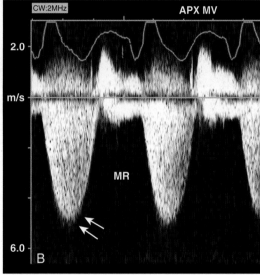

Fig. 14.15 **Acute valve regurgitation.** Regurgitation due to endocarditis often has an acute onset. (A) Acute aortic regurgitation shows a dense signal with a steep deceleration slope due to rapid equalization of aortic and LV pressures in diastole. (B) With acute mitral regurgitation, an early fall-off from peak velocity is due to an increased LA systolic pressure and v wave. *AR,* Aortic regurgitation; *MR,* mitral regurgitation.

□ LV systolic function may be impaired, without LV dilation, with acute severe aortic regurgitation due to endocarditis, possibly due to the effects of systemic infection, combined with a shift to the steep segment of the LV pressure volume curve.

Step 7: Look for Other Complications of Endocarditis

■ More than one cardiac valve may be affected, due either to primary infection at more than one site or by direct extension of infection to adjacent structures.

■ Septic coronary artery emboli, resulting in myocardial infarction, occur in 10% of patients.

■ Endocarditis may occur at intracardiac sites other than valve leaflets, including a mitral or tricuspid valve chord, a Chiari network or Eustachian valve, or the RA wall in a region abraded by the tip of a central catheter.

■ A pericardial effusion may be present, either as a nonspecific sign of systemic infection or due to direct extension of infection.

❖ KEY POINTS

□ Once a vegetation has been detected on one valve, careful evaluation for infection of other valves is needed.

□ The presence of a regional wall motion abnormality in a patient with endocarditis is consistent with a coronary embolus from a valve vegetation.

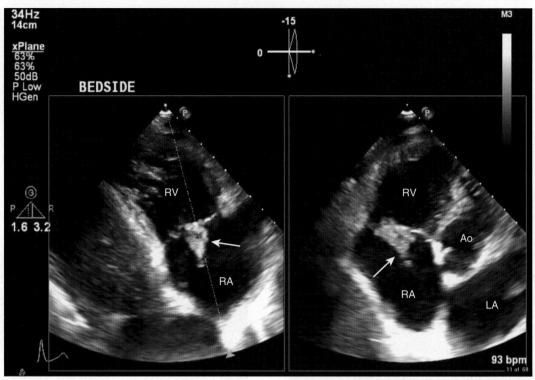

Fig. 14.16 Tricuspid valve vegetation. TTE biplane imaging in an RV inflow view shows an irregular mass attached to the tricuspid valve leaflets with prolapse into the RA in systole. In real time, the mass oscillated rapidly, independent of valve motion. This finding is consistent with a valvular vegetation. *Ao,* Aorta.

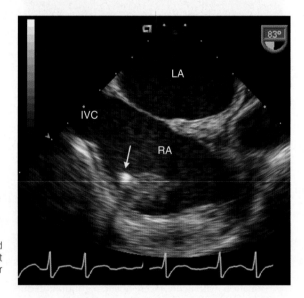

Fig. 14.17 Infected pacer lead. This TEE bicaval view shows a pacer lead *(arrow),* traversing the RA chamber with an attached echogenic mass that showed independent mobility. The appearance is consistent with vegetation or a thrombus. *IVC,* Inferior vena cava.

❑ Intracardiac sites subject to injury (such as the RA wall in a patient with a central catheter or the tricuspid valve in a patient with an indwelling right heart catheter) should be carefully examined for evidence of infection (Fig. 14.16).

SPECIAL SITUATIONS

Right-Sided Endocarditis

■ Only 6% to 13% of febrile intravenous drug users have endocarditis.

■ In intravenous drug users, infection affects the right side of the heart (predominantly the tricuspid valve) in 75% of cases (Fig. 14.17).

■ Most cases of right-sided endocarditis in drug users are due to *Staphylococcus aureus,* and persistent infection or abscess formation requiring surgery occurs in less than 25% of cases.

■ Pulmonary emboli due to right heart vegetations may result in elevated pulmonary pressures.

■ Left-sided involvement occurs in 25% to 35% of endocarditis cases in patients with a history of intravenous drug use.

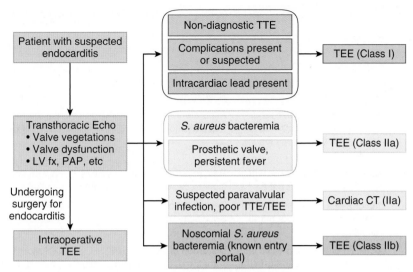

Fig. 14.18 Flow chart for the suggested role of echocardiography in the diagnosis of endocarditis. TTE is the initial step in evaluation of patients with a concern for endocarditis based on clinical or bacteriological findings. However, TEE often is needed in addition to transthoracic images as indicated in this algorithm. The Class of recommendation refers to the AHA/ACC 2014/17 recommendations for valvular heart disease. Class I is "indicated," Class IIa is "reasonable," and Class IIb "may be considered." *CT,* Computed tomography; *PAP,* pulmonary artery pressure. *(From Otto CM:* Textbook of clinical echocardiography, *ed 6, Philadelphia, 2018, Elsevier.)*

- TTE often is adequate for evaluation of tricuspid valve endocarditis, but TEE may be needed to exclude left heart involvement.

Prosthetic Valves

- Blood cultures should be drawn before any antibiotic therapy in febrile patients with a prosthetic heart valve.
- TEE is indicated in all patients with a prosthetic heart valve and positive blood cultures.
- TEE should be considered in patients with a prosthetic heart valve and suspected endocarditis, because transthoracic imaging is inadequate to exclude prosthetic valve infection.
- More than 50% of patients with prosthetic valve endocarditis require surgical intervention.

Pacer/Defibrillator Leads

- Blood cultures should be drawn before any antibiotic therapy in febrile patients with an intracardiac device.

- If pacer/defibrillator leads are not optimally seen by transthoracic imaging, TEE should be performed.
- Vegetations on the pacer wire are detected in less than 25% of cases on transthoracic imaging but are seen in more than 90% on TEE when infection is present (Fig. 14.18).
- The differential diagnosis of a mobile mass on a pacer lead includes thrombus. Thrombus and vegetation cannot be distinguished by echocardiography.

Staphylococcus aureus Bacteremia

- TEE is reasonable in patients with persistently positive blood cultures for *Staphylococcus aureus*, even if the transthoracic study is negative.
- In patients at high risk for a TEE study, an alternate approach is to repeat the TTE study in 5-10 days to look for evidence of new valve dysfunction.

THE ECHO EXAM

Echo Findings in Endocarditis

Finding	Definition	TTE	TEE
Valvular vegetations	Mass attached to leaflet with independent motion	Sensitivity 50%-80% Specificity 90%-100%	Sensitivity 90%-100% Specificity 90%-100%
Leaflet destruction	New or worsening valve regurgitation due to loss of normal coaptation with valve closure or chordal rupture	Accurate for detection and quantitation of regurgitation	May better define mechanism of regurgitation
Leaflet perforation	Disruption in leaflet tissue with a hole in the center or base	Regurgitation detected but loss of structure difficult to identify	3D TEE shows discontinuity in leaflet
Abscess	Infected area adjacent to valve, usually in the aortic or mitral annulus	Sensitivity low Specificity 90%-100%	Sensitivity 90%-100% Specificity 90%-100%
Aneurysm	Localized dilation of a valve leaflet, aortic sinus or aortic-mitral intervalvular fibrosa	Distortion of aortic sinus anatomy, outpouching of mitral leaflet, space between aortic annulus and anterior mitral leaflet	TEE more sensitive for detection of aneurysm
Pseudoaneurysm	Contained cardiac or aortic rupture, most often around aorta or at LV base	Abnormal echodense or echo lucent area around aorta or posterior to LV	TEE more sensitive for diagnosis but CT imaging often needed
Fistula	Abnormal communication between cardiac chambers or great vessels	Color or CW Doppler may show abnormal flow signal with timing and velocity diagnostic for location	TEE images allow visualization of location and size of intracardiac fistula
Prosthetic valve dehiscence	Detachment (partial) of the prosthetic valve from the annular tissue	Paravalvular regurgitation is typical Abnormal motion of valve is diagnostic but rare	TEE more sensitive for evaluation of prosthetic mitral valves Combination of TTE (anterior aspect of valve) and TEE (for posterior aspect) needed for aortic prosthetic valves

CT, Computed tomography.

SELF-ASSESSMENT QUESTIONS

Question 1

Which of the following indications for echocardiography least contributes to a definite diagnosis of endocarditis as per the Duke modified criteria?

A. Bacteremia
B. Systemic embolic events
C. Cardiac murmur
D. Fever
E. Immunologic phenomenon

Question 2

A 39-year-old man presents to the emergency department with lethargy and fatigue that has been progressive for several weeks. He has no prior cardiac history. Three months ago, he had developed a cough and was diagnosed with a community-acquired pneumonia. He had completed at least two courses of oral antibiotic therapy, prescribed for ongoing symptoms, by his physician before presentation. The following images (parasternal long-axis 2D view and a spectral Doppler tracing from the apical view) are obtained (Fig. 14.19).

The most likely diagnosis is:

A. Aortic to left atrial fistula
B. Aneurysm of the aortic-mitral intervalvular fibrosa
C. Aortic sinus aneurysm
D. Ventricular septal defect
E. Unrepaired tetralogy of Fallot

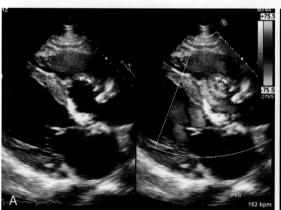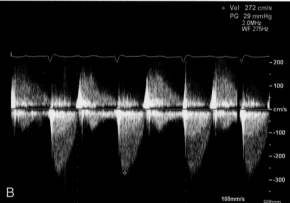

Fig. 14.19

Question 3

A 57-year-old man presents with complaints of dizziness and shortness of breath. Three months prior he had infectious endocarditis with severe mitral regurgitation that required extensive debridement and mitral valve replacement. Currently there is no fever, normal white blood cell count, and negative blood cultures. An echocardiogram is obtained with representative subcostal (Fig. 14.20) and apical 2-chamber views, with zoomed color Doppler. Which of the following best explains the patient's presentation?

A. Pseudoaneurysm
B. Pericardial abscess
C. Pleural effusion
D. Mitral valve dehiscence

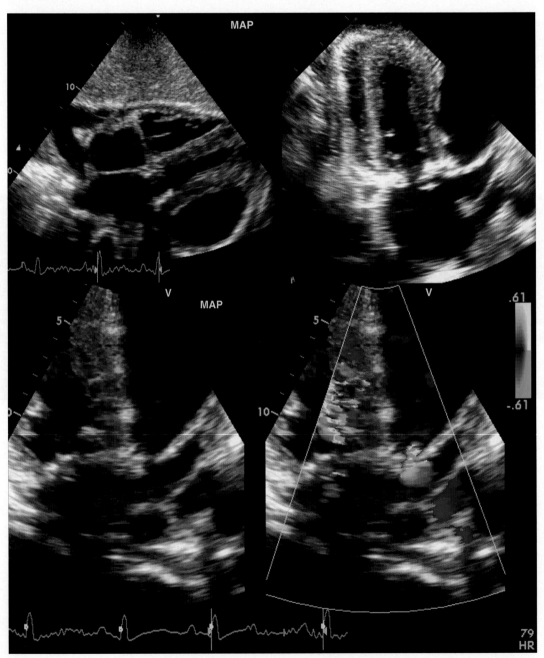

Fig. 14.20

Question 4

TTE was requested in a 69-year-old man with end-stage liver disease and a fever. He has no history of cardiac disease and blood cultures are negative (Fig. 14.21).

The most likely diagnosis is:
- **A.** Bacterial endocarditis
- **B.** Lambl excrescence
- **C.** Papillary fibroelastoma
- **D.** Nonbacterial thrombotic endocarditis
- **E.** Ultrasound artifact

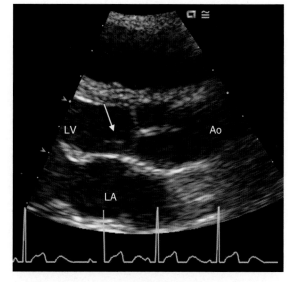

Fig. 14.21

Question 5

A 73-year-old man with a prior history of bioprosthetic aortic valve replacement for aortic stenosis now presents with fever, chills, and serial blood cultures positive for *Streptococcus viridans*. He has been successfully initiated on intravenous antibiotic therapy and a TEE is ordered. The following image is obtained (Fig. 14.22). Based on the data provided, you conclude that the patient has now developed which complication of endocarditis?
- **A.** Paravalvular abscess
- **B.** Prosthetic valve stenosis
- **C.** Aortic pseudoaneurysm
- **D.** Aortic regurgitation
- **E.** Ventricular septal defect

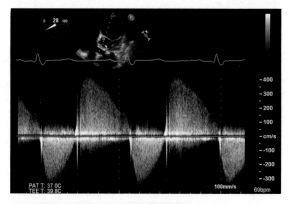

Fig. 14.22

Question 6

A 44-year-old man presents with a several-day history of fevers, tachycardia, and fatigue. A transthoracic echo is obtained. Based on the image shown (Fig. 14.23), what additional findings would you expect on subsequent clinical evaluation?
- **A.** Progressive AV block on electrocardiogram
- **B.** Oxygen saturation step-up from RA to RV on right heart catheterization
- **C.** Pulse pressure 75 mm Hg on blood pressure cuff
- **D.** Prominent internal jugular venous pulsation on physical exam

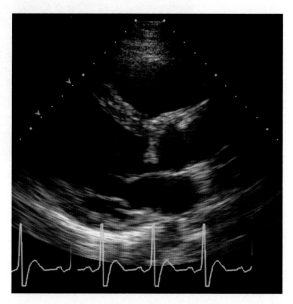

Fig. 14.23

Question 7

A 49-year-old woman with a bicuspid aortic valve presented with fever and syncope. A TEE echocardiogram is shown (Fig. 14.24). What is the most likely cause of syncope in this patient?

    A. Pericardial tamponade
    B. Acute mitral regurgitation
    C. Aortic dissection
    D. Atrioventricular heart block

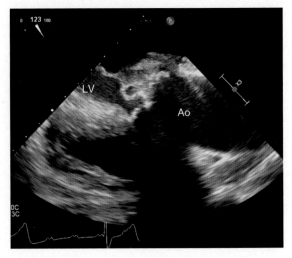

Fig. 14.24

Question 8

A 62-year-old man with a history of bioprosthetic valve replacement presented with acute shortness of breath, hypotension, and fevers. Four sets of blood cultures grew gram-positive cocci in clusters. An emergent echocardiogram was performed parasternal long-axis views in diastole and systole shown in Fig. 14.25. Which of the following is most likely?

    A. Paravalvular regurgitation
    B. Septic pulmonary embolism
    C. Mitral annular abscess
    D. Pericardial tamponade

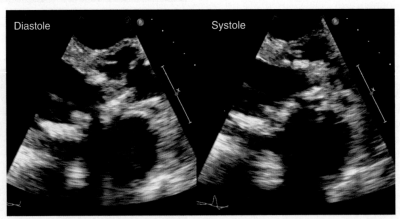

Fig. 14.25

Question 9

A 62-year-old man is admitted to the intensive care unit with hypotension and pulmonary edema. After endotracheal intubation and stabilization, a bedside echocardiogram is performed. This Doppler signal is recorded from an apical window (Fig. 14.26).

The most likely diagnosis is:
A. Moderate mitral stenosis
B. Severe aortic stenosis
C. Ventricular septal rupture
D. Severe pulmonary hypertension
E. Acute mitral regurgitation

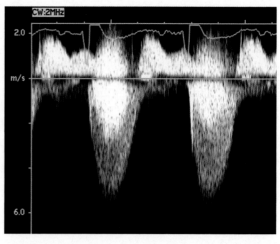

Fig. 14.26

Question 10

A 24-year-old woman presents for evaluation of a murmur. She has a history of aortic valve endocarditis complicated by an aortic annular abscess for which she underwent homograft aortic valve replacement 3 months ago.

The findings in this parasternal short-axis view (Fig. 14.27) and the CW Doppler recording of the flow disturbance are most consistent with:
A. Aortic regurgitation
B. Ventricular septal defect
C. Aorta to LA fistula
D. Perforated anterior mitral leaflet
E. Aortic annular abscess

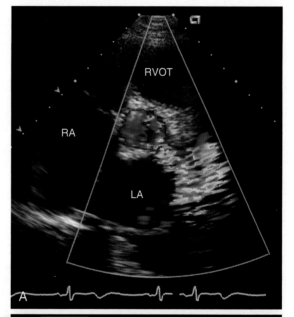

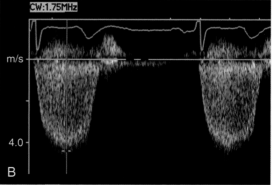

Fig. 14.27

Question 11

A 32-year-old woman with severe lupus nephritis presents with progressive shortness of breath for 3 months. The patient had a temporary dialysis catheter removed 2 weeks prior to presentation. The patient is afebrile and had no growth from blood cultures drawn at the time of catheter removal. The patient had an echocardiogram with moderate to severe mitral regurgitation with findings shown in Fig. 14.28. The most likely etiology for the patient's symptoms is which of the following?

A. Culture-negative infective endocarditis
B. Non-bacterial thrombotic endocarditis
C. Valvular myxoma
D. Mitral annular calcification

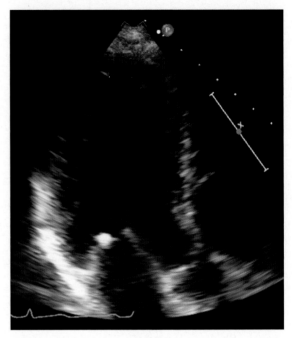

Fig. 14.28

Question 12

A 29-year-old man presented with fever, acute kidney injury, and bacteremia. Physical examination revealed a new holosystolic murmur, and transthoracic echocardiogram reported mitral regurgitation. A transesophageal echocardiogram during systole with color Doppler (and zoomed 3D mitral valve from the LA perspective) (Fig. 14.29) was obtained. Which of the following is the etiology of the mitral regurgitation?

A. Flail leaflet
B. Annular abscess
C. Leaflet perforation
D. Annular dilatation

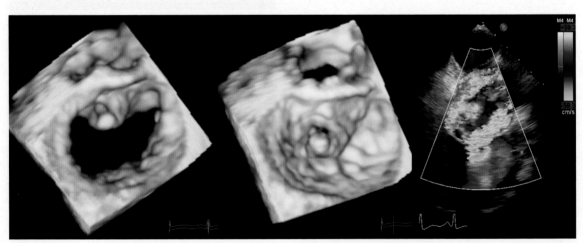

Fig. 14.29

ANSWERS

Answer 1: C

The Duke criteria for endocarditis diagnosis are grouped into major and minor diagnostic criteria initially described in 1994 and then revised ("modified") in 2000. A definite diagnosis of endocarditis is present for one of the following three conditions: presence of two major criteria, *or* presence of one major and three minor criteria, *or* presence of five minor criteria. Although a new or changing heart murmur is an important clinical finding in patients with endocarditis, murmur characteristics are not a component of the Duke criteria.

Major criteria for endocarditis diagnosis are:
1. Bacteremia with a typical endocarditis organism (such as *Staph.* or *Strep.* species) with two positive blood cultures drawn at least 12 hours apart
2. Echocardiographic evidence of endocarditis (such as a large vegetation, abscess, or dehisced prosthetic valve)

Minor criteria for endocarditis diagnosis are:
1. Predisposing condition (such as a prosthetic valve), or prior known endocarditis
2. Fever
3. Evidence of systemic embolic events
4. Immunologic phenomenon (such as glomerular nephritis or Osler nodes)
5. Positive blood cultures that do not meet the major criterion

Answer 2: C

This patient has no known prior cardiac history but has a markedly abnormal echocardiogram. The aortic valve is bright and thickened with an oblique closure plane consistent with a bicuspid aortic valve. In this case, the leaflet was thickened additionally due to vegetation, not optimally shown in the images provided. The parasternal long-axis view shows distortion of the aortic sinuses. There is a large sinus of Valsalva aneurysm at the right coronary sinus that protrudes into the RV outflow tract. Color Doppler flow into this aneurysm does not demonstrate a fistulous connection or rupture of the sinus, which, if present, would show flow in both systole and diastole (answer A). A ventricular septal defect would show abnormal systolic flow on the RV side of the septum (answer D). An aneurysm of the aortic-mitral intravalvular fibrosa would be seen in the region between the aortic and mitral valves (answer B). An unrepaired tetralogy of Fallot is characterized by a ventricular septal defect, enlarged aorta, and RV outflow obstruction. In this case, CW Doppler from the apical view shows aortic valve flow with a dense regurgitant jet with a steep deceleration slope, indicative of a rapid decrease in the diastolic aortic pressure gradient to nearly baseline at end-diastole. There is a mildly elevated anterograde velocity of 2.7 m/s, which is indicative of increased volume flow across the valve, rather than significant stenosis.

Answer 3: A

The patient has a large pseudoaneurysm (pAn); there is a large echolucent space from a contained rupture with communication at the base of the LA adjacent to the LA appendage. The zoomed color Doppler shows a turbulent color flow near the LA appendage, which would not be consistent with a walled-off abscess (answer B). The large fluid collection is leading to abnormal contours of the LV anterior and anterolateral walls, which is not seen with a pleural effusion (answer C). The prosthetic mitral valve is seen in a normal position without evidence of paravalvular regurgitation, making dehiscence unlikely (answer D). Multimodality imaging with magnetic resonance imaging (MRI) in this patient (Fig. 14.30) demonstrates communication of blood flow *(arrow)* between the large pseudoaneurysm (pAn) and left atrium (LA), resulting in external compression of the LV.

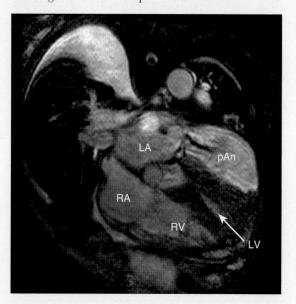

Fig. 14.30

Answer 4: B

A faint linear echodensity is seen in the LV outflow tract with a normal aortic valve and normal size LV and LA. This appearance is most consistent with a Lambl excrescence—a small filamentous structure, more often seen on the ventricular side of the valve, a normal variant that increases in prevalence with age. Endocarditis typically results in larger vegetations on the downstream side of the valve (LV side of aortic valve) in association with leaflet tissue destruction resulting in valve regurgitation. A papillary fibroelastoma is a benign tumor attached to the valve leaflet that appears as a mobile mass; although typically an incidental finding, a larger papillary fibroelastoma can be associated with thrombosis and adverse clinical events. Nonbacterial thrombotic endocarditis typically appears as a globular mass (or masses) attached to the upstream side (aortic side of aortic valve) in patients with systemic inflammatory disorders. These vegetations tend to be multiple, sessile masses on the leaflets. This might be an ultrasound artifact given the smooth linear appearance, but there is no obvious structure between the mass and transducer that might cause a reverberation artifact.

Answer 5: D

This CW Doppler signal was recorded from a midesophageal window at an image plane rotation angle of 28°. The guide image shows an oblique view of the aortic valve and LV outflow tract in the midportion of the image. The LA is adjacent to the transducer and the LV is not well seen. The Doppler tracing shows an early peaking systolic signal with a peak velocity of ≈3 m/s. There is a dense diastolic signal with a steep deceleration slope directed towards the transducer. The aortic root is not well visualized, but there is no clear fluid collection or echolucency adjacent to the aortic valve to suggest an abscess or pseudoaneurysm. The Doppler signal is not consistent with ventricular septal defect (VSD), which would show a high velocity systolic left-to-right shunt flow, not the bidirectional flow shown. Although the signal is not optimally aligned with LV outflow, the anterograde velocity is increased, at least 3 m/s, which should raise suspicion of prosthetic valve stenosis. However, the signal is early peaking (a normal flow pattern). In this case, the relatively mild increase in anterograde velocities is due to increased transvalvular flow from the significant aortic regurgitation. The aortic regurgitant signal is nearly as dense as the anterograde signal, and the steep deceleration slope suggests rapid equalization of the diastolic pressure gradient between the aorta and the LV.

Answer 6: C

This patient has abnormal thickening and asymmetry of the aortic valve consistent with a large vegetation, and it is likely that he has significant aortic regurgitation. This would manifest clinically with a widened pulse pressure (difference between systolic and diastolic blood pressures). Progressive atrioventricular (AV) nodal block on electrocardiogram (ECG) may occur in the setting of intramyocardial abscess extension with involvement of the conduction system. This parasternal view does not show a paravalvular abscess (typically shown as an echodense or echolucent region adjacent to the affected valve). Paravalvular abscess

is a more common manifestation of endocarditis associated with prosthetic valves. Patients with intramyocardial extension of an abscess to the point of interventricular septal rupture or rupture from the aorta to RV would have oxygenated blood entering the RV via the defect. On right heart catheterization, this would manifest as a step-up in oxygen saturation in blood sampled from the RV relative to the RA. Prominent internal jugular venous pulsation is a clinical examination finding in patients with severe tricuspid regurgitation, not seen in this case.

Answer 7: D

The patient presents with symptoms of infection and bradycardia. The TEE image demonstrates a cardiac abscess with both echolucent cystic and echodense thickness changes in the aortic annulus and intravalvular fibrosa, consistent with endocarditis. The most likely cause of syncope is high-grade atrioventricular heart block due to the abscess as seen on the rhythm strip in the echo image. Cardiac abscesses require debridement and valve replacement with cardiac surgery for curative treatment. TEE provides superior imaging to diagnose a paravalvular abscess and should be considered when there are high-risk features, such as fever and new-onset heart block. Only a small segment of the mitral valve is included in this image, but there is no evidence for acute mitral regurgitation. The aorta is slightly enlarged, but a dissection flap is not seen. There are no findings to indicate a pericardial effusion or tamponade. Incidentally, extensive shadowing distal to the aortic valve indicates severe aortic valve calcification, so she likely has bicuspid valve disease with underlying aortic stenosis as well.

Answer 8: A

The images show a bioprosthetic aortic valve with extensive vegetations and probable valve dehiscence. The bioprosthetic struts can be seen in the correct annular position in diastole but exhibit significant anterior movement and annular separation into the aortic root during systole. Paravalvular regurgitation is likely, as the prosthetic valve is no longer attached to the annulus circumferentially. However, diagnosis of paravalvular regurgitation may require TEE, because shadowing from prosthesis may obscures the color Doppler signal from the transthoracic windows. Septic pulmonary embolism (answer B) is a complication of right-sided (not left-sided) endocarditis. Prosthetic aortic valve endocarditis is associated with aortic (not mitral) annular abscess formation (answer C). Endocarditis rarely is complicated by a significant pericardial effusion or tamponade (answer D). When present, an effusion may be purulent due to rupture of a mitral annular abscess into the pericardial space.

Answer 9: E

This high-velocity systolic signal directed away from the apex might be due to aortic stenosis, mitral regurgitation, tricuspid regurgitation (if severe pulmonary hypertension is present), or a ventricular septal defect. All of these are possible with this clinical presentation; for example, this patient could have a postmyocardial infarction ventricular septal defect or papillary muscle rupture. This signal can be identified as mitral regurgitation based on the timing relative to the QRS (starts early) and associated diastolic flow signal. In diastole, an LV filling curve is seen with an E and A wave, with velocities typical of left (not right) heart filling. The systolic signal begins and ends exactly at the end and beginning of the diastolic flow signal, confirming this is mitral regurgitation, not aortic stenosis, which would have slight gaps in the onset and offset of flow due to isovolumic contraction and relaxation. In fact, the denser aortic signal can be seen "underneath" the mitral regurgitant signal on the first beat. The shape of the velocity curve is suggestive of *acute* regurgitation, with a rapid decline in velocity in late systole, instead of the more rounded waveform of chronic regurgitation. With acute regurgitation, the rise in LV pressure (or v wave) as the regurgitant flow fills the small noncompliant chamber results in a smaller pressure difference (and lower velocity) between the LV and LA. Endocarditis can present as pulmonary edema or cardiogenic shock if there is valve destruction with severe regurgitation, as in this example. Echocardiography reliability identifies the valve dysfunction and may demonstrate the cause of regurgitation—for example, vegetations consistent with endocarditis or a wall motion abnormality and papillary muscle rupture consistent with myocardial infarction. Mitral stenosis can present acutely if there is a concurrent medical issue (such as infection or anemia) with increased cardiac demand, but Doppler would show the typical *diastolic* flow signal. A high-velocity tricuspid regurgitant jet due to pulmonary hypertension is longer in duration than mitral regurgitation, and the associated flow in diastole is lower-velocity tricuspid, not mitral, inflow. It can be challenging to separate a ventricular septal defect signal from mitral regurgitation, but duration typically is longer, and the mitral inflow signal is usually not seen in diastole. Instead, low-velocity left-to-right flow across the septal defect may be seen in diastole along with the high-velocity systolic jet.

Answer 10: D

These findings are consistent with a perforated anterior mitral leaflet. The color Doppler image demonstrates a flow disturbance entering the LA from either the aorta or the LV outflow tract; it is difficult to be certain of the position of this image plane relative to the aortic valve in the short-axis plane. The corresponding long-axis view showed the flow disturbance originating at the base of the anterior mitral leaflet. Review of the operative report showed that the aortic homograft was trimmed to retain a segment of the anterior mitral leaflet base, which was used to repair the native mitral valve. The perforation is between the homograft and native leaflet tissue. The CW Doppler is diagnostic showing a high-velocity systolic waveform consistent with mitral regurgitation. Although the Doppler signal for a ventricular septal defect might be similar, there usually is a low-velocity diastolic component because of the slight diastolic pressure difference between the ventricles, and the color flow image is not consistent with a ventricular septal defect. An aortic to LA fistula would exhibit high-velocity systolic *and diastolic* flow due to the higher aortic, relative to LA, diastolic pressure. An aortic annular abscess may have areas of flow, but the CW Doppler velocity is low and the color signal is localized to the area adjacent to the valve. Aortic regurgitation is a likely complication of endocarditis but, of course, is a diastolic flow signal from the aorta into the LV.

Answer 11: B

The patient has several echocardiographic features of nonbacterial thrombotic endocarditis. There is a small echodense vegetation on the atrial side of the mitral valve at the coaptation point with minimal mobility. In the clinical setting of lupus without other signs of infection, a Libman-Sacks endocarditis is most likely. Culture negative infectious endocarditis (answer A) is uncommon and most often associated with previous antibiotic use. There are not enough Duke Criteria (fever, immunologic phenomena, vascular phenomena) present to support a diagnosis of infectious endocarditis. Although a valvular myxoma (answer C) may rarely occur, these are more often mobile and located within the atrial wall with a characteristic pedunculated mass and narrow stalk. Mitral annular calcification (answer D) can have a round and bright echogenic appearance but would be more commonly found in older individuals. The lesion shown is in the leaflet coaptation, not in the annulus.

Answer 12: C

The patient has endocarditis with bacteremia and vegetation with perforated leaflet of the anterior mitral valve with severe regurgitation. A mobile vegetation can be seen in the anterior leaflet. 3D imaging of the mitral valve is useful for localization of vegetations and perforations. There is no pathology or flail of the posterior leaflet seen (answer C). Annular dilation (answer D) would be expected in chronic heart failure with LV dilation and is usually a centrally oriented mitral jet. Mitral abscess (answer B) would demonstrate echogenic thickness or cystic structure most commonly around the annulus.

15 Cardiac Masses and Potential Cardiac Source of Embolus

BASIC PRINCIPLES

- The first step in evaluation of a cardiac mass on echocardiography is to determine if the findings are due to an ultrasound artifact or an actual anatomic finding (Fig. 15.1).
- A prominent normal cardiac structure of a normal anatomic variant may be mistaken for an abnormal mass (Table 15.1).
- Ultrasound has limited utility for determination of tissue type; diagnosis of a cardiac mass is based on location, attachment, appearance, and any associated abnormalities.

❖ KEY POINTS

- Image quality for evaluation of a cardiac mass is optimized by using:
  - Highest transducer frequency with adequate tissue penetration
  - Acoustic access adjacent to the structure of interest (e.g., transthoracic apical for ventricular thrombi versus transesophageal echocardiography [TEE] for atrial thrombi)
  - Visualization of the motion of the mass with the cardiac cycle
  - Use of a narrow sector and zoom mode once a mass is identified
  - Careful gain and processing adjustments (excessive or inadequate gain can obscure a mass)
  - Off-axis views from standard image planes
- A detailed knowledge of cardiac anatomy and normal variants allows recognition of structures that may mimic a cardiac mass.
- Echocardiography cannot identify the etiology of a cardiac mass based on appearance. A differential diagnosis for the echocardiographic finding is based on the location, appearance, size, mobility, physiologic effects, and other findings associated with the mass.

- Clinical data and other echocardiographic findings often provide clues about the identity of a cardiac mass (e.g., a left atrial mass in a patient with severe rheumatic mitral stenosis likely is an atrial thrombus).

STEP-BY-STEP APPROACH

Step 1: Left Atrial Thrombi

- Left atrial thrombi most often form in the atrial appendage, particularly in patients with atrial fibrillation (Fig. 15.2).

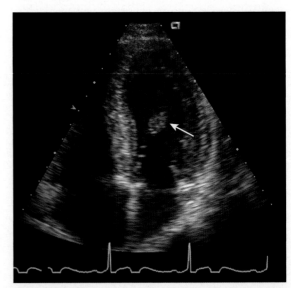

Fig. 15.1 **Normal cardiac structure.** In this apical 4-chamber view, an apparent mass *(arrow)* is seen in the LV chamber. Given the relationship of this mass to the anterior mitral leaflet, this most likely is a normal papillary muscle tip, seen in oblique view. This diagnosis can be confirmed by scanning posteriorly to show its connection to the lateral LV wall.

TABLE 15.1	Structures That May Be Mistaken for an Abnormal Cardiac Mass
Left atrium	Dilated coronary sinus (persistent left SVC) Raphe between left superior pulmonary vein and LA appendage Atrial suture line after cardiac transplant Beam-width artifact from calcified aortic valve, aortic valve prosthesis, or other echogenic target adjacent to the atrium Interatrial septal aneurysm
Right atrium	Crista terminalis Chiari network (Eustachian valve remnants) Lipomatous hypertrophy of the interatrial septum Trabeculation of RA appendage Atrial suture line after cardiac transplant Pacer wire, Swan-Ganz catheter, or central venous line
Left ventricle	Papillary muscles LV web (aberrant chordae) Prominent apical trabeculations Prominent mitral annular calcification
Right ventricle	Moderator band Papillary muscles Swan-Ganz catheter or pacer wire
Aortic valve	Nodules of Arantius Lambl excrescences Base of valve leaflet seen *en face* in diastole
Mitral valve	Redundant chordae Myxomatous mitral valve tissue
Pulmonary artery	LA appendage (just caudal to pulmonary artery)
Pericardium	Epicardial adipose tissue Fibrinous debris in a chronic organized pericardial effusion

SVC, Superior vena cava.
From Otto CM: *Textbook of Clinical Echocardiography*, ed 6, Philadelphia, 2018, Elsevier.

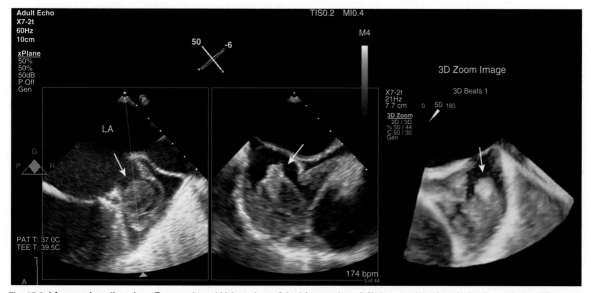

Fig. 15.2 **LA appendage thrombus.** Transesophageal biplane views of the LA appendage *(left)* shows an irregular echodensity consistent with an atrial thrombus *(arrows)* in a patient with atrial fibrillation. The 3D zoom image *(right)* shows the relationship of the thrombus to the atrial appendage in more detail.

- Thrombi may be seen in the body of the left atrium (LA) with severe stasis of blood flow (e.g., with mitral stenosis).
- TEE is required to exclude LA thrombi when clinically indicated.

❖ KEY POINTS

- Transthoracic echocardiography (TTE) is not sensitive for the diagnosis of LA thrombi due to the distance between the transducer and LA (limiting image quality at that depth) and the small size and location in the atrial appendage of most thrombi.
- The LA appendage may be visualized on transthoracic imaging in a parasternal short-axis view or in an apical 2-chamber view, but image quality often is limited.
- TEE images of the LA appendage are obtained from a high esophageal position. Evaluation includes:
  - Use of a high transducer frequency (typically 7 MHz)
  - A narrow image sector and zoom mode
  - Visualization in at least two orthogonal views, typically in views rotated to 0° and 60° (Use of simultaneous biplane imaging with a three-dimensional [3D] probe is optimal.)
  - Pulsed Doppler recording of atrial appendage flow with the sample volume about 1 cm from the junction of the atrial appendage with the LA chamber
- The normal Doppler velocity with atrial contraction is more than 0.4 m/s; lower velocities in sinus rhythm suggest contractile dysfunction.
- The LA appendage has normal trabeculations that are distinguished from thrombus by their continuity with and echogenicity similar to the appendage

wall, as well as their lack of independent mobility (Fig. 15.3).
- Reverberation artifact from the ridge between the left upper pulmonary vein and LA appendage may hinder definitive exclusion of an appendage thrombus.

Step 2: Left Ventricular Thrombi

- Left ventricular (LV) thrombus formation occurs in regions of blood flow stasis or low-velocity flow.
- LV thrombi most often form in an akinetic or dyskinetic apex after myocardial infarction (Fig. 15.4).

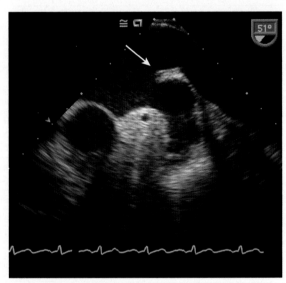

Fig. 15.3 **Normal atrial appendage anatomy.** Transesophageal imaging of the LA appendage at about 50° using a 7-MHz transducer frequency. The normal ridge between the LA appendage and left superior pulmonary vein is clearly seen *(arrow)*. The LA appendage was imaged in several planes to evaluate for possible thrombus. The small circular echolucent structure seen between the LV outflow tract and LA is a cross section of the circumflex coronary artery.

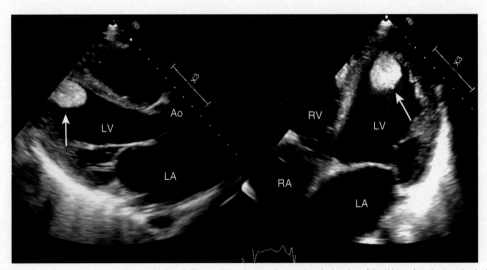

Fig. 15.4 **LV thrombus.** In a low parasternal long-axis view *(left)*, an echogenic mass is seen in apical region of the LV. In a foreshortened apical view *(right)*, the large echogenic mass is seen in an akinetic apex consistent with LV thrombus. *Ao,* Aorta.

- LV thrombi also are seen in patients with severely reduced LV systolic dysfunction.

❖ **KEY POINTS**

- ❏ TTE from the apical window is the optimal approach to detection of LV thrombi, with a sensitivity of 92% to 95% and a specificity of 86% to 88%.
- ❏ Detection of LV apical thrombi is enhanced by:
  - ❏ A steep left lateral decubitus patient position on a stretcher with an apical cutout
  - ❏ Use of a high transducer frequency (typically 5 to 7 MHz)
  - ❏ Standard and oblique image planes of the apex, especially medial angulation from a lateral transducer position
  - ❏ A shallow depth setting
- ❏ Myocardial trabeculations are differentiated from thrombi by their linear shape with an echodensity similar to and attachment to the myocardium (Fig. 15.5).
- ❏ Left echo contrast is helpful in identifying thrombus when image quality is suboptimal.
- ❏ Transesophageal imaging is not sensitive for diagnosis of LV apical thrombi, because the apex is in the far field of the image and the true apex may not be included in the image plane.

Step 3: Right Heart Thrombi

- RA thrombi may be seen in patients with central lines that abrade the RA wall.
- Thrombi also may form on permanent pacer leads in the right atrium (RA) or right ventricle (RV).

- Peripheral venous thrombi may embolize to the right heart and become entangled in the tricuspid valve chords or a RA Chiari network (Fig. 15.6).

❖ **KEY POINTS**

- ❏ Normal echogenic structures in the RA that may be mistaken for a thrombus include:

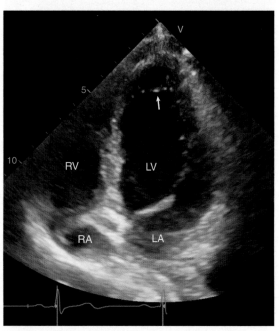

Fig. 15.5 **LV web.** A thin bright linear echodensity is seen in the LV apex that connects with myocardium at both ends and is not associated with wall motion abnormalities. This finding is consistent with an LV "web" or aberrant trabeculation and is a normal variant. Often slightly off-axis views (as in this example) are needed to show the connections of the web to the myocardium at both ends.

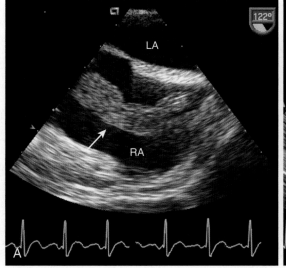
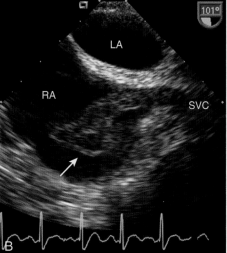

Fig. 15.6 **Thrombus in transit.** (A) In this TEE long-axis view of the RA, a large, echogenic, tubular, mobile mass *(arrow)* is seen. (B) Slight medial turning of the TEE probe demonstrates that the mass *(arrow)* originates from the region of the superior vena cava *(SVC)*. By imaging in multiple planes, the attachment of this mass to a chronic indwelling catheter was demonstrated. The location, clinical setting, and appearance of the mass are most consistent with thrombus.

❏   Eustachian valve or Chiari network (Fig. 15.7)
❏   Crista terminalis (Fig. 15.8)
❏   Eustachian valves and Chiari networks are thin filamentous structures that extend from the region of the inferior vena cava (IVC) toward the superior

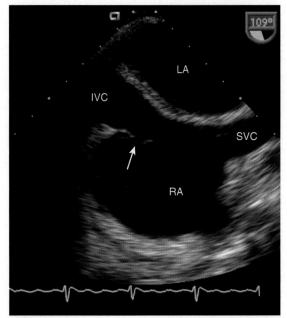

Fig. 15.7 **Eustachian valve.** In this TEE bicaval view, a linear mobile echo originating from the junction of the inferior vena cava *(IVC)* and RA is seen, consistent with a normal eustachian valve. In some patients, this embryologic remnant is more extensive, forming a network of filamentous strands extending from the region of the inferior to the superior vena cava *(SVC).* This finding, called a *Chiari network,* may appear on TTE imaging as bright mobile echoes with chaotic motion in the RA often best appreciated in parasternal short-axis, RV inflow, and subcostal 4-chamber views.

vena cava (SVC). The bright mobile echoes of a Chiari network may look similar to echo contrast in the RA.

❏   The RA and RV are examined in parasternal short-axis and RV inflow views, in the apical 4-chamber view, and from the subcostal window.

❏   Transesophageal imaging provides improved visualization of the right heart when thrombi are suspected.

Step 4: Nonprimary Cardiac Tumors

■   Nonprimary cardiac tumors are 20 times more common than primary cardiac tumors.

■   Nonprimary tumors can involve the heart by:
   ○   Direct extension
   ○   Metastatic spread of disease
   ○   Production of biologically active substances
   ○   Side effects related to treatment of the primary tumor

■   Nonprimary cardiac tumors most often involve the pericardium but also may invade the myocardium. They rarely appear as intracardiac masses (Fig. 15.9).

❖   **KEY POINTS**

❏   The most common nonprimary cardiac tumors, in order of frequency, are:
   ❏   Lung
   ❏   Lymphoma
   ❏   Breast
   ❏   Leukemia
   ❏   Stomach
   ❏   Melanoma
   ❏   Liver
   ❏   Colon

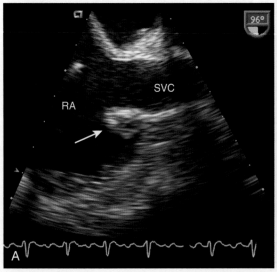
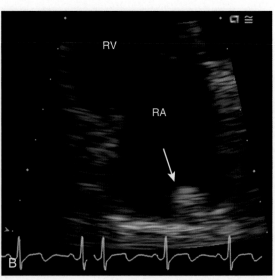

Fig. 15.8 **Crista terminalis.** (A) This TEE long-axis image of the superior vena cava *(SVC)* and RA demonstrates the crista *(arrow),* the ridge at the junction of the trabeculated and smooth segments of the RA wall. (B) The crista terminalis often is seen in the transthoracic apical 4-chamber view as a slight bump on the superior aspect of the RA wall *(arrow).*

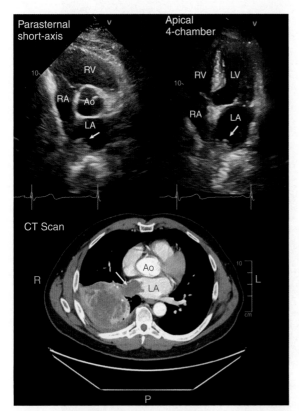

Fig. 15.9 Direct extension of non-cardiac tumor. In the parasternal short-axis view *(top left)*, a mass *(arrows)* is seen in the LA that appears to be protruding from the right upper pulmonary view. The apical 4-chamber view *(top right)* confirms an irregular mass protruding from the right upper pulmonary vein with some areas of independent mobility. A computed tomography (CT) scan done later that day *(bottom)* better shows the mass protruding into the LA by direct extension from a large lung tumor. *Ao,* Aorta.

❏ All these tumors may involve the pericardium by direct extension (breast, lung) or by metastatic spread, presenting with a pericardial effusion, sometimes with tamponade physiology.

❏ Renal cell carcinoma may extend up the IVC into the RA and may be removed surgically en bloc with the primary tumor.

❏ Carcinoid heart disease is characterized by thickening and shortening of the right heart valve leaflets, resulting in pulmonic and tricuspid regurgitation (Fig. 15.10).

❏ Some forms of chemotherapy affect myocardial function, so periodic monitoring of ejection fraction by echocardiography often is recommended.

❏ Radiation therapy that included cardiac structures in the treatment field may have very late (20 years or greater) adverse cardiac effects, including valve disease, accelerated coronary atherosclerosis, pericardial constriction, and myocardial fibrosis.

❏ TTE in standard views usually is adequate for evaluation of nonprimary cardiac tumors, but TEE provides improved image quality when needed.

❏ 3D imaging may be helpful in defining the relationship of the mass to other cardiac structures.

Step 5: Primary Cardiac Tumors

■ Primary cardiac tumors in adults usually are histologically benign.

■ Benign cardiac tumors result in adverse clinical outcomes due to both:
  ○ Obstruction of blood flow
  ○ Embolization

■ Primary cardiac tumors most often present on echocardiography as an intracardiac mass.

❖ **KEY POINTS**

❏ The most common primary cardiac tumors in adults, in order of frequency, are:
  ❏ Myxoma (Fig. 15.11)
  ❏ Pericardial cyst
  ❏ Lipoma
  ❏ Papillary fibroelastoma (Fig. 15.12)
  ❏ Angiosarcoma (malignant)
  ❏ Rhabdomyosarcoma (malignant)

❏ Myxomas most often are seen in the LA (75% of cases), attached by a narrow stalk to the center of the interatrial septum. Myxomas less often are seen in the RA, LV, and RV.

❏ A pericardial cyst is a single or multilobed sac lined by mesothelium that communicates with the pericardial space. Pericardial cysts are rare but, when present, most often are seen adjacent to the RA.

❏ Papillary fibroelastomas typically are small masses attached to the downstream side of a cardiac valve. The appearance is similar to a vegetation (except that vegetations usually are on the upstream side of the valve), but blood cultures are negative and clinical signs of endocarditis are absent.

❏ Lipomatous hypertrophy of the interatrial septum is common, with a typical appearance of sparing of the fossa ovalis. If in doubt, computed tomographic imaging confirms adipose tissue.

❏ Malignant primary cardiac tumors are rare, usually seen as an intracardiac mass.

❏ The goals of echocardiography in patients with a cardiac tumor are:
  ❏ Define the location and extent of tumor involvement
  ❏ Evaluate obstruction or regurgitation due to the tumor
  ❏ Evaluate any associated pericardial effusion and signs of tamponade

❏ Often both transthoracic and transesophageal imaging are needed to fully evaluate a cardiac tumor. Masses located in the LA may be missed on transthoracic imaging (Fig. 15.13).

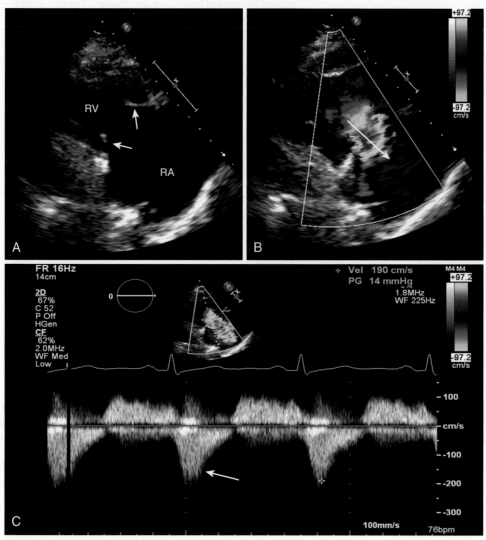

Fig. 15.10 Carcinoid heart disease. (A) In a RV inflow view the shortened thickened tricuspid leaflets *(arrows)* are pathognomonic for a diagnosis of carcinoid disease. (B) Color Doppler shows a wide jet of tricuspid regurgitation. (C) CW Doppler shows low velocity forward and reverse flow *(arrow)* across the tricuspid valve consistent with severe regurgitation and normal pulmonary pressures.

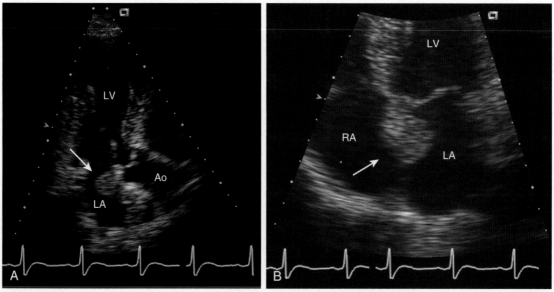

Fig. 15.11 Atrial myxoma. The location and smooth contour of this LA mass, seen in an apical long-axis view (A) and a 4-chamber view (B), is consistent with an atrial myxoma. *Ao,* Aorta.

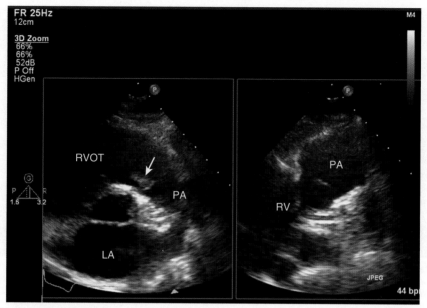

Fig. 15.12 Pulmonic valve papillary fibroelastoma. In a biplane parasternal view, a small mobile mass *(arrow)* is seen attached to the pulmonic valve but with independent motion. The patient had no systemic symptoms, and blood cultures were negative. The size and shape of this mass have been stable on annual examinations over the past 5 years suggesting a diagnosis of papillary fibroelastoma. *RVOT,* Right ventricular outflow tract.

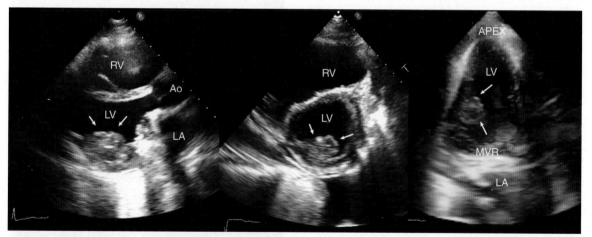

Fig. 15.13 Primary cardiac tumor. Recurrent primary malignant cardiac sarcoma with recurrence 4 years after prior resection and mechanical mitral valve replacement. The long-axis view *(left)* shows a large mass *(arrows)* involving the posterior LV wall and protruding into the LV chamber. The mitral valve prosthesis causes reverberations and shadowing. The parasternal short-axis view *(center)* shows the medial-lateral size of the mass *(arrows)*. 3D imaging *(right)* provides further visualization of the size and location of the LV mass. *Ao,* Aorta; *MVR,* mitral valve replacement.

Step 6: Vegetations

- Vegetations are infected or noninfected masses of platelets and fibrin debris, typically attached to a valve leaflet.
- The vegetations of nonbacterial thrombotic endocarditis are small and attached to the downstream (compared with upstream with infective vegetations) side of the valve (Fig. 15.14).
- Infective vegetations are discussed in Chapter 14.

❖ KEY POINTS

- ❏ The most critical step in evaluation of a patient with an intracardiac mass, especially a valve vegetation, is to obtain blood cultures for possible infective endocarditis.
- ❏ Like infective endocarditis, nonbacterial thrombotic endocarditis is diagnosed based on a combination of clinical and echocardiographic findings.
- ❏ TEE is more accurate for diagnosis of nonbacterial valve vegetations compared with transthoracic imaging.
- ❏ Valve involvement by noninfected vegetations is seen in patients with systemic inflammatory diseases (i.e., systemic lupus erythematosus) and some malignancies.

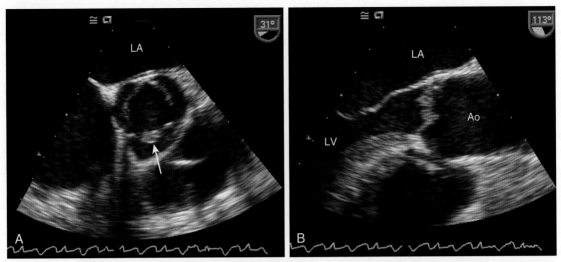

Fig. 15.14 **Nonbacterial thrombotic endocarditis.** A small mass *(arrow)* is seen on the right coronary cusp of the aortic valve on this TEE short-axis image (A) with the long-axis view (B) showing small masses at the leaflet base and at the leaflet tip. These masses showed independent motion in real time suggestive of vegetations. The patient had no clinical signs of endocarditis and blood cultures were negative, so these findings may be due to nonbacterial thrombotic endocarditis. *Ao,* Aorta.

Step 7: Benign Valve-Associated Lesions

- Nodules of Arantius are small nodules at the central coaptation points of the semilunar valves.
- Lambl excrescences are thin, mobile, linear echodensities seen on the downstream side of a valve, most commonly the aortic valve.
- Calcification of the posterior mitral annulus is common in the elderly.

❖ KEY POINTS

- ☐ Nodules of Arantius typically are more prominent with age on the aortic side of the valve.
- ☐ Lambl excrescences also are more common in older patients, are most often seen in the LV outflow tract, and may be mistaken for a vegetation. They less often are seen on the LA side of the mitral valve.
- ☐ Caseous calcification of the mitral annulus is a rare variant of mitral annular calcification, appearing as a smooth, round periannular mass with a central echolucent zone by echocardiography.

Step 8: Patent Foramen Ovale

- A small communication (patent foramen ovale) between the RA and LA is present in 20% to 30% of adults.
- In some patients, a patent foramen ovale is associated with a contour abnormality of the septum

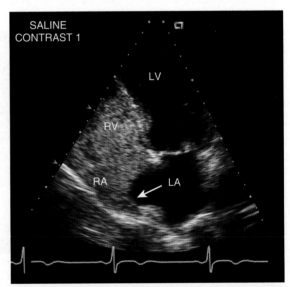

Fig. 15.15 **Atrial septal aneurysm.** An atrial septal aneurysm is seen in this apical 4-chamber view with saline contrast used to opacify the right heart. The atrial septum deviates from left to right in the region of the fossa ovalis with a radius of more than 15 mm at the maximum curvature point.

with bulging from the midline more than 15 mm (atrial septal aneurysm) (Fig. 15.15).
- There is a higher prevalence of patent foramen ovale in patients with a cryptogenic stroke.

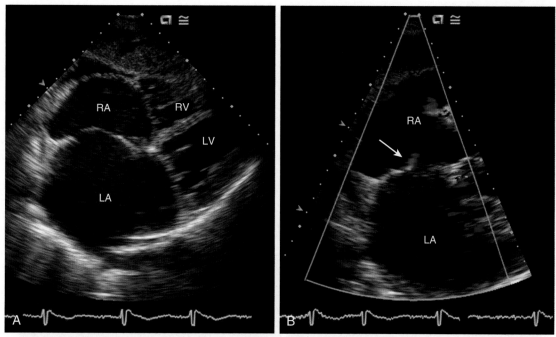

Fig. 15.16 **TTE of patent foramen ovale.** (A) In a subcostal 4-chamber view the atrial septum bulges toward the RA. (B) Color Doppler demonstrates a small jet of flow *(arrow)* from left to right across the interatrial septum consistent with a patent foramen ovale.

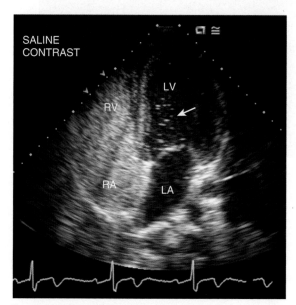

Fig. 15.17 **Saline contrast study.** Saline contrast study in an apical 4-chamber view in a patient with a systemic embolic event shows a small amount of contrast *(arrow)* in the left heart within three beats of contrast appearance in the right heart consistent with a patent foramen ovale.

❖ **KEY POINTS**

☐ Shunting at the atrial level is sometimes seen with color Doppler but often requires a saline contrast injection for detection (Figs. 15.16 and 15.17).

☐ A patent foramen ovale allows blood flow from RA to LA when RA pressure exceeds LA pressure.

In some patients, shunting occurs at rest; in others, a right-to-left shunt is seen only after Valsalva maneuver to transiently increase RA pressure.

☐ Appearance of echo contrast in the LA within three beats of right heart opacification is consistent with a patent foramen ovale. Later appearance of contrast (after three to five cycles) may be due to transpulmonary passage.

☐ Longer digital clip lengths, which include entry of contrast into the right heart and at least five beats after RA opacification, are needed for evaluation of a saline contrast study. Review of videotaped images may be needed to include an adequate number of cardiac cycles with each injection.

☐ At least two saline contrast injections are needed—one at rest and one with Valsalva maneuver. However, accuracy is optimized with at least four contrast injections, two at rest and two with Valsalva.

☐ Saline contrast studies are sensitive for detection of a patent foramen ovale but do not provide accurate size estimates, because the amount of shunting depends on timing, relative pressures, and other factors in addition to size of the defect.

☐ TEE is more sensitive than transthoracic imaging for detection of a patent foramen ovale (Fig. 15.18). In patients with chronically elevated RA pressures (such as severe pulmonary hypertension with right heart failure), persistent right-to-left shunting may result in arterial oxygen desaturation.

☐ Echocardiography (TEE or TTE) can be used to guide percutaneous closure of a patent foramen ovale (Fig. 15.19).

Step 9: Evaluation for Other Cardiac Sources of Embolus

- Echocardiography requested to evaluate for a cardiac source of embolus should include a saline contrast study for detection of patent foramen ovale.
- A careful examination for cardiac thrombi, tumors, valvular vegetations, and aortic atheroma, often with TEE, is needed when a cardiac source of embolus is suspected (Table 15.2).

❖ KEY POINTS

- ❑ If atrial fibrillation is present, an LA thrombus is a likely cause of clinical events, even if not detected on TEE.

- ❑ Embolic events in patients with mechanical prosthetic valves must be presumed to be related to the prosthetic valve, regardless of echocardiographic findings.
- ❑ Aortic atheroma, detected on TEE, are associated with an increased prevalence of embolic events.
- ❑ TEE to evaluate for a cardiac source of embolus is recommended in patients with:
  - ❑ Abrupt occlusion of a major peripheral or visceral artery
  - ❑ Unexplained embolic stroke in patients younger than 60 years old
  - ❑ Whenever clinical management would be altered based on the echocardiographic findings

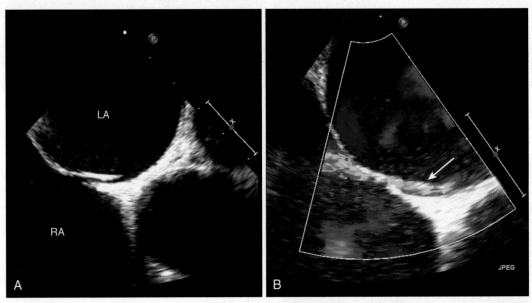

Fig. 15.18 TTE of patent foramen ovale. (A) TEE in a patient with a cryptogenic stroke shows the typical "flap valve" appearance of a patent foramen ovale on 2D imaging with (B) color Doppler demonstrating a narrow red flow signal *(arrow)* in the slit-like orifice.

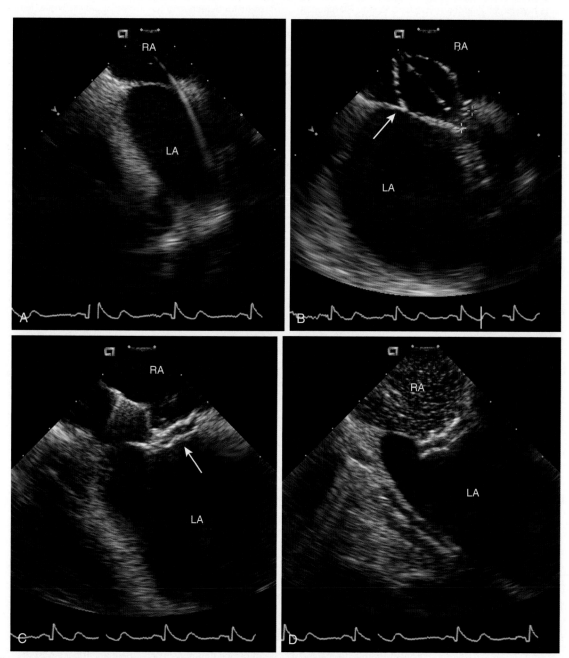

Fig. 15.19 Intracardiac echocardiographic guidance of percutaneous closure of a patent foramen ovale. The transducer tip (top of the sector) is in the RA, with the septum in the midfield and LA in the far field of the images. (A) The guiding catheter has been passed through the patent foramen ovale. (B) A sizing balloon is inflated to measure the defect size. (C) The closure device is in position but still attached to the catheter seen in the RA. (D) The guiding catheter has been removed and contrast injected into the right heart. The parallel linear echoes of the closure device are seen positioned on the atrial septum with no evidence for residual shunting.

TABLE 15.2	European Association of Echocardiography Recommendations for Echocardiography in Diagnosis and Management of Cardiac Sources of Embolism		
Clinical Condition	**TTE**	**TEE**	**Comments**
Acute myocardial infarction	Evaluate LV and RV function and detect LV thrombus	Not useful for detection of LV thrombus	Contrast may improve detection of LV thrombus on TTE
Cardiomyopathy	Evaluate LV and RV dysfunction, detect LV thrombus		Contrast may improve detection of LV thrombus on TTE
Atrial fibrillation	Detect underlying structural heart disease To indicate, guide, and follow-up invasive surgical procedures	Required to exclude atrial thrombus in guiding cardioversion, pre-ablation, recurrent embolism, and to determine risk of future embolism	
Detection of PFO	May be sufficient to detect PFO with good image quality, saline contrast with Valsalva maneuver	Highest sensitivity for detection and evaluation of PFO	Factors that suggest an association between stroke and PFO include (1) a temporal relationship with a venous thrombosis, (2) younger age (<55 years) and absence of other causes, (3) associated atrial septal aneurysm, and (4) large spontaneous or provokable right-to-left shunt
Aortic atherosclerosis	Suprasternal TTE may help identify arch atheromas	TEE may be indicated when TTE images are suboptimal or when plaque characterization is needed	
Cardiac masses	Recommended for patients with clinical syndromes suggesting a cardiac mass or patients with conditions known to predispose to mass formation Recommended for follow-up after mass removal if recurrence is likely	TEE is appropriate when TTE is nondiagnostic	
Endocarditis	Recommended as first step in evaluation of endocarditis	Recommended when TTE is negative and clinical likelihood is high, with prosthetic valves or when TTE provides inadequate imaging	Repeat TTE or TEE recommended in 7-10 days if initial study is negative but clinical likelihood remains high
Prosthetic valves	TTE must be performed in patients with a prosthetic valve and embolic event.	TEE also must be performed in patients with a prosthetic valve and embolic event, even if TTE is negative	Repeat TTE or TEE is recommended for follow-up after thrombolytic or anticoagulant therapy
Intracardiac devices	TTE is recommended in patients with a device and a pulmonary emboli event or when paradoxical embolus is suspected	TEE is also used for diagnosis of device thrombosis or infection	Intracardiac devices include permanent pacemakers and implantable cardioverters defibrillators

PFO, Patent foramen ovale.
Data from Pepi M, Evangelista A, et al: Recommendations for echocardiography use in the diagnosis and management of cardiac sources of embolism: European Association of Echocardiography (EAE) (a registered branch of the ESC). *Eur J Echocardiogr* 11:461-476, 2010.
From Otto CM: *Textbook of Clinical Echocardiography*, ed 6, Philadelphia, 2018, Elsevier.

THE ECHO EXAM

Echocardiographic Findings Associated With Systemic Embolism

Potential Embolic Source	Clinical Setting	Echocardiographic Findings	Caveats
Patent foramen ovale (PFO)	• Cryptogenic stroke	• Saline contrast shows right-to-left shunt at the atrial level; best visualized in TEE	• PFO present in 20%–30% of people
LA thrombus	• Atrial fibrillation—before cardioversion, AF ablation, or mitral commissurotomy	• LA mass, most often located in LA appendage, often mobile	• TEE required for diagnosis of LV thrombus because of low sensitivity of TTE
Endocarditis	• Bacteremia • Clinical criteria for endocarditis	• Valve vegetations with valve destruction	• TEE often needed in addition to TTE
Prosthetic valve thrombosis	• Mechanical or bioprosthetic valve	• Mobile mass attached to leaflets or sewing ring • Valve obstruction or regurgitation	• A prosthetic valve is always a potential embolic source, even when echo findings are absent
LV thrombus	• Apical akinesis after myocardial infarction • Global hypokinesis with dilated cardiomyopathy	• Echodense mass in LV apex	• Best seen on TTE apical views with high-frequency transducer • TEE has low sensitivity
Aortic atherosclerosis	• Evaluation for stroke or intraoperative evaluation of aorta for graft placement	• Typical atheroma	• Aortic arch visualization suboptimal on TEE • Intraoperative direct placement of a sterile probe on the aorta is an option
Non-bacterial thrombotic endocarditis	• Systemic inflammatory disease	• Valve masses with less independent motion than typical vegetations	• Blood cultures are needed to exclude infective endocarditis
Lipomatous hypertrophy of the atrial septum	• Benign incidental finding	• Bright, smooth thickening of the interatrial septum with sparing of the fossa ovalis	• Echo appearance is typical, but CT allows tissue characterization if diagnosis is unclear
Papillary fibroelastoma	• Cryptogenic stroke or incidental echo finding	• Highly mobile small mass, usually attached to valve, often with a stalk	• Blood cultures are needed to exclude infective endocarditis
Atrial myxoma	• TIA or stroke	• Well-circumscribed mass attached to atrial septum, most often in LA	• Best seen on TEE, but initial diagnosis often with TTE imaging
Secondary cardiac tumors	• Direct extension of lung or breast cancer into heart, or metastatic disease	• Pericardial effusion and tumor involvement is most common	• Further evaluation for a specific diagnosis is needed
Malignant primary cardiac tumors	• Rare in adults	• Intracardiac mass with invasion of chamber walls	• Imaging with CMR imaging or CT provides better definition of the site and extent of tumor involvement

AF, Atrial fibrillation; *CMR,* cardiac magnetic resonance; *CT,* computed tomography; *TIA,* transient ischemic attack.

Distinguishing Characteristics of Intracardiac Masses

Characteristic	Thrombus	Tumor	Vegetation
Location	• LA (especially when enlarged or associated with MV disease) • LV (in setting of reduced systolic function or segmental wall abnormalities)	• LA (myxoma) • Myocardium • Pericardium • Valves	• Usually valvular • Occasionally on ventricular wall or Chiari network
Appearance	• Usually discrete and somewhat spherical in shape or laminated against LV apex or LA wall	• Various: Circumscribed or irregular	• Irregular shape, attached to the proximal (upstream) side of the valve with motion independent from the valve
Associated findings	• Underlying cause usually evident • LV systolic dysfunction or segmental wall motion abnormalities (exception—eosinophilic heart disease) • MV disease with LA enlargement	• Intracardiac obstruction depending on site of tumor • Clinically: Fevers, systemic signs of endocarditis, positive blood cultures	• Valvular regurgitation usually present

MV, Mitral valve.

SELF-ASSESSMENT QUESTIONS

Question 1

The echocardiograms in Fig. 15.20 were obtained in four different individuals for evaluation of a stroke. Which patient has a potential cardiac source of emboli?

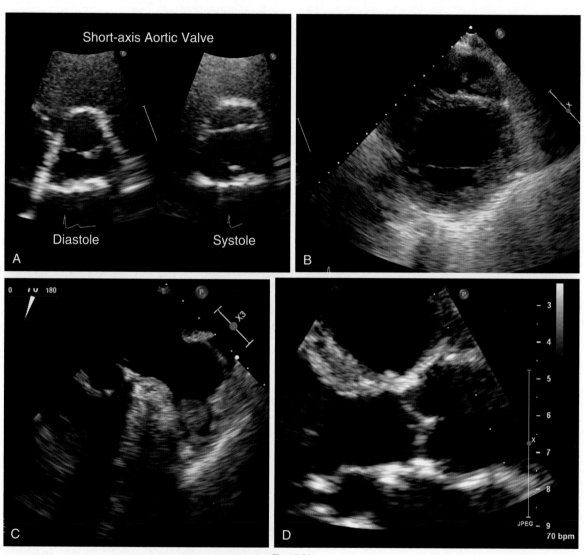

Fig. 15.20

Question 2

What is the most likely diagnosis for the mass *(arrow)* seen in this echocardiographic image (Fig. 15.21)?

- **A.** Central venous catheter
- **B.** Pacer lead
- **C.** Moderator band
- **D.** Apical thrombus

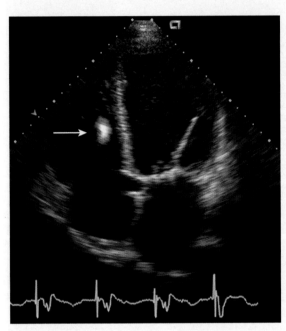

Fig. 15.21

Question 3

A 52-year-old woman suffered an acute stroke with left-sided weakness. The patient was afebrile with no other medical history. A transesophageal echocardiogram was obtained (Fig. 15.22). Which of the following best explains the findings demonstrated?

- **A.** Infectious endocarditis
- **B.** Lambl excrescences
- **C.** Thrombus
- **D.** Atrial fibrillation
- **E.** Papillary fibroelastoma

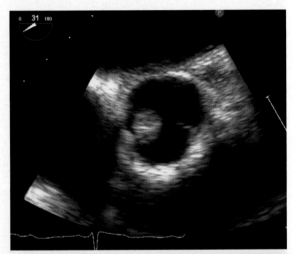

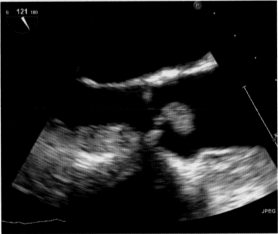

Fig. 15.22

Question 4

TEE was requested before elective cardioversion in a patient with symptomatic atrial fibrillation. The following finding *(arrow)* was identified on the transesophageal study (Fig. 15.23).

Based on this image, the most appropriate next step is:

A. Cancel cardioversion procedure

B. Proceed with cardioversion

C. Delay cardioversion and repeat TEE after 4 weeks of anticoagulation therapy

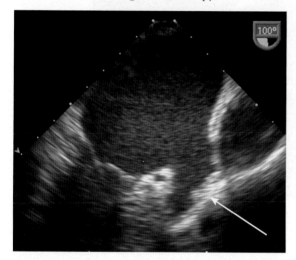

Fig. 15.23

Question 5

Doppler data were recorded during an elective TEE in an outpatient (Fig. 15.24).

This Doppler recording is most consistent with:

A. Normal sinus rhythm

B. Atrial fibrillation

C. Atrial flutter

D. Ventricular tachycardia

E. Ventricular fibrillation

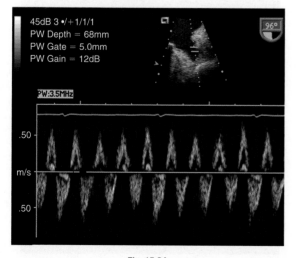

Fig. 15.24

Question 6

A 36-year-old woman presents for clinical evaluation. She describes a history of cough, intermittent fevers, and joint pain lasting for several months. A TTE is ordered and the following image is recorded (Fig. 15.25):

Based on the echocardiographic appearance of the finding, which one of the following recommendations would you make?

A. Parenteral antibiotic therapy

B. Cardiac magnetic resonance (CMR) imaging

C. Intravenous anticoagulation therapy

D. Cardiac surgery referral

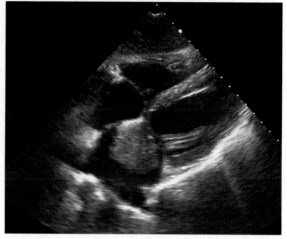

Fig. 15.25

Question 7

This M-mode tracing was obtained in a patient referred for evaluation of an embolic stroke (Fig. 15.26).

This finding is most consistent with:

A. Normal

B. Mitral stenosis

C. Aortic stenosis

D. Atrial septal aneurysm

E. Atrial myxoma

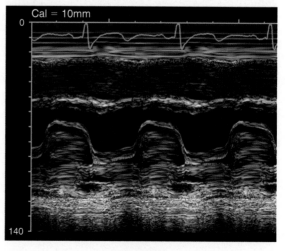

Fig. 15.26

Question 8

A 39-year-old woman is referred for TEE for two episodes of transient aphasia. Color Doppler imaging shows the following flow pattern (Fig. 15.27).

This finding is most consistent with:

A. Eustachian valve
B. Atrial myxoma
C. Crista terminalis
D. Thebesian valve

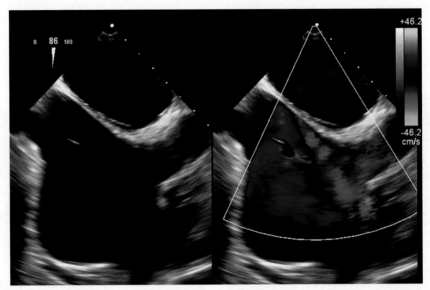

Fig. 15.27

Question 9

A 58-year-old male patient presents with progressive dyspnea. The image obtained (Fig. 15.28) suggests which of the following:

A. Atrial myxoma
B. Bacterial endocarditis
C. Intracardiac thrombus
D. Papillary fibroelastoma

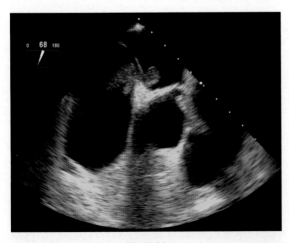

Fig. 15.28

Question 10

TEE is requested to evaluate for a potential cardiac source of embolus in a 73-year-old woman with a transient ischemic event (Fig. 15.29).

This finding is diagnostic of:

A. Atrial septal aneurysm
B. Patent foramen ovale (PFO)
C. Atrial myxoma
D. Lipomatous hypertrophy
E. Atrial septal occluder device

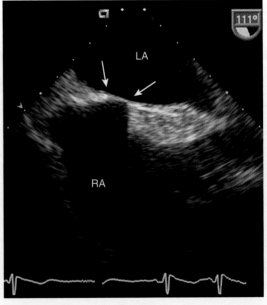

Fig. 15.29

Question 11

A 41-year-old woman presents with cardiopulmonary symptoms and a TTE is ordered. The following image is obtained (Fig. 15.30).

The most likely origin of this mass is:
- **A.** Intracardiac
- **B.** Pericardial
- **C.** Abdominal
- **D.** Intracranial

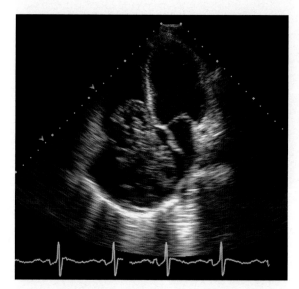

Fig. 15.30

Question 12

A 71-year-old woman presented with shortness of breath and weight loss of 3 months duration. An echocardiogram reported normal RV and LV size and function. An RV modified apical 4-chamber view demonstrated a cardiac mass (Fig. 15.31). The cardiac mass is most likely which of the following?
- **A.** Myxoma
- **B.** Malignant tumor
- **C.** Apical thrombus
- **D.** Papillary fibroelastoma
- **E.** Moderator band

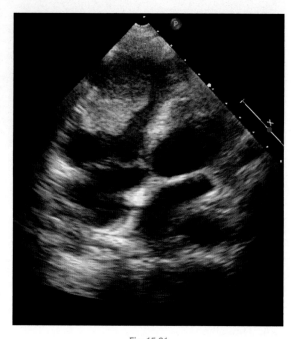

Fig. 15.31

Question 13

A 42-year-old woman had sudden onset of changes in vision. Ophthalmic examination revealed a central retinal arterial occlusion. A transesophageal echocardiogram was requested to evaluate for cardioembolic sources. An M-mode (Fig. 15.32) and 2D bicaval view at one cardiac cycle after right atrial opacification with agitated saline is shown. Which of the following best describe the findings?

A. Lipomatous hypertrophy

B. Secundum atrial septal defect

C. Pulmonary arteriovenous malformation

D. Interatrial septal aneurysm with patent foramen ovale (PFO)

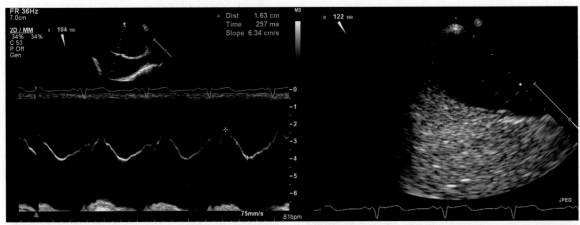

Fig. 15.32

Question 14

A 78-year-old man underwent echocardiography to evaluate LV function 1 month after an acute anterior myocardial infarction. The patient had a previously normal echocardiogram 3 months prior to his infarction. The patient had new septal and apical akinesis with an ejection fraction of 25%. The finding in Fig. 15.33 is most likely which of the following?

A. Thrombus

B. LV web

C. Primary cardiac tumor

D. Ring-down artifact

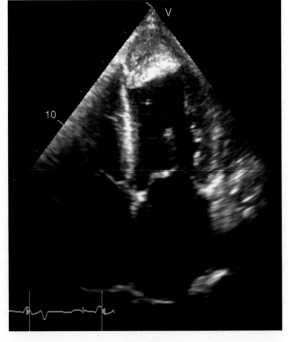

Fig. 15.33

ANSWERS

Answer 1: C

Patient C demonstrates a TEE zoomed view of the LA appendage with thrombus. LA appendage thrombus should be distinguished from normal trabeculations based on its size, mobility, and slightly different echogenicity compared to the appendage wall. The other images consist of normal variants. Patient A demonstrates small nodules at the central coaptation of the aortic valve consistent with nodules of Arantius, a benign valve-associated lesion. Patient B has a thin bright linear echo connecting at different ends in the myocardium consistent with a normal LV web variant. Patient D has a small Lambl excrescence, a small, thin linear echo most commonly seen on the aortic valve.

Answer 2: B

This bright dense "mass" seen in the RV is a pacer lead. This diagnosis can be confirmed by reviewing the clinical history (or asking the patient) and by imaging in other views to demonstrate the length of the pacer lead as it traverses the RA and RV. A central venous catheter should be in the superior vena cava (SVC) or RA; in the rare event that a central catheter extends into the RV, the thickness of the catheter is less than the metallic pacer leads. The moderator band is a normal muscle band closer to the RV apex, extending from the free wall to septum, with an echodensity similar to the rest of the myocardium. Ventricular thrombi are unusual in the RV but, when present, have an echodensity similar to myocardium and occur in regions of myocardial dysfunction. Peripheral venous thrombi may embolize to the heart and lodge in the RV or tricuspid valve apparatus, with a tubular shape reflecting formation in a peripheral vein.

Answer 3: E

The figure demonstrates an aortic valve during diastole with a 1 cm mass attached to the downstream side of the aortic valve. Large papillary fibroelastoma may be associated with the risk of stroke from potential thromboembolic events. The differential for papillary fibroelastoma includes valvular vegetations, but the patient has no reported infectious findings, and infectious endocarditis lesions are more often located upstream of the valve (answer A). Lambl excrescences (answer B) are more typically thin, mobile linear masses that are seen in normal older adults.

Thrombus (answer C) may be seen on prosthetic valves, but the valvular mass representing thrombus alone would be unlikely in an otherwise healthy adult. Atrial fibrillation is a common cause for stroke but would more likely demonstrate thrombus in the left atrial appendage. The rhythm strip in Fig. 15.2 demonstrates a normal rhythm.

Answer 4: B

This TEE image taken at 100° view shows an enlarged LA. The left atrial appendage is well seen and there is prominent trabeculation present *(arrow)*. Given the absence of thrombus, the elective cardioversion should proceed in this symptomatic patient. Trabeculations are differentiated from thrombus typically by higher echogenicity (brighter), continuity with the atrial wall, and contractile motion, although in patients with atrial fibrillation, contractile motion of the trabeculae will be decreased compared with patients in sinus rhythm. Multiple views of the left atrial appendage are needed to show continuity of trabeculations with atrial myocardium. In patients with a prominent ridge between the left atrial appendage and left upper pulmonary vein, acoustic shadowing of the appendage may hinder definitive evaluation for thrombus. Characteristic appearance of thrombus is one of blood stasis, with increased density at the tip of the appendage. When a thrombus is present, several weeks or months of anticoagulation are appropriate before re-evaluation for resolution of thrombus.

Answer 5: C

This Doppler signal was recorded in the left atrial appendage, seen in the 2D image in the 90° view, with the Doppler sample volume about 1 cm into the appendage. Regular flow in and out of the atrial appendage at a rate about 300 bpm is seen with a velocity about 0.5 m/s, in both directions. This is consistent with atrial flutter with typical atrial (and appendage) contractions at a rate of 300 bpm. Normal sinus rhythm results in flow out of the atrial appendage following the P-wave on the electrocardiogram with a single velocity peak of at least 0.4 ms/s with each cardiac cycle. Atrial fibrillation results in rapid, irregular, low-velocity flow waves from the atrial appendage. Ventricular tachycardia and ventricular fibrillation affect the contraction of the LV, not the LA, and usually are associated with hemodynamic compromise.

Answer 6: D

This image was taken from a 4-chamber subcostal view. There is a large atrial myxoma in the LA, with attachment along the interatrial septum. The mass abuts the mitral valve and nearly obliterates the LA. Most myxomas (70% to 80%) occur in the LA, with an attachment point at the interatrial septum. Generally, myxomas are the most common primary cardiac tumor. They are benign, derived from multipotential mesenchymal cells, and are more common in women. Clinical presentation may be asymptomatic or there may be an array of symptoms such as dizziness, cough fever, cachexia, and arthralgias. Large myxomas may occlude LV inflow and present with symptoms analogous to mitral valve obstruction, such as syncope, dyspnea, or palpitations. Additional cardiac imaging is not needed; echocardiography was diagnostic, and a referral to cardiac surgery for resection is indicated. Cardiac thrombi occur in areas of blood stasis, such as the left atrial appendage in atrial fibrillation or the LV apex with aneurysm. Isolated thrombi in the main chamber of the LA is unlikely and intravenous anticoagulation is not indicated. The mass is more consistent with myxoma than a vegetation in its size and septal attachment point. While antibiotic therapy should be considered, the correct intervention is surgical resection.

Answer 7: E

This is an M-mode tracing of the mitral valve, with the structures seen, from anterior to posterior including the RV, septum, mitral valve, and posterior LV wall. An aortic valve M-mode would show the parallel walls of the aorta anterior to the LA. An atrial septal aneurysm is not usually seen well by M-mode given the orientation of the atrial septum relative to the chest wall. The diastolic slope of the anterior leaflet is flat, as is seen with mitral stenosis, but leaflet excursion and E-point septal separation are normal. In addition, there are multiple parallel echoes moving with the mitral valve, seen filling the space between the anterior and posterior leaflets in diastole. This finding is consistent with a mass, most likely a left atrial myxoma *(arrow)* prolapsing in the mitral orifice in diastole, as confirmed on 2D imaging (Fig. 15.34).

Answer 8: A

The Eustachian valve overlies the inferior vena cava (IVC), lies at the junction of the IVC and RA, and is variable in size, length, and prominence in individuals.

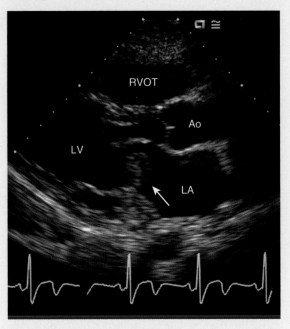

Fig. 15.34

In the image provided, it protrudes into the RA and displaces color Doppler flow (absence of color in the left side of the image). The function of the eustachian valve was to direct intrauterine flow of oxygenated blood from the IVC to the fossa ovalis. The crista terminalis is the embryologic line of union between the trabeculated appendage and the RA. When echo imaging planes go through the midportion of the crista terminalis, a prominent junction line appears as a circular echodensity along the right atrial wall. An atrial myxoma is a benign cardiac tumor, most commonly in the LA with an attachment point on or near the interatrial septum. The thebesian valve is a membranous structure that originates at the superior vena cava, at the orifice of the coronary sinus. It is highly variable in size among individuals and is not commonly seen.

Answer 9: C

The TEE image provided was taken from an upper esophageal view of the base of the heart. In the midportion of the image, the aortic sinuses are seen cut in cross section. The take-off of the left main coronary artery is seen originating at the top of the aorta, and the take-off of the right coronary artery is seen originating at the bottom of the aorta. Just above the aorta, the interatrial septum is seen, and there is a large thrombus in transit crossing a patent foramen ovale.

The thrombus diameter is ≈1 cm, consistent with a proximal deep vein thrombosis vessel diameter. In this patient, there was heavy thrombus burden throughout the right heart and pulmonary artery, consistent with prior pulmonary embolism. He had recently been in a motor vehicle accident and was in recovery when he developed progressive dyspnea.

Answer 10: D

In this TEE bicaval view of the LA and RA, the atrial septum appears intact with a normal thin fossa ovalis *(between arrows)* but with marked thickening and increased echodensity of the rest of the septum, diagnostic for lipomatous hypertrophy of the interatrial septum. This benign normal variant is commonly seen, with prevalence increasing with age and body mass index. Although the fossa ovalis appears relatively thin, it is normal thickness and is not deviated toward either side. The definition of an atrial septum aneurysm is deviation by 1.5 cm or more, which the image does not demonstrate. A patent foramen ovale may or may not be present, but diagnosis requires color Doppler and a saline contrast injection. If a secundum or primum atrial septal defect were present, the right heart chambers would be enlarged and there would be a discontinuity in the atrial septum. With a sinus venosus atrial septal defect, the septum might appear intact in this view, but the right heart would still be enlarged. An atrial septal occluder device results in prominent echo densities on both sides of the fossa ovalis, in a shape consistent with the specific device implanted.

Answer 11: C

The image from the apical 4-chamber view shows a heterogenous, large mass occupying the RA and RV. Although the most common primary cardiac tumors are myxomas, typically originating in the LA, secondary cardiac tumors are much more common. Identification of an intracardiac mass should prompt clinical evaluation for an extracardiac malignancy source. Secondary tumors may originate from a variety of places, but are most commonly related to the lungs, kidneys, melanoma, or hematologic disorders (such as lymphoma or leukemia). A primary pericardial source is rare. Of the options listed, the most likely source is abdominal. Additional imaging in this patient confirmed a uterine mass. Echocardiographic imaging from the subcostal view showed tumor invading the heart from the inferior vena cava (dilated to 3.2 cm),

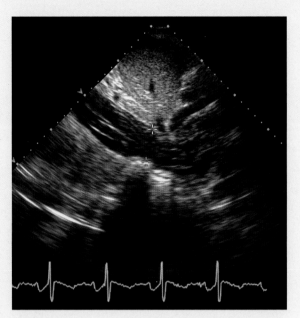

Fig. 15.35

marked with asterisks in the image below, and filled with tumor (Fig. 15.35).

Answer 12: B

There is a large irregular contoured myocardial mass in the right lateral free wall projecting into the RV. The patient has associated systemic symptoms with weight loss associated with advanced malignancy. While definitive diagnosis of a malignancy requires pathologic examination from a biopsy, malignant cardiac tumor characteristics should be distinguished from other benign tumors, thrombus, and normal cardiac structures. A myxoma (answer A) is most commonly located in the LA attached to a stalk at the center of the interatrial septum. An apical thrombus (answer C) may have similar appearance but is uncommon in the RV and would be associated with regional wall motion abnormalities. Papillary fibroelastomas are small benign tumors most often arising on valvular tissue. A moderator band (answer E) is a normal cardiac structure in the RV that has a small trabecular muscle bundle from the ventricular septum to the base of the papillary muscle. This patient was found to have metastatic melanoma. Nonprimary cardiac tumors more often invade pericardial structures, but myocardial invasion may occur with melanoma and lymphoma.

Answer 13: D

The patient has an interatrial septal aneurysm with bulging of the fossa ovalis region greater than 15 mm. Interatrial septal aneurysms are associated with very high rates of fenestrations. A patent foramen ovale is confirmed, with agitated saline demonstrating microbubbles in the LA in less than three cardiac cycles. Color Doppler as well may visualize the patent foramen ovale by transesophageal echocardiogram when the flap valve is open (Fig. 15.36). Lipomatous hypertrophy (answer A) of the interatrial septum may appear as a mass involving the superior and inferior fatty portions of the septum while sparing the fossa ovalis region. A secundum atrial septal defect (answer B) would demonstrate a larger defect in the center of the septum (see Chapter 17). A pulmonary arteriovenous malformation would lead to transpulmonary shunting, which could not explain agitated saline in the LA appearing in under three cardiac cycles.

Answer 14: A

The patient has a LV thrombus, an apical mass with distinct contour that has a more echogenic appearance than the underlying myocardium. LV thrombi occur in regions of blood stasis (such as in an akinetic or aneurysmal cardiac apex). An LV web (answer B) would be a thin trabeculae that moves with the myocardium. A primary cardiac tumor is less likely than thrombus in the clinical scenario and would not have formed within 3 months' time. A near-field "ring-down" artifact can frequently be misinterpreted for LV thrombus but would not appear more echogenic. Improving near-field resolution with a higher-frequency transducer, scanning across the apex from different views, and echo-contrast can help distinguish artifact from true LV thrombus when needed.

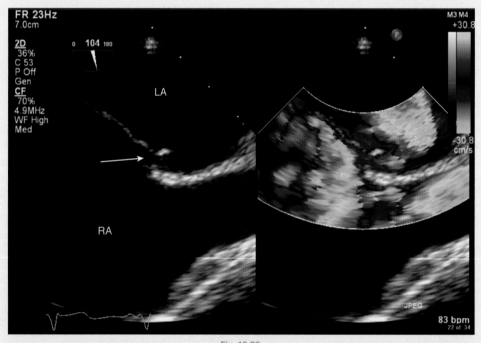

Fig. 15.36

16 Diseases of the Great Arteries

BASIC PRINCIPLES

- A systematic approach is needed for echocardiographic evaluation of the great arteries.
- Transesophageal echocardiography (TEE) is more sensitive than transthoracic imaging for detection of aortic aneurysm and dissection.
- Wider field of view tomographic imaging techniques, including chest computed tomography (CT) or cardiac magnetic resonance (CMR) imaging, provide optimal evaluation of the great vessels.

❖ KEY POINTS

- ❑ Many segments of the aorta and pulmonary artery can be visualized on transthoracic imaging, but:
  - ❑ Evaluation of branch pulmonary arteries and the branching of systemic arteries from the aorta often is not possible.
  - ❑ Ultrasound imaging artifacts must be distinguished from an intraluminal dissection flap.
- ❑ The colloquial term *aortic root* includes the aortic annulus, sinuses of Valsalva, sinotubular junction, and ascending aorta.
- ❑ When the echocardiogram is nondiagnostic or equivocal, additional imaging techniques should be recommended, based on the clinical signs and symptoms.

STEP-BY-STEP APPROACH

Transthoracic Echocardiography

- Examination of the aorta is based on visualization of several segments from different acoustic windows.

- The sequence suggested here follows the sequence of a standard transthoracic study; other exam sequences may be appropriate with an acute clinical presentation.

Step 1: Record Blood Pressure

- Aortic disease often presents as a medical/surgical emergency; appropriately trained health care providers should be available during the study.
- Blood pressure is recorded at the beginning of the study, because findings may change with altered loading conditions.

❖ KEY POINTS

- ❑ When time is of the essence, limited imaging and Doppler data should be focused on the specific clinical question.
- ❑ It may be appropriate to proceed directly to TEE when aortic dissection is suspected; the echocardiographer should consult with the referring provider to ensure that the most appropriate test is performed in a timely manner.

Step 2: Aortic Sinuses and Ascending Aorta

- The aortic sinuses are seen in the standard and high parasternal long-axis view (Fig. 16.1 and Fig. 16.2).
- Diameter measurements are reported at end-diastole for the aortic annulus, sinuses of Valsalva, and sinotubular junction and in the mid-ascending aorta (Fig. 16.3).
- Color Doppler allows detection of aortic regurgitation and evaluation of the flow pattern in the ascending aorta.

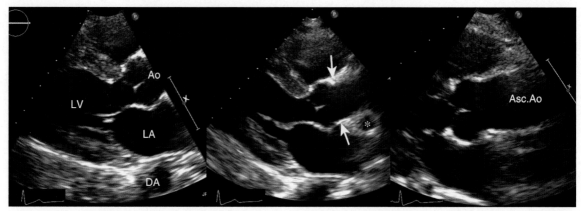

Fig. 16.1 Parasternal imaging of the aorta. In a typical parasternal long-axis view *(left)*, only part of the aortic sinuses are seen. With the transducer moved up an interspace *(center)*, the sinotubular junction *(arrows)* now is seen along with a few centimeters of the ascending aorta. The right pulmonary artery often can be seen posterior to the ascending aorta *(asterisk)*. From an even higher interspace, additional segments of the ascending aorta *(Asc. Ao)* are visualized. The image is zoomed *(right)* to improve resolution of the aortic sinuses, sinotubular junction, and ascending aorta for accurate measurements. *Ao*, Aorta; *DA*, descending thoracic aorta.

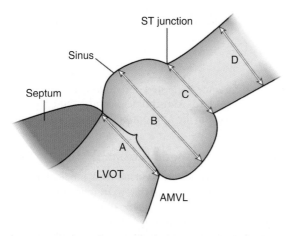

Fig. 16.2 Aortic diameter measurements. In addition to standard measurement at the (A) annulus and (B) sinuses of Valsalva, (C) the sinotubular junction and (D) mid-ascending aorta are measured when the aorta is dilated as shown in this schematic illustration. *AMVL*, Anterior mitral valve leaflet; *LVOT*, left ventricular outflow tract; *ST*, sinotubular.

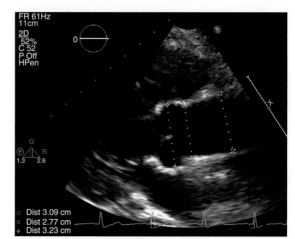

Fig. 16.3 Example of aortic measurements. Diameter is measured at the sinuses, sinotubular junction, and mid-ascending aorta at end-diastole. Current guidelines recommend a leading-edge to leading-edge measurement, but many centers continue to measure from the inner white–black border of the anterior wall to the black–white border of the posterior aortic wall, because reproducibility is higher and for comparison with prior studies. Care is needed to ensure that the image plane is centered in the aorta and that measurements are perpendicular to the long axis of the vessel. An off-center image plane will underestimate aortic size; conversely, oblique measurements will overestimate aortic size.

❖ **KEY POINTS**

❑ After recording the standard parasternal long-axis view of the aortic sinuses, the transducer is moved up one or more interspaces to visualize as much of the ascending aorta as possible.

❑ The sinotubular junction is defined as the top of the sinuses of Valsalva and is recognized by the acute angle at the transition from the curved sinuses to the tubular ascending aorta.

❑ Aortic dimensions are measured on two-dimensional (2D) images from the inner white–black border to the inner black–white border of the aortic lumen.

❑ Comparison of measurements on serial studies or by different modalities should be made at the same time point in the cardiac cycle.

❑ In comparing measurements from different modalities (CT and MRI), both imaging physics

differ and measurement norms may vary, leading to apparent discrepancies.

Step 3: Descending Thoracic Aorta

■ The midportion of the descending thoracic aorta can be visualized from the parasternal long-axis view, posterior to the left atrium (LA), by rotating the image plane clockwise to obtain a longitudinal view of the aorta (Fig. 16.4).

■ The descending thoracic aorta also can be imaged from the apical 2-chamber view by lateral angulation of the image plane (Fig. 16.5).

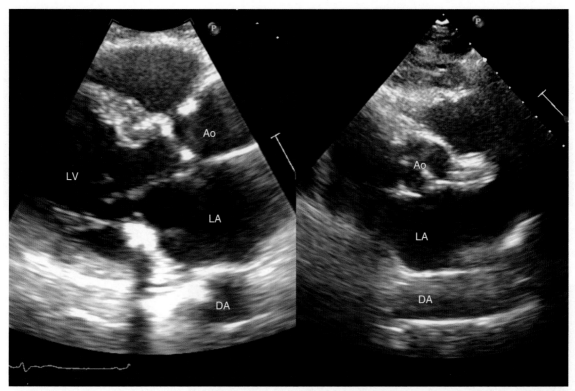

Fig. 16.4 **Parasternal views of descending aorta.** In a Marfan patient, the descending aorta is seen posterior to the LA. A long-axis view of the descending thoracic aorta can be obtained by rotating the transducer clockwise into a parasternal short-axis plane. *Ao,* Aorta; *DA,* descending aorta.

- Color Doppler is helpful in distinguishing image artifacts from an intraluminal flap in these views.

❖ **KEY POINTS**

  - Dilation of the descending aorta and dissection flaps can be identified in these views when image quality is adequate.
  - Only some segments of the descending thoracic aorta are visualized, so significant pathology may be missed.
  - The aorta is in the far field of the image in these views, limiting evaluation for aortic atheroma.
  - In patients with a large left pleural effusion, the descending aorta can be imaged from the posterior chest wall, using the pleural effusion as an acoustic window.

Step 4: Proximal Abdominal Aorta

- The proximal abdominal aorta is seen in the subcostal view by medial angulation from the inferior vena cava (IVC) image plane (Fig. 16.6).
- Holodiastolic flow reversal is seen in the proximal abdominal aorta in patients with severe aortic valve regurgitation (see Fig. 12.5).

❖ **KEY POINTS**

  - Diameter of the proximal abdominal aorta is routinely measured in patients with aortic disease, such as Marfan syndrome.

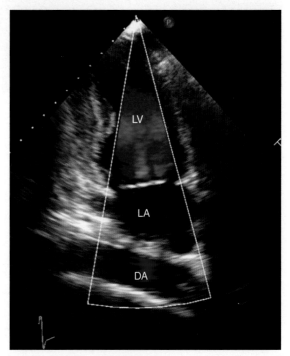

Fig. 16.5 **Apical views of descending aorta.** The descending thoracic aorta can be imaged from the apical 2-chamber view with lateral angulation of the image plane. *DA,* Descending aorta.

  - With a normal pattern of flow, antegrade systolic flow is followed by early diastolic flow reversal due to coronary blood flow, mid-diastolic

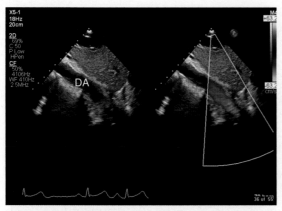

Fig. 16.6 Proximal abdominal aorta. From the subcostal window, the image plane is turned medially from the inferior vena cava (IVC) to visualize the aorta in a long-axis view. Color Doppler *(right)* shows normal laminar antegrade flow in systole. *DA,* Descending aorta.

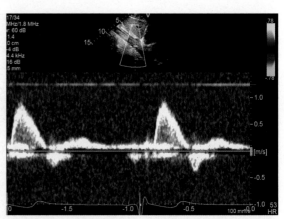

Fig. 16.7 Normal flow in the proximal abdominal aorta. There is antegrade flow in systole, brief early diastolic reversal *(arrow)*, low-velocity forward flow in mid-diastole, and then a slight flow reversal at end-diastole.

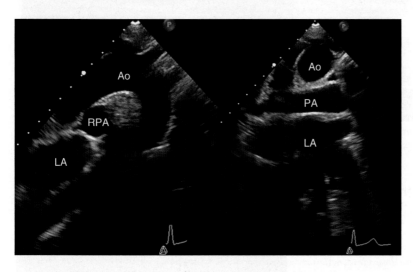

Fig. 16.8 Aortic arch. From the suprasternal notch position *(left)*, a long-axis view of the aortic arch shows segments of the ascending and descending thoracic aorta, the arch, and the origins of the head and neck vessels. The right pulmonary artery is seen under the curve of the arch. In the short-axis view of the arch *(right)*, the LA and pulmonary veins are seen inferior to the right pulmonary artery. *Ao,* Aorta; *PA,* pulmonary artery; *RPA,* right pulmonary artery.

low-velocity antegrade flow, and a very brief late diastolic flow signal due to elastic recoil of the aorta (Fig. 16.7).

- In order to detect the holodiastolic flow reversal seen with severe aortic regurgitation, the filters are adjusted to show low-velocity flow.
- Holodiastolic flow reversal also is seen with other aortic diastolic flow abnormalities (such as a patent ductus arteriosus, surgical systemic-to-pulmonary shunt [e.g., Blalock-Taussig shunt], or aorto-pulmonary window) or other large arteriovenous communication (such as an upper extremity dialysis fistula in patients with end-stage renal disease).

Step 5: Aortic Arch

- The aortic arch is visualized in long- and short-axis views from the suprasternal notch window (Fig. 16.8)
- Pulsed Doppler recordings of flow in the proximal descending aorta show holodiastolic flow reversal when moderate to severe aortic regurgitation is present (Fig. 16.9). The normal flow pattern is shown in Fig. 16.10.

❖ KEY POINTS

- The aortic arch is measured in its midsection, where the ultrasound beam is perpendicular to the aortic walls.
- The descending aorta appears to "taper," even when normal, due to the oblique plane of the ultrasound image compared with the curvature of the aorta.
- The distance from the aortic valve that holodiastolic flow reversal persists correlates with regurgitant severity. Thus, reversal in the proximal descending aorta is seen with moderate regurgitation, but reversal in the abdominal aorta indicates severe regurgitation.
- The right pulmonary artery is seen in cross-section, under the arch, in the long-axis view of the aortic arch.
- A longitudinal view of the left pulmonary artery can be obtained by leftward rotation and angulation of the image plane.

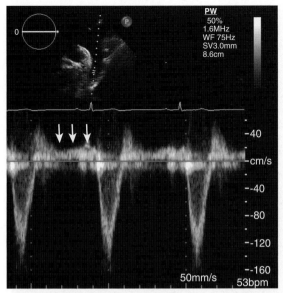

Fig. 16.9 Holodiastolic aortic flow reversal. In a patient with severe aortic regurgitation, holodiastolic flow *(arrows)* is seen in the descending thoracic aorta. The diastolic flow signal is above the baseline from the end of ejection up to the start of the next ejection period.

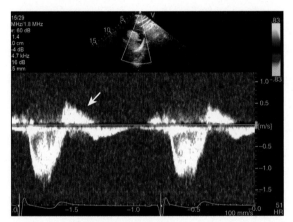

Fig. 16.10 Normal descending aortic flow. Normal flow in the descending thoracic aorta shows early diastolic flow reversal *(arrow, corresponding to diastolic coronary blood flow)*, low-velocity forward flow in mid-diastole, and slight reversal at end-diastole. This patient had no aortic regurgitation.

Step 6: Decide if TEE or Other Imaging Procedures Are Needed

■ Echocardiographic interpretation should first describe the imaging and Doppler findings, along with a differential diagnosis for these findings. The level of confidence in any diagnosis should be indicated.

■ Second, the interpretation should indicate any areas of uncertainly and suggest additional diagnostic procedures in consultation with the referring physician.

❖ **KEY POINTS**

❏ Complete evaluation of the aorta may require additional imaging procedures, including:
  ❏ TEE
  ❏ Chest CT

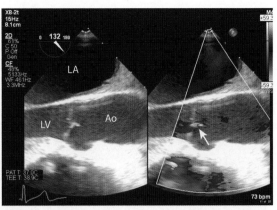

Fig. 16.11 TEE long-axis view of the ascending aorta. This view is obtained from a high TEE probe position at about 120° to 140° rotation. The aortic valve, sinuses, sinotubular junction, and ascending aorta are visualized. Only trace aortic regurgitation *(arrow)* is present on color Doppler flow imaging. *Ao*, Aorta.

  ❏ CMR imaging
  ❏ Cardiac catheterization with aortography
❏ Selection of the most appropriate diagnostic modality depends on several clinical factors, including the differential diagnosis, acuity of symptoms, concurrent diseases, and local expertise in imaging.

Transesophageal Echocardiography

Step 1: Aortic Sinuses and Ascending Aorta

■ Long-axis views of the ascending aorta provide excellent image quality for detection of aortic dilation or dissection.

■ Short-axis images provide confirmation of findings and are helpful in distinguishing artifact from intraluminal abnormalities.

■ Color Doppler evaluation of the flow pattern in the aorta helps identify dissection flaps.

❖ **KEY POINTS**

❏ The long-axis view typically is obtained at 120° rotation, but there is individual variability, so the image plane should be adjusted to show the ascending aorta in a long-axis orientation (Fig. 16.11).

❏ From the long-axis view, the transducer is moved up in the esophagus to image as much of the ascending aorta as possible.

❏ Slow medial and lateral turning of the image plane from the long-axis view may identify abnormalities not seen in the centered long-axis view.

❏ The short-axis view is used to provide an orthogonal image plane. The short-axis view should be recorded from the aortic valve level to as high as possible in the ascending aorta (Fig. 16.12).

❏ Color Doppler in long- and short-axis views may show flow in two lumens when a dissection is present.

❏ The mid- and distal ascending aorta may be better seen by decreasing the rotation to about 100° and slightly withdrawing the probe.

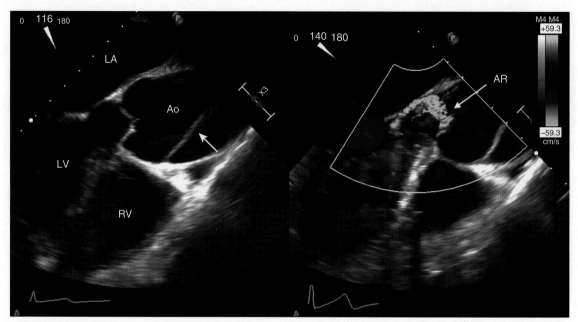

Fig. 16.12 Aortic dissection. In a long-axis TEE view *(left)*, the ascending aorta is dilated with a linear echo in the lumen with undulating motion in real time consistent with a dissection flap. Color Doppler *(right)* shows an eccentric jet of aortic regurgitation with a vent contracta width of 4 mm. The cause of valve regurgitation most likely is dilation of the sinotubular junction, distorting the normal aortic commissural relationships. *Ao,* Aorta.

❑ The distal ascending aorta just proximal to the arch is often not well seen due to the interposed air column (trachea) between the esophagus and aorta.

❑ Imaging artifacts commonly seen in the ascending aorta often include linear reverberations from the aorta itself or adjacent structures. Artifacts are distinguished from anatomic abnormalities by examination in at least two imaging planes; their location, appearance, and pattern of motion relative to the aortic wall; and correlation with color Doppler flow patterns.

Step 2: Aortic Valve Anatomy and Function

■ The presence of aortic valve disease prompts careful evaluation for associated disease of the aortic sinuses and ascending aorta (Tables 16.1 and 16.2).

■ Conversely, aortic disease may result in secondary aortic valve regurgitation.

❖ **KEY POINTS**

❑ The risk of aortic dilation and dissection is higher in patients with a congenitally bicuspid or unicuspid valve, compared with those with a trileaflet valve (Fig. 16.13).

❑ Aortic disease may result in aortic regurgitation either due to dilation of the aortic sinuses and central non-coaptation of the leaflets or due to extension of a dissection flap into the valve, resulting in a flail leaflet.

❑ Aortic valve anatomy and function is evaluated with 2D imaging and color Doppler in a long-axis view at about 120° rotation and in the short-axis view at about 30° rotation.

❑ Additional scanning medially and laterally from the long-axis view and superiorly and inferiorly from the short-axis view also is helpful.

Step 3: Descending Thoracic Aorta

■ The descending thoracic aorta is well visualized on TEE by turning the image plane posteriorly.

■ The short-axis view is recorded with the transducer slowly withdrawn from the transgastric level to the high esophagus (Fig. 16.14).

■ The aortic arch is visualized from the high TEE position by turning the image plane medially with inferior angulation.

❖ **KEY POINTS**

❑ Long-axis views of the descending aorta supplement short-axis views and are helpful for evaluation of any abnormal findings. However, the long-axis view alone may miss abnormalities that are located medial and lateral to the image plane.

❑ Color flow provides visualization of flow in the true and false lumens when dissection is present.

❑ Color flow also is helpful in distinguishing image artifacts from dissection flaps and atheroma.

❑ When the aorta is tortuous, care is needed to distinguish intraluminal abnormalities from an oblique image plane.

TABLE 16.1 Normal Echocardiographic Valve Annulus and Great Vessel Dimensions in Adults

Range	Range	Indexed to Body Surface Area	Upper Limit of Normal Aorta (End-Diastole)*
Annulus diameter (cm)	1.4–2.6	1.3±0.1 cm/m^2	<1.6 cm/m^2
Diameter at leaflet tips (cm)	2.2–3.6	1.7±0.2 cm/m^2	<2.1 cm/m^2
Ascending aorta diameter	2.1–3.4	1.5±0.2 cm/m^2	
Arch diameter (cm)	2.0–3.6		
Mitral Annulus			
End-diastole (cm)	2.7±0.4		
End-systole (cm)	2.9±0.3		
Pulmonary Artery			
Annulus diameter (cm)	1.5–2.1		
Main PA (cm)	0.9–2.9		
Inferior Vena Cava Diameters			
(1-2 cm from RA junction) (cm)	Normal <1.7 cm		

PA, Pulmonary artery.

*See Chapter 16 in *Textbook of Clinical Echocardiography* for a more detailed approach to normalization of aortic dimensions for age and body size. Data from: Roman MJ, Devereux RB, Kramer-Fox R, O'Loughlin J: Two-dimensional echocardiographic aortic root dimensions in normal children and adults, *Am J Cardiol* 64(8):507-512, 1989; Pini R, Roman MJ, Kramer-Fox R, Devereux RB: Mitral valve dimensions and motion in Marfan patients with and without mitral valve prolapse. Comparison to primary mitral valve prolapse and normal subjects, *Circulation* 80(4):915-924, 1989; Schnittger I, Gordon EP, Fitzgerald PJ, Popp RL: Standardized intracardiac measurements of two-dimensional echocardiography, *J Am Coll Cardiol* 2(5):934-938, 1983; Kircher BJ, Himelman RB, Schiller NB: Noninvasive estimation of right atrial pressure from the inspiratory collapse of the inferior vena cava, *Am J Cardiol* 66:493-496, 1990.

TABLE 16.2 Normal Aortic Root Diameters by Age

Normal aortic root diameter by age for men with BSA of 2.0 m^2						
	Age (y)					
	15–29	**30–39**	**40–49**	**50–59**	**60–69**	**≥70**
Mean normal (cm)	3.3	3.4	3.5	3.6	3.7	3.8
Upper limit of normal (cm) (95% CI)	3.7	3.8	3.9	4.0	4.1	4.2

Add 0.5 mm per 0.1 m^2 BSA above 2.0 m^2 or subtract 0.5 mm per 0.1 m^2 BSA below 2.0 m^2.

BSA, Body surface area; *CI,* confidence interval.

Normal aortic root diameter by age for women with BSA of 1.7 m^2						
	Age (y)					
	15–29	**30–39**	**40–49**	**50–59**	**60–69**	**≥70**
Mean normal (cm)	2.9	3.0	3.2	3.2	3.3	3.4
Upper limit of normal (cm)	3.3	3.4	3.6	3.6	3.7	3.9

Add 0.5 mm per 0.1 m^2 BSA above 1.7 m^2 or subtract 0.5 mm per 0.1 m^2 BSA below 1.7 m^2.
Data from Devereux RB, de Simone G, Arnett DK, et al: Normal limits in relation to age, body size and gender of two-dimensional echocardiographic aortic root dimensions in persons ≥15 years of age, *Am J Cardiol* 110:1189-1194, 2012.

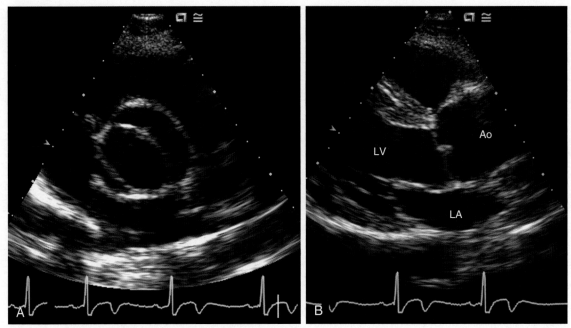

Fig. 16.13 Bicuspid aortic valve disease. Transthoracic imaging of a bicuspid aortic valve in short-axis (A) often is associated with dilation of the aortic sinuses or ascending aorta as seen in the corresponding long-axis view (B). *Ao,* Aorta.

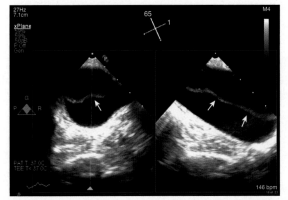

Fig. 16.14 TEE imaging of the descending thoracic aorta. TEE biplane images shows an aortic dissection flap *(arrows)* separating the true and false lumens. Color Doppler often shows multiple fenestrations in the flap with flow between the true and false lumens.

SPECIAL CONSIDERATIONS

Chronic Aortic Dilation

- There are many causes of aortic dilation, including (Table 16.3):
  - Hypertension
  - Atherosclerosis
  - Familial aortic aneurysm
  - Marfan syndrome and other connective tissue disorders
  - Aortic dilation associated with congenital unicuspid and bicuspid aortic valves
  - Inflammatory diseases of the aorta, including tertiary syphilis, giant cell arteritis, and Takayasu arteritis
  - Systemic inflammatory diseases, including ankylosing spondylitis
- Echocardiography provides accurate measurement of the aortic sinuses and ascending aorta and often provides anatomic clues about the cause of disease.

❖ KEY POINTS

- ❑ Hypertensive aortic dilation usually is mild and accompanied by left ventricular (LV) hypertrophy, aortic valve sclerosis, and mitral annular calcification.
- ❑ Marfan syndrome is characterized by loss of the normal acute angle at the sinotubular junction. Early in the disease this finding may be subtle; late in the disease the aortic sinuses appear globular with no discernible sinotubular junction (Fig. 16.15).
- ❑ Aortic dilation associated with congenital valve abnormalities is independent of valve hemodynamics.

TABLE 16.3   Aortic Disease: Clinical Echocardiographic Correlates

	Clinical Correlation	Echocardiographic Findings	Imaging Recommendations
Hypertensive heart disease	Chronic hypertension is associated with mild aortic dilation.	Dilation of the ascending aorta with normal sinuses and STJ is typical.	TTE imaging from a high interspace allows measurement of the ascending aorta.
Aortic atherosclerosis	Atherosclerosis is associated with mild aortic dilation. Aortic atheroma may cause systemic emboli, especially with large protruding atheroma with mobile thrombus.	Focal irregular thickening of the aortic wall with areas of calcification. Associated thrombus is seen as a mobile echodensity.	TEE is needed for evaluation of aortic atheroma.
Bicuspid aortic valve disease	Associated aortopathy in some patients with an increased risk of progressive dilation and dissection.	Enlargement of the aortic sinuses and/or the ascending aorta, usually with a preserved STJ.	CT or CMR imaging is recommended for evaluation of the ascending aorta if not fully imaged by echocardiography.
Marfan (and Loeys-Dietz) syndrome	Aortic dilation, ectopia lentis, skeletal features, family history	Dilated sinuses with enlargement (or effacement) of the STJ. Long anterior mitral leaflet with prolapse.	Aortic imaging (TTE or CMR imaging) recommended every 6-12 months. CMR imaging recommended annually in patients with Loeys-Dietz, from cerebrovascular circulation to pelvis. TTE recommended in first-degree relatives of patients with thoracic aneurysm/dissection or known genetic mutation.
Systemic inflammatory disease (ankylosing spondylitis, etc.)	Arthritis with systemic inflammation. Aortic involvement in about 20% of patients.	Dilated, thick-walled aorta with characteristic thickening extending onto base of the anterior mitral valve leaflet.	TTE appropriate when aortic regurgitant murmur is present. Routine surveillance not recommended.
Syphilitic aortitis	Aneurysm of the ascending aorta is seen 10-25 years after initial spirochetal infection.	Dilated aorta with calcification. May involve proximal coronary arteries.	Rare in North America or Europe.
Takayasu or giant cell arteritis	Loss of distal artery pulses in patients under age 40 years (Takayasu) or over age 50 years (giant cell). Elevated systemic inflammatory markers.	Dilation of thoracic aorta and abdominal aorta.	TTE and TEE show aortic dilation; aortic walls may be thickened and irregular.
Aortic dissection	Acute onset of chest pain, often described as tearing. May radiate to neck or back.	Intimal flap with flow in true and false lumen. Type A dissection involves ascending aorta; type B dissection is limited to descending thoracic aorta.	TEE, CMR imaging, or CT recommended in patients at high risk of aortic dissection. Choice of procedures depends on patient variables and availability of each imaging modality.
Intramural hematoma	Acute presentation with chest or back pain.	Crescent-shaped thickening of aortic wall. May be localized.	Intramural hematoma may be seen on TTE, but TEE has a higher sensitivity for this diagnosis.
Aortic pseudoaneurysm	Typically seen after complex aortic valve surgery or endocarditis.	Echo-free space adjacent to aorta. Flow from aortic lumen in and out of the pseudoaneurysm may be seen.	TEE, CT, and/or CMR imaging is needed to evaluate known or suspected aortic pseudoaneurysm.

Continued

TABLE 16.3 Aortic Disease: Clinical Echocardiographic Correlates—cont'd

	Clinical Correlation	Echocardiographic Findings	Imaging Recommendations
Traumatic aortic disease	Deceleration injury can result in aortic rupture, most often at the ligamentum arteriosus (45%) or the ascending aorta (23%).	Disruption of the aorta at the junction between the arch and the descending thoracic aorta may be difficult to appreciate on TTE or TEE.	CT recommended for diagnosis. Delayed diagnosis may result in pseudoaneurysm at the aortic isthmus.
Sinus of Valsalva aneurysm	Isolated congenital sinus of Valsalva aneurysms may be a smooth dilation of one sinus or may have a "wind sock" appearance. Aneurysms due to endocarditis are associated with thickening of the aortic wall and abscess formation.	Rupture may occur into the RV outflow tract from the left coronary cusp, into the RA from the right coronary cusp, or into the LA from the noncoronary cusp.	Both color and spectral Doppler are helpful in determining which chamber is affected by a ruptured sinus of Valsalva aneurysm.

CMR, Cardiac magnetic resonance; *CT,* computed tomography; *STJ,* sinotubular junction.

- Aortic dilation due to an inflammatory process usually is characterized by increased thickness of the aortic walls.
- In ankylosing spondylitis, the increase in aortic wall thickness extends into the base of the anterior mitral valve leaflet, with the appearance of a subaortic "bump" in a long-axis view.
- Takayasu arteritis typically involves the aortic arch and branches, resulting in areas of stenosis and dilation, but the descending aorta also may be involved.

Aortic Dissection

Step 1: Use the Basic Approach for Evaluation of the Aorta to Identify the Dissection Flap

- The characteristics of a dissection flap (Fig. 16.16) are:
  - A thin, linear, mobile intraluminal echo
  - Motion independent of the aortic walls
  - Separation of the lumen into two channels
- Sites where there is communication between the true and false lumens may be identified with color Doppler.
- An ascending aortic dissection usually requires surgical intervention, so it is especially important to determine if a dissection flap is present in the ascending aorta.
- TEE is more sensitive than transthoracic imaging for detection of aortic dissection and should be the initial echo procedure when this diagnosis is suspected.

❖ KEY POINTS

- Imaging artifacts may be mistaken for a dissection flap. Approaches to avoiding a false positive diagnosis include imaging the flap in more than one imaging plane, demonstrating flow in two separate lumens, and demonstrating the three key characteristics of a dissection flap.

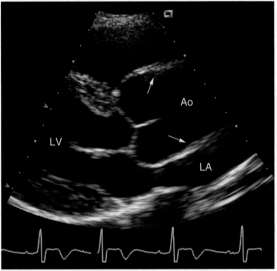

Fig. 16.15 Effacement of the sinotubular junction. In patients with Marfan syndrome, the normal acute angle between the curved sinuses and tubular ascending aorta at the sinotubular junction is attenuated *(arrows)*, resulting in a "water balloon" appearance of the aorta. *Ao,* Aorta.

- There may be more than one entry site from the true into the false lumen, and multiple exit sites may be detected distally (see Fig. 16.14).
- The false lumen may be thrombosed. In this situation, the flap does not move and the false lumen is filled with an irregular echodensity, which is consistent with thrombus.
- Localized dissection into the aortic wall may result in a crescent-shaped intramural hematoma without a dissection flap (Fig. 16.17).
- Outcomes with intramural hematoma and dissection are similar.
- Extraluminal, periaortic hematoma in association with aortic dissection is a poor prognostic marker.

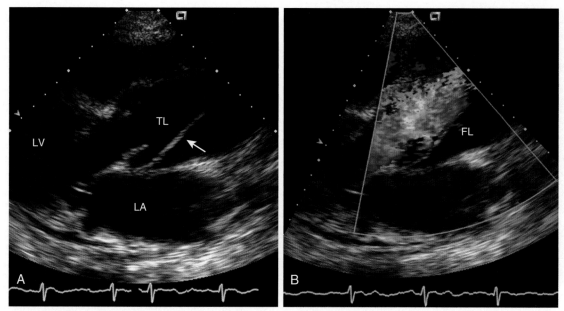

Fig. 16.16 TTE view of aortic dissection. (A) Transthoracic parasternal long-axis view showing a linear echo in the lumen of a dilated ascending aorta consistent with a dissection flap *(arrow)* separating the true lumen *(TL)* from the false lumen *(FL)*. In real time, this linear echo showed motion separate from the motion of the aortic wall and was seen in multiple image planes. (B) Color Doppler shows flow only in the true lumen.

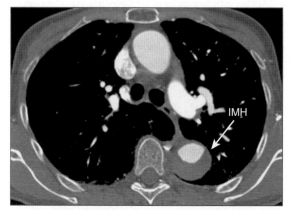

Fig. 16.17 Intramural hematoma in the descending thoracic aorta on chest CT. These findings can be seen on TEE but may be difficult to distinguish from atheromatous or extra aortic disease. *IMH,* Intramural hematoma.

Step 2: Look for Complications of Aortic Dissection

- Complications of aortic dissection include:
  - ○ Pericardial effusion
  - ○ Aortic regurgitation
  - ○ Extension of the dissection flap into a coronary artery
  - ○ Involvement of arteries that arise from the aorta
- Echocardiography may detect the central complications of aortic dissection, but evaluation of branch vessels typically requires other imaging techniques.

❖ KEY POINTS

- ❏ Pericardial effusion may be due to rupture of the dissection into the pericardial space. Because the effusion is acute, tamponade physiology may be present with only a small effusion.
- ❏ Aortic regurgitation may be due to aortic dilation with central non-coaptation of the leaflets or due to a flail leaflet from extension of the dissection flap into the valve (Fig. 16.18).
- ❏ Extension of a dissection flap into the coronary artery may be visualized on transthoracic echocardiography (TTE) or TEE imaging in some cases. More often, the key finding is a regional wall motion abnormality due to ischemia in the myocardium supplied by the dissected vessel.
- ❏ The proximal segments of the left carotid and subclavian and right brachiocephalic artery may be seen by echocardiography in some cases. However, accurate evaluation of these vessels and more distal arteries (renal, mesenteric, etc.) requires other imaging approaches.

Sinus of Valsalva Aneurysm

- Congenital sinus of Valsalva aneurysms are irregularly shaped, thin-walled outpouchings of the sinus.
- Rupture into adjacent chambers results in a fistula from the aorta into the right ventricle (RV), right atrium (RA), or LA, depending on which sinus is affected.
- Acquired sinus of Valsalva aneurysms usually are due to endocarditis and typically have a rounded symmetric shape (Fig. 16.19).

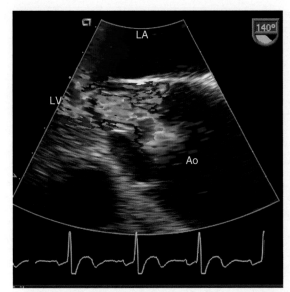

Fig. 16.18 Severe secondary aortic regurgitation. The aortic dissection flap has extended into the aortic valve leaflet, resulting in severe regurgitation. *Ao,* Aorta.

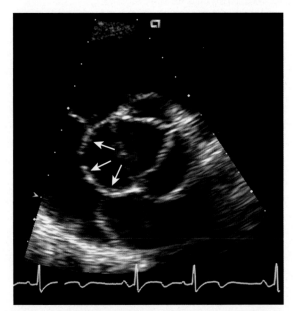

Fig. 16.19 Sinus of Valsalva aneurysm. This short-axis view of the aortic valve shows the valve leaflets open to a triangular shape in systole. There is asymmetric dilation of the sinuses of Valsalva, most prominently involving the noncoronary sinus *(arrows),* consistent with a sinus of Valsalva aneurysm.

❖ **KEY POINTS**

◻ Rupture of a right coronary sinus aneurysm is into the RV, left coronary sinus into the LA, and noncoronary sinus into the RA.

◻ Flow in the fistula from the aorta is continuous with high-velocity flow in both systole and diastole, reflecting the systolic and diastolic pressure differences between the aortas and receiving chamber.

◻ Acquired aneurysms due to infection may extend below the aortic valve, into the base of the septum. Imaging in long-axis views helps determine the level and extent of involvement.

Aortic Pseudoaneurysm

■ An aortic pseudoaneurysm is a contained aortic rupture (Fig. 16.20).

■ Pseudoaneurysms may occur after aortic surgery due to dehiscence at the proximal or distal anastomosis or at a coronary reimplantation site.

❖ **KEY POINTS**

◻ A pseudoaneurysm is detected as an echolucent space adjacent to the aorta. The pseudoaneurysm may be echodense if hematoma is present.

◻ A pseudoaneurysm should be suspected when a paraaortic mass is found in a patient with recent or remote surgery on the ascending aorta.

◻ Although often initially diagnosed by echocardiography, evaluation of the size and origin of the pseudoaneurysm often requires a wide field of view imaging approach, such as CMR imaging or CT.

Atherosclerotic Aortic Disease

■ Aortic atheromas may be detected on TEE imaging of the ascending and descending thoracic aorta and are a marker of coronary disease (Fig. 16.21).

■ Atheroma that protrude into the aortic lumen and atheroma associated with mobile thrombus are associated with an increased risk of embolic events.

❖ **KEY POINTS**

◻ Atheroma is identified as irregular focal areas of thickening of the aortic wall, with or without associated calcification.

◻ Images of the aortic arch are limited, even with TEE, but atheroma may be detected from a high esophageal position in some cases.

Persistent Left Superior Vena Cava

■ A persistent left superior vena cava (SVC) is a normal variant in which left upper extremity venous return enters the RA via the coronary sinus.

❖ **KEY POINTS**

◻ A dilated coronary sinus is seen in cross section, posterior to the LA, in long-axis views, and in long axis with posterior angulation from a 4-chamber view.

◻ The persistent left SVC may be directly visualized in some cases; Doppler flow shows low-velocity antegrade systolic and diastolic flow.

◻ A persistent left SVC can be confirmed with saline contrast injection into the left upper extremity venous system, where saline contrast opacifies the coronary sinus before entering the RA.

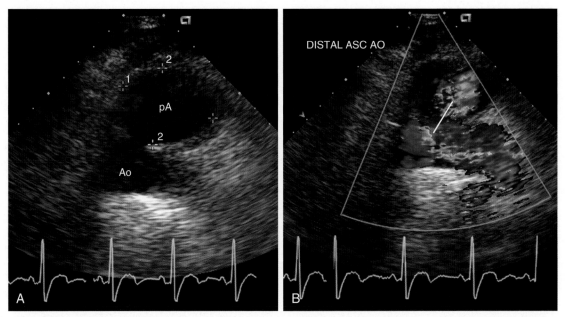

Fig. 16.20 **Aortic pseudoaneurysm.** In a patient with a Dacron tube graft replacement of the ascending aorta, an abnormal echolucent space is seen adjacent to the ascending aorta, near the distal anastomosis site. (A) The 3.5- by 4.5-cm diameter (measurements *1* and *2* shown) space appears lined by thrombus. (B) Color Doppler demonstrates flow from the aorta into this space, consistent with a contained aortic rupture or pseudoaneurysm. *Ao,* Aorta; *DISTAL ASC AO,* distal ascending aorta; *pA,* pseudoaneurysm.

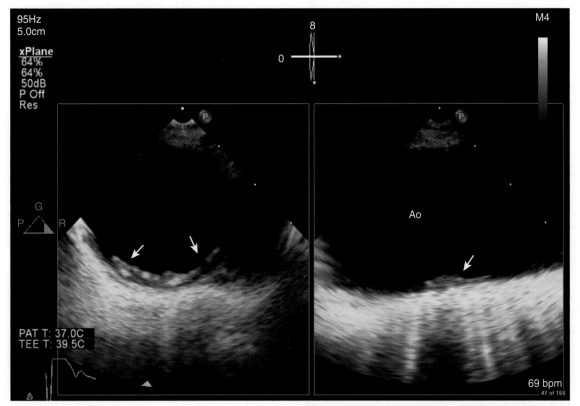

Fig. 16.21 **Aortic atheroma.** TEE biplane imaging shows the short-axis *(left)* and long-axis *(right)* views. The irregular thickening of the aortic wall with an area of calcification (with shadowing) is consistent with an aortic atheroma. Sequential images of the entire descending thoracic aorta were recorded as the transducer was withdrawn in the esophagus, with the image plane turned medially and angulated inferiorly to show the aortic arch and ascending aorta, before withdrawing the probe at the end of the TEE study. *Ao,* Aorta.

Pulmonary Artery Abnormalities

Clinical Concerns

- Isolated abnormalities of the pulmonary artery are rare; most pulmonary artery disease is associated with congenital heart disease (Fig. 16.22).
- Idiopathic dilation of the pulmonary artery is an uncommon abnormality in which a dilated pulmonary artery is seen in the absence of other congenital lesions.
- Thrombus in the pulmonary artery may be seen on transesophageal or transthoracic imaging in some cases, but echocardiography is not an accurate approach to diagnosis of pulmonary embolism.

❖ **KEY POINTS**

- Abnormalities of the pulmonary artery associated with other congenital heart disease include pulmonary artery dilation and branch pulmonary artery stenosis.
- Pulmonary artery dissection is rare.

Basic Echocardiographic Approach

- The pulmonary artery is visualized in the transthoracic short-axis view by angulation superiorly to demonstrate the bifurcation of the main pulmonary artery.
- Images also can be obtained in the transthoracic RV outflow view.
- TEE imaging of the pulmonary artery is challenging and requires high esophageal views.

- Color, pulsed, and continuous-wave (CW) Doppler allow detection of pulmonic regurgitation and abnormal pulmonary artery flow patterns.

❖ **KEY POINTS**

- In adults, visualization of the lateral wall of the pulmonary artery is difficult due to limitation of the acoustic window by the adjacent lung.
- Pulmonary artery diameter measurements are mainly helpful in adults with congenital heart disease, and may be better made by other imaging techniques.
- A small amount of pulmonic regurgitation is normal and is characterized by a narrow jet on color Doppler and a low-intensity, low-velocity spectral Doppler signal.
- With pulmonary hypertension, the pulmonic regurgitant velocity is increased, reflecting the elevation of pulmonary diastolic pressure, and there is a shortened time-to-peak velocity and mid-systolic deceleration in the antegrade flow signal.
- With branch pulmonary artery stenosis, a high-velocity signal may be detected with spectral Doppler, even when image quality is suboptimal (Fig. 16.23).
- With a patent ductus arteriosus, the diastolic flow from the descending aorta into the pulmonary artery is seen with color and spectral Doppler.
- Full evaluation of the main pulmonary artery and branches in patients with congenital heart disease usually requires CMR or CT imaging.

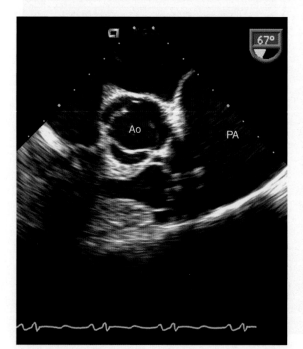

Fig. 16.22 Severe dilation of the pulmonary artery. TEE in a patient with congenital heart disease in a short-axis view of the aortic valve shows a severely dilated pulmonary artery. *Ao,* Aorta; *PA,* pulmonary artery.

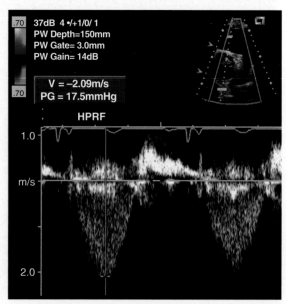

Fig. 16.23 Branch pulmonary artery stenosis. Stenosis of the distal right pulmonary artery in this patient with a repaired tetralogy of Fallot is demonstrated using high-pulse repetition frequency *(HPRF)* Doppler to localize the origin of the high velocity jet.

THE ECHO EXAM

Examination of the Aorta

Aortic Segment	Modality	View	Recording	Limitations
Aortic sinuses	TTE	Parasternal long-axis	Images of sinuses of Valsalva, aortic annulus, and sinotubular junction	Shadowing of posterior aortic sinuses
	TEE	High esophageal long-axis	Standard long-axis plane by rotating to about 120°-130°	
Ascending	TTE	Parasternal long-axis	Move transducer superiorly to image sinotubular junction and ascending aorta	Only limited segments visualized, variable among patients
	TTE Doppler	Apical	LVOT and ascending aorta flow recorded with pulsed or CW Doppler from an anteriorly angulated 4-chamber view	Velocity underestimation if the angle between the Doppler beam and flow is not parallel
	TEE	High esophageal long-axis	From long-axis view, move transducer superiorly to image ascending aorta	The distal ascending aorta may not be visualized
Arch	TTE	Suprasternal	Long- and short-axis views of aortic arch	Descending aorta appears to taper as it leaves the image plane
	TEE	High esophageal	From the short-axis view of the initial segment of the descending thoracic aorta, turn the probe toward the patient's right side, and angulate inferiorly	View not obtained in all patients; the aortic segment at the junction of the ascending aorta and arch may not be visualized
Descending thoracic	TTE	Parasternal and modified apical views	Rotate from long-axis view to image thoracic aorta in long axis posterior to LV From apical 2-chamber view, use lateral angulation and counter-clockwise rotation to image aorta	Depth of thoracic aorta on TTE limits image quality TEE usually needed for diagnosis
	TTE Doppler	Suprasternal	Descending aorta flow recorded with pulsed Doppler from SSN view	Low wall filters needed to evaluate for holodiastolic flow reversal
	TEE	Short-axis aorta	Sequential short-axis views of the aorta from the level of the diaphragm to the arch with the image plane turned posteriorly and the transducer slowly withdrawn	Long-axis views allow further evaluation of abnormal findings
Proximal abdominal	TTE	Subcostal	Long axis of proximal abdominal aorta	Only the proximal segment is visualized
	TTE Doppler	Transgastric	Proximal abdominal aorta flow recorded with pulsed Doppler	Low wall filters needed to evaluate for holodiastolic flow reversal
	TEE	Transgastric	From the transgastric position, portions of the abdominal aorta may be seen posteriorly	Does not allow evaluation of entire abdominal aorta

LVOT, Left ventricular outflow tract; *SSN*, suprasternal notch.

Key Features of Aortic Diseases

Aortic Dissection

Dissection flap	In aortic lumen True and false lumen	Independent motion Entry sites Thrombosis of false lumen
Intramural hematoma		
Indirect findings	Aortic dilation Aortic regurgitation Coronary ostial involvement Pericardial effusion	

Complications of Aortic Dissection

Aortic regurgitation	Due to aortic root dilation Due to leaflet flail	
Coronary artery occlusion	Ventricular fibrillation Acute myocardial infarction	
Distal vessel obstruction	Carotid (stroke) Subclavian (upper limb ischemia)	
Aortic rupture	Into the pericardium Into the mediastinum Into the pleural space	Pericardial effusion Pericardial tamponade Pleural effusion Exsanguination

Sinus of Valsalva Aneurysm

Congenital	Complex shape Protrusion into RV outflow tract Fenestrations	
Acquired	Infection or inflammation Symmetric shape Communication with aorta Potential for rupture	

Aortic Atheroma

	Complex ($\geq$4 mm or mobile) Associated with:	Coronary artery disease Cerebroembolic events

SELF-ASSESSMENT QUESTIONS

Question 1

A 74-year-old man with hypertension, chronic obstructive pulmonary disease, and chronic kidney disease had sudden sharp chest pain. Transthoracic imaging had poor image quality and nondiagnostic due to underlying pulmonary disease. Based on the TEE image shown (Fig. 16.24), what is the most likely diagnosis?

   A. Hypertensive heart disease
   B. Aortic aneurysm with imaging artifact
   C. Ankylosing spondylitis
   D. Aortic dissection

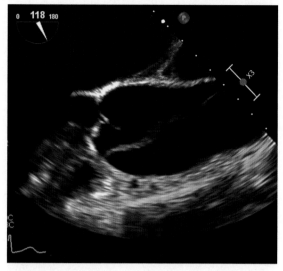

Fig. 16.24

Question 2

A transthoracic echocardiogram is ordered for a newly diagnosed murmur. No valvular abnormalities or dysfunction is identified. Doppler interrogation of the thoracic aorta reveals the following (Fig. 16.25). You conclude that the most likely diagnosis is:

   A. Aortic coarctation
   B. Aortic regurgitation
   C. Patent ductus arteriosus
   D. Aortic atherosclerosis

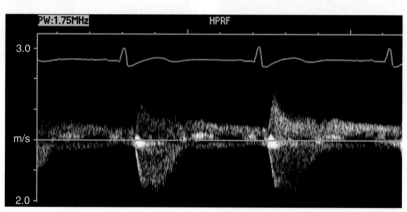

Fig. 16.25

Question 3

Identify each structure on this TEE image (Fig. 16.26):

A _____
B _____
C _____
D _____
E _____

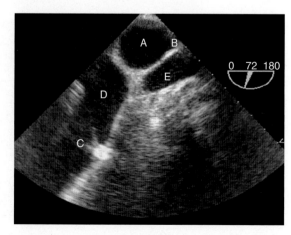

Fig. 16.26

Question 4

Identify the structures (Fig. 16.27, numbered *1* to *4*) by matching them with the following list:

- **A.** Descending aorta
- **B.** Ascending aorta
- **C.** Left ventricle
- **D.** Left atrium
- **E.** Right pulmonary artery
- **F.** Left pulmonary artery
- **G.** Brachiocephalic vein
- **H.** Azygous vein

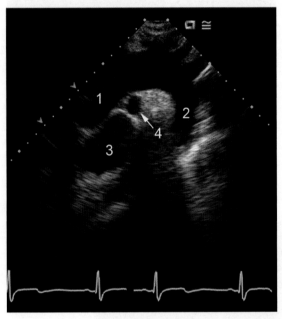

Fig. 16.27

Question 5

A patient is referred for an echocardiogram. During scanning, the following image is obtained (Fig. 16.28).

Additional imaging is suggested to confirm the diagnosis. You recommend:

- **A.** Transpulmonary microbubble contrast study
- **B.** Repeat imaging following Valsalva maneuver
- **C.** 3D TEE imaging
- **D.** Imaging from left supraclavicular window

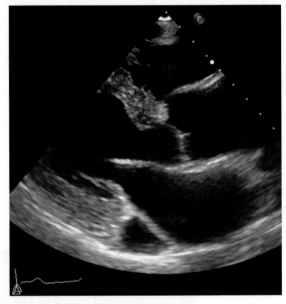

Fig. 16.28

Question 6

A 54-year-old man presents to the emergency department following a motor vehicle accident. A TEE is ordered and the following image is obtained (Fig. 16.29). Based on this study, you make the following diagnosis:

- **A.** Intramural hematoma
- **B.** Aortic dissection
- **C.** Penetrating aortic atheroma
- **D.** Aortic transection

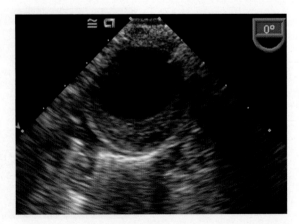

Fig. 16.29

Question 7

Several echocardiographic findings may be associated with an ascending aortic dissection. Which of the following is least likely of a complication of acute aortic dissection?

A. Pericardial effusion
B. Periaortic hematoma
C. Myocardial infarction
D. Mitral regurgitation

Question 8

A 56-year-old man with a long history of hypertension presented to the emergency department with the sudden onset of severe tearing chest pain. His electrocardiogram (ECG) showed only nonspecific ST changes. Urgent echocardiography at the bedside was performed (Fig. 16.30). Based on the clinical history and this image, the echocardiographic exam should next focus on:

A. Calculation of LV ejection fraction
B. Evaluation of regional ventricular systolic function
C. Imaging of the ascending aorta
D. Measurement of tricuspid regurgitant (TR) jet velocity
E. Respiratory variation in RV and LV diastolic filling

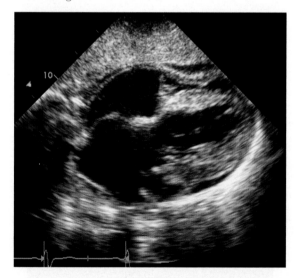

Fig. 16.30

Question 9

A 32-year-old asymptomatic man with a history of sudden death in the family was sent for TTE due to a systolic murmur (Fig. 16.31). Which of the following diagnoses is most likely?

A. Congenital sinus of Valsalva aneurysm
B. Marfan syndrome
C. Aortic atherosclerosis
D. Aortic dissection
E. Hypertrophic cardiomyopathy

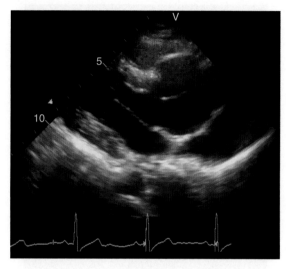

Fig. 16.31

Question 10

The most likely diagnosis in the 56-year-old man with this aortic flow signal (Fig. 16.32) is:

A. Aortic coarctation
B. Aortic regurgitation
C. Patent ductus arteriosus
D. Branch pulmonary stenosis
E. Persistent left superior vena cava

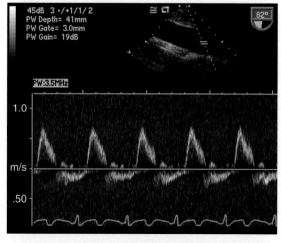

Fig. 16.32

Question 11

Match each image and clinical scenario to the most likely diagnosis.

Diagnosis:
  A. Aortic aneurysm
  B. Aortic dissection
  C. Aortic intramural hematoma
  D. Aortic pseudoaneurysm
  E. Complex aortic atheroma
  F. Normal variant
  G. Penetrating atherosclerotic ulcer
  H. Persistent left superior vena cava
  I. Pulmonary artery thrombus
  IMAGE 1 (Fig. 16.33)
  IMAGE 2 (Fig. 16.34)
  IMAGE 3 (Fig. 16.35)
  IMAGE 4 (Fig. 16.36)
  IMAGE 5 (Fig. 16.37)
  IMAGE 6 (Fig. 16.38)

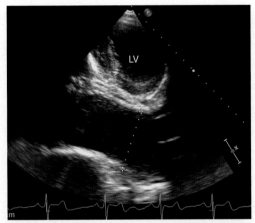

Fig. 16.33 A 74-year-old smoker with palpable abdominal mass.

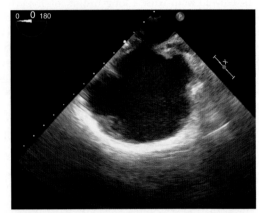

Fig. 16.36 A 69-year-old woman with hypotension and back pain.

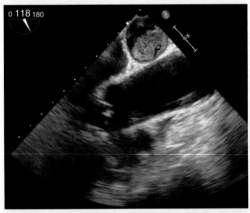

Fig. 16.34 A 62-year-old woman with sudden shortness of breath.

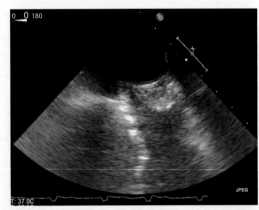

Fig. 16.37 A 51-year-old man undergoing TEE with cardioversion for atrial fibrillation.

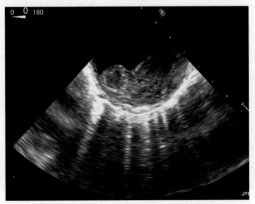

Fig. 16.35 An 83-year-old man with a stroke.

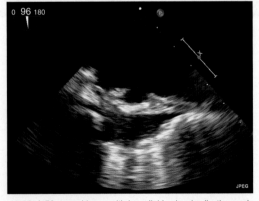

Fig. 16.38 A 58-year-old man with hyperlipidemia, claudication, and prior coronary artery bypass surgery.

ANSWERS

Answer 1: D

Fig. 16.24 shows a thin, linear, mobile intraluminal echo with separation of the lumen in two channels. Real-time imaging showed motion independent of the aortic walls. These three features are characteristic of a dissection flap. Additional short-axis views of the descending thoracic aorta confirmed the diagnosis with imaging the dissection flap in a second plane (Fig. 16.39) and color Doppler showing flow in both lumens (Fig. 16.40) confirming that the flap was not an imaging artifact (answer B). Ankylosing spondylitis is a systemic inflammatory disorder that may lead in aortic root and anterior mitral valve leaflet thickening with regurgitation (answer C). Hypertensive heart disease (answer A) does not describe the clinical picture and is more often used to describe chronic changes seen with hypertension (e.g., LV hypertrophy and mild aortic root dilation).

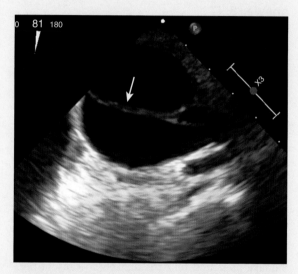

Fig. 16.39

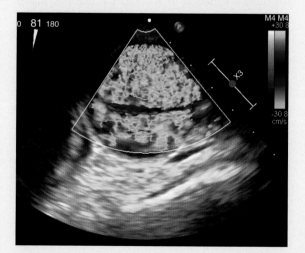

Fig. 16.40

Answer 2: C

The Doppler tracing was taken of the descending thoracic aorta from the suprasternal notch. Systolic flow is directed away from the transducer. In both systole and diastole, there is continuous flow directed toward the transducer. This is consistent with a patent ductus arteriosus, where flow is directed from the descending thoracic aorta to the pulmonary artery. Flow is continuous because of lower pressure in the pulmonary vasculature relative to the aorta. Aortic coarctation, if significant, would result in increased anterograde velocity and continued anterograde flow during diastole (away from the transducer), "diastolic run-off." With aortic regurgitation of at least moderate severity, holodiastolic flow reversal may be present. However, with aortic regurgitation, there is a demarcation between systole (flow directed away from the transducer) and diastole (flow directed toward the transducer). Additionally, the clinical vignette described no echocardiographic findings of valvular abnormalities or dysfunction. Aortic atherosclerosis does not typically affect the Doppler signal in diastole. If significant atherosclerosis is obstructive, this may affect anterograde (systolic) velocities.

Answer 3:

The view is an upper esophageal view with some retroflexion showing the distal aortic arch (answer A) in short axis. The subclavian artery (answer B) can be seen branching from the aortic arch in this view. The pulmonic valve (answer C) and main pulmonary artery (answer D) can have a parallel alignment allowing for Doppler interrogation if needed. The structure shown in answer E is the innominate (left brachiocephalic) vein running anteriorly alongside the subclavian artery. The high esophageal view may not be fully tolerated in all patients and may require deep or general sedation to obtain. This view was taken during an intraoperative cardiac procedure with general anesthesia.

Answer 4:

This suprasternal notch long-axis view of the aortic arch shows the following matches:
1. B. Ascending aorta
2. A. Descending aorta
3. D. Left atrium
4. E. Right pulmonary artery

The LV is not well seen in this view. The right pulmonary artery is seen in cross-section under the aortic arch, but the image plane does not include the left pulmonary artery. The azygous vein arises from the inferior vena cava, courses superiorly adjacent to the spine receiving the drainage of the intercostal veins, and then enters the superior vena cava above the right mainstem bronchus. When normal in size, it is rarely seen by echocardiography and lies medial to the descending thoracic aorta.

Answer 5: D

This parasternal long-axis view shows a dilated coronary sinus in the atrioventricular groove just posterior to the mitral valve. This finding is consistent with a persistent left-sided superior vena cava, which drains into the coronary sinus. 2D imaging from the left supraclavicular window showed both a normal right-sided and a persistent left-sided superior vena cava. At first glance, a dilated coronary sinus might be mistaken for the descending thoracic aorta in cross section, but the descending aorta is external to the pericardial, located more distally and superiorly compared to the coronary sinus in this view.

If this diagnosis is suspected, an agitated saline contrast study can confirm the diagnosis. For an agitated saline study, intravenous access is placed in the left upper extremity. Following injection of saline, a persistent left superior vena cava is present if contrast opacifies the coronary sinus before the right-sided chambers. Answer A is incorrect; transpulmonary microbubble contrast traverses the pulmonary circulation and is used to opacify LV endocardial borders. 3D imaging of the interatrial septum may be helpful if an atrial septal defect is suspected, but the image shown suggests a tubular, vascular structure rather than a septal defect. Imaging following a Valsalva maneuver would not be helpful for diagnosis of a persistent left superior vena cava.

Answer 6: A

The image is a short-axis view of the descending thoracic aorta taken at 0°. The aortic lumen is echolucent. In the far field, there is crescentic thickening of the wall (hematoma), which encompasses half of the diameter of the aorta and is echodense relative to the lumen. No clear dissection flap is seen. Aortic atherosclerosis typically lies along the aortic wall. Prominent atherosclerotic lesions may protrude into the lumen of the aorta, but the wall is not smooth, as seen in this image. Atherosclerosis is also echodense (calcium), commonly with acoustic shadowing of the far field. An aortic transection shows as a discontinuity of the aorta from long-axis views. Periaortic hematoma is present with Doppler imaging showing flow outside the aortic border.

Answer 7: D

Proximal propagation of an ascending aortic dissection to the aortic root may extend to the coronary arteries and aortic valve. If the outer wall of the aorta is disrupted from the dissection, periaortic hematoma or pericardial effusion will be seen. Propagation down a coronary artery may occlude the vessel leading to myocardial infarction. Involvement of the dissection to aortic valve may cause faulty leaflet coaptation and aortic regurgitation. Mitral regurgitation is not a direct complication of aortic dissection.

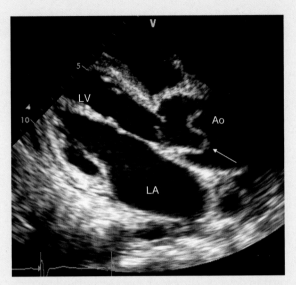

Fig. 16.41

Answer 8: C

This patient's clinical history is strongly suggestive of acute aortic dissection, and the presence of a small pericardial effusion is an ominous sign, suggesting partial rupture into the pericardium. The immediate next step should be evaluation of the ascending aorta, which in this patient showed a definite dissection flap *(arrow)* on a TTE parasternal long-axis view (Fig. 16.41).

When aortic dissection is suspected and transthoracic imaging is not diagnostic, prompt additional imaging (computed tomography angiography or TEE) is recommended as urgent surgical intervention is indicated. In a clinically stable patient, quantitative evaluation of ventricular function is appropriate, but if the patient is unstable, a qualitative assessment of function (visual estimate) is reasonable. Pulmonary embolism may result in an acute elevation in pulmonary pressures, but it is unlikely to cause a pericardial effusion. Tamponade physiology, resulting in respiratory variation in RV and LV diastolic filling, can occur with aortic dissection but would be evident clinically as a low blood pressure or pulsus paradoxus, and treatment requires identification of the underlying cause—aortic dissection in this case.

Answer 9: B

The patient has characteristic echocardiographic findings of Marfan syndrome. There are dilated aortic sinuses with effacement of the sinotubular junction ("water balloon" appearance) and a long, redundant anterior mitral valve leaflet. Marfan syndrome is an inherited connective tissue disease that may affect multiple organ systems. Diagnosis is based on a combination of family history, genetic testing, aortic findings, and other systemic connective tissue features. The most common life-threatening complication is aortic dissection, but there is no evidence of a dissection flap and the patient is asymptomatic. A congenital sinus of Valsalva aneurysm is more typically seen as a complex "wind sock" appearance of irregular, mobile echoes protruding from the sinus into another cardiac chamber. The patient is young to have aortic atherosclerosis, which would appear as focal irregular thickening of the aortic wall with calcifications. Hypertrophic cardiomyopathy can be associated with family histories of sudden cardiac death and enlargement of the mitral valve leaflets; however, aortic aneurysms are not associated with hypertrophic myocardial disease. In this image, septal wall thickness is normal.

Answer 10: B

This pulsed Doppler recording in a long-axis view of the descending aorta on TEE shows antegrade flow in systole with reversal of flow for the full duration of diastole (e.g., holodiastolic). This flow signal indicates continuous retrograde diastolic flow in the descending aorta, which is consistent with a communication from the aorta to a chamber or vessel with a lower diastolic pressure. Possible diagnoses include aortic regurgitation (aorta to LV) or a patent ductus arteriosus (aorta to pulmonary artery), but aortic regurgitation is most likely given the patient's age. This diagnosis can be confirmed by color and CW Doppler evaluation of the aortic valve and by confirming the absence of diastolic flow in the main pulmonary artery. With aortic coarctation, the systolic velocity is higher than normal, and there is continuous forward flow in diastole. Branch pulmonary stenosis would result in high-velocity systolic flow in the right or left pulmonary artery, which are not seen in this view. A persistent left superior vena cava would have a typical venous flow pattern with low-velocity antegrade systolic and diastolic flow and is associated with an enlarged coronary sinus, as the left superior vena cava usually drains into the RA via the coronary sinus.

Answer 11:

IMAGE 1: Answer A, Aortic aneurysm
This transthoracic apical 2-chamber view angulated laterally shows the descending thoracic aorta posterior to the LV with enlargement to 5.5 cm, diagnostic of an aortic aneurysm.

IMAGE 2: Answer I, Pulmonary artery thrombus
This TEE long-axis view of the ascending aorta shows the right pulmonary artery filled with a large irregular echogenic mass consistent with a thrombus (e.g., pulmonary embolism). The linear echodensity within the aortic lumen is consistent with a beam-width artifact.

IMAGE 3: Answer E, Complex aortic atheroma
The patient has several risk factors for atherosclerotic disease, and complex aortic atheroma is associated with an increased risk of stroke. This TEE short-axis view of the descending thoracic aorta demonstrates an irregular-shaped protruding border with extensive thickening that was diffusely seen through the aortic arch and descending aorta.

IMAGE 4: Answer D, Aortic pseudoaneurysm
In a TEE short-axis view of the descending thoracic aorta, the aortic shape is irregular, rather than circular, with a discontinuity in the aortic wall at the top of the image and a second echolucent space consistent with a contained aortic rupture.

IMAGE 5: Answer F, Normal variant
This TEE short-axis view of the descending thoracic aorta shows a crescent-shaped echodensity, but the aortic valve is intact and the echo density is outside the aorta, which is most consistent with adipose tissue within the hemiazygos sheath. A normal healthy intimal wall can be seen along with the echo-bright adventitial boundary. The fat is outside of the adventitial layer and surrounded by a small pleural effusion. This normal variant is distinguished from an intramural hematoma by the epiaortic (rather than intraluminal) location.

IMAGE 6: Answer G, Penetrating atherosclerotic ulcer
In this long-axis view of the descending thoracic aorta a large atheroma is present with a crater-like outpouching within the atheromatous aortic wall.

17 The Adult With Congenital Heart Disease

BASIC PRINCIPLES

Identification of Cardiac Chambers and Vessels

- Identification of the chambers, great vessels, and their connections is the first step in echocardiographic evaluation of the patient with congenital heart disease (see The Echo Exam).

❖ KEY POINTS

- ❏ The right ventricle (RV) and left ventricle (LV) are distinguished based on the atrioventricular valve anatomy and position, the presence or absence of a moderator band, and the presence or absence of a muscular infundibular region (Fig. 17.1).
- ❏ The size and location of the ventricular chamber is not reliable for distinguishing the anatomic LV from RV.
- ❏ The RV tends to have a more triangular shape, whereas the LV is more ellipsoid, but shape can be unreliable when severe dilation is present.
- ❏ The aorta and pulmonary artery are identified by their distal anatomy; the pulmonary artery bifurcates into right and left pulmonary arteries, whereas the aorta supplies the head and neck arteries via the arch (Fig. 17.2).
- ❏ In addition to anatomic definitions, the ventricle that pumps oxygenated blood into the aorta

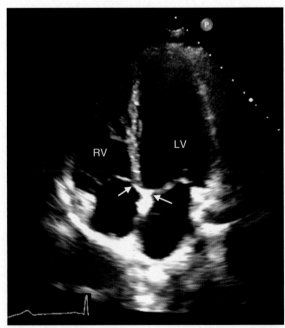

Fig. 17.1 **Identify the ventricles.** The anatomic RV and LV are identified in the apical 4-chamber view based on morphologic features that include a more apical position of the tricuspid versus mitral annulus *(arrows)* and the moderator band and trabeculations in the RV. The atrioventricular valves are associated with the correct anatomic ventricle, even when atrial or great vessel connections are discordant. Mitral and tricuspid valve anatomy were confirmed in other views.

is called the *systemic ventricle*, and the ventricle that pumps systemic venous return into the pulmonary artery is called the *pulmonic ventricle*.

Valve Stenosis and Regurgitation

- Valve stenosis and regurgitation are evaluated using the same methods as for acquired valve disease.

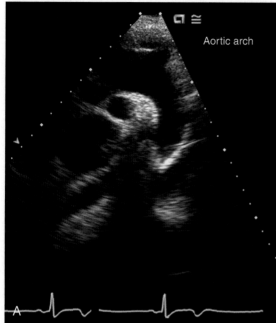

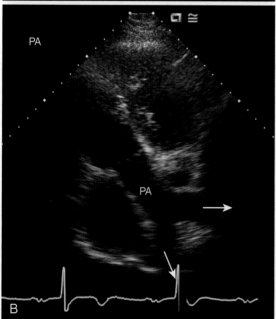

Fig. 17.2 Identify the great arteries. (A) The aortic arch, in a suprasternal notch view, is identified by the arch and head and neck vessels. (B) The pulmonary artery *(PA)*, from an apical transducer position angulated anteriorly from the 4-chamber view, is identified based on its bifurcation to the main PA branches *(arrows)*.

❖ **KEY POINTS**

- ❏ Congenital valve stenosis may be valvular, subvalvular, or supravalvular.
- ❏ Delineation of the level of obstruction using pulsed and color Doppler is necessary, in addition to continuous-wave (CW) Doppler measurements.

Intracardiac Shunts

- Intracardiac shunts are detected and quantitated using multiple Doppler modalities.
- The effects of shunting on chamber size and function are critical elements in assessment of shunt size.

❖ **KEY POINTS**

- ❏ Intracardiac shunts are detected based on the presence of a flow disturbance on the downstream side of the shunt with color or pulsed Doppler.
- ❏ The velocity and shape of the CW Doppler signal across an intracardiac shunt reflects the pressure difference across the shunt and is a key factor in determining shunt location.
- ❏ The pulmonic-to-systemic flow ratio is calculated based on transpulmonic stroke volume and transaortic stroke volume.
- ❏ A significant shunt results in enlargement of the chambers exposed to volume overload and may result in systolic ventricular dysfunction.

Complex Disease

- Most patients with congenital heart disease should be evaluated at centers with established Adult Congenital Heart Disease programs.

❖ **KEY POINTS**

- ❏ This chapter includes a basic approach for simple conditions or patients with a well-established diagnosis.
- ❏ More complex cases require additional data acquisition by sonographers and physicians with expertise in congenital heart disease.

STEP-BY-STEP APPROACH

Basic Transthoracic Echo Exam

- A structured study sequence is needed to ensure that all the images and Doppler flows needed for diagnosis are recorded.
- Most adult echocardiography laboratories acquire images and Doppler data in a similar sequence as for a standard adult study.
- With complex disease, the sonographer and physician work together during image acquisition to ensure the needed data are obtained.

Step 1: Review the Clinical History

- Review the details of any previous surgical or percutaneous procedures.

- Obtain reports (and images when possible) of any previous diagnostic tests.
- Determine the specific objectives of the current examination.

❖ **KEY POINTS**

- ❑ Knowledge of previous procedures and diagnostic studies ensures the current exam provides additional information and focuses on the key clinical issues.
- ❑ Complete evaluation of the adult with congenital heart disease often requires multiple diagnostic modalities; the echocardiographic examination provides only part of the needed information.

Step 2: Acquire Imaging and Doppler Data

Parasternal Long-Axis View

- The position and angle of the transducer needed to obtain a long-axis view help identify an abnormal cardiac position in the chest (dextroversion or dextrocardia).
- Great vessel morphology and location are evaluated in the long-axis view.
- The connections of the great vessels to the ventricles are determined.
- Doppler is used to evaluate for valve regurgitation, areas of stenosis, and intracardiac shunts.

❖ **KEY POINTS**

- ❑ Three-dimensional (3D), biplane imaging or single-plane imaging with medial and lateral angulation of the transducer shows the relationship of the great vessels to each other and to the ventricular chambers.
- ❑ The pulmonary artery normally is anterior and runs perpendicular to the aorta; an anteriorly located aorta that lies parallel with the pulmonary artery suggests transposition of the great vessels (Fig. 17.3).
- ❑ The transducer is moved up one or more interspaces to follow the great vessel(s) seen in the long-axis view, allowing differentiation of the aorta from the pulmonary artery.
- ❑ Ventricular and atrial septal defects (ASDs) can be identified with color Doppler while slowly scanning from lateral to medial in the long-axis image plane and from apex to base in the short-axis plane. 3D color imaging may be helpful if a high frame rate is possible.
- ❑ Standard measurements of great vessels and cardiac chambers are recorded in the long-axis view.
- ❑ When the heart or great vessel position is abnormal, transducer location for image acquisition is recorded, because this information cannot be determined from the images themselves.
- ❑ An enlarged coronary sinus suggests a persistent left superior vena cava. If needed, this can be confirmed with intravenous administration of saline contrast via the left upper extremity; after

injection, contrast will appear in the coronary sinus before it drains into the right atrium (RA).

Parasternal Short-Axis View

- The short-axis view shows the relationship of the semilunar (aortic and pulmonic) valves (Fig. 17.4).
- Basal ventricular size, systolic function, and septal motion are evaluated.

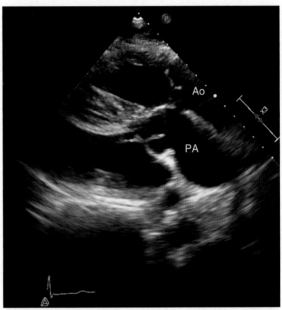

Fig. 17.3 Anteriorly located aorta (Ao). In this parasternal long-axis image of a patient with complete transposition of the great arteries, the anterior–posterior locations of the aorta (larger and anterior) and pulmonary artery *(PA)* (smaller and posterior) are opposite the normal position, and the vessels lie parallel to each, rather than in the normal perpendicular relationship.

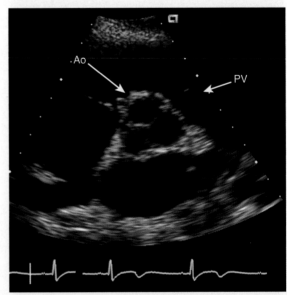

Fig. 17.4 Normal aortic and pulmonary artery positions. The normal aortic valve *(Ao)* and pulmonic valve *(PV)* planes are perpendicular to each other so that the aortic valve is seen in short axis when the pulmonic valve is seen in long axis. Normally, the most anterior great vessel at the base of the heart is the pulmonary artery.

- Ventricular septal defects (VSDs) and ASDs are demonstrated using color Doppler.
- A cleft anterior mitral valve leaflet, commonly associated with primum ASDs, may be seen from a parasternal short-axis view of the mitral valve.

❖ **KEY POINTS**

- ❑ The normal relationship of the aortic and pulmonic valve planes is perpendicular to each other. When both are seen in short-axis view in the same image plane, transposition of the great vessels is present (Fig. 17.5).
- ❑ The anterior-posterior and medial-lateral locations of the aorta and pulmonary artery at the base are evaluated; the aortic root is anterior to the pulmonary artery when transposition is present.
- ❑ ASDs and VSDs typically are well seen in the short-axis view.
- ❑ The location of a VSD relative to the aortic valve helps distinguish a membranous from subpulmonic (or supracristal) defect.
- ❑ Pulsed and CW Doppler interrogation of any abnormal color flow signal is helpful for diagnosis based on the time course and velocity of flow.

Parasternal Right Ventricular Inflow and Outflow Views

- The RV inflow view is helpful for evaluation of the RA, pulmonary atrioventricular valve, and annulus (Fig. 17.6).

- CW Doppler measurement of atrioventricular valve regurgitant velocity allows measurement of RV (or pulmonary) systolic pressure.
- The RV outflow view allows visualization of RV outflow obstruction at the subvalvular, pulmonic valve, or supravalvular level.
- Doppler evaluation allows localization of the level of RV outflow obstruction and calculation of the gradient between the ventricle and pulmonary artery.

❖ **KEY POINTS**

- ❑ Standard RV inflow and outflow views may be difficult to obtain when transposition is present.
- ❑ Slow angulation from the long-axis view toward the RV inflow view, using color Doppler, may be helpful for diagnosis of ASD and VSD.
- ❑ When right (or pulmonic) ventricular outflow tract obstruction is present, ventricular systolic pressure does *not* equal pulmonary systolic pressure; instead, the transpulmonic gradient is subtracted from ventricular systolic pressure to determine pulmonary systolic pressure (Fig. 17.7).
- ❑ Evaluation of RV outflow obstruction requires color and pulsed Doppler to determine the anatomic location of the increase in velocity and CW Doppler to measure the peak velocity.

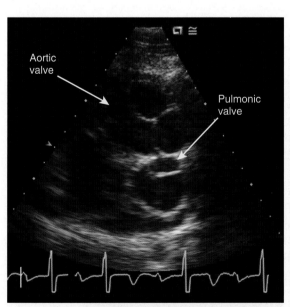

Fig. 17.5 Abnormal aortic and pulmonary artery positions. With transposition of the great arteries, the aorta is anterior to the pulmonary artery with a side-by-side (instead of crisscross) relationship of the great arteries. The semilunar valves are both in the same image plane so that the aortic and pulmonic valves are both seen in cross section in a short-axis view.

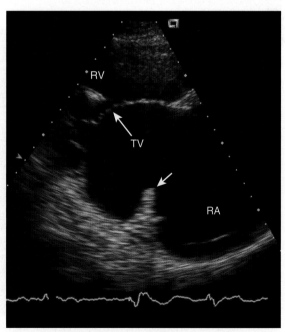

Fig. 17.6 Ebstein anomaly. The RV inflow view in a patient with Ebstein anomaly of the tricuspid valve *(TV)* shows the apical displacement of the septal leaflet from the annulus *(short arrow)*, with the atrialized portion of the RV between the annulus and leaflet attachment level.

Apical Views

- The morphology, size, and function of both ventricles are evaluated in the 4-chamber, 2-chamber, and long-axis views.
- The atrioventricular valves are evaluated using two-dimensional (2D) imaging, color Doppler, and CW Doppler.

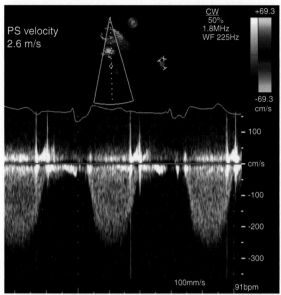

Fig. 17.7 **Mild stenosis of a transcatheter bioprosthetic pulmonic valve.** In a patient with tetralogy of Fallot who had undergone transcatheter bioprosthetic pulmonic valve replacement for severe pulmonic regurgitation, CW Doppler from the parasternal window shows an antegrade velocity of 2.6 m/s, consistent with mild stenosis, but no regurgitation is seen.

- Anterior angulation from the 4-chamber view often allows imaging of the connection from each ventricle to the great vessels (Fig. 17.8).
- Ventricular inflow and outflow signals are recorded using pulsed and CW Doppler.

❖ KEY POINTS

- ❑ The normal transducer orientation is used to ensure correct identification of the location and anatomy of each ventricle.
- ❑ The apical view often allows recognition of the anatomic RV based on the shorter distance from the annulus to the apex, compared with the LV, as well as presence of the moderator band.
- ❑ The atrioventricular valves are evaluated using standard Doppler approaches.
- ❑ With anterior angulation to image the great vessels, the bifurcation of the pulmonary artery and the curve of the aortic arch may be visualized, helping with identification of the ventricular to great vessel connections.
- ❑ With posterior angulation, the size and location of the coronary sinus are evaluated.
- ❑ Atrial anatomy and size may be evaluated, although the distance of these chambers from the transducer may limit detailed evaluation, particularly in patients with an interatrial baffle repair.
- ❑ Evaluation of the interatrial septum may be limited by ultrasound dropout, because the atrial septum is parallel to the ultrasound beam.

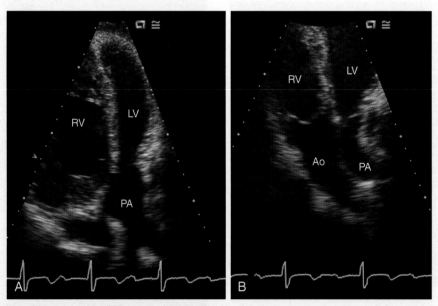

Fig. 17.8 **Transposition of the great arteries (TGA).** In this patient with TGA, from the apical 4-chamber view, the transducer is angulated anteriorly to show the pulmonary artery *(PA)* with its bifurcation (A) and then the ascending aorta *(Ao)*, which has coronary ostia and an arch in the far field (B). This view is helpful for documenting which ventricle ejects into each great vessel. In this patient with transposition of the great vessels and an interatrial baffle repair, the RV ejects into the anteriorly located aorta and the LV ejects into the more posteriorly located pulmonary artery.

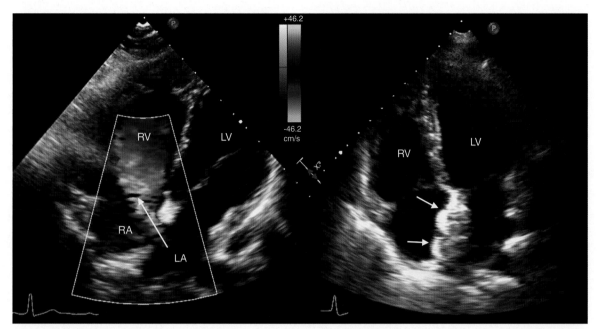

Fig. 17.9 Secundum atrial septal defect. In a modified apical 4-chamber view *(left)*, color Doppler shows a wide jet of flow from LA to RA across the center of the atrial septum. The RV is dilated due to volume overload from the left-to-right shunt. In a standard 4-chamber view after placement of a transcatheter atrial septal occluder device *(right)*, the bright echoes and thick atrial septum *(arrows)* are consistent with the expected position of the device. RV size has normalized with correction of the RV overload.

Subcostal Views

- The subcostal 4-chamber view allows evaluation of the interatrial septum (Fig. 17.9).
- RV size and systolic function often are best evaluated from the subcostal view.
- The entrance of the inferior vena cava provides clear identification of the RA chamber.

❖ KEY POINTS

- ❏ The ultrasound beam is perpendicular to the interatrial septum from the subcostal view so that ultrasound dropout, simulating an atrial defect, is less likely. This view is optimal for 2D and color Doppler detection of an ASD or patent foramen ovale.
- ❏ In adults, the free wall of the RV may not be well seen in apical views. The subcostal view provides a more standard image plane of the RV, with the ultrasound beam perpendicular to the RV free wall, and thus is more reliable for evaluation of RV size and function.
- ❏ The junction of the inferior vena cava and RA provides anatomic information on atrial situs, in addition to allowing estimation of RA pressure.

Suprasternal Notch Views

- A standard transducer orientation allows identification of aortic arch position and anatomy.
- Aortic coarctation is evaluated (or excluded) based on CW Doppler descending aortic flow (Figs. 17.10 and 17.11).

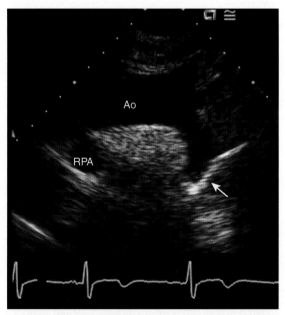

Fig. 17.10 Aortic arch imaging. The suprasternal notch view is used to evaluate aortic coarctation. However, on 2D imaging even a normal descending aorta *(Ao)* appears to taper *(arrow)*, because the curvature of the vessel results in an oblique plane through the vessel. *RPA,* Right pulmonary artery.

- Images and pulsed Doppler flows in the superior vena cava are useful in many types of congenital heart disease.

❖ KEY POINTS

- ❏ A right-sided aortic arch may be missed if the transducer or image orientation is reversed.

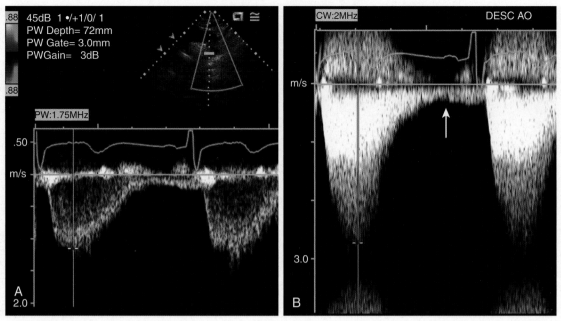

Fig. 17.11 Doppler flows in aortic coarctation. Flow is recorded using pulsed Doppler in the descending aorta proximal to the coarctation (A) and with CW Doppler as blood passes through the narrowed segment (B). When a severe coarctation is present, there is persistent antegrade flow in diastole *(arrow)* due to a higher diastolic pressure proximal, compared with distal, to the coarctation.

- ❑ Normal systolic and diastolic flow in the descending aorta excludes a diagnosis of aortic coarctation.
- ❑ The superior vena cava typically is to the right of the ascending aorta. Flow patterns are diagnostic if obstruction is present or when the superior vena cava flow has been redirected into the pulmonary artery.
- ❑ The right pulmonary artery is seen inferior to the arch. When ultrasound penetration is optimal, the left atrium (LA) and pulmonary veins also may be identified.
- ❑ The branch pulmonary arteries may be seen in the parasternal short-axis view in some patients.
- ❑ An aortic to pulmonary artery shunt may be evaluated from the suprasternal notch view in some cases (e.g., patent ductus arteriosis, aortic to pulmonary window).

Step 3: Estimate Pulmonary Pressure

- ■ In the absence of pulmonic stenosis, RV (and pulmonary) systolic pressure is calculated by the standard approach based on tricuspid regurgitant jet velocity and estimated RA pressure (Fig. 17.12).
- ■ With complex congenital heart disease, estimation of pulmonary pressures depends on the exact cardiac anatomy.

❖ KEY POINTS

- ❑ When pulmonic stenosis is present, pulmonary systolic pressure is estimated by subtracting the transpulmonic gradient the RV systolic pressure, using the pulmonic stenosis (V_{PS}) and tricuspid regurgitant jet (V_{TR}) velocities:

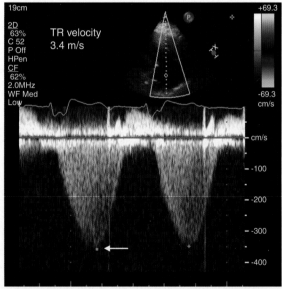

Fig. 17.12 Elevated RV, but not pulmonary, systolic pressure. This tricuspid regurgitation *(TR)* jet shows a maximum velocity of 3.4 m/s, consistent with an RV to RA systolic pressure difference of 46 mm Hg, or an estimated RV systolic pressure of 56 mm Hg, assuming an RA pressure of 10 mm Hg. However, this patient has mild stenosis of her bioprosthetic pulmonic valve (shown in Fig. 17.7), so the RV-to-pulmonary artery (PA) systolic gradient must be subtracted from the estimated RV pressure to estimate PA systolic pressure. Thus, estimated PA systolic pressure is 56 mm Hg – 27 mm Hg = 29 mm Hg.

$$\text{Estimated PA systolic pressure} = 4(V_{TR})^2 - 4(V_{PS})^2$$

- ❑ With a large unrestricted VSD and Eisenmenger physiology, pulmonary artery and aortic pressures are equalized, even if there is no tricuspid regurgitation.

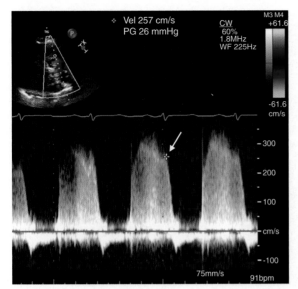

Fig. 17.13 **Pulmonic regurgitant velocity.** The end-diastolic pulmonic regurgitant velocity reflects the diastolic pulmonary artery (PA)-to-RV pressure gradient, which is 26 mm Hg in this case. Assuming an RV diastolic pressure of 10 mm Hg, estimated PA diastolic pressure is 26 mm Hg + 10 mm Hg = 36 mm Hg, which is consistent with moderate pulmonary hypertension.

- ❏ With tricuspid atresia and Fontan physiology (direct connection of systemic venous return to the pulmonary artery), pulmonary pressures are low with a venous type blood flow pattern.
- ❏ Pulmonary diastolic pressure can be estimated from the end-diastolic pulmonic regurgitant velocity, plus an estimate of RV diastolic pressure (Fig. 17.13).
- ❏ The velocity through a VSD reflects the instantaneous LV-to-RV systolic pressure difference.

Step 4: Review and Report Study Results

- ■ Most adult congenital disease studies are reported in the standard format with additional sections for the congenital findings.
- ■ The report describes the anatomy and physiology, with an indication of the level of certainty of each finding, depending on data quality.
- ■ The echocardiographic findings are interpreted in view of the clinical history, previous surgical procedures, and current clinical indication.

❖ **KEY POINTS**

- ❏ The findings in most patients with congenital disease can be described using a standard report format; however, with complex congenital heart disease, a more detailed narrative description is needed.
- ❏ The echocardiographic study should not be used to deduce the surgical history; instead, the surgical history should be reviewed to ensure the echocardiographic study provides a complete evaluation.
- ❏ The echocardiographic study should seek to answer the specific clinical question articulated by the referring physician.

- ❏ The current study should be compared with previous examinations (with side-by-side review of images when possible).

Step 5: Determine Remaining Anatomic/ Physiologic Questions

- ■ Initial evaluation of simple congenital heart disease and follow-up studies of more complex disease may require only transthoracic echocardiography.
- ■ Additional diagnostic procedures often are needed for evaluation of complex congenital heart disease.

❖ **KEY POINTS**

- ❏ Transthoracic echocardiography often cannot fully evaluate atrial-level anatomy and flow in patients with Fontan physiology or an interatrial baffle repair, due to the distance of the transducer from the structures of interest (Fig. 17.14).
- ❏ Extracardiac connections, such as arterial-to-pulmonary shunts, are difficult to assess by transthoracic echocardiography.
- ❏ Previous surgical procedures may result in shadowing or reverberations due to prosthetic valves, conduits, or patch material.
- ❏ Evaluation of branch pulmonary artery stenosis usually requires other diagnostic approaches.
- ❏ Quantitation of RV volumes and systolic function is problematic with standard echocardiographic approaches.
- ❏ These areas of uncertainty or issues that cannot be addressed by echocardiography are identified at the end of the study with suggestions for appropriate additional diagnostic approaches.

Basic Transesophageal Approach

Step 1: Assess the Risk of TEE and Institute Appropriate Modifications in the Study Protocol

- ■ The risk of conscious sedation is higher in some patients with congenital heart disease.
- ■ Additional monitoring and sedation by an anesthesiologist may be needed in some cases.

❖ **KEY POINTS**

- ❏ Risk of sedation is highest in patients with cyanosis, severe pulmonary hypertension, or Eisenmenger physiology.
- ❏ Concurrent pulmonary or other medical conditions also may be present that increase procedural risk.
- ❏ Baseline oxygen saturation is assessed before beginning the procedure, because patients may have significant chronic desaturation due to an intracardiac shunt.
- ❏ When risk is high or uncertain, a cardiac anesthesiologist should be asked to assist with the procedure.

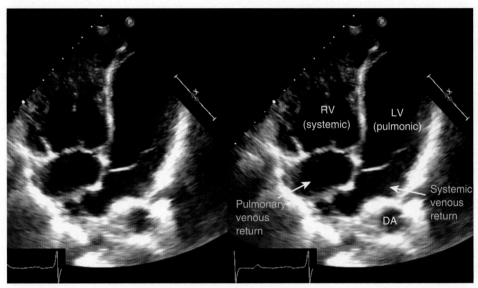

Fig. 17.14 **Interatrial baffle.** Apical 4-chamber view of a patient with complete transposition of the great arteries (d-TGA) and an interatrial baffle repair. The systemic ventricle (anatomic RV) fills from the pulmonary venous return arm of the baffle. The systemic ventricle has an appropriate size and wall thickness for a systemic ventricle, but the moderator band and more apical position of the tricuspid valve insertion identify it as an anatomic RV. The pulmonic (anatomic left, LV) ventricle fills from the systemic venous return arm of the baffle. The pulmonic ventricle (anatomic LV) is relatively normal in size and systolic function. If there is concern for baffle obstruction or leak, TEE or cardiac magnetic resonance imaging provides better visualization of the atrial baffle. *DA*, Descending aorta.

❏ All health care providers involved in the study (e.g., physician, nurse, and sonographer) should understand and review any potential risks.

Step 2: Determine the Objectives of the TEE Study

■ In consultation with the referring physician, the clinical data and transthoracic echocardiogram are reviewed to determine the specific areas of interest on the transesophageal echocardiography (TEE) study.

■ A complete TEE study is performed whenever possible, putting priority on key elements if study length is constrained.

❖ **KEY POINTS**

❏ TEE provides better visualization of posterior structures, such as the atrial septum, pulmonary veins, and interatrial baffle repairs (Fig. 17.15).

❏ 3D imaging allows better visualization of the shape of the defect and accurate measurement of defect size (Fig. 17.16).

❏ TEE provides improved images when prosthetic material shadows posterior structures from the transthoracic approach.

❏ Anterior and extracardiac structures (such as systemic venous return conduits, branch pulmonary stenosis, and arterial to pulmonic shunts) may be difficult to visualize on TEE (Fig. 17.17).

❏ Be sure all individuals involved in the TEE study understand the study objectives.

Step 3: TEE Imaging Sequence

■ The standard imaging sequence, described in Chapter 3, is appropriate for adults with congenital heart disease.

■ The examiner should ensure that all cardiac structures are evaluated by imaging and Doppler, preferably in at least two orthogonal views.

❖ **KEY POINTS**

❏ Start with the standard TEE 4-chamber, 2-chamber, long-axis rotational series of images to provide an overview of cardiac anatomy.

❏ Follow a checklist to ensure all structures are evaluated:
  ❏ Systemic and pulmonic ventricles (including anatomic identity, location, great vessel connections, and systolic function)
  ❏ Aorta and pulmonary artery (including size, location, and connections to the ventricles)
  ❏ Aortic and pulmonic valves (including anatomy and Doppler flows)
  ❏ Systemic and pulmonic atrioventricular valves (anatomy and function)
  ❏ Left and right atria (or interatrial baffle, Fontan conduit, etc.)
  ❏ Atrial septum and ventricular septum
  ❏ Location and flow patterns in all four pulmonary veins
  ❏ Superior and inferior vena cava
  ❏ Coronary sinus
  ❏ Descending aorta

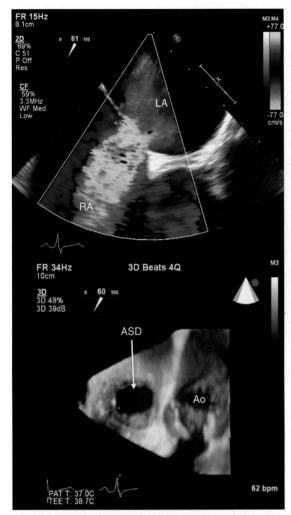

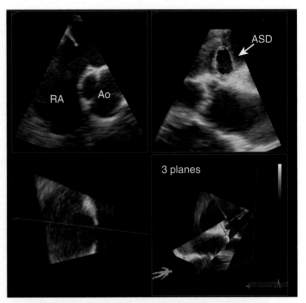

Fig. 17.16 **3D measurement of atrial septal defect (ASD) size.** From a 3D volumetric data acquisition in the same patient as in Fig. 17.15, the image planes are adjusted to provide a planar view of the ASD *(arrow)*, which allows accurate measurement of the area of the ASD and diameter for planning a transcatheter closure. *Ao,* Aorta.

- Anomalous pulmonary venous drainage into the RA or cavae also results in right-sided volume overload.
- Both the anatomic size of an ASD (measured directly) and the physiologic effects (based on the amount of flow across the defect) are useful measures of disease severity.

❖ **KEY POINTS**

- ❏ A secundum or primum ASD may be visualized on transthoracic imaging in parasternal short axis, apical 4-chamber, and subcostal 4-chamber views (see Fig. 17.9).
- ❏ Color Doppler evidence of transatrial flow avoids mistaking echo dropout from an ASD, but care is needed to distinguish normal superior and inferior vena cava inflow from flow across the atrial septum.
- ❏ A primum ASD may be accompanied by a cleft anterior mitral leaflet (Fig. 17.18).
- ❏ An endocardial cushion defect is the association of a primum ASD with an adjacent VSD, often with associated abnormalities of the atrioventricular valves.
- ❏ A sinus venosus ASD may be difficult to visualize on transthoracic imaging and often is suspected based on unexplained right-sided enlargement; on TEE imaging in the bicaval view with the probe rotated slightly rightward, the defect is seen at the junction of the superior vena cava with the RA. Anomalous pulmonary venous return may also be seen.

Fig. 17.15 **TEE imaging of atrial septal defect.** *Top,* 2D TEE shows a secundum ASD with left-to-right flow seen on color Doppler. *Bottom,* A 3D image better shows the shape and size of the defect. *Ao,* Aorta.

- ❏ Transgastric views may provide alternate views of the ventricles, atrioventricular valves, and aortic and pulmonic valves.
- ❏ Before completing the study, ask the nurse and sonographer if any imaging views or Doppler flows have been missed and if they have any other suggestions.

SPECIAL CONSIDERATIONS IN COMMON CONDITIONS

Atrial Septal Defect

- RV volume overload due to an ASD results in the characteristic findings of RV enlargement and paradoxical septal motion.
- ASDs are classified as:
  - ○ Secundum (center of atrial septum)
  - ○ Primum (adjacent to the atrioventricular valves)
  - ○ Sinus venosus (near junction of superior or inferior vena cava)

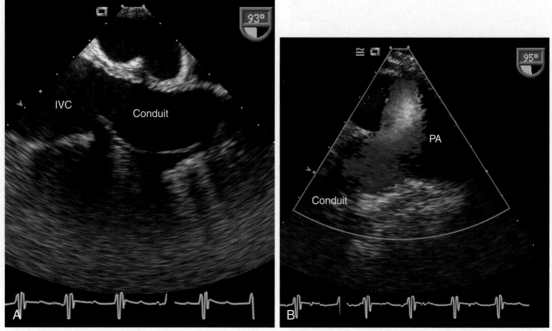

Fig. 17.17 **Tricuspid atresia with Fontan conduit.** The conduit from the inferior vena cava *(IVC)* to the pulmonary artery *(PA)* is seen on TEE in a vertical image plane by turning the probe toward the patient's right side. The junction of the IVC and the conduit (A) is seen and then the probe is slowly withdrawn in the esophagus, keeping the conduit centered in the image plane (B) to show the flow from the conduit into the pulmonary artery.

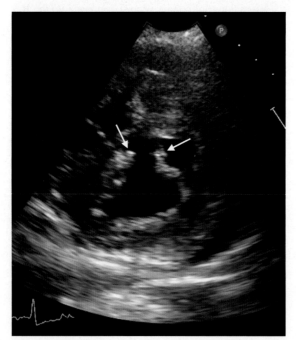

Fig. 17.18 **Cleft anterior mitral valve.** In a parasternal short-axis image, the differing maximal excursion of the medial and lateral aspects of the cleft leaflet *(arrows)* are seen.

❑ The presence of RV dilation mandates a careful search for an ASD or anomalous pulmonary venous return using 2D imaging, color Doppler, and an intravenous saline contrast study.

❑ When visualized, the diameter of the ASD should be directly measured from two images or on 3D imaging.
❑ Shunt flow, defined as the ratio of pulmonary blood flow (Qp) to systemic blood flow (Qs), is determined by calculating stroke volume in the pulmonary artery and aorta, with a ratio of more than 1.5:1 considered significant.
❑ Transesophageal imaging is more sensitive than transthoracic imaging for detection of a sinus venosus ASD or anomalous pulmonary venous return.

Ventricular Septal Defect

- VSDs are classified as:
  ○ Membranous (from just beneath the aortic valve to under the septal tricuspid leaflet)
  ○ Supracristal (from just beneath the aortic valve to under the pulmonic valve)
  ○ Inlet (between the mitral and tricuspid valves)
  ○ Muscular (anywhere in the muscular part of the ventricular septum)
- Large uncorrected VSDs result in severe pulmonary hypertension early in life with equalization of pulmonary and systolic pressures and bidirectional shunting (Eisenmenger physiology).
- Small VSDs are associated with a high-pressure difference (and high velocity) between the LV and RV in systole.

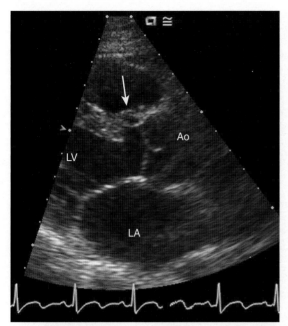

Fig. 17.19 **Ventricular septal defect imaging.** In a patient referred for a systolic murmur, the region of the membranous septum *(arrow)* appears abnormal in the standard parasternal long-axis view. *Ao,* Aorta.

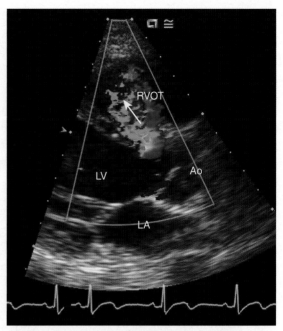

Fig. 17.20 **Ventricular septal defect (VSD) color Doppler flow.** In the same patient as in Fig. 17.19, color Doppler confirms left-to-right flow consistent with a membranous VSD. *Ao,* Aorta; *RVOT,* right ventricular outflow tract.

❖ **KEY POINTS**

❑ The anatomic site of a VSD is detected using the combination of 2D imaging (Fig. 17.19) and color Doppler to demonstrate systolic turbulence on the right side of the ventricular septum (Fig. 17.20).

❑ The VSD is confirmed using CW Doppler to demonstrate the high-velocity systolic ejection type Doppler curve (Fig. 17.21).

❑ The peak velocity of the VSD jet is related to the left to RV systolic pressure difference as stated in the Bernoulli equation:

$$\Delta P = 4V^2$$

❑ A low-velocity diastolic signal also may be seen corresponding to the diastolic pressure difference between the LV and RV.

❑ With Eisenmenger physiology, a large VSD is seen on 2D imaging with bidirectional flow on color and spectral Doppler. RV and LV size and wall thickness are similar and the velocities in the mitral and tricuspid regurgitation jets are equal (Fig. 17.22).

Patent Ductus Arteriosus

■ Most patent ductus arteriosus (PDAs) are diagnosed and treated early in life, with only rare cases diagnosed in adults.

■ Continuous systolic and diastolic flow into the main pulmonary artery is the key findings in adults with a PDA.

❖ **KEY POINTS**

❑ Color Doppler of the main pulmonary artery shows the diastolic flow from the PDA originating near the pulmonary artery bifurcation (Fig. 17.23).

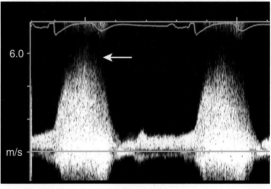

Fig. 17.21 **Ventricular septal defect CW Doppler.** In the same patient as in Fig. 17.20, the CW Doppler recording shows a very high-velocity signal *(arrow)* consistent with a small defect and a large systolic pressure gradient between the LV and RV in systole. There also is low-velocity left-to-right flow in diastole.

❑ Pulsed Doppler evidence of continuous flow in the pulmonary artery is diagnostic; this flow differs from pulmonic regurgitation by being distal to the pulmonic valve, and the diastolic components extend into systole (Fig. 17.24).

❑ Diastolic flow reversal also may be seen in the descending thoracic aorta and should not be mistaken for aortic regurgitation.

Aortic Coarctation

■ An aortic coarctation results in an increased systolic velocity and persistent diastolic antegrade flow in the descending thoracic aorta (Fig. 17.25).

■ Descending aortic flow is recorded with CW Doppler from the suprasternal notch view.

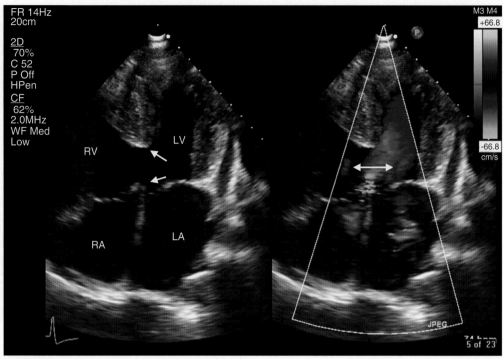

Fig. 17.22 **Eisenmenger ventricular septal defect (VSD).** With a large VSD, as seen in this low parasternal 4-chamber view in a patient with trisomy 21 *(left)*, Eisenmenger physiology is present with equalization of RV and LV pressures, significant systemic oxygen desaturation, and cyanosis. Color Doppler *(right)* shows unobstructed, low-velocity right-to-left and left-to-right flow.

❖ KEY POINTS

- ❏ Doppler may underestimate the severity of coarctation due to nonparallel intercept angle between the eccentric jet and ultrasound beam.
- ❏ When the proximal velocity is also increased, the proximal velocity should be included in the pressure gradient (ΔP) calculation:

$$\Delta P = 4 \left(V_{max}^2 - V_{prox}^2 \right)$$

- ❏ Imaging of the coarctation is rarely possible by transthoracic imaging in adults; TEE may be helpful in selected cases.
- ❏ Further evaluation of aortic coarctation with computed tomographic imaging or cardiac catheterization typically is needed.

Ebstein Anomaly

- ■ Ebstein anomaly is characterized by apical displacement of one or more tricuspid valve leaflets (Fig. 17.26; and see Fig. 17.6).
- ■ Imaging the tricuspid annulus and leaflets in parasternal RV inflow and apical 4-chamber views usually is diagnostic.
- ■ The segment of the RV between the annulus and displaced leaflet is "atrialized;" that is, ventricular myocardium is physiologically part of the atrial chamber.

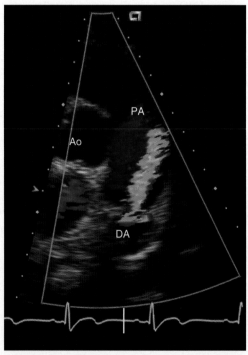

Fig. 17.23 **Patent ductus arteriosus.** In a parasternal short-axis image of the pulmonary artery *(PA)*, a color jet of diastolic flow is seen entering the PA near its bifurcation, with the flow originating from the descending aorta *(DA)* just posterior to the PA. *Ao,* Aorta.

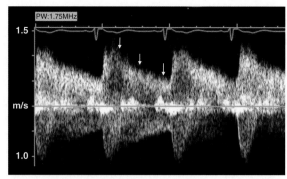

Fig. 17.24 CW Doppler of patent ductus arteriosus. There is continuous flow from the aorta into the pulmonary artery with the shape and velocity reflecting the pressure difference between the two vessels. For example, the increased systolic velocity corresponds to the increase in systemic blood pressure during systole.

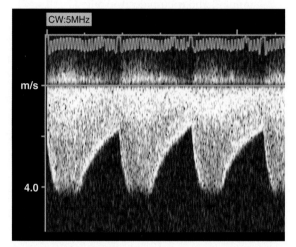

Fig. 17.25 Aortic coarctation. CW Doppler flow in the descending aorta shows an antegrade velocity greater than 4 m/s consistent with a pressure gradient of at least 64 mm Hg (possibly higher if the intercept angle is not parallel to blood flow). Persistent antegrade flow in diastole confirms severe obstruction.

❖ **KEY POINTS**

❑ Ebstein anomaly may be isolated or associated with an ASD and is common (about 15% to 40%) in patients with congenitally corrected transposition of the great vessels (see later section).

❑ Ebstein anomaly is often associated with ventricular preexcitation due to an accessory atrioventricular pathway (e.g., Wolf-Parkinson-White syndrome).

❑ In the apical 4-chamber view, a distance greater than 10 mm between the mitral and tricuspid leaflet insertions is diagnostic of Ebstein anomaly.

❑ Ebstein anomaly typically results in moderate or severe tricuspid regurgitation.

Complex Congenital Heart Disease

Tetralogy of Fallot

■ Tetralogy of Fallot is characterized by:
  ○ A membranous (anteriorly misaligned) VSD

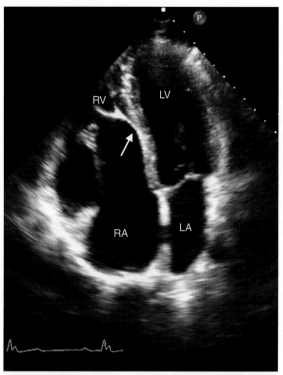

Fig. 17.26 Ebstein anomaly. Severe apical displacement of the septal tricuspid valve leaflet *(arrow)* is seen in an apical 4-chamber view.

  ○ An aorta that straddles the ventricular septum *and*
  ○ RV outflow obstruction *resulting in*
  ○ RV hypertrophy
■ Most adults with tetralogy of Fallot have undergone previous surgical repair with VSD closure and relief of RV outflow obstruction (Fig. 17.27).
■ The most common long-term issue after tetralogy of Fallot repair is severe pulmonic regurgitation with progressive RV enlargement and eventual dysfunction.
■ Patients with tetralogy of Fallot usually have mild dilation of the aortic sinuses.

❖ **KEY POINTS**

❑ RV outflow obstruction may be subvalvular, valvular, or supravalvular or may occur at more than one site, including branch pulmonary artery stenoses.

❑ Occasionally an adult patient with an untreated tetralogy of Fallot will be diagnosed by echocardiography, because the RV outflow obstruction prevents pulmonary hypertension.

❑ Severe pulmonic regurgitation typically is low velocity with a to-and-fro flow pattern by pulsed, CW, and color Doppler that may be overlooked due to the absence of turbulence (Fig. 17.28).

❑ Additional evaluation with cardiac magnetic resonance imaging often is needed for quantitation of RV size and function.

Congenitally Corrected Transposition of the Great Arteries

- The pathway of blood flow with transposition of the great arteries (L-TGA) is:
  - Systemic venous return to the RA, then into the LV and out the pulmonary artery.
  - Pulmonary venous return to the LA, then into the RV and out the aorta.
- Some patients with L-TGA remain undiagnosed until adulthood, because the flow of oxygenated and unoxygenated blood is physiologic, even though the anatomic RV serves as the systemic ventricle.

- Defects commonly associated with L-TGA include a VSD, pulmonic stenosis, Ebstein anomaly of the systemic (tricuspid) atrioventricular valve, and complete heart block.

❖ **KEY POINTS**

- L-TGA also is called *ventricular inversion*, because the pattern of blood flow is normal other than the reversed positions of the ventricles (and the associated atrioventricular valves).
- Typically, the aortic annulus is anterior and to the left (the *L* in L-TGA) of the pulmonic valve.
- L-TGA is evident on echocardiography based on the systemic ventricle having the anatomic features of an RV (moderator band, apical annulus, and tricuspid valve) (Fig. 17.29).

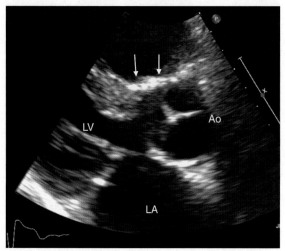

Fig. 17.27 Tetralogy of Fallot. Parasternal long-axis view in a typical patient with repaired tetralogy of Fallot. The basal septum is intact but has increased echogenicity *(arrows)* consistent with a ventricular septal defect patch repair; and the aorta *(Ao)* is mildly enlarged and slightly overrides the septum.

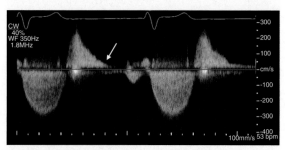

Fig. 17.28 Severe pulmonic regurgitation. CW Doppler signal of severe pulmonic regurgitation in a patient with repaired tetralogy of Fallot and persistent pulmonic regurgitation after surgical pulmonic valvotomy. The retrograde flow in diastole has a signal density similar to antegrade flow, consistent with similar volume flow rates. The diastolic deceleration slope is steep and reaches the baseline before the end of diastole *(arrow)*, which is consistent with equalization of diastolic pulmonary artery and RV pressures.

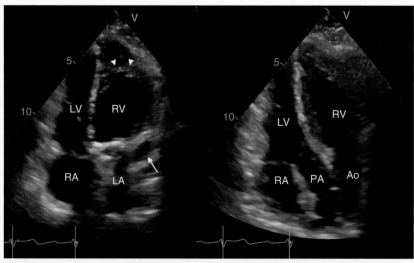

Fig. 17.29 Congenitally corrected transposition of the great arteries ventricular inversion. In the apical 4-chamber view *(left)*, pulmonic ventricle is the anatomic LV, filling from the RA. The systemic ventricle is the anatomic RV filing from the LA. The moderator band *(arrowheads)* is seen in the anatomic RV. The LA is identified by the prominent atrial appendage *(arrow)*. When the transducer is angulate anteriorly from the apical 4-chamber view *(right)*, the image plane now shows the side-by-side parallel great vessels with the pulmonary artery *(PA)* arising from the anatomic LV and the aorta *(Ao)* arising from the anatomic RV. The PA is identified by bifurcation into right and left branches; the Ao is identified by the arch vessels.

- The atrioventricular valves are associated with each ventricle, so the systemic atrioventricular valve is the tricuspid valve, and the pulmonary atrioventricular valve is the mitral valve.
- Long-term systolic dysfunction of the systemic ventricle may complicate L-TGA.
- Dextroversion (apex pointed toward the right) or mesocardia often is present with L-TGA, which limits acoustic access due to the retrosternal cardiac position.

Complete Transposition of the Great Arteries

- Complete transposition of the great arteries (d-TGA) requires intervention at birth to provide mixing between the separated pulmonic and systemic blood flow circuits.
- d-TGA then is treated by redirection of blood flow in childhood with:
  - An interatrial baffle repair that redirects systemic and pulmonary venous inflow to restore a normal pattern of circulation, but with the anatomic RV serving as the systemic ventricle (Mustard or Senning repair) *or*
  - More recently, an arterial switch procedure with the aorta and pulmonary artery transected and reconnected to the correct ventricles.
- The aorta is anterior and the great vessels are parallel to each other when d-TGA is present (see Figs. 17.3 and 17.4).
- With an interatrial baffle repair, a major long-term issue is systolic dysfunction of the systemic (anatomic right) ventricle.
- With an arterial switch repair, a few patients develop systemic semilunar valve regurgitation, particularly of the neo-aortic valve with dilation of the proximal "aortic" root (Fig. 17.30).

❖ KEY POINTS

- With an interatrial baffle repair, the circulatory pattern of oxygenated and unoxygenated blood is normal, but the systemic ventricle is the anatomic RV, and the pulmonic ventricle is the anatomic LV (Fig. 17.31).
- The atrioventricular valves are associated with each ventricle, so the systemic atrioventricular valve is the tricuspid valve, and the pulmonic atrioventricular valve is the mitral valve.
- Atrial baffle leaks and stenosis are difficult to evaluate by transthoracic imaging, typically requiring TEE or other imaging approaches.
- A lower Nyquist limit (i.e., signal aliasing at a lower velocity) and use of variance mode on the color display enhance detection of baffle leaks.
- With an arterial switch procedure, the neoaorta—the systemic semilunar valve and sinuses—was the anatomic pulmonic valve. The coronary arteries also were transposed to the neoaorta.

- Branch pulmonic stenosis can occur after an arterial switch repair related to moving the pulmonary artery anteriorly during the repair procedure.

Fontan Physiology With Tricuspid Atresia

- Fontan physiology refers to a direct valveless surgical connection from the systemic venous return to the pulmonary artery, without an intervening RV.
- A Fontan repair is used for patients with only a single functional ventricle, including those with tricuspid atresia (Fig. 17.32).

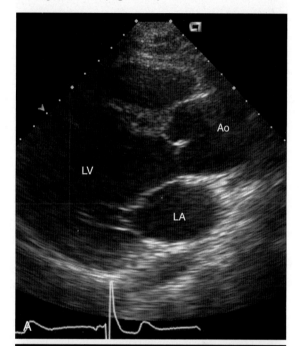

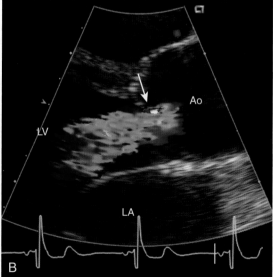

Fig. 17.30 Transposition the great arteries (d-TGA). This 19-year-old man with complete TGA underwent a great vessel switch repair as an infant. The ventricular to great vessel relationships now are relatively normal as seen in this long-axis view. However, the sinuses of the transposed pulmonic valve (neo-aorta) are dilated to 4.6 cm (A) and central "aortic" regurgitation is present (B), with a vena contracta width of 0.5 cm. *Ao,* Aorta.

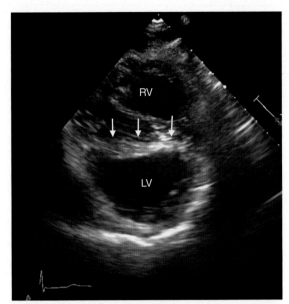

Fig. 17.31 **Transposition the great arteries (d-TGA).** Short-axis view of the ventricles in a patient with TGA and an interatrial baffle repair. The RV is located anteriorly but serves as the systemic ventricle and is appropriately dilated and hypertrophied but with a moderator band and prominent trabeculation. The smaller, posteriorly located LV is the low-pressure pulmonic ventricle with septal flattening *(arrows)* in diastole (and systole) reflecting the higher pressure in the systemic ventricle (anatomic RV) compared to the pulmonic ventricle (anatomic LV).

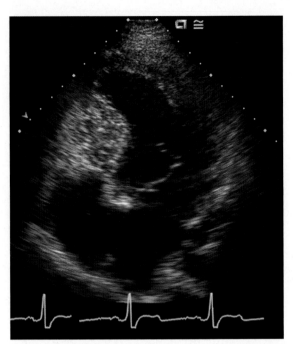

Fig. 17.32 **Single ventricle physiology.** Apical view in a patient with tricuspid and pulmonic atresia shows only one ventricle and atrioventricular valve. The tricuspid valve is absent, with the small residual RV chamber (not visible in this view) communicating with the LV via a ventricular septal defect. The right and left atria are connected by a large atrial septal defect. Pulmonary blood flow in this patient is provided by a right subclavian artery to pulmonary artery shunt.

- Flow in a Fontan conduit is driven by the pressure gradient from the systemic venous return to the pulmonary artery, with a flow pattern similar to a normal systemic venous inflow (Fig. 17.33).

❖ **KEY POINTS**

- There are many variations of the Fontan procedure:
  - Early Fontan repairs connected the RA to the pulmonary artery. These patients often have a severely enlarged RA with significant arrhythmias and may have obstruction of the pulmonary veins posterior to the dilated atrium.
  - More recent repairs include a direct connection of the superior vena cava to the right pulmonary artery with the inferior vena cava connected to the pulmonary artery by a conduit. This repair leaves the small residual RA (with the coronary sinus) in communication with the LA via an ASD.
- Transthoracic and transesophageal echocardiographic evaluation of a Fontan conduit is challenging and depends on the exact surgical repair and location of the conduit (see Fig. 17.17).
- Valved conduits connecting the RV to the pulmonary artery are used for other types of complex congenital heart disease. These patients do not have Fontan physiology, because the RV provides pulsatile systolic pulmonary blood flow.

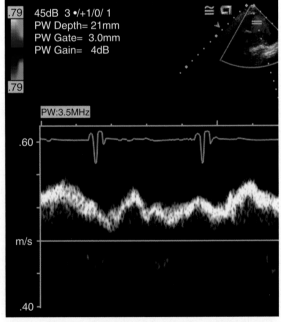

Fig. 17.33 **Fontan conduit flow.** The flow pattern is similar to systemic venous flow, with low-velocity forward flow in systole and diastole, because pulmonary blood flow is driven by systemic venous pressure in the absence of the pumping action of a RV.

THE ECHO EXAM
Adult Congenital Heart Disease

Categories of Congenital Heart Disease

Congenital Stenotic Lesions

Subvalvular
Valvular
Supravalvular
Great vessels (e.g., aortic coarctation)

Congenital Regurgitant Lesions

Ebstein anomaly
Cleft mitral valve

Abnormal Intracardiac Communications

Atrial septal defect
Ventricular septal defect
Patent ductus arteriosus

Abnormal Chamber and Great Vessel Connections

Transposition of the great arteries (d-TGA)
Congenitally corrected transposition (L-TGA or CCTGA)
Tetralogy of Fallot
Tricuspid atresia
Truncus arteriosus

Approach to the Echocardiographic Examination in Adults With Congenital Heart Disease

Before the Examination

Review the clinical history.
Obtain details of any prior surgical procedures.
Review results of prior diagnostic tests.
Formulate specific questions.

Sequence of Examination

Identify cardiac chambers, great vessels, and their connections.
Identify associated defects, and evaluate the physiology of each lesion.
Regurgitation and/or stenosis (quantitate as per Chapters 11 and 12)
Shunts (calculate $Q_p:Q_s$)
Pulmonary hypertension (calculate pulmonary pressure)
Ventricular dysfunction (measure ejection fraction if anatomy allows)

After the Examination

Integrate echo and Doppler findings with clinical data.
Summarize findings.
Identify which clinical questions remain unanswered, and suggest appropriate subsequent diagnostic tests.

Clues to the Identification of Cardiac Structures in Adults With Congenital Heart Disease

Structure	Anatomic feature	Echo Approach
Right atrium	• Inferior vena cava enters RA	• Start with subcostal approach to identify RA
Right ventricle	• Prominent trabeculation • Moderator band • Infundibulum • Tricuspid valve • Apical location of annulus	• Apical 4-chamber view to compare annular insertions of two ventricles • Parasternal view for valve anatomy and infundibulum
Pulmonary artery	• Bifurcates	• Parasternal long-axis view or apical 4-chamber view angulated very anteriorly
Left atrium	• Pulmonary veins usually enter LA	• TEE imaging for pulmonary vein anatomy
Left ventricle	• Mitral valve • Basal location of annulus • Fibrous continuity between anterior mitral leaflet and semilunar valve	• Apical 4-chamber view and parasternal long- and short-axis views
Aorta	• Gives rise to aortic arch and arterial branches	• Start with parasternal long-axis view and move transducer superiorly to follow vessel to its branches

SELF-ASSESSMENT QUESTIONS

Question 1

A 23-year-old asymptomatic woman is referred for echocardiography to evaluate a murmur (Fig. 17.34). The most likely diagnosis is:

A. Aortic coarctation
B. Bicuspid aortic valve
C. Ventricular septal defect
D. Ebstein anomaly
E. Pulmonic stenosis

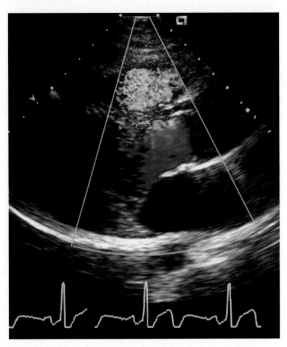

Fig. 17.34

Question 2

Regarding the patient in Question 1, the maximum velocity in the CW Doppler signal is expected to be closest to which of the following?

A. 1 m/s
B. 2 m/s
C. 3 m/s
D. 4 m/s
E. 5 m/s

Question 3

Identify the two cardiac chambers and two valves numbered in Fig. 17.35:

1. _____
2. _____
3. _____
4. _____

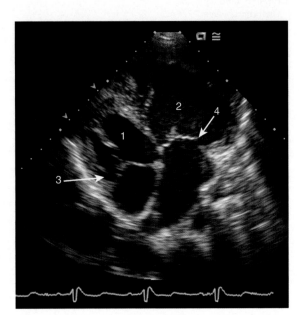

Fig. 17.35

Question 4

A transthoracic echocardiogram is obtained in a recent immigrant who has not previously seen a cardiologist. The only abnormal finding on clinical exam is a systolic murmur. Parasternal long-axis view reveals a large ventricular septal defect (VSD) with an overriding great vessel. The most useful next step in evaluation is measurement of:

A. Doppler velocity across the VSD
B. The pulmonic to systemic shunt ratio
C. Transaortic flow velocity
D. Transpulmonic flow velocity
E. Velocity of tricuspid regurgitation

Question 5

A 27-year-old woman undergoes echocardiography for a murmur during pregnancy and is found to have an ASD. The following measurements are made:

Pulmonary Artery

Velocity	1.8 m/s
Velocity-time integral (VTI$_{RVOT}$)	36 cm
Diameter	2.6 cm

LV Outflow

Velocity	1.1 m/s
Velocity-time integral (VTI$_{LVOT}$)	25 cm
Diameter	2.2 cm

Mitral Valve

Velocity-time integral (VTI$_{MV}$)	11 cm
Annulus diameter	3.3 cm

Calculate the pulmonic to systemic shunt ratio:

Question 6

A 52-year-old man with history of a VSD presents for a follow-up echocardiogram. Vital signs include a blood pressure of 120/68 mm Hg and a heart rate of 70 bpm. On transthoracic imaging, peak systolic velocity across the VSD is 4 m/s, and peak systolic velocity across the pulmonary valve is 2 m/s.

What is the estimated pulmonary arterial systolic pressure?

A. 80 mm Hg
B. 64 mm Hg
C. 56 mm Hg
D. 40 mm Hg

Question 7

A 45-year-old woman who underwent childhood surgical repair of tetralogy of Fallot now presents with decreased exercise tolerance. CW Doppler interrogation from a parasternal window is provided (Fig. 17.36).

What is this Doppler tracing consistent with?

A. Valvular pulmonary stenosis
B. Residual VSD flow
C. Pulmonary artery branch stenosis
D. Pulmonic regurgitation
E. Infundibular pulmonic stenosis

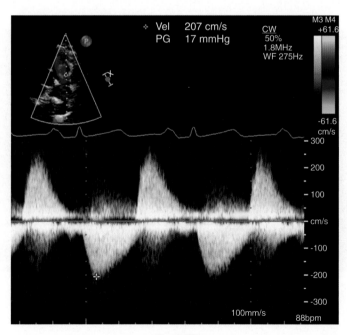

Fig. 17.36

Question 8

The most likely diagnosis in the patient with the imaging and Doppler data shown in Fig. 17.37 is:

   A. Anomalous left coronary artery from the pulmonary artery (ALCAPA)

B. Aortic regurgitation
C. Coronary artery fistula
D. Patent ductus arteriosus
E. Ventricular septal defect

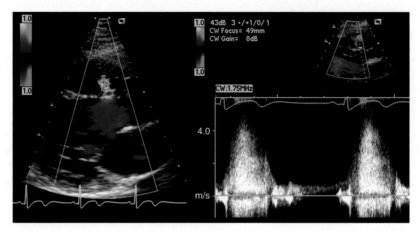

Fig. 17.37

Question 9

The most likely diagnosis in the patient with the color and CW Doppler data shown in Fig. 17.38 is:

   A. Aortic coarctation
   B. Aortic regurgitation

C. Atrial septal defect
D. Patent ductus arteriosus
E. Ventricular septal defect

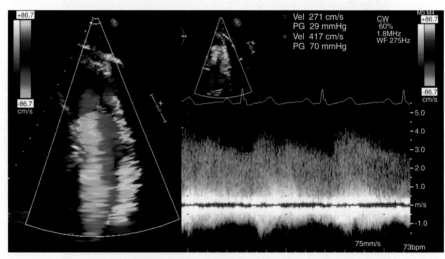

Fig. 17.38

Question 10

Echocardiography is requested in a 24-year-old woman with complex congenital heart disease with palliative surgery in childhood. Her aortic and mitral valves show normal function with no significant regurgitation, but this Doppler flow tracing is recorded (Fig. 17.39). This finding is most likely due to:

A. Severe tricuspid regurgitation
B. Anomalous pulmonary venous return
C. Aortopulmonary window
D. Aortic coarctation
E. Branch pulmonary stenosis

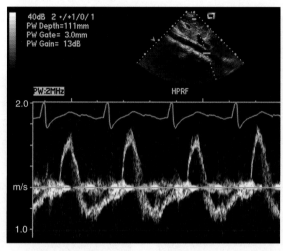

Fig. 17.39

Question 11

This echocardiographic image (Fig. 17.40) was obtained in a patient with congenital heart disease with a prior surgical repair.

The most likely diagnosis in this patient is:
A. Atrial septal defect
B. Cor triatriatum

C. Ebstein anomaly
D. Tetralogy of Fallot
E. Transposition of the great arteries

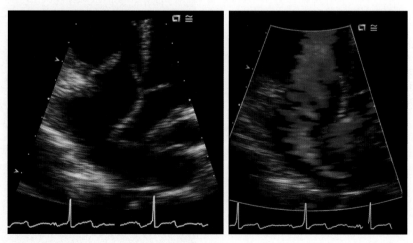

Fig. 17.40

Question 12

An echocardiographic image is obtained (Fig. 17.41).
   What is the most likely diagnosis?
   A. Bicuspid aortic valve
   B. Mitral valve prolapse
   C. Shone complex
   D. Subaortic membrane
   E. Aortic coarctation

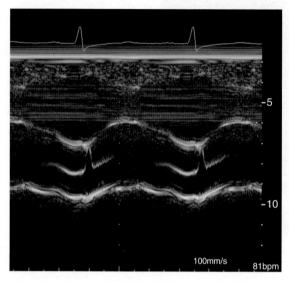

Fig. 17.41

Question 13

A 49-year-old patient with complex congenital heart disease presents for routine follow-up transthoracic echocardiogram, and the following image in systole is obtained (Fig. 17.42).
   These findings are most consistent with:
   A. Tetralogy of Fallot
   B. Ebstein's anomaly
   C. L-loop transposition of the great arteries
   D. Complete atrioventricular canal

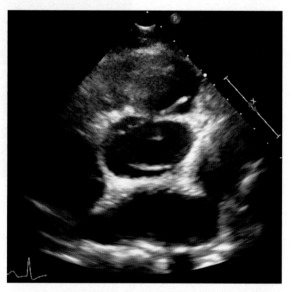

Fig. 17.42

Question 14

A 55-year-old patient with dyspnea is referred for echocardiography. The following image is obtained (Fig. 17.43).
   What is the most likely diagnosis?
   A. Partial anomalous pulmonary venous return
   B. Cor triatriatum
   C. Unroofed coronary sinus
   D. Sinus venosus atrial septal defect

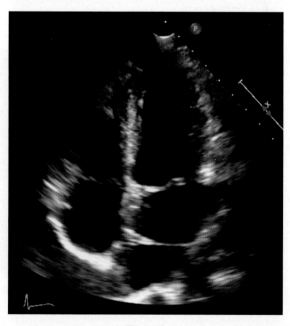

Fig. 17.43

Question 15

A 35-year-old patient with congenital heart disease presents for follow-up and a transthoracic echocardiogram is obtained (Fig. 17.44).

Based on the image provided, the patient's diagnosis is most consistent with?

A. Ebstein anomaly
B. LV noncompaction
C. D-loop transposition
D. RV dysplasia

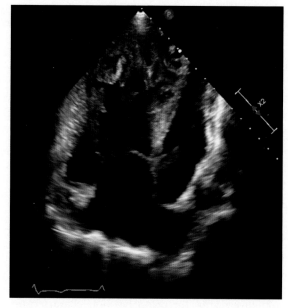

Fig. 17.44

ANSWERS

Answer 1: C

In this parasternal long-axis view, turbulent flow is seen in systole (mitral valve closed, aortic valve open) in the RV outflow tract. This is most likely due to a membranous VSD. Aortic coarctation would result in high-velocity flow and turbulence in the descending thoracic aorta, which is not seen on this image. A bicuspid valve would be associated with an asymmetric aortic valve, systolic doming of the leaflets, and (possibly) an increased flow velocity in the ascending aorta. Ebstein anomaly is associated with tricuspid regurgitation with a flow jet in the RA. Pulmonic stenosis would result in turbulent flow distal to the pulmonic valve, not in the RV outflow tract.

Answer 2: E

This patient has an asymptomatic small VSD. The restrictive size of the defect has flow characteristics similar to a stenotic valve so that the velocity in the defect reflects the systolic pressure difference between the LV (about 120 mm Hg with a normal systolic blood pressure) and RV (about 20 mm Hg in the absence of pulmonary hypertension). Thus, based on the Bernoulli $4V^2$ equation, the 100 mm Hg pressure difference between the LV and RV is equivalent to a velocity of 5 m/s.

Pulmonary (and RV) systolic pressure should be normal in this patient with only a small volume of flow across the defect. Eisenmenger physiology, or equalization of systemic and pulmonary pressures, only occurs with larger VSDs that result in equalization of LV and RV systolic pressures due to unrestricted flow between the ventricles in systole. Eisenmenger physiology typically occurs early in life and is associated with significant clinical symptoms and physical examination findings; echocardiography would not show turbulence in the RV outflow tract, because the flow velocity across the defect is low in this situation.

Answer 3

1. Anatomic LV
2. Anatomic RV
3. Mitral valve
4. Tricuspid valve

This is an apical 4-chamber view in a patient with congenitally corrected transposition of the great vessels. The transducer is in the normal orientation at the apex, with the anatomic RV on the right and the anatomic LV on the left of the image. The RV is the systemic ventricle, with the interatrial baffle directing pulmonary venous return to the RV, which then ejects into the aorta. The atrioventricular valves go with the corresponding ventricles so that the anatomic RV has a tricuspid valve. The tricuspid valve annulus usually is slightly more apical than the mitral valve annulus (as seen on this image), so this is a reliable feature for

identifying the RV. Occasionally, the tricuspid and mitral valve annulus are at the same level so that other features must be used for anatomic identification of the ventricular chambers. The presence of a moderator band is reliable for identification of the RV, but the degree of trabeculation is not reliable. The normal triangular shape, smaller size, and thinner walls of the RV are all altered when the anatomic RV serves as the systemic ventricle. With systemic pressures, the RV appropriately enlarges, hypertrophies, and changes shape, similar to an anatomic LV. The location of the RV and LV in the chest is abnormal in some patients with complex congenital heart disease and is not a reliable indicator of anatomy.

Answer 4: D

The most likely diagnosis is an unrepaired tetralogy of Fallot with a ventricular septal defect, overriding aorta, pulmonic stenosis, and RV hypertrophy. With a large VSD, the flow between the RV and LV will be unrestricted with equal systolic pressure (and low velocity flow) between the chambers. The patient would be cyanotic with Eisenmenger syndrome if there was no obstruction to RV outflow. Given the absence of cyanosis and the presence of a systolic murmur, he most likely also has pulmonic stenosis so that measurement of transpulmonic flow velocity would be most helpful. The pulmonic-to-systemic shunt ratio would not be helpful, would be difficult to calculate given pulmonic stenosis, and is not a major factor in clinical decision making at this point. The transaortic flow velocity reflects aortic valve function and likely would be normal. The tricuspid regurgitant velocity reflects RV systolic pressure, which is equal to LV systolic pressure in this patient, but does not indicate pulmonary pressure.

Answer 5: Q_p: Q_s = 2:1

The shunt ratio is calculated from the ratio of pulmonary flow (Q_p), measured in the RV outflow tract, and systemic flow (Q_s), measured in the LV outflow tract. At each site, cross-sectional area is calculated as the area of a circle:

$$CSA_{RVOT} = \pi \, (D/2)^2 = 3.14(2.6/2)^2 = 5.3 \text{ cm}^2$$

$$CSA_{LVOT} = \pi \, (D/2)^2 = 3.14(2.2/2)^2 = 3.8 \text{ cm}^2$$

Flow at each site then is calculated:

$$Q_p = CSA_{RVOT} \times VTI_{RVOT} = 5.3 \text{ cm}^2 \times 36 \text{ cm}$$
$$= 191 \text{ cm}^3 \text{ or mL}$$

$$Q_s = CSA_{LVOT} \times VTI_{LVOT} = 3.8 \text{ cm}^2 \times 25 \text{ cm}$$
$$= 95 \text{ cm}^3 \text{ or mL}$$

So that:

$$Q_p : Q_s = 191/95 = n \, 2 : 1$$

These calculations are consistent with a large shunt that likely is associated with right-sided heart enlargement and will require further evaluation and consideration of closure after pregnancy.

The transmitral volume flow rate should equal transaortic flow, in the absence of aortic or mitral regurgitation, and might provide an alternate site for calculation of systemic blood flow.

$$Q_{MV} = CSA_{MV} \times VTI_{MV} = 8.5 \text{ cm}^2 \times 11 \text{ cm}$$
$$= 94 \text{ cm}^3 \text{ or mL}$$

In this case, there is only a slight (1 mL) difference between transaortic and transmitral flow rates, which is within measurement error. Transmitral flow is rarely used for shunt ratio calculations, because reproducible measurement of mitral annulus diameter is problematic.

Answer 6: D

RV systolic pressure is obtained by subtracting the pressure gradient across the ventricular septal defect (VSD) (64 mm Hg) from systemic systolic pressure (120 mm Hg), to yield 56 mm Hg. From this, the pressure gradient across the pulmonic valve (16 mm Hg) is subtracted to provide the pulmonary arterial systolic pressure estimation—40 mm Hg.

Answer 7: D

The Doppler tracing is taken from the parasternal short-axis view, evaluating the RV outflow tract across the pulmonic valve. In diastole, there is a dense regurgitant jet, which comes to the baseline prior to the end of diastole, consistent with equalization of pulmonary artery and RV diastolic pressures. The peak systolic velocity is 2.1 m/s, which is not consistent with either valvular or infundibular pulmonic stenosis. The systolic peak velocity is also not consistent with systemic pressures, as would be seen with residual VSD flow.

Answer 8: E

In the parasternal long-axis view *(left)* a small color jet is seen with flow crossing the septum from left to right. The location is on the LV side of the aorta valve, and the CW Doppler signal *(right)* shows high-velocity systolic flow from left to right, with an ejection type velocity curve, consistent with a small ventricular septal defect (VSD) with normal LV and RV pressures. Low-velocity, passive, left-to-right flow in diastole also is present, consistent with higher LV than RV diastolic pressures.

An anomalous left coronary artery arising from the pulmonary artery (ALCAPA) is an unusual anomaly in which the direction of flow in the left coronary artery is reversed, with coronary flow supplied by the normal right coronary then going retrograde in the left coronary and emptying into the pulmonary artery. These patients usually have significant coronary ischemia, resulting in heart failure. Echocardiography shows an abnormal diastolic flow signal in the pulmonary artery. Aortic regurgitation occurs in diastole, and color flow would be directed into the LV. A coronary artery fistula may arise from either coronary artery with drainage into the right heart in over 90% of cases. Coronary flow is increased with continuous diastolic and systolic flow when a fistula is present. A patent ductus arteriosus results in continuous diastolic and systolic flow in the pulmonary artery.

Answer 9: D

The color Doppler image *(left)* shows the pulmonary artery in a parasternal RV outflow view with a diastolic flow disturbance along the lateral wall of the pulmonary artery. CW Doppler confirms continuous high-velocity systolic and diastolic flow consistent with a patent ductus arteriosus from the descending aorta (high pressure in systolic and diastole) to the low-pressure pulmonary artery.

Aortic regurgitation would occur only in diastole with characteristic diastolic flow curve from the aorta to LV. An ASD results in low-velocity back-and-forth flow between the RA and LA with flow predominantly from right to left, as long as pulmonary pressures are not severely elevated. A VSD results in high-velocity systolic flow from the LV to the RV, with an ejection type curve similar in shape and velocity to mitral regurgitation but slightly longer in duration.

Answer 10: C

This is a Doppler recording of flow from the transthoracic subcostal view in the proximal abdominal aorta with normal antegrade systolic flow and abnormal holodiastolic flow reversal. Retrograde diastolic flow in the aorta may be due to any communication from the proximal aorta into a lower-pressure vessel or chamber; classically, this finding is seen with severe aortic regurgitation. Other causes of aortic diastolic flow reversal include a systemic arterial to pulmonary arterial shunt, such as a Blalock-Taussig shunt. This patient had pulmonary atresia and single-ventricle physiology with pulmonary blood flow supplied by a surgically created aortic-to-pulmonary window, which accounts for the flow pattern seen in the aorta. Severe tricuspid regurgitation causes systolic flow reversal in the inferior vena cava or hepatic veins. Anomalous pulmonary venous return may enter the inferior vena cava or RA junction and would show a typical low-velocity systolic and diastolic filling pattern. Aortic coarctation results in continued forward flow in the aorta in diastole, as well as an increased systolic velocity. Branch pulmonary stenosis results in a high systolic velocity, and the pulmonary artery is not seen on this subcostal view.

Answer 11: E

This is an apical 4-chamber view, magnified to focus on the atrium and atrioventricular valves. The 2D images show a linear echo across the atrial region with color Doppler showing laminar blood flow through this channel and then across an atrioventricular valve into a ventricle. These images are consistent with an interatrial baffle surgical repair (Mustard or Senning) for d-TGA. The baffle directs systemic venous return to the pulmonary artery via the anatomic LV and pulmonary venous return to the aorta via the anatomic RV. This corrects blood flow to the pulmonary and systemic circuits but leaves the anatomic RV as the systemic ventricle. Although patients with this surgical procedure are still seen, the current approach for surgical repair is an arterial switch (Jatene) procedure.

There is an apparent defect in the atrial septum because of the anatomy of the baffle repair, but there is no intracardiac shunt and no evidence for volume overload of the pulmonic ventricle. Cor triatriatum is a partial membrane across the LA chamber, with normal ventricular and great vessel relationships. In Ebstein anomaly, the anatomic tricuspid valve (the systemic atrioventricular valve in this case) is displaced apically, whereas this image shows the atrioventricular valve insertions at the same level. Tetralogy of Fallot includes a VSD, an enlarged aorta, and RV outflow obstruction with RV hypertrophy—none of which are seen on these images.

Answer 12: D

The M-mode tracing shown is of the aortic valve in a patient with subaortic membrane. During systole, there is brief leaflet opening with early sustained closure. In hypertrophic cardiomyopathy, following systolic opening of the aortic valve, LV outflow obstruction in mid-systole decreases forward flow, with partial closure of the aortic valve. Then, as LV systolic pressure rises and overcomes dynamic obstruction, the aortic valve opens in late systole, giving an M-shaped appearance of aortic valve motion. The mitral valve is not shown on the image provided. Shone complex is an array of congenital abnormalities comprised of left heart obstructive defects, including aortic coarctation, aortic valve and subvalvular stenoses, and mitral stenosis (due to two leaflets attached to one papillary muscle, termed *parachute mitral valve*). There is not enough imaging data to confirm a diagnosis of Shone complex. A diagnosis of aortic coarctation cannot be made from an M-mode tracing of the aortic valve.

Answer 13: A

This patient has L-loop (congenitally corrected) transposition of the great arteries (TGA). Parasternal short-axis view at the level of the great vessels shows short-axis views of the aortic and pulmonic valves in the same

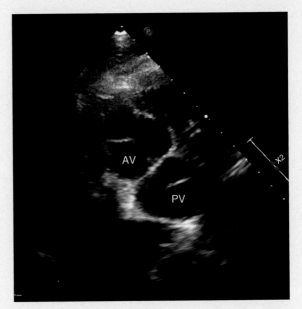

Fig. 17.45

imaging plane, with the aortic valve anterior and leftward relative to the pulmonic valve. L-loop TGA is an acyanotic defect in which the morphologic LV and RV are transposed, in addition to transposition of the great vessels. In complete TGA (D-loop), orientation of the aortic and pulmonic valves are also in the same plane, but short-axis views of the heart, in contrast to L-loop TGA, show the aortic valve anterior and rightward relative to the pulmonic valve (Fig. 17.45). For the other lesions, tetralogy of Fallot, Ebstien's anomaly, and complete atrioventricular canal, there is normal orientation of the aortic valve and pulmonary valves—not in the same plane, typically offset by approximately 70 to 90 degrees—with a short-axis view of one valve concurrently showing a long-axis view of the other.

Answer 14: B

Cor triatriatum is a congenital heart malformation where the atrium is divided by a thin membrane, resulting in three atrial chambers. Cor triatriatum more commonly occurs in the LA compared to the RA, and the membrane may be fenestrated or more complete. Accordingly, clinical presentation can vary from asymptomatic to significant LV inflow obstruction (similar to mitral stenosis). Partial anomalous pulmonary venous return is suspected in patients with right heart failure and pulmonary hypertension, and it is best diagnosed with TEE or tomographic imaging, such as cardiac computed tomography or magnetic resonance. The coronary sinus is not visualized in the apical 4-chamber view presented in this patient, and the atrial septum is intact.

Answer 15: C

This patient has transposition of the great arteries, with prior history of surgical atrial baffle (Mustard) procedure. In the apical 4-chamber view, the atrial baffle is seen crossing the atrial plane, directing flow to the morphologic right (systemic) ventricle via the tricuspid valve. The hypertrophied, systemic RV is also severely dilated. Ebstein anomaly is not present; the tricuspid valve is not apically displaced relative to the mitral valve. The morphologic LV (subpulmonic) is small and not hypertrophied.

18 Intraoperative and Interventional Echocardiography

STEP-BY-STEP APPROACH

- Transesophageal echocardiography (TEE) is increasingly used to guide surgical and transcatheter cardiac procedures (Table 18.1).
- TEE performance and interpretation occur simultaneously, with immediate communication of results to the physician performing the surgical or percutaneous procedure.
- More detailed information on intraoperative TEE is provided in *Intraoperative and Interventional Echocardiography: Atlas of Transesophageal Imaging*, 2nd edition, by Don Oxorn and Catherine Otto (Elsevier, 2018).

❖ KEY POINTS

- ❑ Time constraints may require a focused examination.
- ❑ Altered loading conditions may affect evaluation of valve and ventricular function.
- ❑ Loading conditions should be matched on baseline and postintervention studies.
- ❑ Urgent decision making based on TEE findings may be necessary.
- ❑ Limitations of the TEE data must be promptly recognized and communicated.
- ❑ Appropriate training and experience are needed for procedural TEE; at many institutions, these TEE studies are performed and interpreted by qualified cardiac anesthesiologists.

Step 1: Preoperative Data Review

- For elective procedures, a complete diagnostic evaluation is performed before the planned intervention to ensure evaluation under normal loading conditions and to allow time for discussion and procedural planning.

- All preprocedure images and diagnostic data should be reviewed, including coronary angiography, hemodynamics, cardiac magnetic resonance (CMR) imaging and computed tomography imaging, as well as echocardiographic data.

❖ KEY POINTS

- ❑ Intraoperative TEE provides:
  - ❑ Confirmation of the diagnosis
  - ❑ Additional information for procedure planning
  - ❑ A baseline study for comparison to postprocedure imaging
  - ❑ Monitoring of left ventricular (LV) function
  - ❑ Guidance for optimization of catheter and device placement
- ❑ Unexpected findings on the baseline procedural TEE may require a change in the planned intervention, consultation with the referring cardiologist, or rescheduling of the procedure.
- ❑ In emergency situations, the baseline procedural TEE may be the primary diagnostic test; in this setting, a complete study should be performed when allowed by time constraints.

Step 2: Hemodynamic Changes and Surgical Instrumentation

- Hemodynamic effects of sedation or anesthesia must be considered in the interpretation of procedural TEE imaging and Doppler data.
- Baseline and postprocedure data should be recorded at similar loading conditions, using volume infusion and pharmacologic agents, if needed, to match hemodynamic parameters.

TABLE 18.1   Indications for Intraoperative or Intraprocedural TEE

Clinical Setting	Procedure	Timing and Goals
Monitoring ventricular function	Before and after cardiopulmonary bypass in high-risk patients	LV volume status, global and regional function
	During noncardiac surgery in high-risk patients	LV volume status, global and regional function
Cardiac surgical procedures	Mitral valve repair	Mechanism and severity of regurgitation
		Functional assessment and complications after mitral valve repair
	Prosthetic valve replacement	Evaluation after valve implantation
		Detection of complications
	Complex surgical valve procedures	Aortic valve resuspension and aortic root repair
		Coronary artery reimplantation
	Endocarditis	Valve involvement and dysfunction
		Assessment after repair or valve replacement
	Hypertrophic cardiomyopathy	LV outflow anatomy before and after myectomy
		Evidence of subaortic obstruction
	Aortic dissection repair	Dissection flap location and flow
		Residual dissection after repair
	Congenital heart disease	Complex anatomy and function before and after surgical repair
Transcatheter interventions	Transcatheter aortic valve implantation (TAVI)	Aortic valve anatomy and function before and after valve implantation
	Transcatheter mitral valve procedures (balloon valvotomy, mitral clip placement, transcatheter mitral valve implantation)	Mitral valve function before and after procedure
	Prosthetic valve dysfunction	Guide and monitor transcatheter closure of paravalvular regurgitation
		Guide valve-in-valve implantation
	Atrial septal defect or patent foramen ovale closure	Baseline size and anatomy of defect
		Residual shunt post-procedure
		Assess for complications
	Septal ablation for hypertrophic cardiomyopathy	Baseline and post-procedure LV outflow obstruction
		Determine optimal site for ablation
Placement of intracardiac devices	Cannula placement	Guide positioning during placement
	Ventricular assist devices	
	Aortic cannulation (avoid atheroma)	
General surgical complications	Loculated pericardial effusion after surgical or transcatheter procedures	Detection, size, and hemodynamic consequences
	Intracardiac air after surgical procedures	Recognition and treatment

From Otto CM: *Textbook of clinical echocardiography,* ed 6, Philadelphia, 2018, Elsevier, p. 509.

❖ **KEY POINTS**

❑ Assessment of hemodynamics and ventricular function is affected by:
  ❑ Positive pressure mechanical ventilation
  ❑ Volume status
  ❑ Myocardial "stunning" (when aortic cross-clamping is necessary)
  ❑ Effects of cardiopulmonary bypass
  ❑ Pharmacologic therapy

❑ Basic hemodynamic parameters (heart rate and blood pressure) should be indicated on the recorded echocardiographic images to ensure matched loading conditions.

❑ When possible, cardiac output, filling pressures, and systemic vascular resistance should also be recorded with the TEE images.

❑ With cardiac surgery, TEE images will be affected by:
  ❑ Inversion of the left atrium (LA) appendage (looks like an LA mass) during mitral valve surgery
  ❑ Reverberations and shadowing by intracardiac cannulas
  ❑ Electronic interference (Fig. 18.1)
  ❑ Intracardiac air (Fig. 18.2)

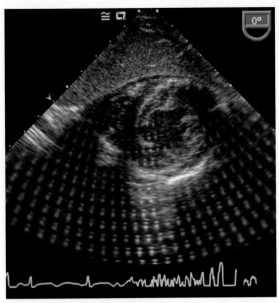

Fig. 18.1 **Electronic artifact.** TEE in the operating room often is complicated by artifacts (such as the electronic interference pattern due to the use of electrocautery), which is seen on this transgastric short-axis view. Diagnostic imaging should be performed when this artifact is absent because it may also affect the color Doppler signal.

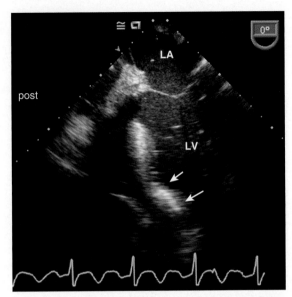

Fig. 18.2 **Intracardiac air.** When weaning from cardiopulmonary bypass, TEE can assist in detection of intracardiac air. In this TEE 4-chamber view, isolated bubbles are seen in the LV chamber along with a denser area (arrows) due to an air collection in the apical aspect of the septum.

Step 3: Baseline Data Acquisition

- A complete systemic TEE (see Chapter 3) is recommended when possible, but time constraints may require a limited study focused on the key diagnostic information.
- Optimal diagnosis is ensured by use of a protocol with a consistent image sequence, and acquisition of images is obtained in standard TEE views.
- Images may be acquired either by:
  - Obtaining all views from each transducer position (high esophageal, midesophageal, transgastric), first with imaging and then with Doppler, or
  - Evaluation of each anatomic structure by both imaging and Doppler in at least two orthogonal views—all four cardiac chambers, all four valves, both great arteries, systemic and pulmonary venous return, atrial appendage, and interatrial septum.

❖ KEY POINTS

- ❑ As with any echocardiographic study, intraoperative and intraprocedural TEE images should be obtained in standard long-axis, short-axis, 2-chamber, and 4-chamber image planes (Fig. 18.3).
- ❑ Three-dimensional (3D) imaging is helpful for evaluation of mitral valve and atrial septal defect anatomy. 3D echocardiographic guidance is essential for some transcatheter procedures.

- ❑ Color Doppler is helpful for evaluation of intracardiac flow patterns, particularly for evaluation of mitral regurgitation. 3D color imaging is useful in selected cases (Fig. 18.4).
- ❑ Pulsed Doppler is useful for evaluation of antegrade pulmonary venous and transmitral flow patterns (Fig. 18.5). The pulsed Doppler signal also may help in identification of anatomic structures when otherwise unclear.
- ❑ Continuous-wave (CW) Doppler is helpful in selected cases, but the possibility of a nonparallel intercept angle (and underestimation of velocity) must be considered due to the constraints on transducer positioning in the esophagus.
- ❑ Interference and technical artifacts that limit image quality may be reduced by repositioning the transducer or pausing electronic devices while images are obtained.
- ❑ Standard instrument presets, including transducer frequency, depth, gain, preprocessing and postprocessing, and sector scan width, may be adequate for some images, but adjustment often is needed during the examination.
- ❑ If the electrocardiogram signal is inadequate or subject to interference, cine loops can be acquired using a set time interval instead of one- or two-beat clips triggered by the electrocardiogram QRS complex.

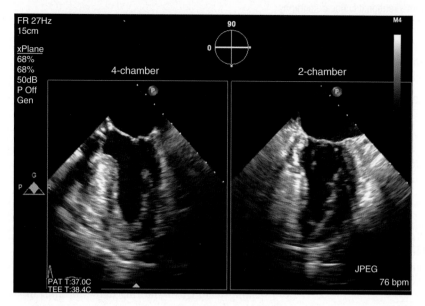

Fig. 18.3 Basic TEE views of the LV. Whenever possible, the intraoperative TEE exam should start with standard 4-chamber, 2-chamber, and long-axis views recorded at a depth to include the LV apex. In this example, biplane imaging is used for simultaneous acquisition of 4-chamber and 2-chamber view. Acquisition of these images takes only 1 to 2 minutes and allows evaluation of LV size, LV regional and global systolic function, and RV size and systolic function.

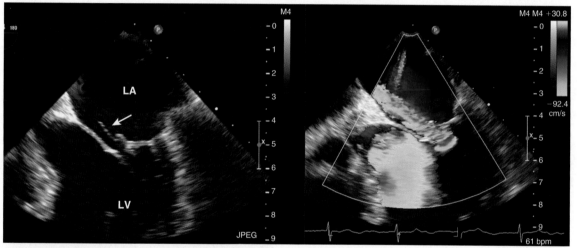

Fig. 18.4 TEE color Doppler imaging. In a patient undergoing surgical mitral valve repair, 2D imaging *(left)* shows a flail posterior mitral leaflet *(arrow)*. Color Doppler *(right)* demonstrates an anteriorly directed mitral regurgitant jet with a wide vena contracta and a large proximal isovelocity surface area radius (color Doppler baseline moved in the direction of flow, toward the transducer).

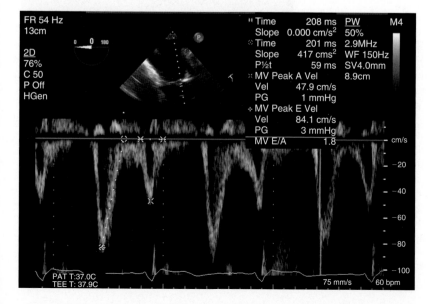

Fig. 18.5 Pulsed Doppler velocity data. LV inflow velocity across the mitral valve is recorded at baseline with a velocity curve similar to that seen on transthoracic imaging except that flow is directly away from the transducer.

❑ The structure of interest should be centered with depth and zoom adjusted to optimize the image.

Step 4: Postprocedure Data Acquisition

■ After the procedure, TEE is repeated to assess the results of the intervention and to evaluate for potential complications.

■ When possible, loading conditions on the postoperative TEE should be similar to the baseline study.

❖ **KEY POINTS**

❑ The postprocedure TEE focuses on the views and Doppler flows needed to evaluate the effect of the procedure; obtaining data in similar views as the baseline study allows direct comparison of the images.

❑ With surgical procedures, the postprocedure TEE is performed after weaning from cardiopulmonary bypass and after restoration of hemodynamics similar to the baseline study.

❑ With percutaneous interventions, TEE data may be used continuously to guide the procedure with repeat evaluations at each stage of the intervention.

❑ Instrument settings should be the same as on the baseline study to avoid differences due to technical factors, rather than to the procedure itself.

Step 5: Interpret and Communicate Findings

■ Unlike a conventional diagnostic TEE, intraoperative and procedural TEE studies are interpreted and reported verbally simultaneously with image acquisition.

■ In addition to the results themselves, the degree of certainty of each finding should be reported.

❖ **KEY POINTS**

❑ TEE findings may prompt a change in surgical plans or additional procedures.

❑ If the findings are equivocal or images are low quality, this information should be communicated to avoid decision making based on inadequate data.

❑ Qualitative data often are adequate for decision making; when quantitative approaches are used, measurements and calculations that can be performed rapidly are preferred.

❑ TEE findings should be documented in the permanent medical record, as well as providing immediate results during the procedure.

❑ Intraoperative and intraprocedural TEE images should be saved, as for any echocardiographic study, to allow comparison with future studies.

INTRAOPERATIVE TEE

Monitoring Left Ventricular Function

■ Intraoperative TEE is useful for continuously monitoring LV function in high-risk patients undergoing noncardiac surgery and for evaluation of LV function after cardiac surgical procedures (see Table 18.1).

■ Images of the LV allow monitoring of:
  ○ Ventricular preload (LV volume)
  ○ Global LV systolic function
  ○ Regional LV function
  ○ Right ventricle (RV) size and systolic function

❖ **KEY POINTS**

❑ In general, the size of the LV chamber reflects filling volume; monitoring allows optimization of preload.

❑ Small LV volumes with adequate filling pressures are seen with restrictive cardiomyopathy, pericardial constraint, severe RV dysfunction, or high contractility states.

❑ The transgastric short-axis view is often used for continuous monitoring of LV size and global and regional function because it includes myocardial segments supplied by the three major coronary arteries (Figs. 18.6 and 18.7).

❑ Standard two-dimensional (2D) TEE images of the LV apex are usually suboptimal, because the LV is typically foreshortened due to the constraints of transducer positioning in the esophagus.

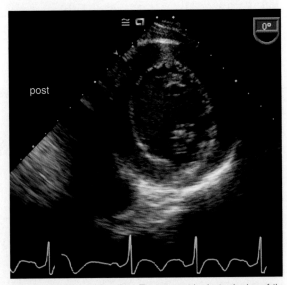

post

Fig. 18.6 LV size and function. The transgastric short-axis view of the LV allows evaluation of overall LV size (reflecting preload or volume status), global ventricular systolic function, and regional dysfunction due to coronary disease.

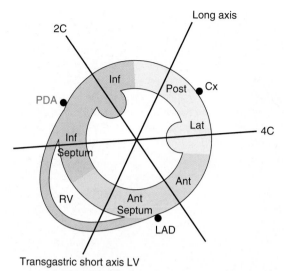

Fig. 18.7 LV regional function. The wall segments seen on the transgastric view, with the corresponding coronary artery supply, are shown on this schematic drawing. *2C,* 2 chamber; *4C,* 4 chamber; *Ant,* anterior; *Cx,* circumflex coronary artery; *Inf,* inferior; *LAD,* left anterior descending coronary artery; *Lat,* lateral; *PDA,* posterior descending coronary artery; *Post,* posterior. *(From Otto CM: Textbook of clinical echocardiography, ed 6, Philadelphia, 2018, Elsevier.)*

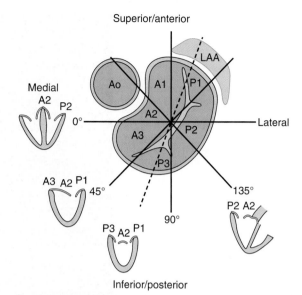

Fig. 18.8 Imaging the mitral valve. Reference view demonstrating the relationship of the TEE rotational imaging planes to the mitral valve with the probe positioned in the standard midesophageal position. *A1, A2, A3,* Anterior mitral leaflet segments; *P1, P2, P3,* posterior mitral leaflet segments. *(From Foster GP, Isselbacher EM, Rose GA, et al: Accurate localization of mitral regurgitant defects using multiplane transesophageal echocardiography, Ann Thorac Surg 65(4):1025-1031, 1998.)*

- 3D LV volumes are recommended for quantitation of LV volumes and ejection fraction.
- Changes in wall motion usually reflect ischemia; other causes include conduction defects, hypovolemia, and myocardial stunning after cardiopulmonary bypass.
- RV dysfunction may be due to ischemia, inadequate cardioplegia, or air embolism into the right coronary artery when separating from cardiopulmonary bypass.

Mitral Valve Repair

- Baseline 2D and 3D TEE allows precise delineation of mitral valve anatomy and the mechanism of regurgitation, which is helpful in planning the surgical repair.
- Postrepair TEE allows evaluation of any residual mitral regurgitation and detection of complications.

❖ **KEY POINTS**

- Mitral valve anatomy is best evaluated using 2D rotational scanning and 3D full volume imaging from a midesophageal position (Fig. 18.8).
  - The central scallops of the anterior (A) and posterior (P) leaflets are seen in the 4-chamber and long-axis views.
  - The lateral (P1) and medial (P2) scallops of the posterior leaflets are seen in the bicommissural view at 60° to 90° rotation.

- Starting in the 4-chamber plane, the lateral scallops of the anterior (A1) and posterior (P1) leaflets can be seen by slightly withdrawing the probe, or tilting superiorly; medial segments (A3 and P3) are seen by advancing the probe or tilting posteriorly.
- From the 2-chamber plane, all three scallops of the anterior leaflet are seen when the probe is turned toward the patient's right and all three scallops of the posterior leaflet are seen when the probe is turned leftward.
- A transgastric short-axis view of the mitral valve, when possible, shows both leaflets.
- 3D images of the mitral valve are recommended in all patients with mitral valve disease. A view showing the LA side of the valve facilitates identification of prolapsing segments and flail chords.
- The direction of the mitral regurgitant jet is helpful in defining the mechanism of regurgitation. Severity of regurgitation is evaluated by (Fig. 18.9):
  - Vena contracta width (2D) or area (3D)
  - CW Doppler signal intensity of regurgitant compared to antegrade flow
  - Pulmonary vein systolic flow reversal (Fig. 18.10)
  - Proximal isovelocity surface area calculation of regurgitant orifice area

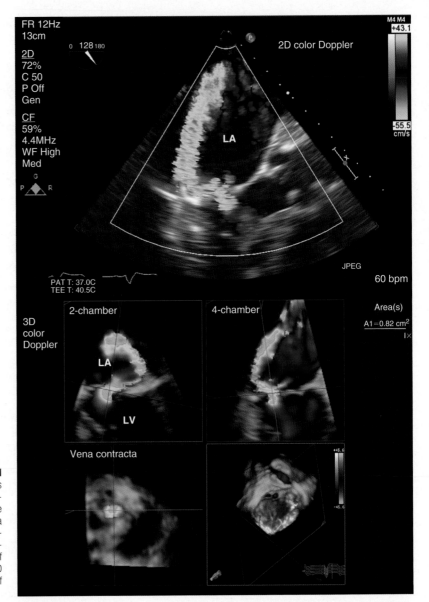

Fig. 18.9 3D Doppler evaluation of mitral regurgitation. Mitral regurgitant severity is evaluated with measurement of vena contracta and calculation of regurgitation orifice area by the proximal isovelocity surface area method, using standard 2D color Doppler imaging. In selected patients, 3D Doppler imaging may be helpful for better visualization of the vena contracta, as shown here with 3D imaging used to obtain a short-axis view of the vena contracta area *(lower left image).*

- Postrepair, anatomic, and functional results are evaluated using the same imaging views and Doppler measures as on the baseline study (Fig. 18.11).
    - Loading conditions (especially blood pressure) should be similar to the baseline study.
    - Use of the same imaging planes facilitates comparison of pre- and postprocedure data.
    - Doppler data are recorded with the same instrument settings to ensure detection of any residual regurgitation.
- The postprocedure TEE includes evaluation for the complications of mitral valve repair:
    - Persistent mitral regurgitation
    - Systolic anterior motion of the mitral leaflet

- Functional mitral stenosis
- Ventricular systolic dysfunction

Aortic or Mitral Valve Replacement

- In patients undergoing aortic or mitral valve replacement, anatomic and functional assessment should be completed before the patient is in the operating room.
- Evaluation of the severity of valve stenosis by TEE is problematic for several reasons, so intraoperative TEE decisions regarding stenosis severity should be avoided (Fig. 18.12).
- The postprocedure TEE allows detection of prosthetic valve dysfunction and assessment of LV systolic function.

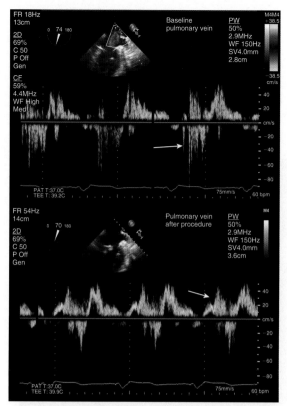

Fig. 18.10 Pulmonary vein flow. In a patient undergoing mitral valve repair, the baseline pulmonary vein flow pattern *(top)* shows systolic reversal *(arrow)*. After valve repair *(bottom)*, systolic flow reversal is no longer present with normal flow into the LA in systole *(arrow)*.

■ Knowledge of the structure and function of each prosthetic valve type is needed for correct interpretation of postprocedure data.

❖ **KEY POINTS**

❑ A parallel alignment between the ultrasound beam and aortic velocity is rarely possible on TEE, resulting in underestimation of stenosis severity.

❑ Direct imaging and planimetry of aortic valve area is limited by reverberations and shadowing due to valve calcification but may be possible with 3D imaging when calcification is not severe.

❑ Mitral stenosis can be evaluated using the Doppler pressure half-time method, because the TEE probe position allows a parallel alignment with antegrade transmitral flow.

❑ A small amount of valve regurgitation is seen with a normally functioning prosthetic valve.

❑ Central regurgitation is common with a bioprosthetic valve; eccentric jets, with a variable pattern of regurgitation depending on valve type, are typical with mechanical valves.

❑ A small amount of paravalvular regurgitation may be seen, but a large paravalvular leak may require immediate correction.

❑ Rarely, retained mitral leaflet tissue impairs normal motion of a mechanical mitral occluder.

❑ Recording images of leaflet/occluder motion and transvalvular Doppler flows in the operating room provides a useful comparison for subsequent studies.

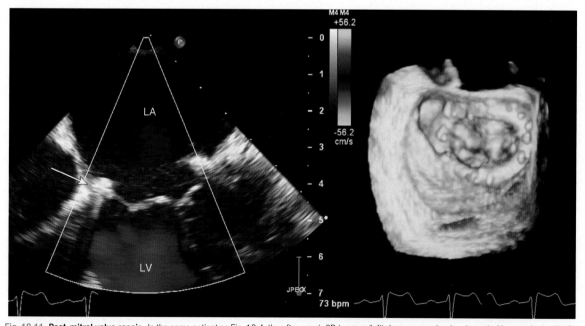

Fig. 18.11 Post-mitral valve repair. In the same patient as Fig. 18.4, the after-repair 2D images *(left)* show an annular ring *(arrow)* with normal mitral leaflet coaptation and no residual regurgitation. The 3D view *(right)* from the LA perspective shows the annular ring with sutures appearing as small bumps along the ring.

Endocarditis

- Intraoperative TEE is essential in assessment of the degree of valve destruction and paravalvular involvement due to endocarditis.
- Postprocedure evaluation in the operating room allows assessment of valve function after repair or replacement and provides a baseline for subsequent imaging studies.

❖ **KEY POINTS**

- ❑ The baseline intraoperative TEE focuses on (Fig. 18.13):
- ❑ Presence and location of vegetations
- ❑ Mechanism of valve dysfunction
- ❑ Severity of regurgitation
- ❑ Paravalvular abscess

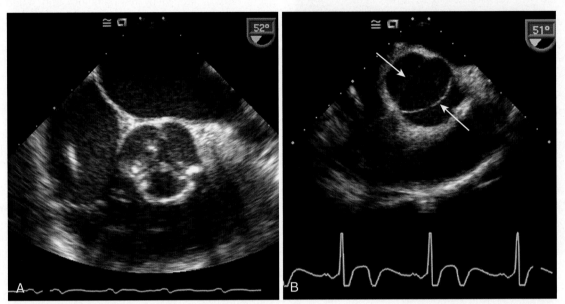

Fig. 18.12 Aortic valve anatomy. TEE short-axis images in two patients with aortic valve disease show a typical calcified trileaflet aortic valve in a 76-year-old patient with severe aortic stenosis showing marked restriction of systolic leaflet opening (A), and a bicuspid valve *(arrows)* in a 28-year-old man with no prior cardiac history who presented with acute aortic dissection (B).

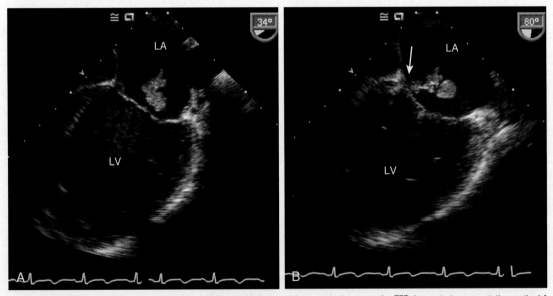

Fig. 18.13 Endocarditis. In a 28-year-old woman who presented with fever and bacteremia, intraoperative TEE demonstrates a vegetation on the LA side of the valve in systole in the 4-chamber view (A), but the attachment site of the vegetation and the mechanism of regurgitation are not well defined. Rotating the image plane toward the 2-chamber plane (B) now demonstrates the attachment of the 2 cm vegetation on the P2 scallop of the posterior leaflet. Color Doppler demonstrated a leaflet perforation adjacent to the vegetation. This information assisted in a successful mitral valve repair (not replacement) in this young woman.

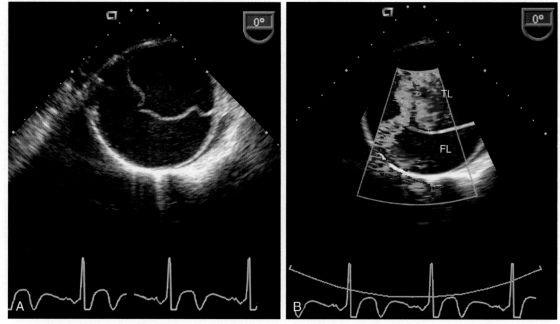

Fig. 18.14 **Aortic dissection.** Intraoperative TEE imaging quickly demonstrates the presence of a dissection flap in the descending thoracic aorta (A) with color Doppler (B) showing a fenestration with flow from the true lumen into the false lumen. *FL,* False lumen; *TL,* true lumen.

❏ Detection of other complications (e.g., fistulas, pseudoaneurysm)

❏ Extensive valve and paravalvular destruction in endocarditis often requires a complex surgical repair; knowledge of the surgical details is needed for correct interpretation of the postprocedure images.

Aortic Disease

■ Atheroma in the ascending aorta can be detected by TEE or epicardial scanning, which allows placement of bypass grafts and aortotomy sites in areas of normal aortic tissue.

■ TEE is essential for accurate diagnosis of the presence and extent of aortic dissection; in urgent cases, diagnostic imaging may be performed in the operating room (Fig. 18.14).

■ TEE distinguishes involvement of the ascending aorta (type A dissection) from a more distal (type B) dissection.

■ Evaluation of aortic regurgitation is a key element of the examination, because dilation of the sinuses or extension of the dissection into the valve can result in valve dysfunction.

❖ KEY POINTS

❏ The ascending aorta often is best visualized using a sterile epicardial transducer to ensure the absence of atheroma at the site of proximal coronary bypass graft anastomoses and at aortotomy sites.

❏ A complete examination for aortic dissection includes:
  ❏ Midesophageal views of the aortic sinuses and ascending aorta
  ❏ Imaging of the descending thoracic aorta in a slow pull-back from the diaphragmatic level to the arch
  ❏ High TEE views of the aortic arch
  ❏ Imaging of the os of the left subclavian artery (which delineates type A and type B dissections)

❏ Color Doppler imaging improves identification of dissection flaps and provides visualization of flow in the true and false lumens.

❏ The aortic valve is examined in standard long- and short-axis views, with color Doppler to detect and quantitate aortic regurgitant severity (Fig. 18.15).

❏ Pulsed Doppler evaluation of descending aortic flow is helpful in evaluation of aortic valve regurgitation.

❏ The coronary arteries are visualized, if possible, because the dissection flap may extend into the (most often, right) coronary ostium.

❏ Other indirect signs of aortic dissection include:
  ❏ Pericardial effusion (from extension into the pericardium, signaling impending aortic rupture)
  ❏ LV regional wall motion abnormalities due to dissection extending into the coronary artery

❏ After surgical repair, a persistent distal dissection flap is common.

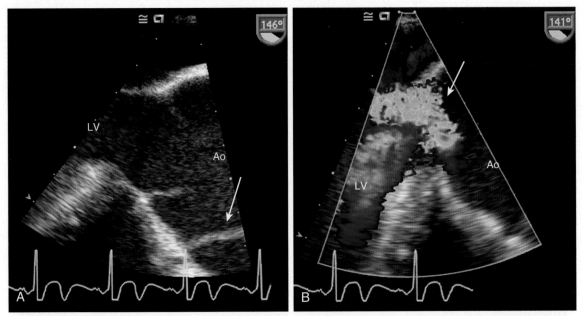

Fig. 18.15 **Complications of aortic dissection.** (A) In the same patient as in Fig. 18.14, the ascending aorta is markedly dilated with a dissection flap *(arrow),* distinct from the open aortic valve leaflets in this image. (B) Color Doppler shows severe aortic regurgitation due to the combination of aortic dilation, dissection, and a bicuspid aortic valve. *Ao,* Aorta.

Hypertrophic Cardiomyopathy

- Hypertrophic cardiomyopathy may be treated surgically by basal septal hypertrophy resection (myectomy) or may be treated percutaneously with catheter-based ablation of basal septal hypertrophy.
- Echocardiography provides evaluation of the pattern of hypertrophy, baseline and postprocedure hemodynamics, and detection of procedural complications.

❖ **KEY POINTS**

- ❏ Imaging allows assessment of the pattern and severity of septal hypertrophy, which is useful in procedural planning.
- ❏ Color Doppler localizes the level of outflow obstruction based on the location of the flow acceleration proximal to the aortic valve plane.
- ❏ CW Doppler alignment with the outflow tract velocity may be difficult by TEE; sterile epicardial scanning in the operating room (transthoracic scanning for percutaneous procedures) is helpful if these data are needed for clinical decision making.
- ❏ After surgical resection, and at each stage of a percutaneous procedure, imaging and Doppler assessment of anatomic and hemodynamic results are documented.
- ❏ Systolic anterior motion of the mitral valve leaflet and accompanying mitral regurgitation may resolve after relief of outflow obstruction.

- ❏ Postprocedure imaging allows detection of complications (such as a ventricular septal defect, which is a rare complication of surgical myotomy-myectomy).

Advanced Heart Failure Therapies

- Left ventricular assist devices (LVADs), transaortic axial flow devices, and total artificial hearts (TAHs) are increasingly used during complex cardiac procedures and long term in patients with severe LV dysfunction.
- The echocardiographer should be familiar with the specific type of LVAD or TAH being used; continual design advances require regular updates on implantation approaches and expected flow patterns (Fig. 18.16).

❖ **KEY POINTS**

- ❏ TEE evaluation is helpful during implantation of an LVAD for:
  - ❏ Placement of inflow and outflow cannula
  - ❏ Ventricular volumes and systolic function
  - ❏ LVAD inflow and outflow velocities and flow patterns
  - ❏ De-airing of the pump before activation
  - ❏ Monitoring and optimizing the position of transaortic axial flow devices (Fig. 18.17)
- ❏ Typically, the LVAD inflow cannula is in the LV apex with the outflow cannula in the proximal ascending aorta.
- ❏ The aortic valve usually remains closed throughout the cardiac cycle, because cardiac output now is directed through the LVAD; significant

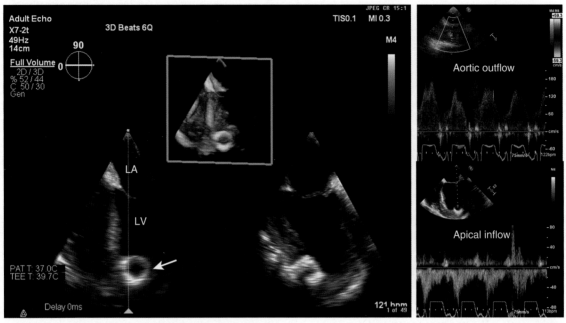

Fig. 18.16 **Left ventricular assist device (LVAD).** Intraoperative TEE in this patient with an LVAD *(left)* shows the inflow cannula in the LV apex *(arrow)* in the 4-chamber, 2-chamber, and 3D views. In a high TEE long-axis view of the ascending aorta *(right, top),* a color Doppler signal is seen with pulsed Doppler confirming continuous flow from the LVAD outflow cannula. The Doppler inflow signal into the apical cannula *(right, bottom)* shows pulsatile flow, which is likely related to LV contraction.

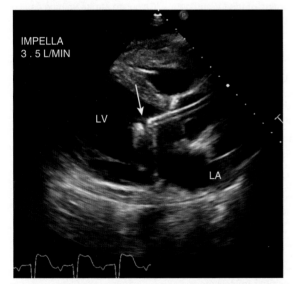

Fig. 18.17 **Transaortic axial flow device.** In the parasternal long-axis view, an axial flow device is seen positioned across the aortic valve to measure the distance from the valve plane to the inflow port *(arrow)* on the cannula.

aortic regurgitation is a contraindication to LVAD placement.

❑ The LV is small (decompressed) when LVAD function is normal. LV contraction reflects the underlying disease process with improvement due to disease resolution, not the LVAD.

❑ LVAD flow may be pulsatile or continuous (also called *axial*); each has a specific expected flow pattern.

❑ Complications of an LVAD that may be detected by echocardiography include:

  ❑ Intracardiac thrombus formation
  ❑ Obstruction of inflow or outflow cannula due to positioning or thrombus
  ❑ Regurgitation of LVAD valves (in some devices)
  ❑ Inadequate flow volumes
  ❑ Pericardial hematoma around the inflow cannula

Heart Transplantation

■ After orthotopic heart transplantation, intraoperative TEE allows evaluation of the anastomoses to the aorta, pulmonary artery, pulmonary veins, and vena cavae.

■ Intraoperative TEE provides a baseline assessment of LV and RV systolic function in the transplanted heart.

❖ **KEY POINTS**

  ❑ Evaluation of LV and RV function in the operating room is helpful in managing acute hemodynamics as the patient is stabilized after heart transplantation. Tricuspid regurgitation may be present early after transplantation if RV systolic dysfunction is present.

Congenital Heart Disease

■ In patients undergoing surgery for congenital heart disease, it is essential that intraoperative TEE be performed by a skilled echocardiographer who is knowledgeable about congenital heart disease anatomy, physiology, and surgical approaches.

❖ **KEY POINTS**

❑ Except for simple corrective procedures, such as closure of an isolated atrial septal defect, intraoperative TEE for congenital heart disease should be performed by echocardiographers with additional training in congenital heart disease.

❑ Additional information on intraoperative TEE for congenital heart disease is available in Chapters 43 to 49 of *The Practice of Clinical Echocardiography*, edited by Catherine Otto (Elsevier, 2017).

TRANSCATHETER AND HYBRID PROCEDURES

Atrial Septal Defect or Patent Foramen Ovale Closure

■ TEE or intracardiac echocardiography (ICE) guidance is used for transcatheter closure of an atrial septal defect or patent foramen ovale (Table 18.2).

■ Baseline images allow visualization of the location, size, and shape of the defect using 2D rotational scanning and 3D imaging.

■ Postprocedure imaging allows evaluation for correct placement of the device and detection of any residual shunt.

TABLE 18.2 Basic Principles for Intraoperative or Intraprocedural TEE

Parameter	View	Additional Imaging	Clinical Pointers
LV Function			
LV volumes	Image LV in mid-esophageal 4-chamber and 2-chamber views, trace at end-systole and end-diastole for LV volume calculation	Acquire multi-beat full volume for 3D measurements	
Cardiac output	Calculate LV outflow tract circular CSA using diameter in mid-esophageal long-axis view. Record pulsed Doppler VTI from transgastric long-axis or apical view	Alternatively use 3D zoom or full volume mode to allow multiplanar reconstruction of the LV outflow tract and planimetry to measure its area	Measurements should be made in systole. Calculate stroke volume as LV outflow CSA times VTI; multiply by heart rate for cardiac output
Ejection fraction	3D or 2D biplane LV volumes and EF from a high TEE 4-chamber and 2-chamber view	Calculate fractional area change using planimetry of midpapillary transgastric short-axis views of the LV in systole and diastole	Use 3D software to calculate volumes and EF
Other measures of global systolic function	Visual assessment of endocardial and myocardial thickening in each myocardial segment	Image mitral valve in midesophageal 4-chamber view to facilitate tissue Doppler imaging of lateral mitral annulus with measurement of S′	
Strain	Measure strain using speckle tracking in the midesophageal views and the transgastric midpapillary view	Recognize that properly identifying the region of interest is of paramount importance	Global longitudinal strain is an alternate measure of global LV systolic function. Target diagrams display regional function
Diastolic function	Image mitral valve in mid-esophageal 4-chamber view to acquire pulsed wave Doppler inflow. Image pulmonary vein to acquire pulsed wave Doppler flow	Image mitral valve in mid-esophageal 4-chamber to facilitate tissue Doppler imaging of lateral mitral annulus	Measure E, A, DT from mitral inflow. Measure E′ and A′ on tissue Doppler. Calculate E/E′
RV Function			
Global RV systolic function	Using the transgastric window, align M-mode parallel to the lateral tricuspid annulus for TAPSE	Using the transgastric window, align tissue Doppler gate parallel to the lateral tricuspid annulus to assess S′	Measure TAPSE and S′
Regional wall motion	Visual assessment of endocardial and myocardial thickening	Measure strain using speckle tracking	Acquire 3D volumes

Parameter	View	Additional Imaging	Clinical Pointers
TABLE 18.2	**Basic Principles for Intraoperative or Intraprocedural TEE—cont'd**		
Position and Function of Intracardiac Devices			
Position of IABP	Image the descending thoracic aorta	Identify the tip of the balloon (suspending its inflation temporarily may help)	Image left subclavian artery Assess distance between balloon tip and left subclavian artery
LVAD inflow cannulae	Image LV in mid-esophageal 4-chamber and 2-chamber views	Assess position of the cannula tip relative to the ventricular walls	Also consider 3D to assess cannula position Color Doppler to assess velocities
LVAD outflow cannula	Image the midesophageal long-axis, and look for cannula entering the ascending aorta	Use color Doppler to assess velocities	
Impella	Image midesophageal long-axis	Assess aortic valve pathology	Asses depth of device into LV Assess mitral valve function
Total artificial heart (TAH)	Use midesophageal 4-chamber to assess mechanical atrioventricular valves Also visualize atria and adjacent pericardial or pleural fluid	Midesophageal long-axis views to look at aortic and pulmonic prosthetic valves	Look for central "cleaning" jets with this type of mechanical valve Be vigilant for atrial compression from effusions
V-V ECMO	Image the cavae and the tricuspid valve using a bicaval view Obtain a transgastric long-axis view of the right heart	Use color Doppler to ensure that outflow from the device goes through tricuspid valve into the RV	
Coronary sinus cannula	View in low midesophageal 4-chamber with retroflexion	View in bicaval with medial turn of probe	
Femoral venous cannula	Bicaval view		

CSA, Cross-sectional area; *ECMO,* extra-corporeal membrane oxygenation; *EF,* ejection fraction; *IABP,* intra-aortic balloon pump; *LVAD,* left ventricular assist device; *TAPSE,* tricuspid annular plane systolic excursion; *VTI,* velocity-time integral; *V-V ECMO,* veno-venous extracorporeal membrane oxygenation.
From Otto CM: *Textbook of clinical echocardiography,* ed 6, Philadelphia, 2018, Elsevier, pp. 520-521.

Transcatheter Aortic Valve Implantation

- TEE monitoring during transcatheter aortic valve implantation (TAVI) is not routinely needed but may be indicated in selected cases (Figs. 18.18 and 18.19).
- TTE evaluation of aortic valve anatomy and severity of stenosis prior to the procedure is essential for clinical decision making.
- Evaluation of the transcatheter valve immediately after implantation is recommended, either with TEE (if being used for procedural monitoring) or with TTE.
- The immediate post-implantation evaluation includes:
  - Visualization of valve position and leaflet motion (Fig. 18.20)
  - Detection and evaluation of paravalvular regurgitation (Fig. 18.21)
  - Measurement of antegrade transvalvular velocity
  - Evaluation of LV systolic function and pulmonary pressures

Transcatheter Mitral Valve Repair

- TEE is used to evaluate patients for transcatheter mitral valve repair with attention to the mechanism of mitral regurgitation and valve anatomy.
- Baseline measurements include annulus dimensions, leaflet tenting distances, and length of width of leaflet non-coaptation.
- TEE guidance is used to monitor positioning of the mitral repair device (Fig. 18.22).
- After the procedure, color and pulsed Doppler allow detection of residual regurgitation and evaluation of antegrade flow velocities (Fig. 18.23).

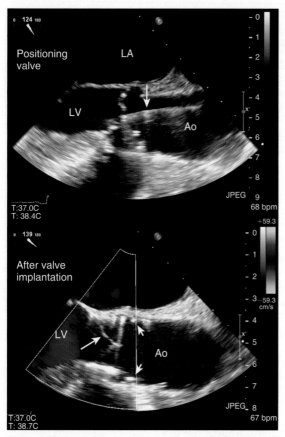

Fig. 18.18 **Guidance of transcatheter aortic valve implantation.** TEE imaging is used during the procedure *(top)* to position the wire *(arrow)* and valve. After valve implantation *(bottom)*, the thin leaflets *(long arrow)* and mesh valve support *(short arrows)* are seen. *Ao,* Aorta.

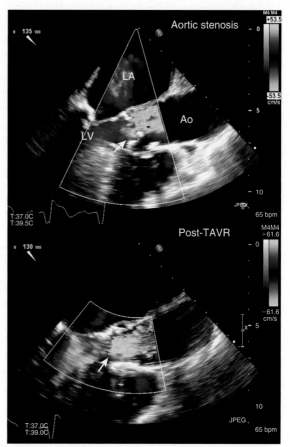

Fig. 18.19 **Aortic stenosis before and after transcatheter valve implantation.** In a long-axis view, the baseline image shows a calcified immobile aortic valve with high-velocity flow beginning at the valve level. The postprocedure image in the same view *(bottom)* now shows laminar low-velocity flow across the prosthetic valve. *Ao,* Aorta.

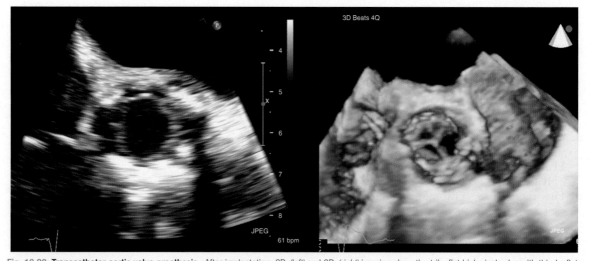

Fig. 18.20 **Transcatheter aortic valve prosthesis.** After implantation, 2D *(left)* and 3D *(right)* imaging show the trileaflet biological valve with thin leaflets and normal systolic opening.

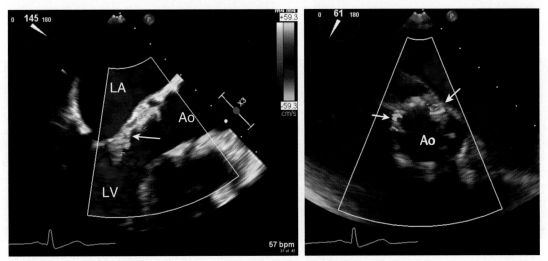

Fig. 18.21 Paravalvular aortic regurgitation after transcatheter aortic valve implantation. TEE long-axis *(left)* and short-axis *(right)* views immediately after placement of a transcatheter aortic valve for severe aortic stenosis show a paravalvular leak *(arrows)* posteriorly, with a second jet located medially seen on the short-axis view. *Ao,* Aorta.

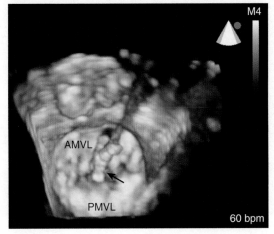

Fig. 18.22 Transcatheter mitral valve repair. Intraprocedural 3D TEE is used to guide the clip device *(arrow)* toward the mitral valve and ensure the device is correctly positioned relative to the specific valve pathology in that patient. *AMVL,* Anterior mitral valve leaflet; *PMVL,* posterior mitral valve leaflet.

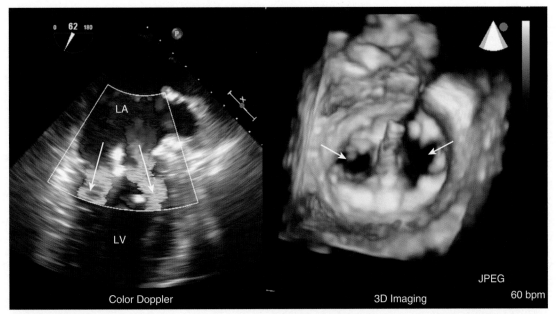

Fig. 18.23 Posttranscatheter mitral valve clip. The anterior and posterior leaflets are now clipped together resulting in two mitral orifices *(arrows)* as seen on color Doppler *(left)* and 3D imaging *(right)*.

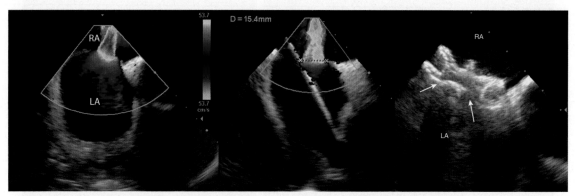

Fig. 18.24 **Intracardiac echocardiographic guidance of atrial septal defect closure.** The intracardiac echocardiography transducer is positioned in the RA showing a large atrial septal defect with a flow jet from the LA to RA *(left)*. A balloon catheter across the defect is used for sizing *(center)*, followed by placement of the atrial septal occluder device *(arrows, right)*. Both color Doppler flow imaging and saline contrast then are used to evaluate for any residual shunting.

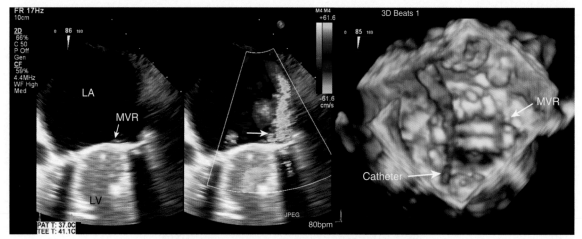

Fig. 18.25 **Paravalvular prosthetic mitral regurgitation.** The 2D image rotation plane *(left)* is adjusted to show the paravalvular jet *(arrow)* lateral to the mitral valve replacement. If possible, acceleration on the LV size of the valve is visualized to precisely locate the defect *(center)*, although this may be challenging due to reverberations from the mechanical prosthetic valve. 3D imaging *(right)* is used during the procedure to guide the catheter *(arrow)* into the paravalvular defect. One device has already been deployed medial to the catheter position. *MVR*, Mitral valve replacement.

Mitral Balloon Valvotomy

- Mitral stenosis often is treated by percutaneous balloon valvotomy rather than by surgical valve replacement using TEE or ICE guidance for positioning of the transseptal catheter and balloon position across the mitral valve.
- Transmitral mean gradient and pressure half-time valve area are monitored after each balloon dilation, along with invasive pressure measurements.
- Doppler evaluation for mitral regurgitation using standard approaches is repeated after each balloon dilation; an increase in regurgitant severity precludes further dilation attempts.
- A small shunt across the atrial septum may be seen after any procedure involving a transseptal puncture (Fig. 18.24).

Transcatheter Closure of Paravalvular Prosthetic Regurgitation

- Newer transcatheter interventions include closure of paravalvular leaks in patients with mechanical valves.

- Echocardiographic imaging is essential during these procedures to:
  - Identify the site, size, and shape of the paravalvular defect (Fig. 18.25)
  - Guide the catheter across the defect for placement of the closure device
  - Ensure the device placement does not affect valve occluder motion (Fig. 18.26)
  - Assess residual regurgitation

Left Atrial Appendage Occluder Placement

- TEE evaluation of LA appendage anatomy and size is used to guide placement of the occluder device.
- Intraprocedural TEE guidance allows correct placement of the device in the LA appendage.
- Repeat TEE early and late after occluder placement is used to evaluate for any residual flow into and out of the LA appendage (Fig. 18.27).

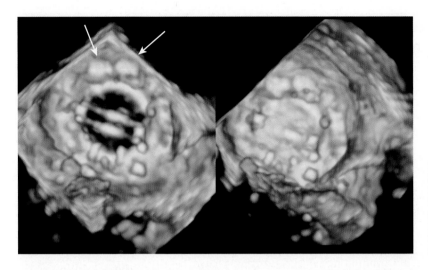

Fig. 18.26 **Postparavalvular leak closure.** 3D imaging from a LA perspective shows a bileaflet mechanical mitral valve in the open position in diastole *(left)* with two small closure devices *(arrows)*. The systolic image with the leaflets closed is shown on the right. The images are rotated compared to the orientation in Fig. 18.25.

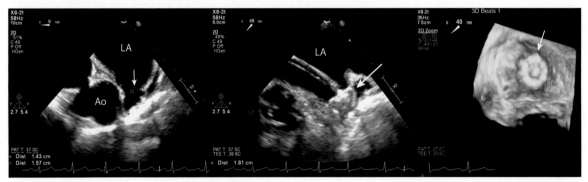

Fig. 18.27   **LA appendage occluder device.**   Procedural guidance during placement of a LA appendage occluder device starts with TEE imaging to determine the size and shape of the atrial appendage *(left)*. The occluder device is positioned in the appendage using TEE imaging guidance *(center)* supplemented with biplane and 3D imaging with as en face view of the device on the right. Color Doppler is used to ensure complete blockage of flow into and out of the appendage.

THE ECHO EXAM

Basic Principles of Intraprocedural TEE

- Establish diagnosis preprocedure when possible.
- The goals of the baseline TEE are to:
  - Confirm the diagnosis.
  - Provide additional information on reparability.
  - Serve as a comparison to postprocedure studies.
  - Assess LV and RV function.
  - Check for other abnormalities.
- Perform a complete study unless there are clinical or time constraints.
- Record postprocedure images at similar loading conditions to those of baseline.
- Communicate and discuss findings at time of study.
- Report TEE findings in medical record, and store TEE images.

Factors That Affect Cardiac Hemodynamics During Surgical or Transcatheter Procedures

Heart rate and blood pressure
Positive pressure mechanical ventilation
Volume status
Myocardial "stunning" secondary to aortic cross-clamping
Effects of cardiopulmonary bypass
Pharmacologic therapy

Imaging for Transcatheter Interventions

Procedure	Procedural Planning	Procedural Guidance*	Postprocedure Evaluation
Transcatheter aortic valve replacement	TTE, CT	TEE optional	TTE
Transcatheter mitral valve repair procedures	TTE, 3D TEE	3D TEE essential	TTE, TEE
Balloon mitral valvotomy	TTE and TEE	TEE or ICE	TTE
Transcatheter closure for paravalvular regurgitation	3D TEE	3D TEE essential	TTE, TEE
Atrial septal defect or patent foramen ovale closure	TTE, 3D TEE	TEE or ICE	TTE, TEE
Septal ablation for hypertrophic cardiomyopathy	TTE	TTE or TEE	TTE
Transcatheter pulmonic valve replacement	TTE, CT	TEE optional	TTE
LA appendage occlusion	TEE, CT	TEE essential	TEE

*In addition to fluoroscopy
ICE, Intracardiac echcocardiography.

Key Data for Intraoperative TEE

Procedure	Pre-procedure	During Procedure	Postprocedure

Mitral valve repair	• Valve anatomy
	• Repairability
	• Regurgitation
	  • Mechanism
	  • Severity
		• Baseline anatomy and regurgitation pre-CPB
		• Residual MR post-CPB
			• Assess for complications
			  • Persistent MR
			  • Mitral SAM
			  • Functional mitral stenosis
			  • Tricuspid regurgitation
			  • Circumflex artery injury
			• LV function

Valve stenosis	• Valve anatomy and calcification • Severity of stenosis • LV function • PA pressures	• Baseline LV function • Baseline valve anatomy and function • Post-CPB assess repaired or prosthetic valve	• Paravalvular regurgitation • LV function
Endocarditis	• Vegetations • Abscess formation • Valve function • LV function • PA pressures	• Baseline valve anatomy and function • Post-CPB valve function	• Baseline postsurgery valve function • LV function
Prosthetic valve dysfunction	• Valve thrombosis • Pannus formation • Paravalvular regurgitation	• Baseline study to guide surgical intervention • Post-CPB assess new prosthetic valve	• Baseline prosthetic valve function • Follow-up depends on residual lesions and valve type.
Aortic dissection	• Confirm diagnosis • Extent of dissection distally • Coronary ostial involvement • Aortic valve function • Pericardial effusion	• Post-CPB document residual dissection flap distal to repair • Assess flow in true and false lumen • Aortic valve function • LV function	• Long-term follow-up of aortic valve and LV function • Residual dissection flap distally
Hypertrophic cardiomyopathy	• Location and severity of septal thickening • Severity of subaortic dynamic obstruction • MR	• Residual subaortic obstruction • Ventricular septal defect • Residual MR	• Long-term hemodynamic results • LV systolic and diastolic function
Congenital heart disease	• Diagnosis of complex anatomy • Surgical planning • Integration with data from other imaging modalities	• Baseline evaluation of each lesion anatomy and hemodynamics • Residual lesions after CPB	• Long-term anatomic and functional results • Ventricular function • Pulmonary pressures

CPB, Cardiopulmonary bypass; *MR*, mitral regurgitation; *PA*, pulmonary artery; *SAM*, systolic anterior motion.

SELF-ASSESSMENT QUESTIONS

Question 1

During weaning from cardiopulmonary bypass in a patient undergoing coronary artery bypass grafting surgery, the following image was obtained (Fig. 18.28). The structure indicated by the arrow most likely is:

A. Air
B. Artifact
C. Cannula
D. Tumor
E. Thrombus

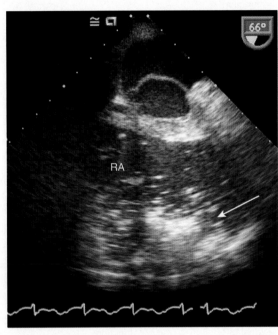

Fig. 18.28

Question 2

An intraprocedural transesophageal echocardiogram is provided for guidance during a LA appendage occluder procedure.

Based on the image provided (Fig. 18.29), your recommendation to the proceduralist would be:

A. Recapture device, move to different position
B. Release device in current position
C. Remove device from current position
D. Redeploy device in current position

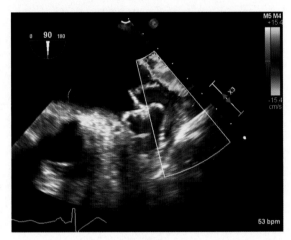

Fig. 18.29

Question 3

In this TEE image (Fig. 18.30), the arrow points at:

A. LA appendage
B. Coronary sinus
C. Left main coronary artery
D. Right coronary artery
E. RA appendage

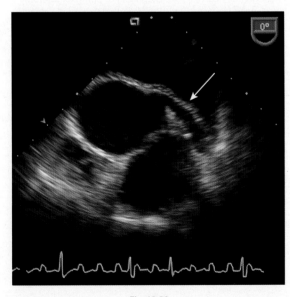

Fig. 18.30

Question 4

3D images are obtained in a patient undergoing a catheter-based valve intervention. The following image of the deployment catheter in the LA is obtained (Fig. 18.31). The echolucent finding *(arrow)* is consistent with:

A. Acoustic shadowing
B. Microbubbles
C. Stitch artifact
D. Vegetation

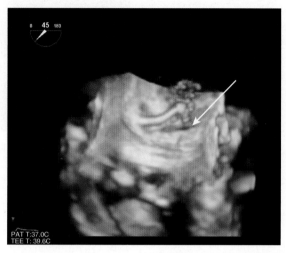

Fig. 18.31

Question 5

This Doppler tracing recording during an intraoperative TEE study shows (Fig. 18.32):

    A. Atrial fibrillation
    B. Atrial flutter
    C. Superior vena caval flow
    D. Coronary artery flow
    E. Pulmonary vein flow

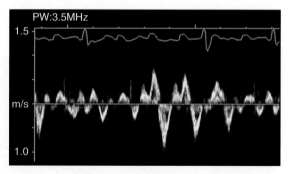

Fig. 18.32

Question 6

You perform a TEE study on a patient who is under evaluation for mitral valve replacement. Cardiac anesthesia is at the bedside and conscious sedation is administered. The probe is advanced through the bite block and oropharynx. The patient is agitated and coughing; the probe cannot be advanced beyond 10 cm. Which of the following is the next step?

A. Refer the patient for barium swallow
B. Withdraw probe and reattempt placement
C. Increase sedation and advance probe further
D. Rotate probe clockwise and retroflex probe tip

Question 7

A 64-year-old man is referred for coronary artery bypass grafting surgery. He has a history of prior cardiac surgery. During his procedure, the following image was obtained (Fig. 18.33). You conclude that his prior procedure was:

A. Coronary artery bypass graft surgery
B. LA appendage exclusion procedure
C. Mitral valve annuloplasty
D. Aortic valve replacement

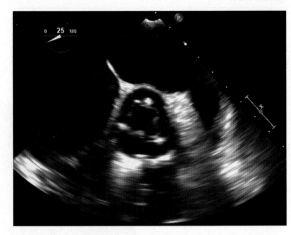

Fig. 18.33

Question 8

A patient with rheumatic mitral valve disease is referred for mitral valvuloplasty. During the pre-procedure TEE, the following images are obtained. Tracing of the mitral inflow Doppler signal provides a diastolic mean gradient of 9 mm Hg at a heart rate of 75 bpm. Based on these images (Fig. 18.34), what additional imaging is needed prior to the valvulo-plasty procedure?

A. 3D imaging of the interatrial septum
B. Quantitation of mitral regurgitation
C. Planimetry of mitral valve orifice area
D. Estimate mitral valve area using pressure half-time

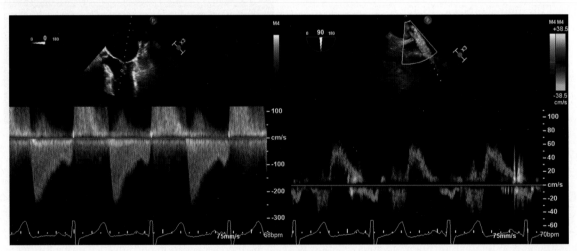

Fig. 18.34

Question 9

A 58-year-old presents to the emergency department with acute, severe chest and upper back pain and was diagnosed with an acute type A aortic dissection. A transthoracic image obtained in the emergency department and an intraoperative TEE recorded at the end of the surgical procedure is shown (Fig. 18.35). The patient has undergone aortic root replacement with:

A. Resuspension of the aortic valve
B. Mechanical aortic valve replacement
C. Bioprosthetic aortic valve replacement
D. Transcatheter aortic valve implantation

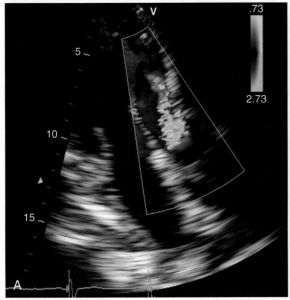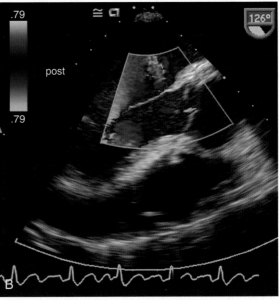

Fig. 18.35

Question 10

What echocardiographic feature is most concerning to result in paravalvular regurgitation post-transcatheter aortic valve placement?

A. Calcification of the LV outflow tract
B. Height of coronary ostia relative to the aortic valve
C. Maximal annular diameter of the aortic valve
D. Increased aortoseptal angulation

Question 11

A patient with severe mitral regurgitation is referred for percutaneous edge-to-edge repair. TEE is utilized to provide intraprocedural guidance, and a systolic imaging is obtained (Fig. 18.36). The most likely etiology and location of the mitral regurgitation is the:

A. Posterior leaflet, medial scallop
B. Posterior leaflet, lateral scallop
C. Anterior leaflet, medial scallop
D. Anterior leaflet, lateral scallop

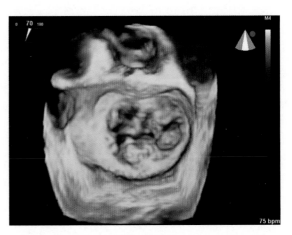

Fig. 18.36

Question 12

Intraprocedural TEE is obtained in a patient during transseptal puncture for a percutaneous edge-to-edge repair procedure. Based on the image obtained (Fig. 18.37), what additional procedure do you anticipate will be needed after completion of the percutaneous edge-to-edge repair?

A. Pericardiocentesis procedure
B. Atrial septal defect (ASD) closure
C. LA appendage occluder device
D. No additional procedure needed

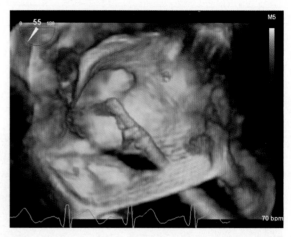

Fig. 18.37

ANSWERS

Answer 1: A

This view of the RA shows microbubbles in the right heart consistent with intracardiac air. The dense mass of echoes indicated by the arrow is an air collection at the superior aspect of the RA, near the RA append-age. Tumor or thrombus is unlikely given the clinical setting and the density of the echo signal. The appear-ance is not suggestive of an artifact. A cannula would show parallel smooth lines; the presence and position of a cannula could be confirmed by direct inspec-tion in the operating room. TEE imaging is helpful in ensuring that all intracardiac air is eliminated before coming off bypass.

Answer 2: D

The LA appendage occluder is well seated in the LA appendage, measuring ≈2 cm in diameter. The tissue ridge between the LA appendage and the left upper pulmonary vein is visualized, with color Dop-pler showing flow into the LA in the upper portion of the image. Between the device and the tissue ridge, there is gap along the device ≈4 mm in diameter (blue Doppler signal), consistent with an under-expanded device. Redeployment in the current position allows for apposition of the device to the entire LA append-age, now measuring 2.4 cm in diameter at this view (Fig. 18.38). The catheter that is used to deploy the device is still attached to the midportion of the device, so recapturing is not needed. The device should not be released in the current position because of the residual gap in place.

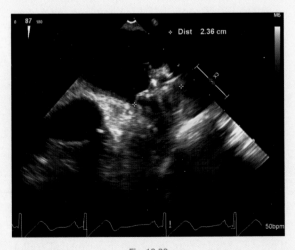

Fig. 18.38

Answer 3: C

This oblique short-axis view at the level of the aortic sinuses, just superior to the aortic valve leaflets, shows the left main coronary artery arising from the left cor-onary cusp (Fig. 18.39).

The LA appendage is just lateral to the coronary artery. The coronary sinus would be seen in a 4-chamber view with posterior angulation or in a low TEE view of the RA and RV. The RA appendage is anterior to the aorta (Ao); in fact, a bit of the RA appendage is seen in this image anterior to the aorta and medial to the RV outflow tract (RVOT).

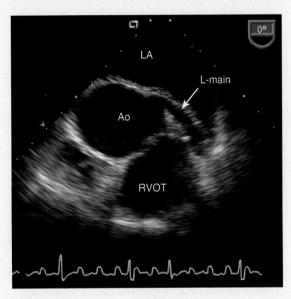

Fig. 18.39

Answer 4: A

This image was taken intraprocedurally in a patient undergoing a percutaneous mitral clip procedure. Device delivery is via a transseptal puncture. In this image, the catheter is seen crossing the interatrial sep-tum with the tip in the LA. As with any ultrasound image, ultrasound does not penetrate through bright reflectors. The field distal to the reflector is acousti-cally shadowed. In this 3D image, there is acoustic shadowing along the length of the catheter, with the largest under the catheter tip where the device is located. Adjacent to the device, injection of saline cre-ates microbubbles just above the catheter tip, which is seen projecting in the top part of the image. A vegeta-tion would appear echodense, not echolucent.

Answer 5: B

This Doppler tracing of flow from the LA appendage into the LA demonstrates regular low-velocity pulsa-tile flow at a rate about 300 bpm, which is consistent with atrial flutter. Atrial fibrillation would result in rapid irregular LA appendage flow signals, usually with an even lower velocity. Flow in the superior vena cava and in the pulmonary vein would show a typical venous flow pattern with systolic and diastolic filling velocities, and a small reversal of flow after atrial contraction. Coronary artery flow occurs predominantly in diastole.

Answer 6: B

This patient is not tolerating the procedure. Coughing during probe placement and difficulty advancing the probe suggests that the probe may be erroneously placed in the trachea. Absence of diagnostic echocardiographic images aids in confirming wrong probe placement. Withdrawing the probe and reattempting placement is the correct answer. When placing the probe, the tip should be midline (not rotated), with the tip slightly anteflexed to aid esophageal intubation. If resistance is encountered during probe placement, the probe should never be advanced further; this may cause esophageal perforation or other patient injury.

Answer 7: D

The image provided is from a midesophageal view taken from the base of the heart. The aortic valve is seen in short axis in the middle of the image. At the juncture of each of the aortic valve cusps, there is a bright echodensity (prosthetic) consistent with valve struts. There are thin, mobile tissue leaflets between the struts. The mitral valve and annulus are not seen in this view. The LA appendage is seen to the right of the aortic valve and is still intact. The tricuspid valve, faint, is seen just to the left of the aortic valve in the image. The interatrial septum is seen at the top-left of the image bisecting one of the aortic valve cusps.

Answer 8: B

The images provided are consistent with severe mitral regurgitation as the dominant valve lesion rather than mitral stenosis. Full quantitation of mitral regurgitation severity is indicated. The mitral inflow Doppler tracing shows an elevated peak early (E wave) velocity over 2.3 m/s with a relatively steep deceleration slope, not consistent with severe stenosis. The image on the right is a Doppler tracing of the right upper pulmonary vein from the bicaval view, showing systolic flow reversal. Planimetry of the mitral valve area may be helpful in determining stenosis severity, but with significant regurgitation this patient is not a candidate for valvuloplasty. When performed, planimetry is a relatively hemodynamically independent assessment of mitral valve area; care should be taken to optimize measurement of the true smallest area of a relatively funnel shaped orifice. Pressure half-time (PHT) is the time for the peak pressure gradient between the LA and LV to reach half its value, but it is dependent on initial peak velocity, which is elevated in this case >2.3 m/s due to mitral regurgitation. PHT will be shortened if LV diastolic pressure rises faster than expected (noncompliant ventricle) or if LA pressure fall faster than expected (noncompliant LA).

Answer 9: A

The intraoperative image shows a normal-appearing aortic valve with thin leaflets and without supporting struts or a sewing ring to suggest either a mechanical or stented bioprosthetic valve. It is possible that a stentless valved conduit may have been used in this case, but it is more likely that the native valve has been resuspended in the aortic graft. With a transcatheter bioprosthetic valve, echodensities along the aortic wall from the valve cage would be seen.

With aortic dissection, aortic regurgitation may be due to an intrinsic anatomic abnormality of the valve (such as a bicuspid aortic valve) or may be due to extension of the dissection into the base of the aortic valve. In this case, aortic regurgitation was due to prolapse of the dissected segment through a normal trileaflet aortic valve. The prolapsing tissue impeded leaflet coaptation, resulting in severe aortic regurgitation. Replacement of the ascending aorta with elimination of the dissection flap restored normal aortic leaflet closure. Thus the aortic valve was resuspended with only mild regurgitation postoperatively.

Answer 10: A

Evaluating the extent of calcification of the left ventricular outflow tract is an important component of pre-intervention TEE imaging. The LV outflow tract is the landing zone of the lower portion of the valve skirt. Focal or nodular calcium deposits increases risk of poor circumferential apposition of the valve stent, resulting in paravalvular aortic regurgitation. A relatively lower height of the coronary ostia and smaller annular diameter increase risk of potential coronary artery obstruction after transcatheter aortic valve placement but do not affect risk of paravalvular regurgitation. Angulation of the LV outflow tract relative to the aortic valve plane (aortoseptal angulation) may present an obstacle to optimal valve positioning but has not been specifically identified as a risk factor for paravalvular regurgitation after transcatheter aortic valve placement.

Answer 11: A

The image provided is a standard enface 3D view of the mitral valve from the atrial side of the valve. By convention, the aortic valve is displayed at the top of the image, with the anterior mitral valve leaflet above the posterior leaflet. In this view, the right side of the image is medial, and the left side of the image is lateral (the os of the LA appendage is also visible just lateral to the mitral valve, on the left side of the image). There is chordal rupture of the most medial scallop of the posterior leaflet, with free chords visible at the valve coaptation. A rotated schematic of the mitral valve in this patient color mapping relative profile changes of the mitral valve is shown in Fig. 18.40 (*red* is prolapsed section).

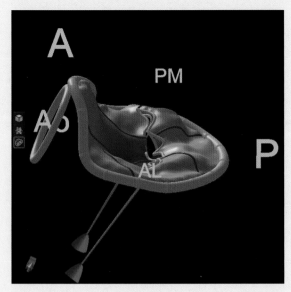

Fig. 18.40

Answer 12: D

This is a 3D image obtained during transseptal puncture. The catheter is seen crossing the interatrial septum. As is the case with any ultrasound imaging, the ultrasound beam cannot penetrate through the catheter, and there is an acoustic shadow distal to the catheter. This should not be misinterpreted as a septal defect. Multiple imaging windows will demonstrate absence of a large defect. The pericardial space is not visualized in this close view, and determination of need for pericardiocentesis cannot be made. Similarly, the LA appendage is not visualized in this view.

Index

Note: Page numbers followed by *f* indicate figure, by *t* table, and by *b* box.